Pharmacology
for Technicians

Understanding Drugs and Their Uses

Fourth Edition

Don A. Ballington, MS
Mary M. Laughlin, MEd, PharmD

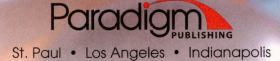

Paradigm
PUBLISHING

St. Paul • Los Angeles • Indianapolis

Acquisitions Editor:	Alison Brown Cerier
Developmental Editor:	Spencer Cotkin
Production Editor:	Bob Dreas
Cover and Text Designer:	Jaana Bykonich
Photo Researcher:	Terri Miller, E-Visual Communications, Inc.
Copyediting, Proofreading, Indexing:	Publication Services, Inc.

Care has been taken to verify the accuracy of information presented in this book. However, the authors, editors, and publisher cannot accept responsibility for Web, e-mail, newsgroup, or chat room subject matter or content, or for consequences from application of the information in this book, and make no warranty, expressed or implied, with respect to its content.

Trademarks: Some of the product names and company names included in this book have been used for identification purposes only and may be trademarks or registered trade names of their respective manufacturers and sellers. The authors, editors, and publisher disclaim any affiliation, association, or connection with, or sponsorship or endorsement by, such owners.

Photo Credits: 4 Archivo Iconografico, S.A./Corbis; **5** (top) Corbis; (bottom) Bettmann/Corbis; **6** Minnesota Historical Society/Corbis; **8** Janeart/Image Bank; **14** ©Brendan McDermid/epa/Corbis; **32** ©iStockphoto.com/ Yin Yang; **42** (top) Ortho-McNeil-Janssen Pharmaceuticals, Inc.; (bottom) ©iStockphoto.com/Sean Locke; **68** Gram's stains Copyright Biodisc, Inc.; **100** Lester V. Bergman/Corbis; **104** SuperStock; **131** ©iStockphoto.com/ Gill Henshall; **140** Michael English/Custom Medical Stock Photos; **166** ©AP Images/PRNewsFoto/Eli Lilly and Company; **224** Custom Medical Stock Photos; **226** ©iStockphoto.com; **236** Courtesy of Dr. Kenneth Nowak; **241** (top) ©iStockphoto.com/mandygodbehear; (bottom) Edward Gallucci/Doctor Stock; **244** ©iStockphoto. com; **245** © Ed Murray/Star Ledger/Corbis; **262** Courtesy of Pfizer Inc., New York, NY; **269** ©iStockphoto.com/ Pamela Moore; **282** ©iStockphoto.com/Rohit Seth; **291** ©iStockphoto.com/creacart; **296** ©iStockphoto.com/ David Pinn; **331** (top) Reprinted with permission of APP Bioscience, Inc. (bottom) Reproduced with permission of Procter & Gamble; **335** ©iStockphoto.com/ranplett; **352** ©iStockphoto.com/Eliza Snow; **370** Custom Medical Stock Photos; **384** Pravachol is a trademark of Bristol-Myers Squibb Company. Used with permission; **397** BSIP/ Photo Researchers, Inc.; **418** Custom Medical Stock Photo, Inc./NMSP; **427** ©iStockphoto.com/Eau Claire Media; **448** ©iStockphoto.com/Andrzej Tokarski; **476** (top) Custom Medical Stock Photo, Inc.; (bottom) Custom Medical Stock Photo, Inc.; **477** Custom Medical Stock Photo, Inc./Michael English, M.D.; **479** Custom Medical Stock Photo, Inc.; **480** Custom Medical Stock Photo, Inc.; **482** Custom Medical Stock Photo, Inc./SPL; **487** (left) SPL/ Custom Medical Stock Photos; (right) J.L. Carlson/Custom Medical Stock Photos; **513** ©Jacob Halaska/Index Stock Imagery/Jupiterimages; **489** Custom Medical Stock Photos; **527** Custom Medical Stock Photo, Inc.; **531** ©iStockphoto.com/art-4-art; **552** Corbis/Mark Gibson; **558** ©iStockphoto.com/Don Bayley; **521** Corbis/Mark Gibson; **566** Hans Reinhard/OKAPIAPhoto Researchers, Inc.; **572** ©iStockphoto.com/sambrogio; **575** (left) CDC/ Laura Rose/photographer: Janice Haney Carr; (right) CDC/Dr. Marshall Fox; **576** (left) CDC/Dr. Fred Murphy; (right) CDC/World Heath Organization; Stanley O. Foster M.D., M.P.H.

We have made every effort to trace the ownership of all copyrighted material and to secure permission from copyright holders. In the event of any question arising as to the use of any material, we will be pleased to make the necessary corrections in future printings. Thanks are due to the aforementioned authors, publishers, and agents for permission to use the materials indicated.

ISBN 978-0-76383-481-4 (text, Study Partner CD, Pocket Guide)
ISBN 978-0-76383-477-7 (text)

© 2010 by Paradigm Publishing, Inc., a division of EMC Publishing, LLC
875 Montreal Way
St. Paul, MN 55102
E-mail: educate@emcp.com
Web site: www.emcp.com

Brief Contents

Contents

Preface

Pharmacology for Technicians, Fourth Edition, supports a comprehensive pharmacology course for students preparing to become pharmacy technicians in community, institutional, and other pharmacy settings. This text offers the tools to achieve the pharmacy technician competencies defined by the American Society of Health-System Pharmacists (ASHP).

The role of the pharmacy technician in today's pharmacy is both challenging and rewarding. Technicians are asked to perform many critical tasks, and it is extremely important that they perform these tasks in the correct way. This text and its Study Partner CD are designed to develop a basic understanding of drug classes and the mechanisms of action for many drugs. Students gain insight into why certain drugs are prescribed for particular disease states. With this essential background information, students are prepared to make informed, intelligent decisions when dispensing drugs and to play an active role in avoiding errors. Issues related to safety are reinforced throughout the book through look-alike and sound-alike drug name sidebars, patient warning stickers, and dosage and dispensing information in the text discussion.

An important goal of *Pharmacology* is to help students develop a commitment to the pharmacy field so that as pharmacy technicians, they remain challenged by this constantly changing topic and motivated to continue learning about the drugs that heal and improve the lives of patients.

Chapter Features: A Visual Walk-Through

Chapter features are designed to help students learn the basic principles of pharmacology, become familiar with the most commonly prescribed drugs, and learn how to use this knowledge to work safely and effectively.

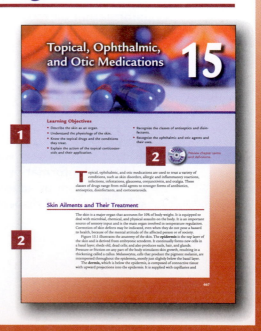

1

LEARNING OBJECTIVES establish clear goals and help focus chapter study.

2

KEY TERMS are bolded and defined in context. Students are encouraged to preview the chapter terms on the Study Partner CD as they begin to study each chapter.

3

Chapters begin with an overview of the anatomy and physiology of the featured body system and the pathology of diseases that affect that system.

4

PHOTOGRAPHS help to relate text content to real life.

5

ILLUSTRATIONS provide additional detail and visual reinforcement of chapter topics.

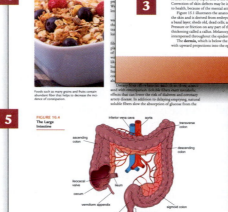

6

DRUG TABLES provide information on most commonly prescribed drugs. Information includes generic and brand names, pronunciation guide for generic names, dosage forms, dispensing status, and, for some drug groups, controlled-substance schedule.

Drugs listed in drug tables are discussed in the text where additional information is provided on mechanism of action, dosage, side effects, and dispensing issues.

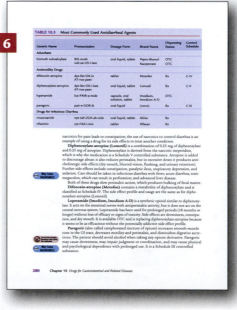

7

Patient WARNING STICKERS in margins provide examples of the types of information pharmacy technician students will share with patients.

8

WARNING SIDEBARS point out potential points of confusion, such as drug names that are spelled alike and pills that look alike.

9

A CHAPTER TERMS section provides a concise list of terms introduced and defined in each chapter.

10

The CHAPTER SUMMARY presents an overview of the key points of the chapter.

11

A DRUG LIST provides a comprehensive list of all of the drugs discussed in the chapter.

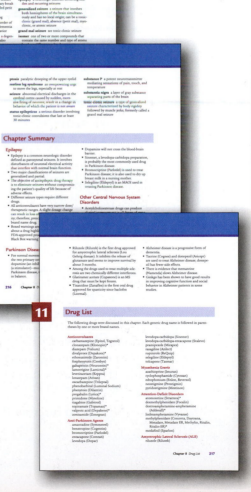

12 The **CHAPTER REVIEW** contains a variety of exercises to help build and assess students' mastery of the content. Topics include **Pharmaceuticals and Body Functions, Diseases and Drug Therapies, Dispensing Medications, Understanding Pharmacology, Phamacology at Work, Internet Research, and What Would You Do?**

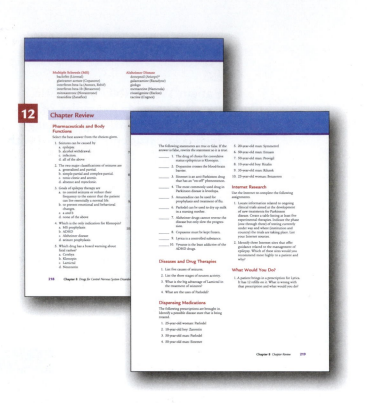

Resources for the Student

To support their study of the textbook, students have access to additional print and electronic resources that enhance the development of technician skills and address different learning styles.

Appendixes

The appendixes provide important reference material, including a list of the most commonly prescribed drugs and their drug categories (Appendix A), a list of look-alike and sound-alike medications and recommendations from the Institute for Safe Medication Practices (ISMP) (Appendix B), abbreviations (Appendix C), the Greek alphabet (Appendix D), and reference lab values that pharmacy technicians encounter at work (Appendix E).

Study Partner CD

The Study Partner CD included with each textbook offers the following tools to support student learning:

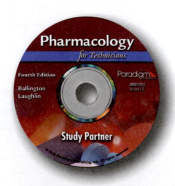

- Chapter Terms and Flash cards
- Matching Activities
- Quizzes in Practice or Reported Modes
- Link to Internet Resource Center

Chapter Terms and Flash Cards help students learn key terminology. Chapter terms include audio plus an image bank of related illustrations.

Interactive Matching Activities offer a fun way for students to check their understanding of chapter content.

Quizzes in Practice mode allow students to perfect their knowledge. In the Reported mode, scores are e-mailed to both the student and the instructor. Both book-level and chapter-specific quizzes are available.

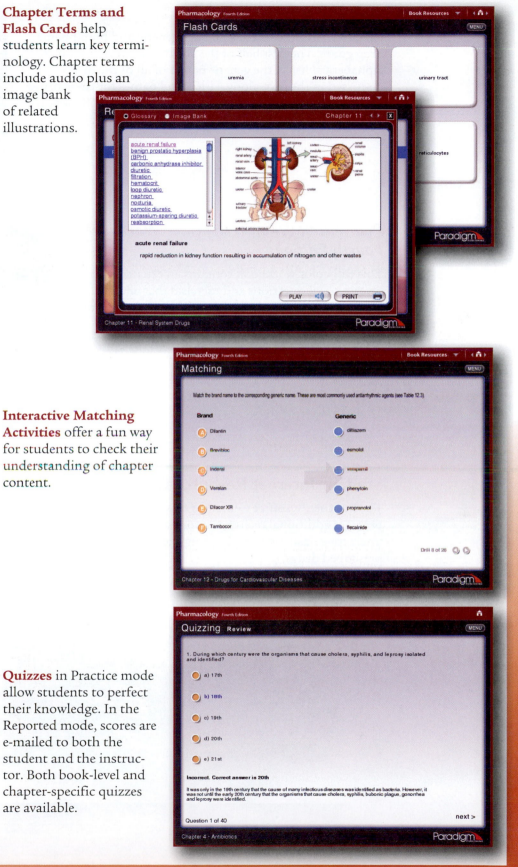

Pocket Guide for Technicians

Packaged with the text is a 96-page generic and brand name drug guide. The first half of the *Pocket Guide* contains an alphabetical list of the generic names of all of the drugs discussed in the text, along with brand names for these drugs. The second half of the *Pocket Guide* contains an alphabetical list of the brand names discussed in the text, along with the generic equivalents.

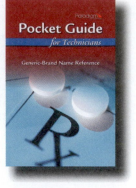

Pharmacology for Technicians Workbook, Fourth Edition

This full-color workbook contains an extensive and diverse set of questions and exercises that allow students to reinforce their knowledge of pharmacology terminology, concepts, and generic and brand drug names.

Student Internet Resource Center

The Internet Resource Center for this title at www.emcp.net/pharmacology4e provides additional reference information and resources, chapter study notes, and interactive flash cards for learning the generic and brand names of the most-prescribed drugs.

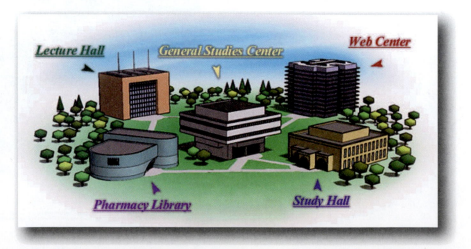

Resources for the Instructor

Pharmacology for Technicians, Fourth Edition, is supported by several tools to help instructors plan their course and assess student learning.

Instructor's Guide with Instructor Resources CD

In addition to course planning tools and suggested syllabi, the *Instructor's Guide* provides chapter-specific teaching hints and answers for all end-of-chapter exercises. The *Instructor's Guide* also provides ready-to-use chapter tests and midterm and final examinations. Included in the package is the Instructor Resources CD, which offers Microsoft® Word documents of all of the resources in the print *Instructor's Guide* as well as PowerPoint® presentations to enhance lectures.

All of the resources from the print *Instructor's Guide* and Instructor Resources CD are available in electronic format on the password-protected instructor section of the Internet Resource Center for this title at www.emcp.net/pharmacology4e.

ExamView Computerized Test Generator

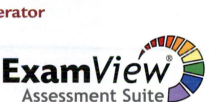

A full-featured computerized test generator on CD offers instructors a wide variety of options for generating both print and online tests. The test bank provides 45 to 50 questions for each chapter. Instructors can create custom tests using the chapter item banks and edit questions or add new items of their own design.

Class Connection

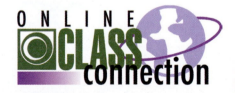

Class Connection is a set of content files for Blackboard and other course management systems. Content includes chapter outlines, PowerPoint presentations, and quizzes.

Textbooks in the Pharmacy Technician Series

In addition to *Pharmacology for Technicians, Fourth Edition,* Paradigm Publishing, Inc. offers other titles designed specifically for the pharmacy technician curriculum:

- *Pharmacology for Technicians Workbook, Fourth Edition*
- *Pharmacy Practice for Technicians, Fourth Edition*
- *Pharmacy Calculations for Technicians, Fourth Edition*
- *Pharmacy Labs for Technicians*

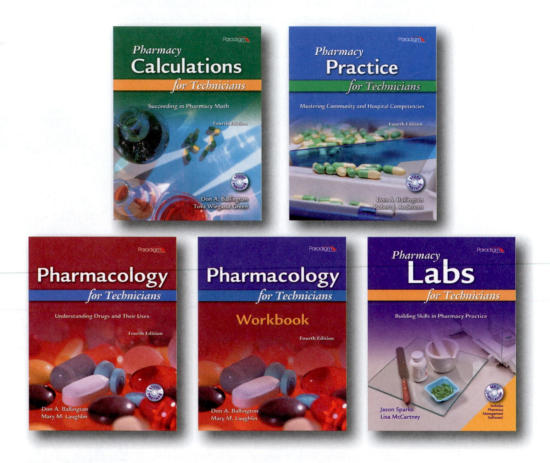

About the Authors

Don A. Ballington, MS, served as program coordinator of the pharmacy technician training program at Midlands Technical College in Columbia, South Carolina for 27 years. He has also served as president of the Pharmacy Technician Educators Council and in 2005 received the council's Educator of the Year award. Mr. Ballington has conducted site visits for pharmacy technician accreditation and helped develop the American Society of Health-System Pharmacists model curriculum. He has also been a consulting editor for the *Journal of Pharmacy Technology*. Over the course of his career at Midlands Technical College, he developed a set of high-quality training materials for pharmacy technicians. These materials became the foundation for Paradigm's Pharmacy Technician series.

Mary M. Laughlin holds a PharmD and an MEd. Dr. Laughlin has been an item writer for both North American Pharmacist Licensure Examination (NAPLEX) and the Pharmacy Technician Certification Exam (PTCE). Currently, she is a PRN pharmacist for Walgreen's in Memphis, Tennessee. Previously, Dr. Laughlin has served as assistant director of the pharmacy at the Regional Medical Center in Memphis and assistant professor of pharmacology and pharmacoeconomics at the College of Pharmacy, located on the campus of the University of Tennessee Health Science Center in Memphis. She has been involved in initiating two pharmacy technician programs in the city of Memphis. In 2002, Dr. Laughlin and her team of pharmacy technicians received the Innovations in Pharmaceutical Care award, presented by the Pharmacy Technician Certification Board (PTCB). Dr. Laughlin serves on the Pharmacy Technician Task Force for the state of Tennessee, and on the advisory board for the pharmacy technician training program at the Tennessee Technology Center at Memphis.

Acknowledgments

The quality of this body of work is a testament to the feedback we have received from the many contributors and reviewers who participated in *Pharmacology for Technicians, Fourth Edition*.

Robert W. Aanonsen, CPhT
Platt College
Tulsa, Oklahoma

Cheryl Aiken, BS Pharm, PharmD, RPh
Hotel Pharmacy, Inc.
Brattleboro, Vermont

Donald Becker, CPhT
San Jacinto College-North Campus
Houston, Texas

Danika Braaten, RPhT, CPhT
Northland Community and Technical
College
East Grand Forks, Minnesota

Verender Gail Brown, CPhT
High-Tech Institute
Orlando, Florida

Linda M. Calvert, CPhT
Front Range Community College
Westminster, Colorado

Nora Chan, PharmD
City College of San Francisco
San Francisco, California

Debborah G. Cummings, CPhT
Southeast Technical Institute
Sioux Falls, South Dakota

Andrea N. Curry, BS, CPhT
Concorde Career College
Memphis, Tennessee

Carla May, RPh
Vance Granville Community College
Henderson, North Carolina

Cathy Dunne
North Orange County Community
College District
Anaheim, California

Michelle C. McCranie, CPhT
Ogeechee Technical College
Statesboro, Georgia

Donna E. Guisado, RDA, BSOM
North-West College
West Covina, California

Ann Oberg, BS, CPhT
National American University
Sioux Falls, South Dakota

Leonard Lichtblau, PhD
University of Minnesota
Minneapolis, Minnesota

Rebecca Schonscheck, CPhT
High-Tech Institute
Phoenix, Arizona

Professor Leonard Lichtblau of the University of Minnesota, Minneapolis, and Judy Peterson of Two Harbors, Minnesota, prepared the quiz materials for the Study Partner CD, the ExamView test bank, and the PowerPoint slides. We thank them for their contributions.

The authors and editorial staff invite your feedback on the text and its supplements. Please reach us by clicking the "Contact us" button at www.emcp.com.

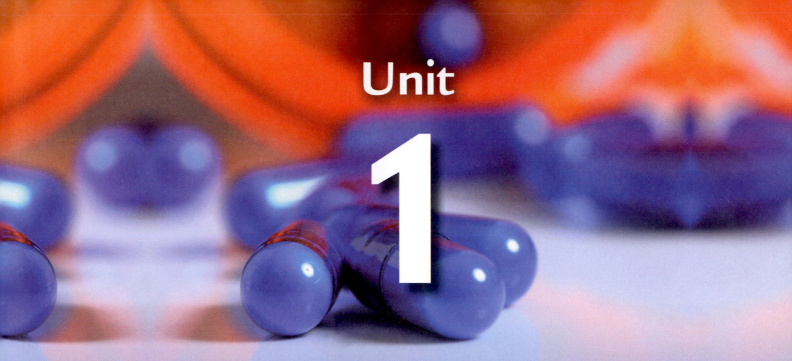

Unit
1

Introduction to Pharmacology

Evolution of Medicinal Drugs

1

Learning Objectives

- Recognize the important contributors, events, and resources in the development of pharmacology through the ages.
- Know what is meant by pharmacology.
- Define what drugs are, identify their sources, and understand how they work.

- Be familiar with the federal laws that regulate drugs and the agencies that administer those laws.
- Be familiar with the procedure for getting a new drug to market.

Preview chapter terms and definitions.

The use of drugs to treat illnesses has changed dramatically since early civilizations first attempted to heal the sick. Pharmacology today is based on solid science and systematic research rather than conventional wisdom and trial and error. During the twentieth century, the discovery of many new drugs revolutionized medical care, and a rational system of laws governing drug manufacture and distribution was developed to protect patients. Under current law, the manufacturers of all new drugs must provide proof that the drugs are effective and safe before they will be approved for marketing.

History of Medicinal Drugs

The study of ancient documents shows that people have been treating physical and mental ailments with medicines for thousands of years. Clay tablets from Babylonia, from the eighteenth century B.C., list more than 500 medicinal remedies. Over the last few centuries, tremendous advances have been made in the understanding of the causes of diseases and their treatments with medicine.

Early humans believed the world was controlled by good and evil spirits. The sick were thought to be victims of evil forces or of a god's anger. Consequently, medical treatment was largely controlled by religious leaders—shamans, or priests and priestesses—who guarded their healing knowledge closely. By their trial and error, folk knowledge of the healing properties of natural substances slowly grew.

Early Remedies

For thousands of years, the only materials that could treat illnesses were substances such as plants and minerals that were easy to gather and found nearby. With time and experience, ancient peoples learned to formulate practical recipes for various treatments. Over 2,000 years ago, Li Che Ten compiled a resource called *Peng T'Sao* that listed over 1000 plants and 8000 recipes that were used for the treatment of illnesses. In 1000 B.C., a Hindu named Susrutas wrote a medicinal work called *The Book of Life*.

Plants and other naturally occurring substances were administered in some of the same ways used today: topically, orally, and rectally. The *Ebers Papyrus*, an Egyptian medical source compiled in approximately 1550 B.C., lists more than 700 different herbal remedies used by healers. These remedies consisted of botanical drugs drawn from the natural environment and used internally, such as castor bean, garlic, and poppy seed. The most common mixtures were laxatives and enemas. The concept of "drug" appears in early Greek records as the word **pharmakon**, which also meant magic spell, remedy, or poison.

The Greek physician Hippocrates (c. 460–377 B.C.) was the first to propose that disease was caused by natural rather than supernatural causes. Although he practiced herbal medicine like his contemporaries, he rejected unsupported theory and superstition in favor of observation and classification, or empirical learning. Hippocrates was also the first to dissect the human body to study the functions of specific organs.

Another Greek physician, Galen (c. A.D. 130–201), lived in Rome and built on Hippocrates' ideas of empirical learning. Using concepts discussed by the philosopher Aristotle, Galen believed disease was caused by an imbalance of one of four "humors"—blood, phlegm, black bile, and yellow bile. Illnesses were cured with an herbal compound of an opposing quality (moist, dry, cold, or warm). Galen's vast writings about these compounds, known as galenicals, influenced medical knowledge for more than 1000 years.

The text *de Materia Medica*, compiled by Dioscorides in the first century A.D., was a major influence on European pharmaceutical knowledge until the sixteenth century. In it, Dioscorides scientifically described and classified 600 plants by substance rather than by the disease they were intended to treat.

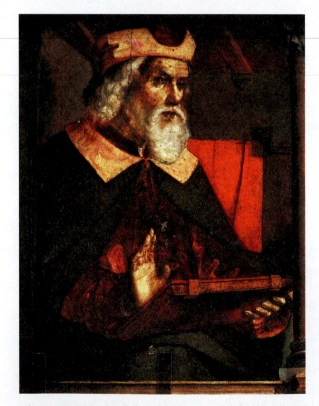

Hippocrates proposed that disease came from natural rather than supernatural causes and was the first to dissect the human body to study the functions of specific organs.

Drugs in the Middle Ages

During the Middle Ages, as the Christian church became a dominating cultural force, the practice of medicine and pharmacy passed again from lay practitioners to religious leaders. Monasteries became centers of treatment and intellectual life. Monks wrote and copied medical texts and grew herb gardens of medicinal plants.

The Swiss surgeon Paracelsus (1493–1541) was the first to challenge the teachings of Galen. He denounced the philosophy of humors in medicine and advocated the use of individual drugs rather

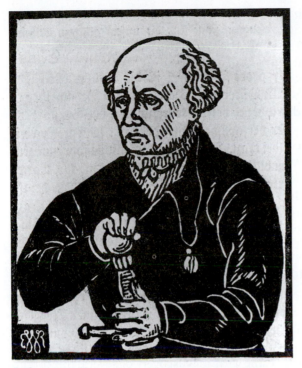

Paracelsus understood that if not dosed correctly, a medicine could easily become a poison.

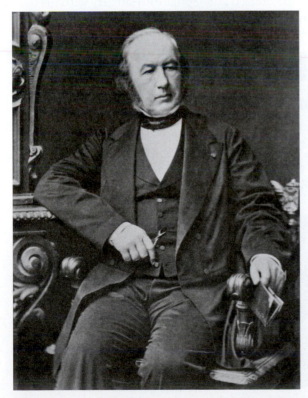

Claude Bernard demonstrated that certain drugs have specific sites of action within the body and used laboratory methods to study drugs.

than mixtures or potions. He reasoned that treating diseases with individual drugs would make it easier to determine which agent helped, which made the patient worse, and how much of a drug was needed. These concepts are still used today.

Near the end of the Middle Ages, the earliest official listings of medical preparations appeared in print. The first was the *Nuovo Receptario,* which was compiled by doctors in Florence, Italy, and was published in 1498. Shortly after that, in 1546, Valerius Cordis published the *Dispensatorium* in Nuremberg, Germany. This type of official listing is often referred to as a **pharmacopoeia.**

Drugs in the Modern Age

During the seventeenth and eighteenth centuries, several advances in pharmacy and chemistry occurred. London physicians eliminated many out-landish drug preparations when the first London pharmacopoeia was compiled in 1618. Some drug mixtures introduced at this time, such as tincture of opium, cocoa, and ipecac, are still used today.

In the nineteenth century, the French physiologist Claude Bernard (1813–1878) advanced the knowledge of how drugs work on the body when he demonstrated that certain drugs have specific sites of action within the body. Because of his use of laboratory methods to study drugs, he is credited with founding the field of experimental **pharmacology**, which is the science of drugs and their interactions with the systems of living animals.

American Pharmacology

Unlike treasure-rich Central and South America, North America held little interest to European settlers during the first century or so after the voyages of Columbus, and early colonies had few medical personnel. As a result, early settlers had to rely on domestic or kitchen medicine from home remedies. As the colonies grew in the eighteenth century, they attracted a broader range of immigrants, including physicians and apothecaries. An **apothecary** was the forerunner of today's pharmacists in England.

Like their European counterparts, most colonial physicians owned a dispensary or pharmacy. They prescribed, prepared, and dispensed drugs imported from Britain. The American Revolution forced American physicians, druggists, and wholesale distributors of drugs to manufacture their own chemically based drugs and to make common preparations of crude drugs. In 1820, the first official listing of drugs in the United States, the *Pharmacopoeia of the United States*, known today as the U.S. Pharmacopeia (USP) was published by the Massachusetts Medical Society, with approval from a national convention of physicians.

During the nineteenth century, in both the United States and Europe, a division between those medical practitioners who treated patients and those primarily interested in preparing medicines emerged. Not until after the American Civil War (1861–1865), however, were the boundaries between the professions of physician and pharmacist clearly drawn. Practitioners who treated patients supported the growth of the pharmaceutical profession because it released them from the responsibility of compounding medicines and stocking a shop. In 1852, the American Pharmaceutical Association (APhA) was formed, partly as a result of encroachment by other medical areas into pharmacy. Through this organization, pharmacists realized the opportunity for individual growth and increased professional stature.

Twentieth-Century Pharmacology

By the second half of the nineteenth century, pharmacology had become a scientific discipline. Following the lead of Oswald Schmiedeberg (1838–1921) at the University of Strasbourg in Germany, several European universities established departments of pharmacology.

Major breakthroughs in medical care came with the discovery of several important drugs. In 1847, Ignaz Philip Semmelweis helped reduce deaths from puerperal fever by requiring those entering maternity wards to scrub their hands first in chlorinated limewater. In the 1860s, Joseph Lister introduced antiseptics into surgery with his use of carbolic acid for cleansing instruments and suture materials.

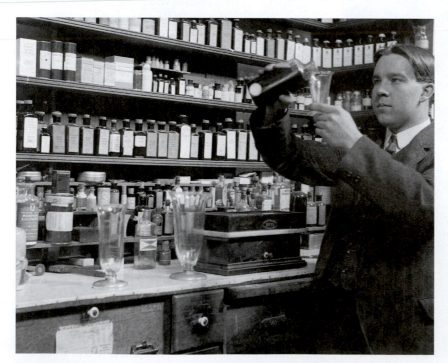

Dr. Emil King prepares medicine in his pharmacy in Fulda, MN, in 1905.

In 1907, Paul Ehrlich, a German bacteriologist, introduced arsphenamine, or Salvarsan, to treat syphilis. This rudimentary antimicrobial was the first chemical agent used to treat an infectious disease. In 1923, Sir Frederick Banting, a Canadian physiologist, and his assistant Charles Best successfully extracted the hormone insulin from the pancreas to create the first effective treatment for diabetes.

In 1935, the first sulfa drug, Prontosil, was introduced by the German Gerhardt Domagk. Ten years later penicillin was discovered by the bacteriologist Sir Alexander Fleming at St. Mary's Hospital in London.

Contemporary Pharmacology Practice

Contemporary pharmacology is a science based on systematic research to determine the origin, nature, chemistry, effects, and uses of drugs. The growth of present-day pharmacologic knowledge has been greatly stimulated by the development of synthetic organic chemistry, which has provided new tools and led to the development of many new therapeutic agents.

As new drugs are introduced, it is essential that those who prescribe them also thoroughly understand them. Various practitioners are essential to carrying out the tasks required for appropriate and effective use of drugs in clinical practice.

The Pharmacist and Pharmacy Technician

A **pharmacist** is licensed to prepare and sell (that is, dispense) drugs and compounds and to fill prescriptions. The primary responsibility of a pharmacist is to make sure that drugs are dispensed properly and used appropriately. The pharmacist is an important professional on the health care team. Furthermore, as pharmacists are being asked increasingly to focus their expertise and judgment on direct patient care and counseling, responsibilities related to dispensing have shifted to the pharmacy technician.

Pharmacists are assisted in these endeavors by the **pharmacy technician**, an equally important member of the healthcare team, who is defined as an individual working in a pharmacy who, under the supervision of a licensed pharmacist, assists in activities not requiring the professional judgment of a pharmacist. Although pharmacy technicians should not counsel patients because doing so requires the judgment of a pharmacist, technicians are involved in all facets of drug distribution. Depending on state law, some of a pharmacy technician's responsibilities could include:

- receiving written prescriptions or requests for prescription refills from patients or their caregivers
- verifying that the information on the prescription is complete and accurate
- counting, weighing, measuring, and mixing the medication
- preparing sterile IVs and chemotherapy compounds
- preparing prescription labels and selecting the containers
- establishing and maintaining patient profiles
- ordering and stocking prescription and over-the-counter (OTC) medications
- assisting with drug studies
- transcribing prescriptions over the telephone
- transferring prescriptions
- tracking and reporting errors
- checking the work of another pharmacy technician in the preparation of medicine carts
- educating nurses and other healthcare professionals about pharmacy-related issues
- obtaining laboratory results for pharmacists
- helping patients with OTC drugs
- making sure patients are counseled by the pharmacist (the technician should always ask whether there are any questions for the pharmacist)
- overseeing and maintaining automated dispensing systems

These areas of responsibility vary tremendously from state to state. For example, in Tennessee a Certified Pharmacy Technician can legally take a prescription over the phone. In some states, a technician can check another technician who picks medications for the unit dose carts. Studies show that technicians who check each other's work—picking medications for unit dose carts—are just as accurate as pharmacists who check a pharmacy technician's work, if not more so.

One of the most efficient measures to prevent medication errors is patient counseling. Even though the technician cannot counsel per se, it is the duty of the technician to make sure the patient understands that the pharmacist is available for counseling. A patient should never leave the facility without being asked whether there are any questions regarding the drugs. Sometimes the technician can respond to these questions by reading information to the patient, but more often the technician will need to get the pharmacist to talk to the patient. One drug-related problem in the United States is noncompliance with the prescription instructions. Patients who understand their medications and know why and how to take them are more likely to take them appropriately.

One responsibility that technicians are claiming across the country is that of overseeing the automated dispensing process, whether it is a robot or a dispensing machine.

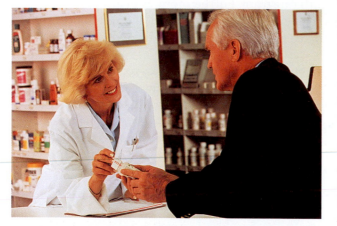

In addition to dispensing medications, the pharmacist plays an important role in instructing patients about side effects of medications, food and drug interactions, and dosing schedules.

As the pharmacy becomes more and more automated, someone must assume the responsibility of overseeing those machines. Technicians who in the past had been relegated to "licking, sticking, and picking" are now involved with complicated computer programs that ensure that safe and effective systems are in place to dispense drugs automatically.

Five organizations—the American Pharmaceutical Association (APhA), the American Society of Health-System Pharmacists (ASHP), the Illinois Council of Health-System Pharmacists (ICHP), the Michigan Pharmacists Association (MPA), and the National Association Boards of Pharmacy (NABP)—have joined to govern the **Pharmacy Technician Certification Board (PTCB)** and to maintain a national certification program. The PTCB develops standards and acts as the nationally recognized credentialing agency. Certified technicians must be recertified every two years by the PTCB. High-quality training and national standards are important because pharmacy technicians with higher qualifications and better skills enable the healthcare team to bring an increased quality of care to the patient, bringing greater value to the pharmacy.

Medicinal Drugs

A **drug** (or a medication) is a medicinal substance or remedy used to change the way a living organism functions. Drug action on a living system is known as **pharmacologic effect**. Drugs are often classified according to their use. A **therapeutic drug** relieves symptoms of a disease, whereas a **prophylactic drug** is used to prevent or decrease the severity of disease. Medications are indicated for numerous uses, such as relief of symptoms, replacement of missing natural chemicals, supplementation, diagnosis of disease, disease prevention, and healing.

Drug Origins and Sources

The study and identification of natural sources for drugs is called **pharmacognosy.** Drugs are derived from a variety of sources: plant parts or products, animals, minerals, chemicals, and recombinant deoxyribonucleic acid (DNA).

Various parts of many plants can be used to make drugs. Examples of drugs that are derived from plants include ergotamine from rye fungi, digoxin from foxglove, and morphine from the opium poppy. Drugs from animal products include thyroid, which is obtained from domestic animal sources. An example of a drug hormone from a mineral is silver nitrate.

Many drugs are produced synthetically from chemical substances. Drugs made synthetically include sulfonamides, aspirin, sodium bicarbonate, and many others. Bioengineered drugs, produced by recombinant DNA technology, are some of the most expensive drugs available; such a drug is also called a **biopharmaceutical.** Current examples are interferon beta-1b (Betaseron), interferon beta-1a (Avonex), and epoetin alfa (Epogen). Table 1.1 provides examples of drug sources along with the corresponding drug names and therapeutic effects.

Drug Names and Classifications

Every drug has three names: a chemical name, a generic name, and a brand name. The **chemical name** describes the chemical makeup of the drug in detail, such as "*para-(N-*acetyl) aminophenol." It is usually long and difficult to pronounce. The **generic name** is a shorter name that identifies the drug without regard to who in particular is manufacturing and marketing the drug, such as "acetaminophen." Also referred to as a USAN (United States Adopted Name), the generic name is not protected by a trademark. It is often a shortened version of the chemical name. The **brand name** or **trade name** is the name under which the manufacturer markets the drug, such as "Tylenol." It is a trademark of a particular company, which has the exclusive right to use that trademark.

The generic name for a drug begins with a lowercase letter, as in "erythromycin," whereas the trade name usually begins with a capital letter, as in "E-Mycin." Both terms refer to the same drug. Several different companies can manufacture the drug denoted by a given generic name, though they use different brand names.

Drug names are developed according to principles of safety, consistency, and logic, while considering the intended use of the drug and existing trade names. The *USP Dictionary of USAN and International Drug Names* describes the process for giving a name to a specific chemical entity. General considerations include safety in using the name

TABLE 1.1 Drug Sources, Drug Names, and Their Therapeutic Effects

Drug Source	Drug Name	Therapeutic Effect
Plant: foxglove	digoxin	Cardiotonic
Animal: stomach of hog and cow	pepsin	Digestive enzyme
Mineral: silver	silver nitrate	Anti-infective
Synthetic: omeprazole	Prilosec	Gastric acid inhibitor
Bioengineering: erythropoietin	Epogen	Stimulator of red blood cell formation

for prescribing, dispensing, ordering, and administering a drug as well as suitability of the name for use in health-related educational programs and publications. Another consideration is the ability to use the name for drug identification and exchange of information internationally.

A request for a drug name is made after an Investigational New Drug (IND) Application has been submitted to the Food and Drug Administration (FDA). Many guidelines direct the naming of a drug.

Alternative Medicine

Americans are spending billions of dollars every year for many different types of **alternative medicine**, including the use of herbs, supplements, and homeopathic remedies. **Homeopathy** is a system of therapeutics in which diseases are treated by giving minute doses of a drug that produces the same symptoms in healthy persons as the disease being treated. This interest in alternative medicine reflects patients' desire to take charge of their own healthcare.

Although some alternative medicine offers real value, it also raises two concerns. One is that legitimate scientific data on alternative medicines is scarce. Determining which supplements work and which do not, which ones are best for which conditions, and the safety and efficacy (that is, how well something works) of each is going to take time and legitimate, well-planned studies. Currently, when more than one formulation is available, there is no way to tell which ones, if any, work at all.

The other concern is that patients frequently do not tell their prescriber and pharmacist that they are taking alternative medicines. This omission can be very dangerous, because interactions can often occur between a prescribed drug and a home remedy. Furthermore, many of these products are not covered by any governmental regulations. Consequently, if a product is made by two different manufacturers, there is no way to know whether one is as strong as the other.

Drug Regulation

The manufacture, sale, and use of drugs are regulated by the U.S. legal system. State and federal laws govern the development, prescribing, and dispensing of drugs, providing a rational system of checks and balances to ensure everyone's safety. These laws have been developed and refined over the past century.

The Food and Drug Administration

In 1906 the Federal Food and Drug Act, often referred to as the Pure Food and Drug Act, was passed as the first attempt by the U.S. government to regulate the sale of drugs or substances that affect the body.

In 1927, the Food, Drug, and Insecticide Administration was formed. In 1930, its name was changed to the **Food and Drug Administration (FDA)**. This agency of the federal government is responsible for ensuring that any drug or food product approved for marketing is safe when used as directed on the label. The FDA controls purity, labeling accuracy, and product safety.

The passage of the Food, Drug, and Cosmetic Act of 1938 initiated the current system of drug regulation in the United States. The act required all new drugs to be proved safe before being marketed. The basic definition of "safe" under this act is "nontoxic" when used in accordance with the conditions set forth on the label. This

act also specifies that every new drug must have been the subject of an approved **New Drug Application (NDA)** before U.S. commercialization. The NDA is the vehicle through which a **drug sponsor**, usually a pharmaceutical company, formally proposes that the FDA approve a new pharmaceutical for sale and marketing in the United States. The NDA will be discussed further later in this chapter.

In 1951, the Durham-Humphrey Amendment established two classes of drugs. A **legend drug** is sold only by prescription and is labeled "Rx only." An **over-the-counter (OTC)** drug may be sold without a prescription.

The FDA has the responsibility of regulating both legend and OTC drugs as well as medical and radiological devices, food, cosmetics, biologics, and veterinary drugs. The FDA does not test drugs itself, although it does conduct limited research in the areas of drug quality, safety, and effectiveness. A company seeking to market a drug is responsible for testing it and submitting evidence that it is safe and clinically effective.

Medication Guides

The FDA requires that **medication guides**, which are specific written information regarding the medication, are to be distributed to patients when certain drugs are dispensed from a retail pharmacy or upon discharge from the hospital. Many retail computer systems are set up to print the medication guide automatically when the drug label is printed. Medication guides may also be obtained from the FDA. Some medication guides are prepared for entire classes of drugs. Examples of such classes of drugs are NSAIDs (non-steroidal anti-inflammatory drugs) and antidepressants. Other medication guides are prepared for specific drugs. Medication guides must be given to patients at *all* dispensings—not just the the first time the drug is dispensed to the patient. (If the package insert is dispensed to the patient, the medication guide is not necessary.) There are approximately 300 drugs for which medication guides are required, and the list is growing.

The technician can play a vital role in making sure that the patient receives the proper medication guide. The technician can also put the guide together with the drug for the pharmacist when the pharmacist verifies the drug. Many different systems can be adopted in order to make this work. It is important for the pharmacist and technician to work together as a team to make sure that the pharmacy is compliant with this federal regulation.

Drug Approval Process

The FDA requires that the manufacturer of any new drug provide evidence of its safety and effectiveness before the drug will be allowed to enter the U.S. market. The drug must be shown to be safe through an intensive testing process that is undertaken by a drug sponsor, which is usually a pharmaceutical company. A drug sponsor must obtain permission from the FDA before testing any new drugs. Any hospital, physician, or researcher involved in experimental drug testing must also get FDA approval.

Drug sponsors are responsible for testing the efficacy and safety of their drugs on animals and, later, on human subjects through controlled clinical trials. Before the clinical testing begins, researchers analyze the main physical and chemical properties of the drug in the laboratory and study its pharmacologic and toxic effects in laboratory animals.

All test results are made available to the FDA through the New Drug Application (NDA), which also specifies proposed labeling for the new drug. The NDA contains details on the entire history of the development and testing of the drug. It documents results of the animal studies and clinical trials; describes components and composition of the drug; explains how the drug behaves in the body; and provides the details of manufacturing, processing, and packaging, with a special emphasis on quality control. The FDA also requires that the NDA include samples of the drug and its labels. A team of FDA physicians, statisticians, chemists, pharmacologists, and other scientists then reviews the contents of the NDA. If the drug is shown to be safe and effective, the FDA will approve it.

Clinical Trials If initial laboratory and animal model research on a particular drug is sufficiently promising, the developer will submit an application to the FDA requesting permission to begin testing the drug on humans. Human testing, referred to as a **clinical trial,** is used to determine whether new drugs or treatments are both safe and effective. Protocols for testing are typically developed by researchers and are subject to the approval of an FDA review board. These protocols describe what type of people may participate in the trial, the schedule of tests and procedures, medications and their dosages, and the length of the study. Throughout the trial phases, participants are monitored to determine the safety and efficacy of the drug. Only about 20% of the drugs that enter clinical trials are ultimately approved for marketing.

During clinical trials, patients are typically separated into two groups. The experimental group receives the drug to be tested, while the control group receives either a standard treatment for the illness or a placebo. A **placebo** is an inactive substance that the patient believes is a medication but that has no pharmacologic effect. In general, neither trial participants nor the study staff know whether a particular participant is in the experimental or the control group. This type of study, which allows for greater objectivity on the part of the investigators, is referred to as a **double blind study**.

Clinical trials of new drugs proceed through four phases:

- **Phase I** The drug is administered to a small group of healthy people (twenty to one hundred) to evaluate its safety, determine a safe dosage range, and identify side effects. Phase I studies assess the most common acute adverse effects and clarify what happens to a drug in the human body.
- **Phase II** The drug is studied in patients who have the condition the drug is intended to treat. At this point, it is determined whether the drug has a favorable effect on the disease state. Short-term placebo-to-drug comparisons are made in double-blind trials to determine the range and response of various doses.
- **Phase III** The drug treatment is compared to commonly used treatments. During this phase, investigators collect information that will allow the drug to be used safely. This phase continues the double-blind, placebo-to-drug comparisons begun in phase II. Dose escalations are used to determine the efficacy of the drug in treating the target disease.
- **Phase IV** Once the drug has been approved for marketing, phase IV studies continue testing it to collect information about its effects in various populations and to identify any side effects associated with long-term use.

The FDA Approval Process In the past, the entire FDA approval process for a drug took from 7 to 10 years. Recently, however, the FDA has taken steps to make urgently needed drugs available sooner. The Prescription Drug User Fee Act of 1992 instituted reforms that shortened the review process for new drugs. This act required that drug companies pay fees upon the submission of NDAs; these funds are used to hire an adequate number of reviewers. Now the FDA must act on standard applications for new drugs within 10 months and act on priority applications for drugs used to treat serious diseases within 6 months.

A classification system helps to determine the order in which applications are reviewed. Priority is given to drugs with the greatest potential benefit. Drugs that offer a significant medical advantage over existing therapies for any given disease state are assigned "priority status." Drugs for life-threatening diseases are considered first.

It is important to remember that no drug is absolutely safe. The FDA's approval is based on a judgment about whether the benefits of a new drug to users will outweigh its risks. The FDA will allow a product to present more of a risk when its potential benefit is great, especially if the product is used to treat a serious, life-threatening condition.

For example, drugs are not tested on pregnant women, but based on all available information, the FDA will classify a drug into one of the five pregnancy categories for use by pregnant patients shown in Table 1.2. The technician needs to be aware of these ratings if a drug is being dispensed to a pregnant patient. Besides protecting the health of the expectant mother or the baby, the information could save the pharmacist, technician, and drug company from a lawsuit.

Postmarketing Surveillance The consumer's well-being is the FDA's most important concern. Public health cannot be safeguarded without procedures to monitor the quality of drugs once they are marketed. The FDA has a branch, the Office of Compliance, which oversees the drug manufacturing process, ensuring that manufacturers follow good manufacturing practices (GMPs) as spelled out in FDA regulations.

In addition to demonstrating that a drug is safe and effective, a manufacturer must adhere to standards set by the United States Pharmacopoeia and the National Formulary (USP-NF) when manufacturing the drug. These standards ensure the strength, quality, effectiveness, and purity of the drug as well as its safety.

Some adverse reactions do not become apparent until after a drug has been approved and has been used by a large number of people. Therefore, postmarketing surveillance (phase IV trials) to ensure that drugs that pose serious safety threats are promptly removed from the market is critical. Professionals and consumers can report serious adverse reactions to MedWatch, the FDA's Medical Products Reporting Program. The purpose of this program is to improve the postmarketing surveillance of medical products and to ensure that new safety information pertaining to drug use is rapidly communicated to the medical community, thereby improving patient care. If a drug poses a health risk, the FDA will remove it from the market even though it has already been approved.

TABLE 1.2   FDA Pregnancy Categories

Catagory	Risk Level
A	No risk
B	Risk cannot be ruled out
C	Caution is advised
D	Is a definite risk
X	Do not use

Removing Drugs from the Market

A drug is considered safe if the FDA determines that the benefits of the drug outweigh the risks when the drug is used by the patients for which it was approved. The drug must also be labeled for use for the indications stated in the approval by the FDA, not for other uses. Any other use is considered unapproved.

"Safe" does not mean "harmless," because *every* drug has risks. When the FDA receives reports of significant adverse events, it evaluates the events to determine their seriousness and the likelihood that they were drug related. Adverse drug events are sometimes so rare that they cannot be predicted. These rare events surface as the drug is prescribed for use with large numbers of people. At other times, a drug turns out to be more toxic than suggested by the clinical trials. When the FDA believes a drug no longer has a place in treatment, it will ask the manufacturer to withdraw the product from the market voluntarily.

Black Box Warning

For drugs that are on the market and have been found to be problematic, but still provide therapy for specific conditions, a **Black Box warning** will be placed on the package insert. This warning alerts prescribers to the known problems associated with the use of the drug. The prescriber must then weigh the advantages of using this drug against the associated risks. Thousands of drugs on the market have Black Box warnings. They are deemed safe enough to continue using, but with known problems.

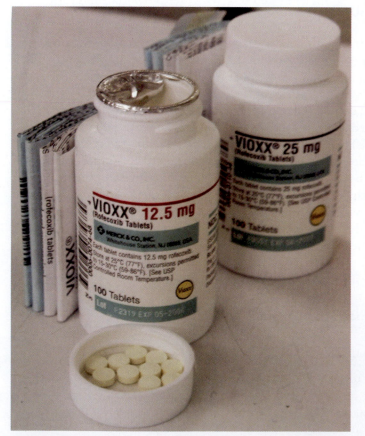

In 2004, Vioxx, a drug used to treat arthritis pain, was voluntarily withdrawn from the market because of a suspected link between the drug and increased heart attack risk.

Controlled Substances

The Controlled Substances Act (Title II of the Comprehensive Drug Abuse Prevention and Control Act of 1970), was designed to combat escalating drug abuse. It promoted drug education and research into the prevention and treatment of drug dependence; strengthened enforcement authority; and designated schedules, or categories, for drugs with a high potential for abuse, according to their probability of abuse. A drug listed on one of these schedules is known as a **controlled substance.**

The **Drug Enforcement Administration (DEA)** was established in 1973 as a branch of the U.S. Justice Department. The DEA is responsible for regulating the sale and use of specified drugs. It works at the national, state, and local levels. Individuals and institutions that handle or prescribe any controlled substances must be registered by the DEA. The prescriber's DEA registry number must be associated with the prescription when it is filled.

TABLE 1.3 Schedules for Controlled Substances

Schedule	Manufacturer's Label	Abuse Potential	Accepted Medical Use	Examples
schedule I	C-I	highest potential for abuse	For research only. Must have license to obtain. No accepted medical use in the United States.	heroin, lysergic acid diethylamide (LSD), marijuana
schedule II	C-II	high possibility of abuse, which can lead to severe psychological or physical dependence	Dispensing is severely restricted. Cannot be prescribed by phone except in an emergency. No refills on prescriptions.	morphine, oxycodone, meperidine, hydromorphone, fentanyl
schedule III	C-III	moderate potential for abuse and addiction	Prescriptions can be refilled up to five times within six months if authorized by a physician.	codeine with aspirin, codeine with acetaminophen, anabolic steroids
schedule IV	C-IV	low abuse potential; associated with limited physical or psychological dependence	Same as for schedule III.	benzodiazepines, meprobamate, phenobarbital
schedule V	C-V	lowest abuse potential	Some sold without a prescription depending on state law; purchaser must be over 18 years and is required to sign a log and show a driver's license.	liquid codeine preparations

Controlled substances are divided among five categories, or "schedules," each with its own set of restrictions imposed on the prescription of such substances. For example, schedule I drugs have the highest potential for abuse and have no accepted medical use. They may be used solely for research purposes. Table 1.3 summarizes the five categories of controlled substance schedules and includes corresponding abuse potential, accepted medicinal uses, and examples of each category.

Generic Drugs

At some stage in the drug development process, a drug sponsor will apply for patent protection. A **patent** protects the drug sponsor's investment in developing the drug by granting the sponsor the sole right to manufacture the drug while the patent is in effect. Under patent protection, the generic and brand names of a drug both belong to the drug sponsor. The manufacturer's proprietary right to the drug expires as soon as the patent expires, leaving other companies free to produce this drug as a nonproprietary, or generic, drug, possibly under their own brand name as well as the generic name. When this occurs, the price differential between the brand-name drug and the generic preparation is frequently substantial.

The substitution of generic drugs for more expensive brands is an important means of reducing healthcare costs, and many insurance companies require the use of generics before they will reimburse patients for drug costs. Some insurance companies actually provide a list of brand-name drugs whose cost they will cover.

Drug companies must submit an Abbreviated New Drug Application (ANDA) to the FDA to obtain approval to market a generic product. In approving a generic drug, the FDA requires many rigorous tests and procedures to ensure that the drug is interchangeable with the innovator drug under all approved indications and conditions of use. The generic drug must meet the following requirements:

- It must contain the same active ingredients as the original brand-name drug.
- It must be identical in strength, dosage form, and route of administration.
- It must have the same use indications.
- It must meet the same batch requirements for identity, strength, purity, and quality.
- It must yield similar blood absorption and urinary excretion curves for the active ingredient.

When the above criteria are met, the generic drug should produce pharmacologic effects similar to the innovator drug (the original brand-name drug).

The FDA has devised an A/B rating system to establish the therapeutic equivalence of generic drugs. The rating indicates whether the agency has judged a drug to be therapeutically equivalent to the innovator drug by meeting the criteria of pharmaceutical equivalence, bioequivalence, labeling, and good manufacturing practices. The FDA has also identified generics that are not therapeutically equivalent. (This information is published in an FDA book referred to as the *Orange Book*.) Although few drugs fall into this category, be aware that such drugs do exist.

Part of the responsibility of the healthcare practitioner is to lower costs without compromising the health of the patient. Healthcare costs have risen at an alarming rate in this country, but pharmaceutical costs have not increased at the same rate—primarily because of generic drugs. Billions of dollars are saved when generics are used.

Over-the-Counter Drugs

Many drugs used in the treatment of disease are over-the-counter (OTC) drugs. These drugs do not require a prescription. Drug companies recognize that consumers' instant recognition of OTC brand names has marketing value and sales potential. Consequently, companies are reluctant to change OTC brand names, even when the ingredients of the drugs change. Thus, drug companies commonly reuse brand names for products with different ingredients. Healthcare professionals are very concerned about this practice, but a loophole in the federal regulations allows it. The confusion created by this practice is potentially very dangerous. For example, Gaviscon, an OTC drug used for alleviating heartburn, previously contained alginic acid. Now it consists of aluminum hydroxide and a magnesium compound. Taking aluminum hydroxide can be very dangerous for a patient who is renally compromised, because it could lead to aluminum toxicity. Patients taking this OTC medication may not know it contains aluminum.

This is one area where the pharmacy technician has tremendous responsibility and can play an important role. Reading the ingredients when helping patients select OTC products is essential. It is also very important to report product problems to the FDA's MedWatch or the Institute for Safe Medication Practices (ISMP). Both can be found online.

Whether it is ideal or not, the reality is that the pharmacy technician is the individual who ultimately guides patients to these drugs. Although pharmacy technicians cannot counsel nor recommend drugs, they certainly need to be able to inform patients what conditions these drugs are used to treat. In most pharmacies OTC drugs are shelved in sections according to vague categories of ailments. For example, drugs for constipation and drugs for diarrhea are in the same section. Although the label contains information, patients are easily confused and often do not understand the medical terms or cannot read the very tiny print on the box. The technician is much better suited than the stock person to help patients find the drugs they are looking for and to describe the use for drugs. In no way could this be construed as counseling. Often it is as simple as reading from the box to an elderly patient who cannot possibly read the very small print on these labels. It is very important that the pharmacy technician is familiar with these drugs.

FDA Food Health Claims

Weighing risks against benefits is the primary objective of the FDA. By ensuring that food products and producers meet certain labeling standards, the FDA protects consumers and enables them to know what they are receiving.

In July 1999, the FDA authorized a new health claim that allows food companies to promote disease-fighting and cancer-fighting benefits of whole grains in various breakfast cereals. Manufacturers of whole grain foods that contain 51% or more whole grain ingredients by weight can now make the following claim: "Diets rich in whole grain foods and other plant foods and low in total fat, saturated fat, and cholesterol may reduce the risk of heart disease and certain cancers." In October 1999, the FDA authorized the use on food labels of health claims for the role of soy protein in reducing the risk of coronary heart disease. Consumers must realize that these products are not substitutes for prescribed medications but are to be used in conjunction with drug therapy.

Chapter Terms

alternative medicine use of herbs, dietary supplements, and homeopathic remedies rather than pharmaceuticals

apothecary forerunner of the modern pharmacists; the name also refers to the shop

Black Box warning information printed on a drug package to alert prescribers to potential problems with the drug

biopharmaceutical a drug produced by recombinant DNA technology

brand name the name under which the manufacturer markets a drug; also known as the trade name

C-I schedule I controlled substance, a drug with the highest potential for abuse, which may be used only for research under a special license

C-II schedule II controlled substance, a drug with a high potential for abuse, for which dispensing is severely restricted and prescriptions may not be refilled

C-III schedule III controlled substance, a drug with a moderate potential for abuse, which can be refilled no more than 5 times in 6 months and only if authorized by the physician for this time period

C-IV schedule IV controlled substance, a drug dispensed under the same restrictions as schedule III but having less potential for abuse

C-V schedule V controlled substance, a drug with a slight potential for abuse; some of which may be sold without a prescription depending on state law, but the purchaser must sign for the drug and show identification

chemical name a name that describes a drug's chemical composition in detail

clinical trial drug testing on humans, used to determine drug safety and efficacy

controlled substance a drug with potential for abuse; organized into five categories or schedules that specify whether and how the drug may be dispensed

double blind study a clinical trial in which neither the trial participants nor the study staff know whether a particular participant is in the control group or the experimental group

drug a medicinal substance or remedy used to change the way a living organism functions; also called a medication

Drug Enforcement Administration (DEA) the branch of the U.S. Justice Department that is responsible for regulating the sale and use of specified drugs, especially controlled substances

drug sponsor the entity, usually a pharmaceutical company, responsible for testing the efficacy and safety of a drug and proposing the drug for approval

Food and Drug Administration (FDA) the agency of the federal government that is responsible for ensuring the safety of drugs and food prepared for the market

generic name a name that identifies a drug independently of its manufacturer; sometimes denotes a drug that is not protected by a trademark; also referred to as a USAN (United States Adopted Name)

homeopathy a system of therapeutics in which diseases are treated by administering minute doses of drugs that, in healthy patients, are capable of producing symptoms like those of the disease being treated

legend drug a drug that may be sold only by prescription and must be labeled "Caution: Federal law prohibits dispensing without prescription" or "Rx only"

medication guide specific information about certain types of drugs that is required by the FDA to be made available to the patient

New Drug Application (NDA) the vehicle through which drug sponsors formally propose that the FDA approve a new pharmaceutical for sale and marketing in the United States

over-the-counter (OTC) drug a drug that may be sold without a prescription

patent a government grant that gives a drug company the exclusive right to manufacture a drug for a certain number of years; protects the company's investment in developing the drug

pharmacist one who is licensed to prepare and sell or dispense drugs and compounds and to fill prescriptions

pharmacognosy the study and identification of natural sources of drugs

pharmacologic effect the action of a drug on a living system

pharmacology the science of drugs and their interactions with the systems of living animals

pharmacopoeia an official listing of medicinal preparations

pharmacy technician an individual working in a pharmacy who, under the supervision of a licensed pharmacist, assists in activities not requiring the professional judgment of a pharmacist

Pharmacy Technician Certification Board (PTCB) a national organization that develops pharmacy technician standards and serves as a credentialing agency for pharmacy technicians

pharmakon a Greek word meaning a magic spell, remedy, or poison that was used in early records to represent the concept of a drug

placebo an inactive substance with no treatment value

prophylactic drug a drug that prevents or decreases the severity of a disease

therapeutic drug a drug that relieves symptoms of a disease

Chapter Summary

History of Medicinal Drugs

- The very concept of an outside force (i.e., drugs) influencing bodily function must be considered one of humanity's greatest advances.
- Humans have used drugs to gain increased control over their lives and to make their lives better and longer. Throughout history, drugs have held a special fascination for humans.
- Pharmacology is a broad term that includes the study of drugs and their actions on the body.
- The twentieth century brought major breakthroughs in medical care. The first antibiotic, sulfa, was soon followed by penicillin.

Contemporary Pharmacology Practice

- Observations of interactions between potent chemicals and living systems contribute to knowledge of biologic processes and provide effective methods for diagnosing, treating, and preventing many diseases. Compounds used for these purposes are called drugs.
- Drugs are derived from sources such as plants, animals, minerals, synthetic materials, and bioengineering advances.
- Billions of dollars are spent every year on alternative medicines. However, there is very little governmental regulation over this industry. These medications can also interact with prescription medications.

Drug Regulation

- Laws govern the drug industry and protect patients' rights.
- Medication guides must be provided to the patient on all dispensings of any drug for which the FDA requires a guide.
- A Black Box warning makes the prescriber aware of any serious problems that have occurred with a drug since it has been on the market.
- The FDA requires that all new drugs be proved effective and safe before they can be approved for marketing.
- Controlled clinical trials, in which results observed in patients receiving the drugs are compared to the results of patients receiving a different treatment, are the best way to determine what a new drug really does.
- When the benefits outweigh the risks, the FDA considers a drug safe enough to be approved.
- Drugs are not tested on pregnant women, but based on all available information, drugs are grouped into safety categories for use during pregnancy.
- Federal law divides controlled substances into five schedules according to their potential for abuse and clinical usefulness: C-I (research only), C-II (dispensing is severely restricted); C-III (can be refilled up to five times in six months if authorized by the physician); C-IV (same restrictions as C-III); C-V (may, depending on state law, be sold without a prescription).
- Generic drugs must be equivalent to the brand-name drugs, and the FDA has devised an A/B rating system to establish this.
- Pharmacy technicians can play an important role in helping patients identify ingredients in OTC medications, especially when it is possible that the ingredients of a previously purchased OTC medication have changed.

FDA Food Health Claims

- The FDA sets food labeling standards to ensure that consumers know what is in the food they are buying.

Chapter Review

Understanding Pharmacology

Select the best answer from the choices given.

1. The word *pharmakon* means
   a. dosing methods.
   b. remedy.
   c. pharmacist in Greek.
   d. none of the above

2. Pharmacognosy is
   a. a broad term that includes the study of drugs and their actions on the body.
   b. the study and identification of natural sources of drugs.
   c. the treatment of disease.
   d. the combined effect of two drugs.

3. Claude Bernard
   a. was a French physiologist who demonstrated that certain drugs have specific sites of action within the body.
   b. grew herbs of medicinal value.
   c. is the father of American pharmacology.
   d. discovered penicillin.

4. Pharmacology is
   a. a broad term that includes the study of drugs and their actions on the body.
   b. the study and identification of natural sources of drugs.
   c. the treatment of disease.
   d. an unusual or unexpected response to a drug.

5. A pharmacy technician should never
   a. take prescriptions over the telephone.
   b. advise patients about the use of their medicine.
   c. mix IV solutions.
   d. maintain patient profiles.

6. The FDA is required to
   a. ensure that a drug is safe and effective.
   b. monitor drug safety after a drug has been approved for sale.
   c. approve drugs in a timely manner.
   d. all of the above

7. Which of the following schedules includes drugs that have no accepted medical use in the United States?
   a. schedule I, C-I
   b. schedule II, C-II
   c. schedule III, C-III
   d. schedule IV, C-IV

8. Which of the following federal laws was designed to prevent drug abuse?
   a. Federal Food and Drug Act
   b. Durham-Humphrey Amendment
   c. Controlled Substances Act
   d. Prescription Drug User Fee Act

9. MedWatch is
   a. a program to shorten the review process for new drugs.
   b. an organization that sets standards for clinical trials.
   c. a system through which healthcare professionals can report adverse drug events.
   d. an organization that registers pharmacists.

10. The FDA's approval of a new drug is based on
    a. the completion of the first three phases of clinical trials.
    b. evidence that a drug is effective in treating the condition for which it was intended.
    c. a judgment that the benefits of a new drug to users will outweigh its risks.
    d. all of the above

The following statements are true or false. If an item is false, rewrite the statement so it is true.

_____ 1. Hippocrates introduced antiseptics to prevent infection.

_____ 2. Dioscorides first dissected the human body to study the function of specific organs.

_____ 3. Paracelsus advocated the use of individual drugs rather than mixtures or potions.

_____ 4. Lister wrote de Materia Medica.

_____ 5. The FDA requires that the manufacturer of any new drug provide evidence of its safety and effectiveness.

_____ 6. The A/B rating system is a system for assessing generic drug equivalence.

_____ 7. Medication guides are Black Box warnings that make the prescriber aware of the hazards of the drug.

_____ 8. The DEA is a branch of the U.S. Justice Department that regulates the manufacturing, distributing, and dispensing of controlled substances.

_____ 9. If two preparations are generically equivalent and their administration yields similar blood absorption and urinary excretion curves for the active ingredient, they are assumed to be therapeutically equivalent and to elicit similar pharmacological effects.

_____ 10. Once a patent expires, the drug may be produced in the generic form. The price differential is considerable when this occurs.

Pharmacology at Work

1. What are the requirements for dispensing schedule II and III prescriptions? Name some examples of each.

2. Describe the four phases in getting a drug to market. What would be the ramifications if the fourth stage were dropped?

3. Explain which requirements must be met before a generic drug is considered to be therapeutically equivalent to the brand. Would you or your family use generics? Why or why not?

Internet Research

Use the Internet to complete the following assignments.

1. Research the career options for trained pharmacy technicians. Write a short (two to three paragraphs) report outlining the qualifications sought by potential employers and explaining how this course will help you succeed in the job market. List at least two Internet sources.

2. Go to the FDA's Web site. Describe two pages within that site that you believe will be of interest to you in your career as a pharmacy technician. How does/will the information contained in those pages affect the marketing of drugs in the United States? List the complete URLs for the pages you selected.

Basic Concepts of Pharmacology

2

Learning Objectives

- Understand receptors and their function in mechanisms of drug actions.

- Appreciate the general principles of pharmacokinetics and the importance of those principles in developing and testing drugs.

- Understand that drugs can have beneficial and harmful effects.

- Become familiar with the common terms used to describe drug interactions.

Preview chapter terms and definitions.

The goal of drug therapy is to produce in the body a response that cures or controls a specific disease or medical condition. Drugs work via a series of processes, which can be described through the science of pharmacokinetics. Pharmacokinetic studies reveal how drugs work in the body and provide critical insight for predicting the effects of each specific drug. An understanding of these processes enables safe and effective treatments to be developed for various diseases.

Drug Actions

Drugs work by a variety of chemical mechanisms. Although detailed understanding of these mechanisms involves an advanced knowledge of biochemistry (the chemistry of the molecules of living organisms) and is beyond the scope of this book, it is important for the pharmacy technician to have a basic understanding of these mechanisms.

The body continually fights to maintain a state of **homeostasis,** or stability, of the organism. Homeostasis is achieved by a system of control and feedback mechanisms that causes the body to keep its living processes in balance. When the body's own processes cannot maintain a healthy state, drugs can be used to help the body restore and maintain this homeostasis. Many drugs exert their powerful and specific actions in the body by working in the same way as the chemical components the body itself uses for control and feedback.

Messengers and Receptors

For the body to maintain healthy control over its processes, it is essential that the cells that perform the various tasks needed for life have the ability to communicate with each other. The principal way in which cells communicate is through the action of chemical messengers. These messengers are chemical substances that cells produce and send out into the extracellular fluids of the body. Histamine, prostaglandin, and bradykinin are some important endogenous chemical messengers (ones that originate within the body). Once the messenger has been released, it can diffuse throughout the extracellular fluid and eventually reach the particular kind of cell that is its target cell. The messenger recognizes and communicates with the target cell via a specific protein molecule, or **receptor**, on the surface of or within the cell. When the messenger molecule binds with the receptor, some effect is produced in the target cell. That effect is the next step in the body's response to the condition that caused the messenger to be produced.

The various types of cells within the body contain different types of receptors, and only certain cell types possess the receptor required to combine with a particular chemical messenger. To bind with a specific cell type, the messenger must have a chemical structure (i.e., the specific geometrical arrangement of atoms) that is complementary to the structure of that cell's receptors. This property of a receptor site is known as **specificity**. For example, the cells involved in immune responses have receptors that are highly specific to molecules on the surfaces of bacteria, viruses, and some cancer cells. Receptors control many important body functions such as blood clotting and smooth muscle contraction, and they also play an important role in the body's protection against injury and infection.

The strength by which a particular messenger binds to its receptor site is referred to as its **affinity** for the site. Affinity is an important concept for understanding how drugs work in the body.

Mechanisms of Drug Action

As mentioned above, drugs often act like the chemical messengers described above to perform their specific actions in the body. Some drugs bind to a particular receptor and trigger the same cellular response as the body's own chemical messenger does. Such a drug is termed an **agonist** of the messenger and enhances the natural reactions of the body.

Other drugs work via a competitive mechanism to block the action of the endogenous messenger. When two substances, such as an endogenous messenger and a drug, have an affinity for the same receptor, they compete for available receptor sites. The number of receptor molecules occupied by each substance depends on the relative concentrations of the two substances as well as their relative affinities for the receptor. A drug that has a similar structure to the endogenous messenger may have a high affinity for the receptor site. When the drug binds to the receptor site, it prevents the endogenous messenger from binding there. If the drug does not trigger the cell's response itself, it inhibits the natural reaction of the body to the messenger. Such a drug is termed an **antagonist**.

Some drugs produce their effects not by interacting with specific receptors but by embedding themselves in cell membranes, which largely consist of chemically nonspecific lipids. A **lipid** is a fatty molecule, which is an important part of the cell wall. Lipids generally repel water. The effectiveness of these drugs is related to their lipid solubility (i.e., how well the lipid dissolves in a fluid) and does not depend on receptor sites. **Solubility** is the ability of a substance to dissolve in a fluid, whether a watery one such as blood or a fatty one such as membrane lipids.

Drugs can also combine with specific molecules in the body other than receptors, such as enzymes, transport proteins, and nucleic acids. Some antidepressants, for example, work by binding to the protein that removes the messenger serotonin from nerve terminals.

Other drugs act without any direct interaction with the cell. For example, drugs can work through an osmotic effect. That is, they can change the amount of water available to flow across a permeable barrier. Mannitol is such a drug. It interferes osmotically with water reabsorption by the kidneys.

Pharmacokinetics

The study of the activity of a drug within the body over a period of time is known as **pharmacokinetics.** Pharmacokinetic research enables scientists to understand how a drug works within the body to affect both normal physiology and disease. Pharmacokinetics involves a series of processes that produce specific effects.

Each drug's pharmacokinetics can be described in terms of four processes of interaction with the body: absorption, distribution, metabolism, and elimination. The overall pharmacokinetic process is sometimes referred to as ADME, an abbreviation for the names of these four processes. An understanding of these processes provides an important framework for researchers who are involved in developing drugs. Figure 2.1 presents a schematic model of these processes.

Absorption   **Absorption** is the process whereby a drug enters the circulatory system. That is, the chemical constituents of the drug are absorbed into the bloodstream. The absorption of a drug depends on its route of administration, its solubility in blood or other bodily fluids, and other physical properties. The form of the drug is an important factor in controlling its solubility. For example, drugs in liquid solution are already dissolved, so they are absorbed more readily than those in solid form.

The most common route of administration is oral. Other routes include intramuscular, subcutaneous, rectal, sublingual, transdermal, inhalation, and epicutaneous (topical) routes. Intravenous and intra-arterial administration do not require absorption, because the drug is immediately present in the systemic blood circulation.

When an oral medication is not given as a solution, its rate of absorption is slowed by the time needed for the tablet or capsule to disintegrate (release the drug) and for the drug to dissolve in the gastrointestinal (GI) tract. Disintegration and dissolution depend on the physical properties of the drug and its dosage form. Factors that affect dissolution include the chemistry of the drug as well as manufacturing variables such as the surface area of the drug particles released from the tablet or capsule. Some drugs interact with gastric contents, such as food. This effect can reduce the amount of drug available for absorption or, more often, increase the amount of time it takes the drug to be absorbed.

The small intestine is the primary site of absorption for many drugs, just as it is the site of absorption for food, because of its large surface area. When drugs are given orally, the degree of movement within the GI tract also affects absorption. The faster the rate of gastric emptying, the more rapid the absorption rate of a drug, because it reaches the vast absorptive surface of the small intestine more quickly.

FIGURE 2.1
The
Pharmacokinetic
Process

The main phases of
drug/body interac-
tions are absorption,
distribution, metabo-
lism, and elimination
(ADME).

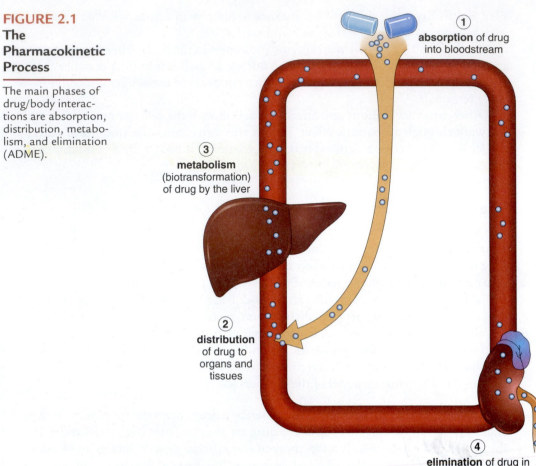

In the small intestine, the drug must cross the cell membranes of the epithelial cells. Membranes are composed of lipids, proteins, and carbohydrates. Pores are small openings or empty spaces in the membrane through which low-weight molecules pass freely. Lipid-soluble molecules, small hydrophilic (water soluble) molecules, and ions readily pass through cell membranes. Some drugs may be metabolized by enzyme action within the epithelial cells before they reach systemic blood.

Distribution   **Distribution** is the process by which a drug moves from the blood-stream into other body fluids and tissues and ultimately to its sites of action. Blood flow is the most important rate limiting factor for distribution of a drug. Three additional factors affect the rate and degree of distribution.

- **Binding to Plasma Proteins**   The biological activity of a drug is related to the concentration of "free" drug in circulation. If a drug molecule binds to a protein in blood plasma, that drug molecule is essentially inactive. An unbound drug molecule, however, is available to reach its site of action. Disease states can also affect protein binding. Renal failure, for example, may result in a loss of plasma proteins (with less available for binding) or in the accumulation of metabolic wastes that could potentially displace some bound drugs. Liver disease may also result in fewer plasma proteins to transport drugs. All of these conditions can therefore increase both the therapeutic and the toxic effects of a drug.

- **Binding to Cellular Constituents** Drugs can bind to proteins other than those in blood plasma, such as proteins in tissues. This type of binding usually occurs when the drug has an affinity for some cellular constituent.
- **Blood-Brain Barrier** The capillaries in the central nervous system (CNS) are enveloped by glial cells, which present a barrier to many water-soluble compounds. This **blood-brain barrier** prevents many substances from entering the cerebrospinal fluid (CSF) from the blood. Therefore, many drugs cannot get to the CNS because they are unable to pass through the blood-brain barrier. Pathologic states such as inflammation will reduce this resistance, and the barrier can become more permeable under such conditions. For example, though general anesthetics easily penetrate this barrier, penicillin cannot penetrate the CNS unless the meninges are swollen.

Metabolism The process in the body by which drugs are converted to other biochemical compounds, and then excreted through metabolic pathways is **metabolism**. A substance into which a drug is converted by metabolism is called a **metabolite** of the drug, and the sequence of chemical steps that convert a drug to a metabolite is called a **metabolic pathway**.

Metabolism converts drugs to more water-soluble (less lipid-soluble) forms. Once in a more water-soluble state, drug metabolites may be more easily excreted by the kidney.

Many factors can alter metabolism and elimination. Disease states, age, and genetic predisposition all affect the way the body metabolizes drugs. In addition, if given together, two drugs may decrease or enhance the metabolism of each other. Some drugs decrease the metabolism of other drugs by competitive or complete **inhibition** of a particular drug-metabolizing enzyme. Other drugs enhance drug metabolism by **induction** of these same enzyme systems.

The two processes of induction and inhibition can control specific enzymes.

- **Induction** The concentration of a particular enzyme can be affected by some drugs, foods, and smoking. Drugs that increase these enzymes can decrease the pharmacologic response to other agents (e.g., phenobarbital increases the metabolism and therefore decreases the effect of warfarin) or to themselves (e.g., some barbiturates stimulate self-metabolism).
- **Inhibition** Some agents can slow or block enzyme activity, which impairs the metabolism of drugs and may increase their concentration and toxic or pharmacologic effects. (e.g. Phenobarbital when combined with opioids or benzodiazepines can severely decrease respiration).

Elimination **Elimination**, the removal of a drug or its metabolites from the body, occurs primarily in the kidney (through urine) and the liver (through feces), but other routes exist. Drugs may be exhaled by the lungs or excreted in perspiration, saliva, and breast milk. The rate at which a drug is eliminated from a specific volume of blood per unit of time is referred to as its **clearance**.

Pharmacokinetic Parameters

An understanding of the pharmacokinetic processes enables researchers to make determinations regarding how a particular drug should be administered to the patient to obtain a specific response. Safe and effective drug therapy requires that a drug is delivered to its target sites in concentrations that will treat the disease state for which it is intended, but without producing a state of toxicity.

A **dose** is the quantity of a drug administered at one time. As greater doses of a drug are given, a greater response will occur, but eventually a point will be reached when either no improved clinical response occurs, or the adverse effects outweigh the beneficial effects. This limitation is called the **ceiling effect**. Figure 2.2 illustrates the typical dose-response curve. Increased dosing beyond the ceiling may result in toxicity, leading to side effects or even death.

Many dosages are fairly universal from patient to patient. In some cases, however, dosage must be individualized to the patient because of variables such as age, size, weight, sex, race, nutritional state, and pregnancy, as well as other drugs the patient may be taking. A determination of individual patient dose and dosing intervals can be made, if necessary, based on the testing of drug concentrations in body fluids such as blood, plasma, and urine. Testing of these fluids over specified time intervals provides an indication of how the patient is metabolizing and eliminating the drug. The lowest level of a drug in the blood is known as the **trough**, and the highest level is the **peak**.

Typically, only a portion of the dose administered becomes biologically active in the body. The fraction of the administered dose that is available to the target tissue is an expression of the drug's **bioavailability**. Drugs taken orally must pass through the intestinal wall and traverse the liver before entering the blood and reaching systemic sites. Metabolism in the liver before a drug reaches the systemic circulation is referred to as the **first-pass effect**. If a drug undergoes considerable first-pass metabolism, its bioavailability will be decreased when it is administered orally. Some drugs have such a substantial first-pass effect that they essentially must be administered by injection.

The **therapeutic range**, also called the therapeutic window, is the range of serum concentrations for a particular drug that provides the optimum probability of achieving the desired response with the least probability of toxicity. Figure 2.3 illustrates the concept of therapeutic range. A defined therapeutic range provides the best chance for successful therapy. Some patients may require concentrations of drug below or above the usual therapeutic range.

Doses and dosing intervals are determined by clinical trials but may need to be adjusted on an individual basis. This is often done based on a blood sample and is particularly beneficial for attaining the desired concentration for a drug with a narrow therapeutic range. When the amount of drug in a patient's blood gives the

FIGURE 2.2
Dose-Response Curve

As greater doses of a drug are given, a greater response is noted until a point is reached when the response no longer improves with increased dosing. This is known as the ceiling effect.

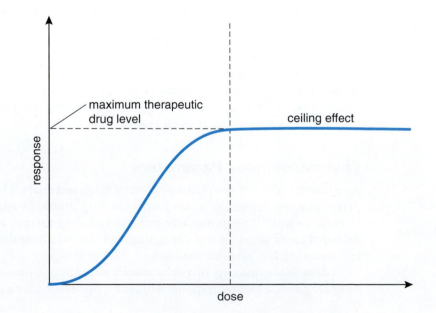

FIGURE 2.3
Therapeutic Range

An optimum dosage range yields beneficial effects without causing toxic effects, whereas underdosing has little benefit on the healing process, and overdosing can lead to toxicity and death.

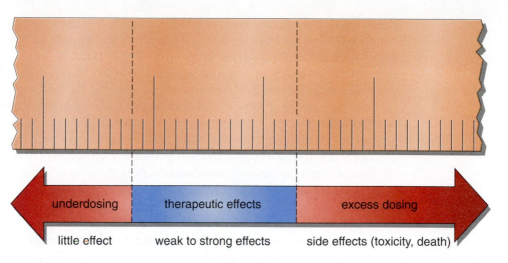

desired response, it is said to be at the therapeutic level. The length of time a drug is at this level is referred to as its **duration of action**. This concept is illustrated by the curve in Figure 2.4.

The time required to achieve therapeutic levels of a drug can be shortened by the administration of a **loading dose**—an amount of a drug that will bring the blood concentration rapidly to a therapeutic level. If a single large dose poses a risk of toxicity, loading can be accomplished by administering the loading amount in a series of doses. The **volume of distribution**, which describes the relationship between the blood concentration attained and the dose of the drug given, is important for prescribing the loading dose.

After the drug concentration has reached a therapeutic level, the patient receives a **maintenance dose** at regular intervals to keep the drug at a therapeutic level. The rate of clearance of the drug is important for calculating the maintenance dose.

Pharmacokinetic Modeling

Pharmacokinetic modeling is a method of describing the process of absorption, distribution, metabolism, and elimination of a drug within the body mathematically. For some drugs, elimination is a **zero-order** process; that is, a fixed quantity of drug is eliminated per unit of time. The best example is alcohol. For the majority of drugs, elimination is said to be **first-order**. That is, a constant fraction of the remaining drug is eliminated per unit of time. The time it takes the body to eliminate half of such a drug is called the **half-life** of the drug and is written $T_{1/2}$. A longer half-life implies a longer

FIGURE 2.4
Duration of Action

Plasma drug concentration must reach a minimum therapeutic level before physiological activity is noted.

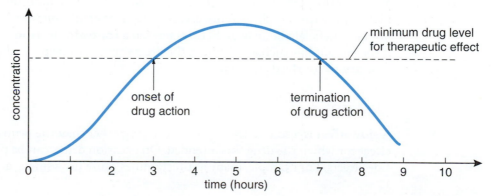

duration of the drug action. It takes about 5 to 7 half-lives to consider the drug "removed" from the body—meaning that only 1% to 3% remains. If the $T_{1/2}$ of a drug is 2 hours, then the drug will be gone in 10 to 14 hours. If the $T_{1/2}$ is 30 hours, then it will take 150 to 210 hours, or 6 to 9 days, to eliminate the drug. A drug with a long half-life may produce effects for days or even weeks after being discontinued.

Studies on drug absorption, distribution, metabolism, and elimination have advanced the concept that the body may be regarded as consisting of different compartments. In the simplest form, a drug passes from one compartment to another in direct proportion to its concentration gradient. Two pharmacokinetic models, based on the compartment theory, have been developed. In the one-compartment model, the drug is distributed into blood volume. This model assumes an instantaneous and homogeneous distribution of the drug throughout the body. In the two-compartment model, the drug is distributed into blood volume and then into body tissue. This more complex model better describes the distribution of many drugs.

Drug Effects

The pharmacokinetic models described above provide critical insight for predicting the effects of each specific drug. Some effects are beneficial, while others can be detrimental or dangerous. Just as each person is different, each person's reaction to a drug may be different. Thus, each patient must be monitored closely to ensure that his or her response to the drug is appropriate.

Beneficial Responses

The desired action of a drug in the treatment of a particular disease state or symptom is referred to as a **therapeutic effect**. The therapeutic effect is the action for which the drug is prescribed. Drugs can act locally or they can act on the body as a whole. A **local effect** is confined to a specific part of the body (e.g., lidocaine, numbing an area for stiches). A **systemic effect**, on the other hand, is a generalized, all-inclusive effect on the entire body (e.g., lowering blood pressure).

Sometimes drugs are prescribed to prevent the occurrence of an infection or disease. In this case, the drug effect is referred to as **prophylaxis**. Patients who will be undergoing surgery will often be administered prophylactic drugs, which will work to prevent the occurrence of infections.

In selecting a drug for an individual patient, the healthcare practitioner considers its medically accepted uses and situations in which it should or should not be given. A disease, symptom, or conditions for which a drug is known to be of benefit is termed an **indication** for the drug; that is, if the patient has the condition, it may be a good idea to prescribe the drug. A disease, symptom, or condition for which the drug will not be beneficial and may do harm is termed a **contraindication** for the drug; that is, if the patient has such a condition, the drug should not be prescribed, even when indications for the drug are present.

Side Effects

A **side effect** is a secondary response to a drug other than the primary therapeutic effect for which the drug was intended. On occasion drugs can be prescribed for their side effects. For example, many antihistamines cause drowsiness, and therefore they are found in many over-the-counter (OTC) insomnia preparations. Sometimes two drugs are prescribed together because the combination has fewer or more tolerable side effects than a high dose of either. Nausea, rash, and constipation are the most common side effects and are usually fairly benign. Others can be very bothersome and even serious.

Allergic Responses An **allergic response** is a local or general reaction of the immune system to an otherwise harmless substance. A substance that produces an allergic response is known as an **allergen**. In general, a molecule that stimulates an immune response, whether allergic or not, is known as an **antigen**.

The first exposure to an allergen generally gives little or no observable response. Rather, what is critical about the initial exposure is the resulting "memory storage" that characterizes active immunity. Upon a subsequent exposure, the body recognizes ("remembers") the antigen and responds with a more potent antibody response. This response can elicit a range of reactions from uncomfortable to life threatening. Some responses start within minutes of exposure; others may be delayed. Exposure to the allergen may cause mild, moderate, or, in some cases, severe inflammation. Some common allergic reactions to drugs include nasal secretions, swelling, wheezing, an excessively rapid heart rate, **urticaria** (hives), **pruritus** (itching), **angioedema** (abnormal accumulation of fluid in tissue), **wheals** (red, elevated areas on body), and, in rare cases, even death.

An **anaphylactic reaction** is a severe allergic response resulting in immediate, life-threatening respiratory distress, usually followed by vascular collapse and shock and accompanied by hives. An **idiosyncratic reaction** is an unusual or unexpected response to a drug that is unrelated to the dose given.

Other Responses to Drugs Drug **dependence** is a state in which a person's body has adapted physiologically and psychologically to a drug and cannot function without it. Dependence should not be confused with **addiction**, which is a dependence characterized by a perceived need to take a drug to attain the psychological and physical effects of mood-altering substances. One sign of addiction is a decrease in psychological well-being and social or vocational functioning. Patients who are being treated for various disease states may become dependent on medications without exhibiting the signs of addiction.

Drug abuse is the use of a drug for purposes other than those prescribed and/or in amounts that were not directed. Abusive use of drugs can be, but is not always, linked to addiction.

After a patient has been taking a drug over a significant period of time, he or she may begin to develop a decreased response to the drug. This decrease in response to the effects of a drug with continued administration is referred to as **tolerance**. As tolerance develops, the dosage of the drug may need to be increased to maintain a constant response.

Drug Interactions

Another reaction to drugs involves **interaction**. One drug can have an effect on the action of another. Foods and other substances such as alcohol and nicotine can also interact with drugs. A common way in which a substance can interact with a drug is by inducing or inhibiting enzymes that metabolize the drug, as described previously. A system of enzymes called cytochrome P-450 contributes to many drug interactions because it plays a key role in oxidizing drugs and other substances.

Grapefruit provides an example of a food-drug interaction. Grapefruit juice contains certain chemicals that inhibit a form of cytochrome P-450 that is found primarily in the intestines. Because of this inhibition, less of the drug undergoes first-pass metabolism, so more active drug is absorbed into the bloodstream, increasing the risk of overdose. The effect of grapefruit juice on intestinal enzymes is partially irreversible; thus, enzyme levels do not return to normal immediately after the juice is cleared from the intestines. Absorption of drugs from the intestines may be affected for up to a day following ingestion of grapefruit juice.

Do not take with grapefruit juice

It is important that the physician and pharmacist have a complete list of all prescription drugs, OTC medications, vitamins, and herbal remedies that a patient is taking so that potential interactions can be recognized and appropriately handled. The pharmacy technician should routinely ask patients for this information.

Table 2.1 describes a number of common drug relationships.

TABLE 2.1   Common Drug Relationships

Drug Relationship	Description
Addition	The combined effect of two drugs is equal to the sum of the effects of each drug taken alone.
Antagonism	The action of one drug negates the action of a second drug.
Potentiation	One drug increases or prolongs the action of another drug, and the total effect is greater than the sum of the effects of each drug used alone. If one drug prescribed alone cannot produce the desired effect, another drug can be prescribed to increase the first drug's potency. This term is used when one of the drugs has little or no action when given alone and the second drug increases the potency of the first drug.
Synergism	The combined effect of two drugs is more intense or longer in duration than the sum of their individual effects. Drugs that work synergistically are usually prescribed together.

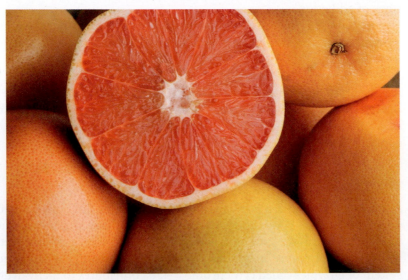

Grapefruit and grapefruit juice interfere with proper absorption of several common drugs.

Chapter Terms

absorption the process whereby a drug enters the circulatory system

addiction a dependence characterized by a perceived need to take a drug to attain the psychological and physical effects of mood-altering substances

affinity the strength by which a particular chemical messenger binds to its receptor site on a cell

agonist drugs that bind to a particular receptor site and trigger the cell's response in a manner similar to the action of the body's own chemical messenger

allergen substance that produces an allergic response

allergic response an instance in which the immune system overreacts to an otherwise harmless substance

anaphylactic reaction a severe allergic response resulting in immediate life-threatening respiratory distress, usually followed by vascular collapse and shock and accompanied by hives

angioedema abnormal accumulation of fluid in tissue

antagonist drugs that bind to a receptor site and block the action of the endogenous messenger or other drugs

antigen a specific molecule that stimulates an immune response

bioavailability the degree to which a drug or other substance becomes available to the target tissue after administration

blood-brain barrier a barrier that prevents many substances from entering the cerebrospinal fluid from the blood; formed by glial cells that envelope the capillaries in the central nervous system, presenting a barrier to many water-soluble compounds though they are permeable to lipid-soluble substances

ceiling effect a point at which no clinical response occurs with increased dosage

clearance the rate at which a drug is eliminated from a specific volume of blood per unit of time

contraindication a disease, condition, or symptom for which a drug will not be beneficial and may do harm

dependence a state in which a person's body has adapted physiologically and psychologically to a drug and cannot function without it

distribution the process by which a drug moves from the blood into other body fluids and tissues and ultimately to its sites of action

dose the quantity of a drug administered at one time

duration of action the length of time a drug gives the desired response or is at the therapeutic level

elimination removal of a drug or its metabolites from the body by excretion

first-order depending directly on the concentration of the drug; elimination of most drugs is a first-order process in which a constant fraction of the drug is eliminated per unit of time

first-pass effect the extent to which a drug is metabolized by the liver before reaching systemic circulation

half-life the time necessary for the body to eliminate half of the drug in the body at any time; written as $T_{1/2}$

homeostasis stability of the organism

idiosyncratic reaction an unusual or unexpected response to a drug that is unrelated to the dose given

indication a disease, symptom, or condition for which a drug is known to be of benefit

induction the process whereby a drug increases the concentration of certain enzymes that affect the pharmacologic response to another drug

inhibition the process whereby a drug blocks enzyme activity and impairs the metabolism of another drug

interaction a change in the action of a drug caused by another drug, a food, or another substance such as alcohol or nicotine

lipid a fatty molecule, an important constituent of cell membranes

local effect an action of a drug that is confined to a specific part of the body

loading dose amount of a drug that will bring the blood concentration rapidly to a therapeutic level

maintenance dose amount of a drug administered at regular intervals to keep the blood concentration at a therapeutic level

metabolic pathway the sequence of chemical steps that convert a drug into a metabolite

metabolism the process by which drugs are chemically converted to other compounds

metabolite a substance into which a drug is chemically converted in the body

peak the top or upper limit of a drug's concentration in the blood

pharmacokinetic modeling a method of describing the process of absorption, distribution, metabolism, and elimination of a drug within the body mathematically

pharmacokinetics the activity of a drug within the body over a period of time; includes absorption, distribution, metabolism, and elimination

prophylaxis effect of a drug in preventing infection or disease

pruritus itching sensation

receptor a protein molecule on the surface of or within a cell that recognizes and binds with specific molecules, thereby producing some effect within the cell

side effect a secondary response to a drug other than the primary therapeutic effect for which the drug was intended

solubility a drug's ability to dissolve in body fluids

specificity the property of a receptor site that enables it to bind only with a specific chemical messenger; to bind with a specific cell type, the messenger must have a chemical structure that is complementary to the structure of that cell's receptors

systemic effect an action of a drug that has a generalized, all-inclusive effect on the body

therapeutic effect the desired action of a drug in the treatment of a particular disease state or symptom

therapeutic level the amount of drug in a patient's blood at which beneficial effects occur

therapeutic range the optimum dosage, providing the best chance for successful therapy; dosing below this range has little effect on the healing process, while overdosing can lead to toxicity and death

tolerance a decrease in response to the effects of a drug as it continues to be administered

trough the lowest level of a drug in the blood

urticaria hives, itching sensation

volume of distribution mathematical relationship between the blood concentration attained and the amount of drug administered

wheals slightly elevated, red areas on the body surface

zero-order not depending on the concentration of the drug in the body; elimination of alcohol is a zero-order process in which a constant quantity of the drug is removed per unit of time

Chapter Summary

Drug Actions

- A receptor is a molecule on the surface of or within a cell that recognizes and binds with specific molecules, producing some effect in the cell.
- By binding to receptors on or within body cells, drugs can mimic or block the action of chemical messengers to exert powerful and specific actions in the body.
- One drug can compete with another drug for its intended receptor.
- Pharmacokinetics is the study of the time course of absorption, distribution, metabolism, and excretion of drugs and their metabolites in relation to the time they are present in the body.
- The pharmacokinetic process is sometimes referred to as ADME.
- The primary sites of elimination are the kidney and the liver. Drugs may also be exhaled by the lungs or excreted in perspiration.

- Testing body fluids over time demonstrates how the body handles the drug.
- The volume of distribution is important for calculating the loading dose, clearance is important for calculating the maintenance dose, and half-life is important for determining the dosing interval.

Drug Effects

- Drug effects include therapeutic effects, adverse reactions, and side effects.
- Drugs can interact with other drugs, food, and the patient's own body.
- Two drugs may be prescribed together because the combination has fewer or more tolerable side effects than a high dose of either.

Chapter Review

Understanding Pharmacology

Select the best answer from the choices given.

1. Responses other than the intended therapeutic one are
   a. side effects.
   b. synergism.
   c. potentiation.
   d. additive.

2. Which term refers to the treatment of disease?
   a. side effects
   b. synergism
   c. therapeutics
   d. addiction

3. Increasing resistance to the usual effects of an established dosage of a drug as a result of continued use is
   a. an idiosyncratic reaction.
   b. an anaphylactic reaction.
   c. tolerance.
   d. dependence.

4. A response that is unusual, unexpected, or opposite from the expected response to a drug is
   a. an idiosyncratic reaction.
   b. an anaphylactic reaction.
   c. tolerance.
   d. dependence.

5. A severe, life-threatening allergic response with breathing difficulty, vascular collapse, and shock, accompanied by urticaria, pruritus, and angioedema is
   a. an idiosyncratic reaction.
   b. an anaphylactic reaction.
   c. tolerance.
   d. dependence.

6. Complete removal of a drug from a specific volume of blood per unit of time is
   a. pharmacokinetics.
   b. bioavailability.
   c. volume of distribution.
   d. clearance.

7. What describes the relationship between the dosage of drug given and the blood concentration attained?
   a. pharmacokinetics
   b. bioavailability
   c. volume of distribution
   d. clearance

8. The degree to which a drug becomes available to the target tissue is
   a. pharmacokinetics.
   b. bioavailability.
   c. volume of distribution.
   d. clearance.

9. A study to understand drug behavior in the human body is
   a. pharmacokinetics.
   b. bioavailability.
   c. volume of distribution.
   d. clearance.

10. A method of describing the process of absorption, distribution, and elimination of a drug within the body is
   a. drug interactions.
   b. disintegration and dissolution.
   c. routes of administration.
   d. pharmacokinetic modeling.

The following statements are true or false. If an item is false, rewrite the statement so that it is true.

_____ 1. Side effects are secondary responses to a drug other than the therapeutic effect.

_____ 2. Potentiation occurs when the combined effect of two drugs is equal to the sum of the effect of each drug taken alone.

_____ 3. Addition is an effect that occurs when a drug increases or prolongs the action of another drug, the total effect being greater than the sum of the two parts.

_____ 4. Half-life is the time required for the drug to eliminate 75% of the drug in circulation at any given time.

_____ 5. GI motility does not affect absorption.

_____ 6. Blood flow is the rate-limiting factor for distribution of a drug.

_____ 7. Pharmacokinetics is the study of the time course of absorption, distribution, metabolism, and elimination of drugs over a period of time.

_____ 8. Only a portion of the dose administered becomes biologically active in the body.

_____ 9. Drugs can pass through the blood-brain barrier quite easily.

_____ 10. When two drugs try to bind to the same receptor, this is called site antagonism.

Pharmacology at Work

1. Explain the statement "Pharmacists must consider the effect the body has on the drug as well as the effect the drug has on the body."

2. Explain the concepts receptor, agonist, and antagonist.

3. Define half-life. If a drug's half-life is six hours, how long would it take to remove the drug from the body?

4. Define ceiling effect and explain its importance in dosing medication.

Internet Research

Use the Internet to complete the following assignments.

1. Go to the National Library of Medicine's PubMed Web site. This site provides a comprehensive index of medical journal articles. Find two journal article abstracts that describe pharmacokinetic studies of new drugs and, for each, list the full citation of the article along with the name(s) of the drug(s) included in the study. Note the abstracts' use of the terms introduced in this chapter (e.g., clearance, half-life, bioavailability) and record an example of one sentence containing such terminology in each of the abstracts. Describe your search strategy.

2. Find a reputable Internet site that will identify medications that interact with grapefruit juice. Print out a list of those medications.

Dispensing Medications

3

Learning Objectives

- Know the components of the prescription, including the commonly used abbreviations.
- Understand the "rights" of correct drug administration.
- Recognize common dosage forms.
- Know the routes of administration.
- Recognize factors that influence the effects of drugs, particularly in the elderly and pediatric populations.

- Understand the immunization process.
- Understand the role of the pharmacy technician in medication safety.

Preview chapter terms and definitions.

Pharmacy technicians play a key role in the dispensing of pharmacologic agents. This role requires a thorough understanding of the components of the prescription and the responsibilities of pharmacy personnel. The prescription includes all the information necessary for the pharmacist to fill the prescription with the correct dosage form and for the patient to take the medication correctly. Two age groups of patients—the elderly and children—have special needs that must be considered in dispensing drugs.

The Prescription

A **prescription** (or an order) is a written or oral directions for medication to be dispensed to a patient. A physician or other licensed practitioner issues a prescription, and it is filled by a pharmacist. When a prescription is issued and dispensed in an institutional setting such as a hospital, it is called an **order**. The term prescription is used in non-institutional settings.

Prescription requirements may vary by state, but typically should contain all of the following:

- the patient's name
- the date the prescription was written
- the **inscription**, which states the name of the drug, dose, and quantities of the ingredients
- the **signa**, often referred to as the "sig," which provides directions to be included on the label for the patient to follow in taking the medication
- an indication of the number of refills allowed, or "no refills" if that is the case
- the signature (handwritten, not stamped) and address of the prescribing physician
- an indication of whether generic substitution is permitted

If the prescription is for a controlled substance, discussed in Chapter 1, the Drug Enforcement Agency (DEA) number of the prescribing physician must be on the prescription.

Figure 3.1 is an example of a prescription with the essential elements labeled. The symbol at the top of the form, ℞ or Rx, is the symbol for prescription. If a medication has this symbol on the container, the medication may not be dispensed unless a prescriber writes an order or prescription for it. It cannot be sold over the counter (OTC).

Pharmacy technicians should always double-check a prescription for accuracy and to ensure that all of the legal requirements have been met. Depending on state laws, the label on the medication container given to the patient must include the patient's name, date the prescription was written, the inscription, the signa, the number of refills, the expiration date, the prescriber's name, the Rx number, and the phone number and address of the pharmacy.

FIGURE 3.1

The Essential Elements of a Prescription

The pharmacy technician should always check these elements.

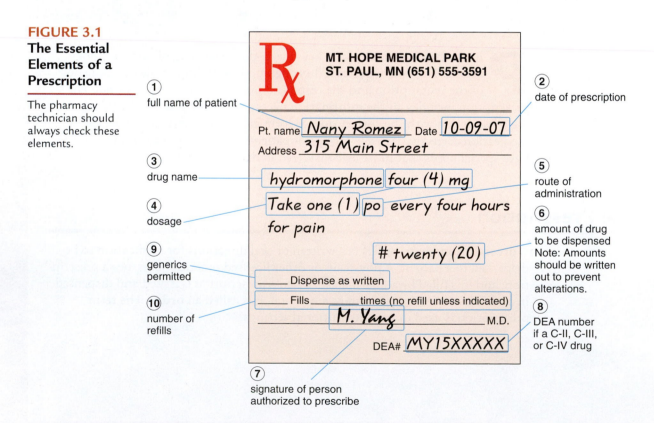

1. full name of patient
2. date of prescription
3. drug name
4. dosage
5. route of administration
6. amount of drug to be dispensed
   Note: Amounts should be written out to prevent alterations.
7. signature of person authorized to prescribe
8. DEA number if a C-II, C-III, or C-IV drug
9. generics permitted
10. number of refills

To fill the prescription safely, the pharmacy technician should be familiar with common abbreviations used in prescriptions, listed in Table 3.1. Although these abbreviations are standard usage for prescribers, pharmacists, and their technicians, the instructions to the patient are not abbreviated but spelled out in full and phrased as simply as possible to ensure proper use of the medication. There is strong evidence to show that abbreviations are the source of many medication errors. When taking a verbal order or prescription, it is recommended that abbreviations *not* be used.

The abbreviations in Table 3.2 have been identified as the cause of many errors and should never be used. Additional dangerous abbreviations are listed at the Institute for Safe Medication Practices (ISMP) Web site. Even though these abbreviations are unapproved, the technician will frequently see them and will need to be able to interpret them in order to fill a prescription.

Most pharmacies give the patient an information sheet with additional details regarding the proper way to take the medication (especially in regard to food intake), possible side effects, and situations in which the prescribing physician should be consulted. Limiting the number of refills allowed without another physician consultation is a way to prevent the patient from encountering severe side effects from the medication.

Warning

Check the ISMP Web site at http:// www.ismp.org for dangerous abbreviations and dose designations.

TABLE 3.1 Abbreviations Used in Writing Prescriptions

Abbreviation	Translation	Abbreviation	Translation
ac	before meals	NKA	no known allergy
am	morning	NKDA	no known drug allergy
bid	twice a day	npo	nothing by mouth
c̄	with	pc	after meals
cap	capsule	PO	by mouth
DAW	dispense as written	prn	as needed
D/C	discontinue	q	every
g	gram*	qh	every hour
gr	grain	q2 h	every 2 hours
gtt	drop	qid	four times a day
h or hr	hour	qs	a sufficient quantity
IM	intramuscular	stat	immediately
IV	intravenously	tab	tablet
L	liter	tid	three times daily
mcg	microgram	ud	as directed
mEq	milliequivalent	wk	week
mL	milliliter		

* The abbreviation gm is sometimes used for gram.

Note: Some prescribers may write abbreviations using capital letters or periods. However, periods should not be used with metrics or medical abbreviations, because they can be a source of medication errors.

TABLE 3.2 Problematic Prescription Abbreviations	
Dangerous Abbreviation	**Correct Form to Use**
μg	microgram or mcg
hs	half strength or hours of sleep, bedtime
qd	every day
qhs	nightly at bedtime
qod	every other day
U	units
$MgSO^4$	magnesium sulfate
MSO^4	morphine sulfate
.2 with no leading zero (often read as 2, creating a tenfold error)	0.2
2.0 with trailing zero (often read as 20, creating a tenfold error)	2

Note: Additional dangerous abbreviations are listed at http://www.ismp.org.

Correct Drug Administration "Rights"

The "rights" of medication administration offer useful guidelines when filling prescriptions for patient medications. The healthcare professionals who are involved in the process from prescribing through administration use these concepts to avoid medication errors. A drug misadventure can occur whenever they are not followed correctly. Figure 3.2 illustrates the concepts, and five of these rights are overviewed below.

- **Right Patient** Always verify the patient's name before dispensing medication. Always use at least two patient identifiers.
- **Right Drug** Always check the medication against the original prescription and the patient's disease state. The medication label contains important information about the drug that will be dispensed to the patient. Figure 3.3 provides an example of a medication label.

FIGURE 3.2
"Rights" for Correct Drug Administration

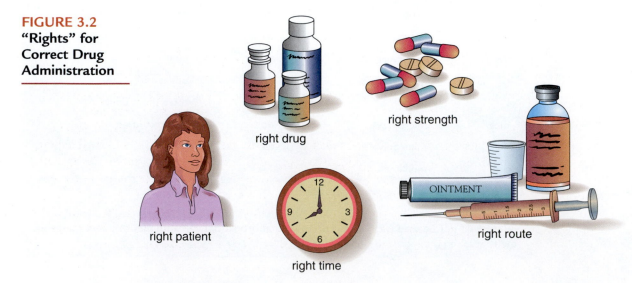

right drug

right strength

right patient

right time

right route

FIGURE 3.3
Medication Label on a Dispensing Container

Important information, such as the drug name, dosage form, dosage strength, precautions, and usual dosage and frequency of administration will be provided on the medication dispensing container.

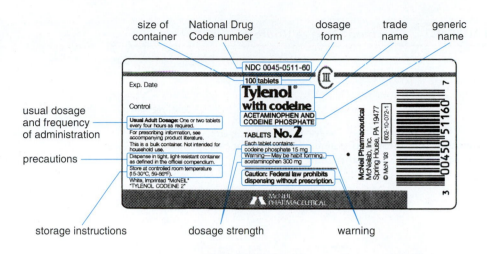

size of container · National Drug Code number · dosage form · trade name · generic name

usual dosage and frequency of administration

precautions

storage instructions · dosage strength · warning

NDC 0045-0511-60
100 tablets

**Tylenol®
with codeine**
ACETAMINOPHEN AND
CODEINE PHOSPHATE
TABLETS **No. 2**

Each tablet contains:
codeine phosphate 15 mg
Warning— May be habit forming.
acetaminophen 300 mg

Caution: Federal law prohibits
dispensing without prescription.

Exp. Date

Control

Usual Adult Dosage: One or two tablets
every four hours as required.
For prescribing information, see
accompanying product literature.
This is a bulk container. Not intended for
household use.
Dispense in tight, light-resistant container
as defined in the official compendium.
Store at controlled room temperature
(15-30°C, 59-86°F).
White, imprinted "McNEIL"
"TYLENOL CODEINE 2"

McNeil Pharmaceutical
McNeilab, Inc.
Spring House, PA 19477
© McN 93   602-10-072-1

McNEIL
PHARMACEUTICAL

- **Right Strength** Check the original prescription for this information and pay attention to the age of the patient.
- **Right Route** Check that the physician's order agrees with the drug's specified route of administration. Many medications can be given by a variety of routes, and the route of administration can affect the medication's absorption.
- **Right Time** Check the prescription to determine the appropriate time for

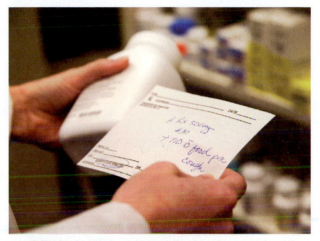

Carefully checking prescriptions is an important responsibilty of the pharmacy technician.

the medication to be administered. Some medications must be taken on an empty stomach (one hour before or two hours after a meal) while others should be taken with food. Sometimes, a certain time span is needed between doses to maintain a therapeutically effective blood level.

Dosage Forms and Routes of Administration

A medicinal agent may be administered in many different forms for convenient and efficacious treatment of disease. The route and dosage form are determined by many factors, including the disease being treated, the area of the body that the drug needs to reach, and the chemical composition of the drug itself. Each drug has its own characteristics related to absorption, distribution, metabolism, and elimination. Drugs are prepared for administration by many conceivable routes, but the primary routes are oral, parenteral, and topical. Table 3.3 lists a few examples of these.

Medications are available in a variety of forms, and frequently a single drug will be available in a number of different forms. Examples of the common drug forms associated with the three primary administration routes are presented in Table 3.4.

TABLE 3.3   Common Dosage Routes

Route	Example
peroral (PO, by mouth)	oral (swallowed) sublingual (under the tongue) buccal (dissolves in the cheek)
parenteral (not through the alimentary canal, but by injection through some other route)	intravenous (vein) intra-arterial (artery) intracardiac (heart) intraspinal/intrathecal (spinal fluid) epidural (fibrous membrane of spinal cord) intrasynovial (joint-fluid area) subcutaneous (beneath the skin) intramuscular (muscle)
topical (applied to surface of skin or mucous membranes)	transdermal (skin surface) conjunctival (conjunctiva) intraocular (eye) intranasal (nose) aural (ear) intrarespiratory (lung) rectal (rectum) vaginal (vagina) urethral (urethra)

The age and condition of the patient often determine the dosage form that will be used. Pediatric and geriatric populations frequently have special needs. These two groups often need liquid dosage forms. Convenience may also play a role in the selection of the appropriate dosage form. Drugs with distinctive sizes, shapes, and colors are inherently easier to identify. Dosage forms that reduce the frequency of administration without sacrificing efficacy are often advantageous and make patient **compliance** (the patient's adherence to the dose schedule and other particular requirements of the specific drug regimen) easier.

Peroral (PO) Routes

The **peroral** (PO) route is the most economical and most convenient way to give medications. This route is commonly referred to as the **oral** route. The term *oral* means that the medication is given by mouth either in solid form, as a tablet or capsule, or in liquid form, as a solution or syrup. Once the medication enters the mouth, it must be swallowed to reach the stomach. Then it must pass to the area of absorption, most commonly the small intestine, although some medications are absorbed in the stomach.

The absorption process takes time and is affected by several factors, including the presence of food (which slows the process) or digestive disorders. It is important to refer to a reliable drug reference guide to determine whether the medication should be given with or without food and whether any specific assessments should be done before dispensing it.

Sublingual (under the tongue) and **buccal** (between the cheek and gum) routes of administration are used when a rapid action is desired, or when a drug is specifically designed to be easily absorbed into blood vessels. The medication enters the bloodstream directly from the richly vascularized mucous membrane of the mouth and

TABLE 3.4   Common Dosage Forms

Route	Primary Dosage Forms
peroral (PO, by mouth)	tablets capsules solutions syrups elixirs suspensions gels powders troches/lozenges
parenteral	solutions suspensions
topical	ointments creams pastes powders aerosols lotions transdermal patches sprays inhalants suppositories enemas emulsions sponges gels

produces its effects more quickly than drugs that are swallowed. This dosage form cannot obtain the same effect if swallowed.

When taking medication by the sublingual route, the patient should hold the tablet under the tongue until it dissolves completely. For buccal administration, the patient should place the tablet between the cheek and gums, close the mouth, and hold the tablet there until it is dissolved. It is important to remind the patient not to drink water or swallow excessively until the tablet is completely absorbed.

Parenteral Routes

Administration of drugs by injection is referred to as the **parenteral** route (meaning "outside of the intestines"). Injections can be painful, and there is a risk of infection at the site of puncture, but parenteral administration may be necessary for several reasons. Some drugs, such as insulin, are inactivated in digestive juices, so swallowing them would be ineffective. Some medications would be inactivated by first-pass metabolism, described in Chapter 2, if they had to pass through the liver before entering the bloodstream, so they are injected directly into the tissues of the body. Parenteral routes also offer the potential for quick absorption of injected medication into the bloodstream and a rapid effect (especially for the intravenous route).

Drugs may be injected into

- a muscle: **intramuscular (IM)**
- a vein: **intravenous (IV)**

- the skin: **intradermal**
- the tissue beneath the skin: **subcutaneous**
- the spinal column: **intraspinal** or **intrathecal**

Topical Routes

Topical medications are applied to the surface of the skin or mucous membranes. The desired effect can be local or **systemic** (affecting the body as a whole). Other topical routes are inhalation, ophthalmic, otic, nasal, rectal, and vaginal.

The **inhalation** route delivers medications to the respiratory system. These medications are intended for one or more of the following purposes: to alter the condition of the mucous membranes, to alter the character of the secretions in the respiratory system, to treat diseases and infections of the respiratory tract, or to produce general anesthesia.

Medications can be administered via the **ophthalmic** route by **instillation** (administration of a medication drop by drop) of a cream, ointment, or drops of a liquid preparation into the conjunctival sac of the eye.

Drugs administered by the **otic** route, into the ear, are used locally to treat inflammation or infection of the external ear canal or to remove excess cerumen (wax) or foreign objects from the canal. Eardrops come in solutions and suspensions. If the patient has a tube in the ear, a suspension rather than a solution should be used. When a prescription for ear drops is dispensed, the technician should always ask whether the patient has an ear tube.

Medications can be administered into the nose by instillation or spray.

Medications that are administered by the rectal route are most commonly in the form of a suppository or as an enema. Suppositories are soft, rounded pieces of cocoa butter, glycerin, or a synthetic base. When inserted into the rectum, they melt at body temperature and release the medication to be absorbed through the walls of the large intestine. The primary advantage of rectal administration is that the medication does not depend on the digestive system to be absorbed into the bloodstream. Therefore, it is frequently used to treat nausea and vomiting. Suppositories can also be used for local effect to treat constipation. Additionally, the rectal route is ideal for treating fever in infants and young children.

Medications given by the vaginal route can be used to treat a **local infection** (restricted to or pertaining to one area of the body) caused by either bacteria or fungi. There can also be some systemic absorption (absorption into the bloodstream) through this route, enabling the medication to circulate throughout the body and affecting other parts of the body.

Factors That Influence Drug Action

A variety of factors can influence the effects of drugs and may require dosage adjustment. Ensuring that patients receive the correct medication, at the correct dosage, and that a newly prescribed medication does not adversely interact with other drugs that a patient is taking are all of paramount importance. Several procedures are in place to help ensure medication safety, and the pharmacy technician plays a role in these.

Children and the elderly may require a reduced dose because of their smaller size or the inability of the liver to metabolize the medication adequately. In these instances, if the dosage is not decreased, it may have toxic effects on the patient. The prescriber can use a variety of formulas when prescribing medications for pediatric or geriatric patients.

Patients with specific diseases may be unable to absorb, metabolize, or excrete various medications. Impaired gastrointestinal function may affect absorption, impaired liver function may affect metabolism, and impaired kidney function may affect elimination. Inadequate nutritional intake may also adversely affect the metabolism of drugs. Therefore, the patient's disease state must be evaluated before medications can be prescribed.

Physicians also consider psychological and genetic factors when prescribing medications. The mental state of a patient can influence the body's ability to release chemical substances needed to absorb or metabolize a drug properly. Genes can also control the release of chemicals and the way the body absorbs or metabolizes various medications. Unfortunately, these factors are less predictable than age, gender, and disease state. Nevertheless, if the patient does not seem to be responding to a medication, these factors should be considered.

Immune responses should also be evaluated for all patients before medications are prescribed. Allergic responses to foods or medications should be documented in the medical record, and each time a new medication is dispensed, the pharmacy technician should ask whether the patient has had any additional allergic responses so that the records can be kept up-to-date.

Special Considerations in Elderly Patients

Elderly patients have special needs in relation to their medications. Aging affects both the chemical reactions that administered drugs undergo in the body (pharmacokinetics) as well as how the body reacts to the drugs (pharmacodynamics). In addition, the elderly not only tend to have more chronic diseases than the young but also tend to use more drugs—both prescription and nonprescription. Four out of five elderly individuals have at least one chronic disease, and many in this age group take numerous medications, three to four times daily. For some elderly patients, medication is often the difference between an independent, ambulatory lifestyle and confinement in a long-term care facility. As a result, geriatric medicine has emerged as a new and important medical specialty of the healthcare system.

Changes in Physiologic Function Aging involves declines in both mental function (ability to continue to meet the demands of daily life) and physiologic well-being (normal functioning of the body). Physiological changes do not occur at the same rate for all individuals, and many changes are not currently predictable. Successful aging is characterized by losses in physiologic function that are **nonpathologic** (not related to disease). Impaired aging represents pathologic (manifestations of disease) changes with greater physiologic loss than in average persons of the same age group.

The following is a list of some of the changes that body systems undergo with aging:

- **Optic Changes** As the lenses of the eye become less elastic, more dense, and yellow, visual acuity is compromised; this can often be improved with corrective lenses. Macular degeneration and cataracts become a problem.
- **Auditory Changes** Hearing loss occurs in all frequencies, but especially in the high ranges. Impairment of sound localization and loudness perception is a problem for many elderly patients. A delay in central processing of auditory messages results in an increase in the time it takes for the person to respond to a question.
- **Gastrointestinal Changes** These changes create many problems, including decreases in saliva production, esophageal motility, hydrochloric acid secretion, absorptive surface, and rate of gastric emptying. Constipation is a daily complaint;

the elderly are often preoccupied with this physiologic function. Overuse of stimulant laxatives is a significant problem for some elderly patients.

- **Pulmonary Changes** Many elderly patients have chronic obstructive pulmonary disease (COPD). Aging brings on increased rigidity of the chest wall, decreased vital capacity (maximum intake and exhalation), and decreased response to hypoxia (reduced oxygen in the blood) and hypercapnia (increased carbon dioxide in the blood). If an elderly patient also has cardiac disease, these functions are further compromised.

- **Cardiovascular Changes** Hypertension and coronary artery disease are major issues to address. Healthy persons at rest have little age-related loss of cardiac output; during exercise, cardiac responses needed to meet the increased oxygen demand are diminished. To compensate, the sympathetic nervous system releases more norepinephrine and epinephrine. As a result, a compensatory increase in stroke volume occurs, and cardiac output is maintained. In elderly patients with cardiac disease, these compensatory mechanisms are impaired, resulting in decreased output.

- **Urinary Changes** Changes pertaining to the fluid excreted by the kidneys can result from a decrease in the number of functioning nephrons (units of the kidney) and in renal blood flow. The elderly have a higher incidence of renal insufficiency (reduced capacity to filter blood). Incontinence (inability to retain urine in the bladder) is often a problem; with these individuals diapers become a necessity. Instability of bladder muscle, overflow, and sphincter weakness are the causes. Diuretics, often necessary medications to treat an existing illness, may aggravate this condition. Urinary retention may be the result of prostate hypertrophy, malignancies, kidney stones, anticholinergic drug intake, or urinary tract infections.

- **Hormonal Changes** Functional changes pertaining to the endocrine system are a natural consequence of aging.

- **Compositional Body Changes** The proportion of total body weight composed of fat increases with age, while lean body mass and total body mass decrease. Albumin (such as the blood plasma protein) production decreases with aging, possibly as the result of poor nutrition, hepatic disorders, or other disease states. Loss in bone density (osteoporosis) causes some loss of height. Arthritis also takes its toll on the skeletal system.

Altered Drug Responses Age-related changes in organ function and body composition can alter the response to medication. The following factors play an important part in selecting a drug and its dosage.

- **Absorption Changes** Changes in GI function with aging may affect dissolution, enzymatic breakdown, and drug ionization. Reduction in the rate of gastric emptying may delay intestinal absorption of some drugs. For most, the rate and extent of absorption are determined by passive diffusion during contact with the surface area of the gut. Reduction in absorptive surface decreases absorption. GI fluid secretion and GI motility also decrease.

- **Distribution Changes** Alterations in body composition, such as protein binding (less protein means more free drug in plasma), affect the distribution of drugs. If a drug is highly protein-bound, it may have enhanced pharmacologic or toxic effects in elderly patients. Other factors that affect distribution are decreases in total body water, lean body mass, and cardiac output.

- **Elimination Changes** Although metabolism occurs in the liver, the kidneys are vital for elimination. Both processes may be altered with aging, with serious effects on blood levels of a drug. Varying degrees of renal and hepatic dysfunction may be present, depending on the patient's disease states, the drugs used, and the degree of successful aging. Elimination by the kidneys is decreased because of reduced filtration rate, blood flow, and tubular secretion. The result of decreased kidney elimination of drug products is an increased half-life that may require a reduction in dose of a drug.

- **Metabolism Changes** During metabolism, a drug is transformed biochemically to a more water-soluble compound. Elderly patients may have impaired metabolism, which decreases clearance and allows the drug to accumulate, sometimes to toxic levels. Normally, blood flow (as measured per minute) decreases about 1% per year as an individual ages, beginning at about age 35 (40% from ages 35 to 75). Decline in liver metabolism occurs as a result of reductions in both enzyme activity and blood flow.

As mentioned, older patients are more likely than younger patients to have chronic diseases requiring long-term treatment. Many take from 3 to 12 medications, and they tend to have a disproportionate number of **adverse drug reactions** (ADRs). Maintaining medication profiles is important in these cases. Almost one-third of ADRs in the elderly are caused by three drugs: Coumadin (warfarin), insulin, and Lanoxin (digoxin). The pharmacy technician must take special care when dispensing these drugs. Always double check the dose and compare it to the profile.

A group of drugs that are especially important to monitor for elderly patients is included in the **Beers List**. This list, which was originally published to provide information on potentially problematic drugs for patients in long term care facilities, is now useful for elderly patients in other settings. The Beers List continues to grow and is periodically revised. Computer data bases commonly contain warnings attached to these drugs. A warning does not mean that the patient should not take the drug, but rather that drugs on this list should be closely monitored in the elderly population. There is also a Canadian list of drugs that should be watched when used in the elderly. Drugs on both lists include Elavil (amitriptyline), reserpine, Persantine (dipyridamole), Mellaril (thioridazine), Thorazine (chlorpromazine), Tranxene (clorazepate), Valium (diazepam), Librium (chlordiazepoxide), and Indocin (indomethacin). There are others but these are especially important.

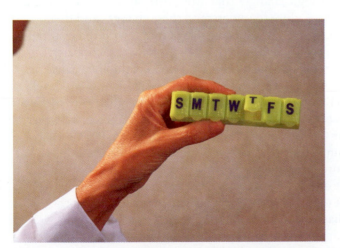

Using tools such as this pillbox will help patients who must take medications daily to remember to take them. The pharmacy technician can help inform patients about such medication management strategies.

Polypharmacy is the term often used to describe concurrent use of multiple medications. ADRs are often the result of overprescribing. Owing to the slowing of drug metabolism with aging, the elderly can often obtain the desired pharmacologic effect with a much lower dose than is normally prescribed. When many drugs are prescribed for a patient, especially when the patient sees more than one physician, the potential for drug interactions or other problems is high.

Aging can also affect cognitive abilities. An inadequate understanding of the need for the medication and the dosage directions for the medication (e.g., whether it is to be taken with or without food) can lead to failure to take the drug, unintentional overdosing, taking the medication for the wrong reason, or taking drugs prescribed for another person. This

TABLE 3.5 Common Adverse Reactions Potentiated in the Elderly

- Central nervous system (CNS) changes (often misdiagnosed as disease manifestations)
- Constipation
- Dermatitis
- Diarrhea
- Drowsiness
- Falls
- GI upset

- Incontinence
- Insomnia
- Rheumatoid symptoms
- Sexual dysfunction
- Urinary retention
- Xerostomia (dry mouth)

failure to adhere to the appropriate drug regimen is referred to as **noncompliance** and is especially prevalent among the elderly. Pharmacy technicians can provide invaluable services in this area. They can make sure the patient gets written information and provide aids to dosing and ways to remember to take medication. Table 3.5 lists adverse drug reactions common among elderly patients.

The elderly population presents a special challenge for the pharmacy technician and will constitute the bulk of the pharmacy practice. As people age, they need more drugs to maintain a healthy lifestyle. Patients visit a pharmacy not because they feel well, but rather because they have health problems; many are ill and/or depressed. They can no longer function as they did when they were younger and it is the technician who often has to deal with this frustration. Technicians must develop skills that enable them to empathize and communicate with elderly patients without sympathy. Successful pharmacy technicians treat elderly patients with respect and understanding.

Special Considerations in Children

Providing drug therapy to children presents a unique set of challenges. As they grow, children undergo profound physiologic changes that affect drug absorption, distribution, metabolism, and elimination. Failure to understand these changes and their effects can lead to underestimating or overestimating drug dosage, with the resultant potential for failure of therapy, severe adverse reactions, or perhaps fatal toxicity.

Age may be the least reliable guide to drug administration in children because of the wide variation in the relationship between age and degree of organ-system development. Height correlates better with lean body mass than does weight. Body surface area may be the best measure because it correlates with all body parameters; however, it is not easily determined. Body weight is most commonly used because of its ease of calculation. Children who are small for their age should receive conservative doses, but larger children may require a dose recommended for the next higher age bracket.

Pediatricians often prescribe an OTC medication for a child without telling the parent how to dose the drug, or they think the dosing instructions will be on the package. A caretaker may purchase the medication only to find that the drug is intended for use in an older child and that appropriate dosage information for a smaller child is not provided with the medication. The pharmacist may have to determine the child's dose for the caretaker. The pharmacy technician should always refer these questions to the pharmacist. Many factors beyond those included in the printed instructions on the box need to be considered before recommending a drug dosage.

The following considerations are important when dosing children.

- Be sure the dosage is appropriate for the child's age. A dose appropriate for a neonate may not be appropriate for a premature infant or a toddler.
- Always double-check all computations.
- Reevaluate all dosages at regular intervals.

Immunization

Immunization is an important part of pediatric medicine. Immunization is a process whereby the immune system is stimulated to acquire immunity to a specific disease. This is generally achieved via the use of a **vaccine**, which is a suspension of whole or microorganisms or parts of them, administered to induce immunity.

There are two types of immunity: active and passive. **Active immunity** develops when a person is exposed to an infectious organism or to an inactivated part of an infectious organism, either through a vaccine or through suffering the disease itself. As a result, the individual develops antibodies that protect the body from that disease. **Passive immunity** results from receiving antibodies that were formed by another person (or animal) having active immunity. A person's immunity to a disease may be determined by measuring the level of circulating antibodies (also referred to as **titer**) to that disease.

Methods for producing and delivering vaccines have changed since their initial discovery. Early vaccines were made from live or weakened ("attenuated") organisms. Many of these vaccines produced questionable results, and some caused serious reactions. Complete organisms are actually not necessary to cause immunity, because the molecule that an antibody recognizes, called its **antigen**, is usually only a small **peptide** (part of a protein) from the surface of the organism. The recent development of recombinant deoxyribonucleic acid (DNA) technology and the success of peptide sequencing and synthesis have helped to develop new and safer vaccines using chemically produced peptide antigens rather than whole organisms. The success of these vaccines depends on the ability of an antibody to recognize and bind to a particular peptide sequence. Synthetic vaccines have two advantages. First, they are quite safe because they do not rely on live or weakened viruses. Second, the antigenic peptides can be synthesized on a large scale.

Development of safe, effective vaccines to prevent infectious diseases has been responsible for the substantial decline in **morbidity** (diseased state or condition) and **mortality** (death rate) associated with smallpox, rabies, diphtheria, pertussis, tetanus, yellow fever, poliomyelitis, measles, mumps, and rubella. Tables 3.6a–c reflect the 2007 recommendations.

In addition to infants and school-age children, for whom immunizations are required, specific populations are at high risk for exposure to infection from diseases normally controlled through the immunization process. These populations include healthcare workers exposed to infected patients, highly mobile individuals such as migrant workers, immigrants who have not been immunized, elderly individuals, persons with debilitating conditions that make them more susceptible, school-age children in situations of increased exposure, and adults with waning immunity who are being exposed to childhood diseases.

Many vaccines present problems with storage and dispensing. Most must be transported and stored at refrigerated temperatures. Some vaccines must be frozen; **Zoster** (to prevent shingles), for example, must remain frozen until 30 minutes before it is injected. **FluMist**, the nasal flu vaccine, is now refrigerated (rather than frozen). **Gardasil**, which prevents some cervical cancers and genital warts, comes in a vial or a syringe. The syringe is very difficult to use, so most health care providers prefer the vial.

TABLE 3.6a   Immunization Schedule

Recommended Immunization Schedule for Persons Aged 0–6 Years—UNITED STATES · 2008

Vaccine	Birth	1 month	2 months	4 months	6 months	12 months	15 months	18 months	19-23 months	2-3 years	4-6 years
Hepatitis B	HepB	HepB				HepB					
Rotavirus			Rota	Rota	Rota						
Diphtheria, Tetanus, Pertussis			DTaP	DTaP	DTaP		DTaP				DTaP
Haemophilus influenzae type b			Hib	Hib	*Hib*	Hib					
Pneumococcal			PCV	PCV	PCV	PCV				PCV	
Inactivated Poliovirus			IPV	IPV		IPV					IPV
Influenza						Influenza (Yearly)					
Measles, Mumps, Rubella						MMR					MMR
Varicella						Varicella					Varicella
Hepatitis A						HepA (2 doses)				HepA Series	
Meningococcal										MCV4	

■ Range of recommended ages   ■ Certain high-risk groups

TABLE 3.6b   Immunization Schedule

Recommended Immunization Schedule for Persons Aged 7–18 Years—UNITED STATES · 2008

Vaccine	7–10 years	11–12 years	13–18 years
Diphtheria, Tetanus, Pertussis		Tdap	Tdap
Human Papillomavirus		HPV (3 doses)	HPV Series
Meningococcal	MCV4	MCV4	MCV4
Pneumococcal		PPV	
Influenza		Influenza (yearly)	
Hepatitis A		HepA Series	
Hepatitis B		HepB Series	
Inactivated Poliovirus		IPV Series	
Measles, Mumps, Rubella		MMR Series	
Varicella		Varicella Series	

■ Range of recommended ages   ■ Catch-up immunization   ■ Certain high-risk groups

TABLE 3.6c   Immunization Schedule

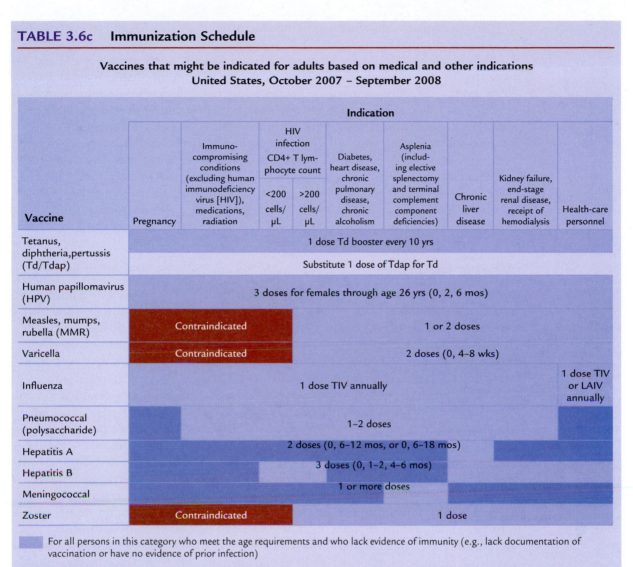

Vaccines that might be indicated for adults based on medical and other indications
United States, October 2007 – September 2008

Vaccine	Indication								
	Pregnancy	Immuno-compromising conditions (excluding human immunodeficiency virus [HIV]), medications, radiation	HIV infection CD4+ T lymphocyte count <200 cells/μL	HIV infection CD4+ T lymphocyte count >200 cells/μL	Diabetes, heart disease, chronic pulmonary disease, chronic alcoholism	Asplenia (including elective splenectomy and terminal complement component deficiencies)	Chronic liver disease	Kidney failure, end-stage renal disease, receipt of hemodialysis	Health-care personnel
Tetanus, diphtheria, pertussis (Td/Tdap)	1 dose Td booster every 10 yrs								
	Substitute 1 dose of Tdap for Td								
Human papillomavirus (HPV)	3 doses for females through age 26 yrs (0, 2, 6 mos)								
Measles, mumps, rubella (MMR)	Contraindicated			1 or 2 doses					
Varicella	Contraindicated			2 doses (0, 4–8 wks)					
Influenza	1 dose TIV annually								1 dose TIV or LAIV annually
Pneumococcal (polysaccharide)	1–2 doses								
Hepatitis A	2 doses (0, 6–12 mos, or 0, 6–18 mos)								
Hepatitis B	3 doses (0, 1–2, 4–6 mos)								
Meningococcal	1 or more doses								
Zoster	Contraindicated			1 dose					

For all persons in this category who meet the age requirements and who lack evidence of immunity (e.g., lack documentation of vaccination or have no evidence of prior infection)

Recommended if some other risk factor is present (e.g., on the basis of medical, occupational, lifestyle, or other indications)

Source: United States Department of Health and Human Services. Center for Disease Control and Prevention.

Immunization for tuberculosis (TB) is mostly used in developing countries with a high incidence of the disease. The vaccine that is used is **BCG** (Bacille Calmette-Guerin), an attenuated form of *Mycobacterium bovis* (one of the strains of the TB bacterium that causes disease in humans). It is used for persons at high risk and those with family members having active TB. A person receiving the vaccine will have positive results on subsequent tuberculin skin tests.

Tdap (a vaccine for tetanus, diphtheria, and pertussis) is recommended for adults. The children's vaccine for these diseases, **DTaP**, contains much more pertussis than older patients need. Be careful not to confuse the two. **Boostrix** is for teenagers and is the only approved vaccine for adolescents that contains the pertussis antigen. It should be shaken vigorously prior to administration. This shot should be given 5 years after the childhood vaccines.

Vaccines should never be mixed in the same syringe with any other medications. If more than one vaccine is administered at the same time, different sites should be selected.

The government is currently stocking vaccine for the *Avian Flu* and trying to anticipate future mutations.

Immunizations should not be given to certain patients, such as those with conditions that depress the ability of the immune system to respond to an antigenic challenge. Even a weakened or attenuated antigen may cause disease in the compromised patient. Live vaccines should not be given if the patient is taking steroids, receiving radiation, or receiving drugs that are immunosuppressive (as is chemotherapy); patients with a current active infection and those who have received immune globulin within the previous three months should also not receive live vaccines. In recent years, some vaccines have begun to be administered in the pharmacy by the pharmacist. For these vaccinations, no prescription is necessary. Because insurance companies will reimburse a pharmacy for some vaccines but not for others, it is important for the pharmacy technician to ensure that correct forms are completed and signed.

Allergic Response

An **allergy** is a state of hypersensitivity of the immune system induced by exposure to a particular substance. Many of these substances occur naturally in the environment, some are seasonal, some occur in food, whereas others occur in pharmaceutical products. In response to an allergy, the body releases chemicals such as **histamine,** which produces symptoms commonly known as the allergic reaction—red, watery eyes; sneezing; urticaria; rash; and bronchiolar constriction—when exposed to these substances. This histamine is designated as H_1 and is treated with antihistamines. Gastric mucosal cells release a different type of histamine, known as H_2, which is treated with the H_2 blockers Axid (nizatidine), Pepcid (fomotidine), Tagamet (cimetidine), and Zantac (ranitidine) (see Chapter 10). Both antihistamines and H_2 blockers are sold over the counter. Most allergic reactions are not serious, and these drugs can be self-prescribed and administered. However, some allergic reactions can be life-threatening.

The pharmacy technician must be very aware that dangerous allergic reactions are a possibility for some medications. One of the most important tasks for the technician is to screen patients for allergies. Allergies must be a part of the patient's medical record, and the technician must always make sure this issue has been addressed before any drugs are dispensed. If the patient has no allergies, "NKA" (no known allergies) should be entered into the record. Under no circumstances should this field be left blank, either in the computer or on the patient chart.

Allergic Diseases

There are many types of **allergic disease**, with a wide range of causes and involving any body system. Hay fever is caused by an allergic reaction of the nasal mucosa to the pollen of trees, grasses, weeds, and molds. It may occur in spring, summer, or fall and may last until frost. Symptoms of allergic rhinitis may last year-round, however, if caused by such allergens as house dust, animal dander, and foods. The mucosa of the upper respiratory tract and conjunctiva become inflamed, with excessive secretion from the nasal mucosa (rhinitis) and the tear ducts (watery eyes). The patient has spells of sneezing, itching and weeping eyes, running nose, and burning in the palate and throat. Asthma may sometimes be a complication. Inhibition of histamine release contributes to relief.

Allergic dermatitis, or eczema, is a noncontagious, itchy rash that often occurs in the creases of the arms, legs, and neck, although it can cover the entire body. It is often associated with allergies.

Contact dermatitis results from direct skin contact with an irritant; animals, plants, chemicals, and minerals are common irritants. Poison ivy is the most common cause of this type of dermatitis.

Urticaria (hives) is an outbreak of itchy welts of varying size. They may develop on the face, lips, tongue, or throat; in the eyes or ears; or internally. Allergies to food or drugs are well-known causes. Long term desensitization programs are often necessary to treat some allergies.

Teaching Patients Medication Management

The pharmacy technician can play an important role in helping patients learn how to manage medications. If the drug does not enter the body or enters it incorrectly, it will not work as desired. The pharmacy technician can positively affect patient compliance by providing clearly written instructions and aids to implement the process.

Federal law requires that the pharmacy collect the patient's history regarding drugs prescribed as well as side effects and adverse reactions experienced by the patient. The pharmacy technician can positively affect patient drug therapy by accurately collecting and recording the patient's medication history in the patient's profile. Information about the prescription drugs ordered and their proper administration must be provided to the patient by the pharmacist filling the prescription. The pharmacist can help the patient understand the administration instructions, as well as any precautions. Specific instructions to emphasize include

- methods for administering the drug
- how to make swallowing easier
- times and time intervals for administration and what to do if a dose is missed
- whether a medication can or should be taken with or without food
- possible side effects and which ones should be reported to the physician
- how long the medication should be taken

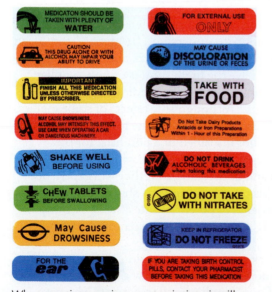

When a patient receives a prescription, it will sometimes include labels that provide instructions for how to self-administer the medication properly. These labels use color and symbols to communicate their message.

It is important that the pharmacy technician explain to patients that the pharmacist is available for any questions or instructions. Also, the technician is allowed to read to the patient the label, medication guide, or educational materials dispensed with the drug—this is *not* counseling and can be very helpful to the patient. However, technicians should read the exact wording of the written information and should bear in mind that they must not offer advice to patients.

In some states, technicians can ensure that patients understand how to read medication labels. Important items to look for include the trade name and/or generic name, the dosage strength, frequency and route of administration, precautions and warnings, and potential interactions. It is important to remember, however, that technicians cannot—by law—counsel patients! Figure 3.5 provides an example of a doctor's prescription and the corresponding medication label that should be affixed to the drug container. The label provides directions that the patient needs to understand and follow.

FIGURE 3.5
Medication Label Information

The information on a prescription, as shown in (a), is translated for the patient as instructions on the medication label, as shown in (b). This label also includes the physician's name and the date the prescription was filled, the drug name, the number of refills, and the pharmacy's address and phone number.

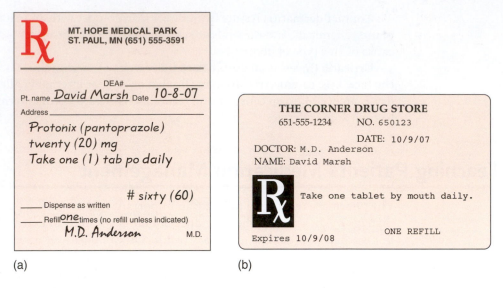

(a)

(b)

Many drugs that are now available over the counter previously required a prescription. This change occurred because the drugs were found to help with common, uncomplicated problems and carry a relatively low risk of adverse effects. However, it is important that patients read the information provided with these drugs to understand their action, interactions, cautions, and possible side effects. OTC drugs can also interfere with the desired effects of prescription drugs ordered by the prescriber. That is why it is important to obtain information about the patient's OTC drug use as well as information about prescription medications.

A medication program can be effective only if the patient or caregiver follows the directions for administration. A regimen may include modifying the lifestyle and keeping medical appointments as follow-up.

When a patient does not comply with the instructions, there may be a relapse or aggravation of the disease. Hospitalization may then be required, causing healthcare costs to rise. The end result may even be the death of the patient.

Reasons why a patient does not comply can be varied and often complex. They include side effects that cause discomfort, failure to understand the disease, confusion caused by cognitive impairment or the complexity of the regimen, and simple forgetfulness. In general, teenagers and the elderly have the highest rates of noncompliance.

Side effects are a common reason for noncompliance. If a medication produces discomfort, the patient may discontinue its use. Although side effects of some medications subside as the drugs are continuously used, it may take time for patients to overcome this obstacle, especially if they are not informed of a potential for these reactions before the medication is administered. Patients may be willing to tolerate some side effects if they are aware of them and understand that they will experience relief over the long term of drug use. For this reason, side effects should be addressed initially. The pharmacist should inform patients of potential side effects. The importance of dosing, what to do if an adverse effect occurs, and how to monitor treatment should all be discussed.

Another problem is that patients may lack adequate information about their disease or their medications. Patients who do not understand how a drug may improve their disease state will be at a higher risk of noncompliance than patients who have some understanding of drug action and can see how the treatment will affect their disease. Patients lacking sufficient knowledge of their disease and the drug therapy for the disease may not take the regimen seriously. Thus, healthcare professionals should educate patients about their disease so that they will understand the drug therapy required. This education should include information about the assumed benefits of the drug regimen, side effects, and the consequences of failing to follow the drug regimen.

Compliance decreases as the number of daily medications and the complexity of the regimen increase. Multiple medications, multiple instructions regarding medications, and a drug that has to be taken at a certain time of the day or several different times of the day, with (or without) food, may all confuse the patient, resulting in poor compliance. The result may be missed doses and a less-than-desired therapeutic response, or an increased risk of adverse drug reactions and hospitalization. With a simpler regimen, there is a greater chance of better patient compliance. Consequently, pharmacists and prescribers should evaluate therapeutic alternatives that ensure patient compliance. Patients with cognitive impairments that affect their ability to understand and follow directions concerning their drugs will be at a higher risk of noncompliance.

Forgetfulness is another reason for lack of compliance. Patients should be encouraged to use various kinds of reminders to aid their memory. Reminders may include taking medications at the time certain daily tasks are performed, placing colored stickers on the calendar after the medication is taken, using pillboxes with daily compartments, setting watches with alarms, or using pill bottle cap alarms or other electronic devices.

Above all, patients should be instructed to monitor their own medication regimens. Pharmacists and pharmacy technicians are in a position to build a trusting relationship in which the patient is generally willing to accept recommendations.

Medication Safety

Ensuring that patients receive the correct medication, at the correct dosage, and that a newly prescribed medication does not adversely interact with other drugs that a patient is taking are all of paramount importance. Several procedures are in place to help ensure medication safety, and the pharmacy technician plays a role in these.

Technician Role

Technicians play a critical role in medication safety. They are an integral part of the medication process, and pharmacists rely heavily on them to catch errors. Properly trained and educated technicians can make a tremendous difference in the quality of care a patient receives.

Technicians must verify the address, date of birth, phone numbers, allergies, and conditions such as pregnancy. Another role of the technician is to make sure the patient gets proper counseling from the pharmacist. This counseling process is very important in minimizing errors.

E-Prescribing

E-prescribing is a process whereby the prescriber enters a prescription into a computer that then communicates directly with the computer at the pharmacy, eliminating the written prescription form. This process can potentially reduce errors and improve patient safety by eliminating illegible prescriptions, and automatically checking for allergies, interactions, dosing errors, and therapeutic duplications. Accidental selection of the wrong drug, dose, or dosage form from the drop-down lists could, however, create a new source of errors. (Prescribers need to make sure that a medically trained person enters the information into the computer.) Presumably, increases in E-prescribing will also lead to fewer errors. Another reason for reluctance to use E-prescribing is the expense of installing appropriate computer programs. The Medicare Modernization Act (MMA) mandates that by 2009, drug plans participating in Medicare D must be consistent with the standards of E-prescribing.

Physical Order Entry

In hospitals, where physicians enter prescriptions into a database, a decrease in errors has been documented. This is physician order entry and is different from E-prescribing. The physician personally enters the order.

Tamper-Resistant Pads

In order for prescribers to file for Medicaid reimbursement, tamper-resistant pads must be used for written prescriptions. If tamper-resistant pads are not used, the technician must call and verify the prescription. This action must be documented on the prescription with the date and time called, the names of the person who verified it and the technician's initials. This regulation should encourage more use of E-prescribing.

Medication Reconciliation

One of the National Patient Safety Goals is to make sure that community and hospital pharmacies share information from patient profiles, a process known as **medication reconciliation**: "The goal is to provide a complete and accurate patient drug profile to each health provider who cares for a patient." Such sharing of health information is allowed under the privacy provisions in Title II of HIPAA (Health Insurance Portability and Accountability Act) and is part of the continuum of care and the effort to improve patient safety as patients move from one level of care to another. Studies show that patients are most at risk at the point of transfers from one level of care to another, where many medication errors occur. This applies both to transitions between hospitals or between hospital and community and to transitions within a hospital, rehab center, nursing home, or other healthcare facility. Hospitals should transmit specific forms with drug regimen information to the patient's next setting. In the future, retail pharmacies will receive greater numbers of calls from providers who need this information. An order to continue medications should never be honored. Rather, the prescribing physician should be contacted for confirmation. Pharmacy technicians will play a major role in making these transitions safer.

Chapter Terms

active immunity protection against disease that occurs as a result of coming into contact with an infectious agent or an inactivated part of such an agent administered by a vaccine

adverse drug reaction reaction to a drug that is harmful to the well-being of the patient

allergic disease a disease caused by an allergic reaction

allergy a state of heightened sensitivity as a result of exposure to a particular substance

antigen the molecule that an antibody recognizes

Beers List a list of drugs for which monitoring is especially important in elderly patients

buccal to be placed between the cheek and the gums

compliance a patient's adherence to the dose schedule and other particular requirements of the specified regimen

E-prescribing the process which allows a prescriber's computer system to talk to the pharmacy's computer system and the medication order/prescription is transmitted to the pharmacy

histamine a chemical produced by the body that evokes the symptoms of an allergic reaction and is blocked by antihistamines

immunization the process by which the immune system is stimulated to acquire protection against a specific disease; usually achieved by use of a vaccine

inhalation administration of a medication through the respiratory system

inscription part of a prescription that identifies the name of the drug, the dose, and the quantities of the ingredients

instillation administration of a medication drop by drop

intradermal to be injected into the skin

intramuscular to be injected into a muscle; abbreviated IM

intraspinal to be injected into the spinal column

intrathecal see intraspinal

intravenous administration of a medication through a vein, thereby avoiding the first-pass effect; abbreviated IV

local infection an infection restricted to or pertaining to one area of the body

medication reconciliation the providing of a complete and accurate drug profile to each health care provider who cares for a patient

morbidity rate of occurrence of a diseased state or condition

mortality death rate from a particular disease

noncompliance failure to adhere to an appropriate drug regimen

nonpathologic not related to disease

ophthalmic to be administered through the eye

oral see peroral (PO)

order a prescription issued in an institutional setting

otic administered in the ear

parenteral administered by injection rather than by way of the alimentary canal

passive immunity protection against a disease as the result of receiving antibodies that were formed by another person or animal who developed them in response to being infected with the disease

peptide a string of amino acid molecules bound together, usually a fragment of a larger protein molecule

peroral (PO) administration of a medication by mouth in either solid form, as a tablet or capsule, or in liquid form, as a solution or syrup; often referred to as oral

polypharmacy the concurrent use of multiple medications

prescription a direction for medication to be dispensed to a patient, written by a physician or a qualified licensed practitioner and filled by a pharmacist; referred to as an order when the medication is requested in a hospital setting

signa part of a prescription that provides directions to be included on the label for the patient to follow in taking the medication

subcutaneous to be injected into the tissue just beneath the skin

sublingual to be placed under the tongue

systemic pertaining to or affecting the body as a whole

titer concentration of an antibody in the bloodstream

topical applied to the surface of the skin or mucous membranes

vaccine a suspension of disease-causing organisms or fragments of them, administered to induce active immunity to the disease

Chapter Summary

The Prescription

- A request for the dispensing of medication to a patient is called an order in a hospital setting; outside the hospital setting it is called a prescription.
- To fill a prescription or order, the pharmacy technician must understand the meanings of abbreviations. Certain abbreviations should not be used on prescriptions or instructions because there is extensive evidence to document them as the source of medication errors.

Correct Drug Administration "Rights"

- The "rights" for correct drug administration are the right patient, the right drug, the right strength, the right route, and the right time.

Dosage Forms and Routes of Administration

- The three primary routes of administration are oral, parenteral, and topical. The pharmacy technician must be familiar with each dosage form. The most common are:

peroral (PO)	parenteral	topical
tablets	intravenous (IV) injections	ointments
capsules	epidural injections	creams
syrups	intramuscular (IM) injections	gels
solutions	subcutaneous injections	suppositories
suspensions		patches
		lotions
		inhalants

Factors That Influence Drug Action

- Altered drug responses in the elderly are due to age-related changes in organ function and body composition. These physiologic changes include visual, auditory, gastrointestinal, pulmonary, cardiovascular, renal, hormonal, and compositional alterations.
- Some special problems of the elderly are poor nutrition, adverse drug reactions, and poor compliance with drug regimens.
- There are some drugs that are especially hazardous when prescribed for elderly patients.
- Empathy and not sympathy is very important for communication with the elderly.
- Body surface area is the best measure to use in determining dosage for children, but it is difficult to ascertain; consequently, weight is most frequently used.

- Immunization is the process whereby the immune system is stimulated to acquire immunity to a specific disease.
- The development of safe and effective vaccines to prevent infectious diseases has been responsible for the substantial decline in morbidity and mortality associated with those diseases.
- There are two types of histamine receptors. Antihistamines block the H_1 receptors. A class of drugs referred to as H_2 blockers blocks the H_2 receptors.
- An important role for the pharmacy technician is determining patient allergies.

Teaching Patients Medication Management

- Patient compliance with the dose schedule and the specific requirements of a drug regimen is important.

- A pharmacy technician can positively influence patient drug therapy by accurately collecting and recording the patient's medication history in the patient profile.
- Pharmacy technicians can help patients understand how to read medication labels.
- Patients should read the information provided with OTC drugs to understand their action, interactions, cautions, and possible side effects.

Medication Safety

- E-prescribing will eliminate poorly written prescriptions.
- Hospitals that use physician order entry (POE) have documented a decrease in errors.
- Medication reconciliation, a national patient safety goal, will prevent many errors.

Drug List

Vaccines
BCG (tuberculosis)
Boostrix (tetanus, diphtheria, pertussis, for adolescents)
DTaP (diphtheria, tetanus, pertussis, for children)
FluMist (influenza)

Gardasil (human papillomavirus—cervical cancer, genital warts)
Tdap (tetanus, diphtheria, and pertussis, for adults)
Zostavax (shingles)

Chapter Review

Understanding Pharmacology

Select the best answer from the choices given.

1. A prescription typically must contain the following parts *except* the
   a. patient's name.
   b. drug and dose.
   c. *signa*.
   d. patient's age.

2. All of the following are "rights" for correct drug administration *except* the right
   a. patient.
   b. drug.
   c. strength.
   d. doctor.

3. Which route of medication administration is the most economical and convenient?
   a. oral
   b. topical
   c. parenteral
   e. none of the above

4. Which drug(s) cause the most ADRs in the elderly?
   a. digoxin
   b. warfarin
   c. insulin
   d. all of the above

5. Immunization has been found to
   a. cure some disease states.
   b. decrease morbidity and mortality associated with specific disease states.
   c. increase morbidity and mortality associated with specific disease states.
   d. none of the above

6. Federal law requires that pharmacists collect
   a. donations for hospitals.
   b. a patient history regarding the drug prescribed.
   c. pharmacokinetic data on animal models.
   d. a list of all the physicians in their state.

7. Which of the following drug forms are administered via the oral route?
   a. tablets
   b. syrups
   c. capsules
   d. all of the above

8. Factors that determine the best route of administration include all of the following, except the
   a. patient's condition.
   b. type of container to be used.
   c. site of desired action.
   d. rapidity of the desired response.

9. A prescription label must have
   a. the patient's and physician's names.
   b. the dosage and how to take the drug.
   c. the address of the pharmacy and date of fill.
   d. all of the above.

10. Parenteral forms
    a. do not pass through the liver before entering the bloodstream.
    b. are inactivated in digestive juices.
    c. are the most common drug forms.
    d. are the most painless way to administer medications.

The following statements are true or false. If an item is false, rewrite the statement so it is true.

_____ 1. It is not necessary for the MD to put a DEA on schedule III and IV drugs.

_____ 2. Abbreviations should *not* be used when taking verbal prescriptions or orders.

_____ 3. In most states, physicians may stamp their name on the prescription.

_____ 4. Elderly people do not spend much money on drugs and are, therefore, unconcerned about the cost.

_____ 5. Constipation is never a problem for the elderly.

_____ 6. It is easy to dose pediatric patients.

_____ 7. Weight is the best method to dose children; however, body surface area is the most used.

_____ 8. Pharmacy technicians play a major role in medication safety.

_____ 9. Many drugs now available OTC once required a prescription.

_____ 10. A drug prepared for the otic route may be used in the eye.

Match the following prescription abbreviations with their correct meaning.

1. qid   _____

2. hs   _____

3. NKDA   _____

4. pc   _____

5. prn   _____

6. IV   _____

7. IM   _____

8. c̄   _____

9. gtt   _____

10. ac   _____

11. NPO   _____

12. po   _____

13. mcg   _____

14. g   _____

15. gr   _____

16. D/C   _____

17. bid   _____

18. tid   _____

19. stat   _____

20. mL   _____

a. four times daily

b. after meals

c. at bedtime

d. no known drug allergy

e. intravenously

f. with

g. as needed

h. intramuscularly

i. before meals

j. drop

k. nothing by mouth

l. by mouth

m. microgram

n. discontinue

o. grain

p. gram

q. milliliter

r. immediately

s. three times daily

t. twice daily

Pharmacology at Work

1. List the components of a prescription.

2. List the components of a medication label on a container given to a patient.

3. List causes for and discuss altered drug response in the elderly.

4. List and explain three things to keep in mind when dosing a child.

Internet Research

Use the Internet to complete the following assignments.

1. Research flu vaccines. Who should get a flu vaccine, and when should they get it? What is the vaccine composed of? Why must the vaccine be given every year? Locate and list at least two sites. Which site(s) were the most helpful to you in answering the questions listed above? Which site(s) would be most useful to an individual concerned about contracting the flu? Which site(s), if any, would be most useful to a scientist studying infectious diseases?

2. Visit the Institute for Safe Medication Practices (ISMP) Web site at http://www.ismp.org and find their current list of dangerous abbreviations. Consider why these abbreviations are considered to be dangerous, and identify other abbreviations that you would recommend to be added to future lists. Also, identify other ways to reduce the potential for misreading medication orders.

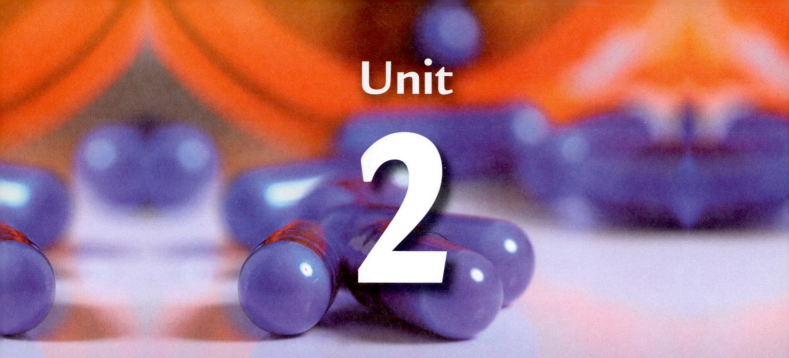

Unit

2

Major Classes of Pharmaceutical Products I

Antibiotics

4

Learning Objectives

- Identify the major types of antibiotics by drug class.
- Know which auxiliary labels to use when dispensing major types of antibiotics.
- Define therapeutic effects, side effects, and administration routes of major antibiotics.

- Use antibiotic and general drug terminology correctly in written and oral communication.

Preview chapter terms and definitions.

Antibiotics are a major class of natural and synthetic pharmaceutical agents that kill or inhibit the growth of infection-causing microorganisms (bacteria). Antibiotics are frequently dispensed for community-acquired infections, which account for more outpatient visits to physicians than any other medical condition. They are also used for infections acquired in the hospital or institutional setting (nosocomial infections).

Fighting Bacterial Infections

Bacteria are single-celled organisms that occur in almost all environments. When bacteria penetrate body tissues, they sometimes establish an **infection**, where their presence or toxins can cause tissue damage. The body's immune system fights back to destroy the bacteria, usually resulting in fever and inflammation. The body can overcome many simple infections, but more serious infections often require the assistance of antibiotics to kill the invaders.

Although infectious diseases have been known to exist for thousands of years, it was not until the nineteenth century that the cause—bacteria—was identified through the work of Louis Pasteur and other scientists. By the early twentieth century, the organisms that cause cholera, syphilis, bubonic plague, gonorrhea, leprosy, and other illnesses had been isolated and identified.

In 1907, German physician Paul Ehrlich patented the drug arsphenamine as a treatment for syphilis. Although this drug marked a breakthrough in eradicating a major infectious disease, it was not until 1936 that the first true antibiotic, sulfanilamide (a sulfonamide), was discovered. When penicillin became widely available in the 1940s, physicians finally had a powerful weapon to use against several common infections, including strep throat, pneumonia, and syphilis. Today a wide variety of antibiotics are used to combat bacteria-caused infections. Each drug is effective against specific kinds of bacteria.

Types of Bacteria

Bacteria are classified in several ways. Broadly, they are grouped into two types based on their need for oxygen. If the bacterium (singular form of *bacteria*) needs oxygen to survive, it is called **aerobic**; if it can survive in the absence of oxygen, it is called **anaerobic**. Both aerobic and anaerobic bacteria can be responsible for infections, including **nosocomial** infections, which are infections acquired by patients while they are in a hospital.

Determining the appropriate antibiotic to use against a specific bacterium requires laboratory testing. A sample of material obtained from the infected area is stained, observed under the microscope, and classified according to two characteristics that help determine the drug to prescribe. The first characteristic consists of the shape and size of the bacterium. Bacteria cells may be round, rod-shaped, curved, or spiral (see Figure 4.1) and range in size from 0.5 micrometer (a micrometer is one-millionth of a meter, sometimes referred to informally as a micron) to 5 micrometers. The second characteristic is the staining property of the bacterium. Depending on their chemical makeup, bacteria change to certain colors during the testing technique called **Gram staining**. If the stain they absorb is purple, the bacteria are gram-positive. If the stain is red, the bacteria are gram-negative. Figure 4.2 provides an example of the Gram stain colors. Table 4.1 lists examples of these two bacteria characteristics and provides an example of a disease for each characteristic.

FIGURE 4.1
Characteristic Bacteria Shapes

(a) Round cocci.
(b) Rodlike bacilli.
(c) Spiral-shaped spirochetes.

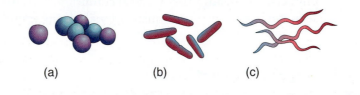

(a)   (b)   (c)

FIGURE 4.2
Gram Stain

(a) Gram-positive bacteria turn a purple color. (b) Gram-negative bacteria appear red.

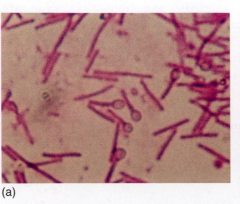
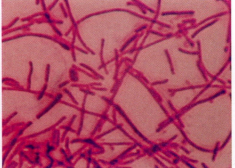

(a)   (b)

TABLE 4.1 Examples of Bacteria Shapes, Gram Stain Results, and Related Diseases

Shape	Gram Stain	Bacteria	Related Diseases
rods	gram-positive	*Corynebacterium*	endocarditis
	gram-negative	*Escherichia coli*	urinary tract infections (UTIs)
cocci	gram-positive	*Staphylococcus*	toxic shock syndrome (associated with tampon use)
	gram-negative	*Neisseria*	gonorrhea
curved or spiral rods	gram-negative	*Campylobacter*	septicemia
spirochetes	gram-negative	*Treponema pallidum*	syphilis

Symptoms of Bacterial Infections

The general signs that an infection may be of bacterial origin are a fever of 101 °F or higher and an increased number of white blood cells (>12,000/mm³). The onset of fever alone, however, is not diagnostic of a bacterial infection. A fever may also be caused by a self-limiting viral illness or by some types of malignancy and autoimmune disorders. In many situations, localizing symptoms or physical findings are necessary to explain the fever.

Antibiotic Treatment and Action

An **antibiotic** is a chemical substance with the ability to kill or inhibit the growth of microorganisms. In developing antibiotics, the challenge is to find a way to kill the invading organism without harming the patient receiving treatment. This mission is easier to accomplish with bacteria than with other kinds of pathogens because many biological processes are unique to bacteria and not shared by humans. Antibiotics work by gaining access to the inside of the bacterial cell and interfering with these unique biological processes in one of six ways.

- preventing folic acid synthesis (sulfonamides)
- impairing cell wall formation (penicillins and cephalosporins)
- blocking protein formation (macrolides, tetracyclines, and aminoglycosides)
- interfering with DNA (deoxyribonucleic acid) formation (quinolones)
- disrupting cell membranes (cyclic lipopeptides)
- disrupting DNA structure (metronidazole)

An antibiotic may be either a **bactericidal agent,** which kills the invading organisms, or a **bacteriostatic agent,** which inhibits the growth or multiplication of bacteria.

Preferably, antibiotic treatment is started after the bacteria have been identified by culturing. The outcome of antibiotic treatment can be evaluated in two ways: (1) the clinical response, meaning the signs and symptoms disappear, or (2) the microbiological response, meaning the organism is completely eradicated. Bacterial infections are contagious until antibiotics have been administered for 24 to 48 hours.

When a patient has a serious or life-threatening infection, an antibiotic treatment must begin immediately. The patient is given a **broad-spectrum antibiotic**, which is effective against multiple organisms. This is referred to as **empirical treatment**.

Side Effects and Dispensing Issues of Antibiotics

The parenteral forms of antibiotics should be mixed exactly as directed by the manufacturers. If mixed inappropriately, the drugs can be ineffective or may cause tissue or vein irritation, renal failure, or even death. When dispensing oral forms of these drugs, it is important to swab the counting tray with alcohol before placing a new drug on the tray so as to prevent cross-contamination, especially with penicillin and sulfa drugs. For example, if a tray used to dispense sulfa is not wiped down before another drug is placed on the tray, sulfa particles could stick to the new drug. This would contaminate the new drug and could result in an adverse reaction if the drug is given to a patient who is allergic to sulfa.

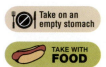

As a general guideline, most antibiotics should be taken on an empty stomach to attain faster absorption. There are exceptions to this rule; for example, nitrofurantoin and cefuroxime. Some antibiotics can cause extreme gastrointestinal (GI) upset. The manufacturer may recommend that these drugs be taken with food. For most antibiotics, however, taking with food slows absorption of the drug. Therefore, the technician should not make this recommendation or place a "take with food" sticker on these drugs unless prompted to do so by the computer or patient handouts.

Another important piece of information about antibiotic agents is that they can interfere with the action of birth control pills and reduce the effectiveness of this contraceptive. The patient should be made aware of this and be warned to use backup contraception during this time.

To maintain consistent drug serum levels, ideally antibiotics should be administered around the clock. An IV administration route can facilitate around-the-clock dosing for very ill patients. Otherwise, spacing the dosage evenly throughout the day will suffice to maintain a relatively constant drug serum level.

Antimicrobial Resistance

Many patients are infected with organisms that were once controlled by antibiotics, including the organisms that cause pneumonia, tuberculosis, and meningitis. New infections are surfacing because many existing drugs are no longer effective. Resistance to antibiotics is developing, largely because of overuse and misuse. Broad-spectrum antibiotics are often prescribed without a specific diagnosis of bacterial infection. Patients, for their part, often do not complete an antibiotic regimen; that is, they stop taking their medication once they begin to feel better. This enables the stronger bacteria to develop a resistant strain. If the infection recurs, it is more difficult to treat. If the mutant strain is passed on to another individual, it is equally difficult to treat. As a result, patients must take more and stronger drugs. If bacteria or fungi resistant to the drugs in use invade the body, a **superinfection**—a new infection complicating the course of therapy of an existing infection—may occur.

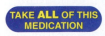

The pharmacy technician's role in preventing overuse of antibiotics is to ensure that all antibiotic prescriptions display an auxiliary label on the bottle that advises the patient to take all of the medication. Because prescriptions for antibiotics have begun to stipulate "dose loading" on the front end, the patient will be instructed that after the initial dose, successive doses are smaller. In any event, it is important that the patient complete the prescribed medication.

Bacteria may become resistant to antibiotic drugs by several different mechanisms. The most frequent form of antibiotic resistance results when bacteria produce enzymes that destroy the molecular integrity of the drug. Beta-lactamase-producing bacteria transform antibiotics such as penicillin and cephalosporin into inactive compounds. Another way that bacteria inactivate antibiotics is by changing the composition of the bacterial membranes or by reducing the number and size of protein molecules in the membrane, preventing the antibiotics from entering the cell. Yet another mechanism by which bacteria render antibiotics ineffective is by developing pumps that flush the antibiotics out of and away from the cell membrane. Finally, other organisms may change the target or binding site.

A bacterial cell may develop antibiotic resistance on its own (mutation), or it may acquire DNA carrying resistance properties from another cell by mechanisms referred to as transduction, transformation, and conjugation.

Major Classes of Antibiotic Drugs

Before 1935, systemic bacterial infections could not be effectively treated with drugs. An infection could be attacked topically with an **antiseptic** (a substance that kills or inhibits the growth of microorganisms on the outside of the body) or a **disinfectant** (an agent that destroys infectious organisms on nonliving objects), but these chemicals could not be used systemically because they were not safe enough. With the discovery of sulfonamides, a new era began. Since that time several additional classes of antibiotics have been discovered. All drugs in each class of antibiotics have some similarities in their molecular structure.

Sulfonamides

Sulfonamides, or sulfa drugs, the oldest antibiotics on the market, are a group of bacteriostatic drugs that are effective against a broad range of microorganisms because they block a specific step in the pathway for making the important biochemical folic acid (vitamin B_9), which is needed in making DNA. The sulfas interfere with PABA (para-aminobenzoic acid) and folic acid formation, thereby destroying the bacteria. They are not harmful to humans because humans do not make their own folic acid and must obtain it from food. Table 4.2 lists the most commonly used sulfonamides and related drugs. Because the sulfa drugs are the oldest antibiotics on the market, the pharmacy technician needs to know both the brand and generic names of these drugs.

In addition to sulfa, several antibacterial agents are used almost exclusively to treat urinary tract infections. One agent is **nitrofurantoin (Macrobid, Macrodantin)**. If

TABLE 4.2   Most Commonly Used Sulfonamides and Related Drugs

Generic Name	Pronunciation	Dosage Form	Brand Name	Dispensing Status
Sulfonamides				
sulfamethoxazole-trimethoprim	sul-fa-meth-OX-a-zole trye-METH-oh-prim	IV, oral liquid, tablet	Bactrim, Bactrim DS, Cotrim, Cotrim DS, Septra, Septra DS	Rx
sulfasalazine	sul-fa-SAL-a-zeen	tablet	Azulfidine	Rx
sulfisoxazole	sul-fi-SOX-a-zole	oral liquid, tablet	Gantrisin	Rx
Related Drug				
nitrofurantoin	nye-troe-fyoor-AN-toyn	capsule, oral liquid	Macrobid, Macrodantin	Rx

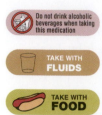

the patient is allergic to sulfa, this is the drug of choice. Its mechanism of action is unknown, but it has a wide antibacterial spectrum. It works better when taken with food. Nausea is the primary side effect, so it is important to take this drug with food. The patient should not drink alcoholic beverages while taking this medication. Nitrofurantoin may turn urine brown and cause false urine glucose tests. Patients should drink large volumes of fluids while on these drugs.

Therapeutic Uses of Sulfonamides Sulfonamides are among the drugs of choice for the following illnesses and some specific bacteria.

- urinary tract infections (UTIs)
- otitis media (middle ear infection), especially in children
- ulcerative colitis
- lower respiratory infections
- prophylaxis in *Pneumocystis carinii* pneumonia in immunocompromised patients

Side Effects and Dispensing Issues of Sulfonamides Sulfa drugs in use today cause fewer allergic reactions than older sulfa drugs did. The most common side effect is a rash. Other side effects include nausea, drug fever (often confused with a recurrent fever from the infection), vomiting, jaundice, blood complications (acute hemolytic anemia, agranulocytosis, and aplastic anemia), and kidney damage. **Stevens-Johnson syndrome**—a reaction that can be fatal, marked by large red blotches on the skin—can occur from use of sulfas. If a rash occurs, the patient should stop taking the drug immediately. Sulfa drugs should have a label warning patients to avoid the sun, which can cause severe skin rashes. Sulfonamides can crystallize in the urine and deposit in the kidneys, resulting in a painful, dangerous condition. To reduce this risk, it is important that a patient taking sulfa drugs maintain an adequate fluid intake of at least six to eight glasses a day. The technician should always place an auxiliary label on sulfonamides and related drugs reminding the patient to drink lots of water or other fluids.

Penicillins

Warning

Penicillin is not the same drug as penicillamine.

Cell wall synthesis

The **penicillin** family is a group of highly effective antibiotics with extremely low toxicity, obtained from the mold *Penicillium chrysogenum*. Manipulating the basic molecular structure of the drug has led to many effective derivatives. Penicillins kill bacteria by preventing them from forming the rigid cell wall needed for survival. The weakened cell wall allows an excessive amount of water to enter the bacterium through osmosis. The cell increases in size and lyses (bursts) as the cell membrane cannot contain the cell contents. Human cells do not have rigid cell walls; therefore, they are not affected by penicillins.

Table 4.3 lists the most commonly used penicillins by generic and brand names and provides the dosage forms for each.

Therapeutic Uses of Penicillin Penicillin is most active against growing and reproducing bacteria, generally gram-positive aerobes and anaerobes. Penicillin and penicillin derivatives are among the drugs of choice for the following illnesses and some specific bacteria.

- abscesses
- beta-hemolytic streptococcus
- meningitis
- otitis media

TABLE 4.3   Most Commonly Used Penicillin Drugs

Generic Name	Pronunciation	Dosage Form	Brand Name	Dispensing Status
amoxicillin	a-mox-i-SIL-in	capsule, oral liquid, tablet	Amoxil	Rx
ampicillin	am-pi-SIL-in	capsule, injection, IV, oral liquid	Principen	Rx
penicillin G	pen-i-SIL-in G	injection, IV	various brand names, also different salts, i.e., potassium, sodium	Rx
penicillin V	pen-i-SIL-in V	oral liquid, tablet	Veetids	Rx

- pneumonia
- respiratory infections
- strep throat
- tooth and gum infections
- sexually transmitted diseases (STDs; syphilis and gonorrhea)
- endocarditis (heart valve infection) due to streptococci

Penicillin and other antibiotics have been shown to reduce risk of disease or death for patients with subacute bacterial endocarditis, an inflammation of the lining of the heart and its valves. These patients are at risk any time a body cavity is invaded.

Preventative dosing, or prophylaxis, is also recommended whenever a patient with certain conditions undergoes any kind of surgical procedure, including normal dental procedures such as filling cavities. The American Dental Association (ADA) released new guidelines for prophylactic therapy in 1997. These guidelines recommend that a single 2 g dose of amoxicillin be administered before dental procedures. For penicillin-allergic patients, 600 mg of clindamycin (Cleocin) or 500 mg of azithromycin (Zithromax) is recommended. This prophylaxis is currently under debate, but many dentists still use it. It is important for the pharmacy technician to be aware of these regimens.

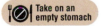
Take on an empty stomach

Side Effects and Dispensing Issues of Penicillins Most drugs in the penicillin group should be taken on an empty stomach with water because food slows absorption, and the acids in fruit juices or colas could deactivate the drug. The most common side effect of these drugs is diarrhea. Penicillin allergy affects 7% to 10% of the population. The allergy may vary from an itchy, very red mild rash to wheezing and anaphylaxis, which can be fatal.

The following are the principal penicillins with their most important side effects and dispensing issues.

- **Penicillin G** is the prototype, but absorption from the gastrointestinal tract is incomplete; therefore, it is supplied only in the injectable form.
- **Penicillin V** is available as a potassium salt, which exhibits greatly enhanced resistance to hydrolysis by gastric acid, so it is the preferred oral form. It is the drug of choice for strep throat. Commonly a more expensive antibiotic is prescribed for strep throat, but the insurance company will not pay for it. In order to treat the patient, the technician will need to make the prescriber aware of the fact that penicillin is the preferred drug.
- **Ampicillin** has a broader antimicrobial spectrum than penicillin G and is available in both oral and injectable forms. It will cause skin rash in a high percentage of

patients with mononucleosis and was formerly used to identify and diagnose this infection, even though the disease is caused by a virus and is not cured by antibiotics. Ampicillin is dosed four times a day.

- **Amoxicillin** is dosed three times a day. Amoxicillin reaches higher concentrations on a milligram per milligram basis than ampicillin, which is why it is used much more frequently.

Resistance to Penicillin Some organisms are resistant to penicillin because of the activity of a group of enzymes (beta-lactamase enzymes). Penicillin is ineffective against staphylococcal penicillinases. Because some organisms are resistant to penicillin, three types of drugs have been developed to compensate for the ineffectiveness of penicillin in specific circumstances (see Table 4.4):

1. Penicillinase-resistant penicillins work against most gram-positive aerobes.
2. Extended-spectrum penicillins are more active than natural penicillins. They are more resistant to inactivation by gram-negative bacteria or are more readily absorbed into the cell membrane of the organism.
3. Penicillin is sometimes combined with other drugs to improve the effect. Certain beta-lactamase inhibitors, such as clavulanate, have been combined with amoxicillin and ticarcillin with therapeutic benefit. **Ampicillin-sulbactam (Unasyn)** works on ampicillin-resistant organisms through sulbactam inhibiting the beta-lactamase enzyme. Diarrhea and nausea are common side effects of **amoxicillin-clavulanate (Augmentin)**. **Ticarcillin-clavulanate (Timentin)** has only an IV dosage form.

TABLE 4.4   Most Commonly Used Resistant Penicillins

Generic Name	Pronunciation	Dosage Form	Brand Name	Dispensing Status
Penicillinase-Resistant Penicillins				
dicloxacillin	dye-klox-a-SIL-in	capsule	Dycil	Rx
nafcillin	naf-SIL-in	injection, IV	Unipen	Rx
oxacillin	ox-a-SIL-in	capsule, injection, IV, oral liquid	(none)	Rx
Extended-Spectrum Penicillins				
carbenicillin	kar-ben-i-SIL-in	tablet	Geocillin	Rx
piperacillin	pi-PER-a-sil-in	injection, IV	(none)	Rx
ticarcillin	tye-kar-SIL-in	injection, IV	Ticar	Rx
Penicillin Combinations				
amoxicillin-clavulanate	a-mox-i-SIL-in klav-yoo-LAN-ate	oral liquid, tablet	Augmentin	Rx
ampicillin-sulbactam	am-pi-SIL-in sul-BAK-tam	injection, IV	Unasyn	Rx
piperacillin-tazobactam	pi-PER-a-sil-in ta-zoe-BAK-tam	IV	Zosyn	Rx
ticarcillin-clavulanate	tye-kar-SIL-in klav-yoo-LAN-ate	IV	Timentin	Rx

Cephalosporins

Warning

Alert the pharmacist and prescriber if a patient who is allergic to penicillin is prescribed a cephalosporin. Even if the prescriber wants the drug dispensed, it is important that this communication be documented in case the person falls into that 1% who does have a cross-reaction.

Antibiotics of the **cephalosporin** family have a mechanism of action similar to penicillins, but they differ in their antibacterial spectrum, resistance to beta-lactamase, and pharmacokinetics. Research now suggests that a person allergic to penicillin has approximately a 1% chance of also being allergic to a cephalosporin. Most computerized drug profile systems place penicillin and cephalosporin in the same category; therefore, if someone has an allergy to either, the computer system will indicate that the patient is allergic to both. Cephalosporins are divided into first-, second-, third-, and fourth-generation agents (see Table 4.5).

The first-generation cephalosporins are similar to the penicillinase-resistant penicillins, but they have greater gram-negative coverage. They are used for mild to moderate **community-acquired** (not acquired in the hospital) infections in ambulatory patients. They can all be taken by mouth, except cefazolin (Ancef), which is only administered intravenously (IV) or intramuscularly (IM, injected deep into the tissue of the muscle). Intramuscular and intravenous injections require longer needles than subcutaneous (SQ, under the skin) injections.

Second-generation cephalosporins have increased activity, especially against *Haemophilus influenzae*, an important pathogen in the pediatric group. Second-

TABLE 4.5   Most Commonly Used Cephalosporins

Generic Name	Pronunciation	Dosage Form	Brand Name	Dispensing Status
First-Generation Cephalosporins				
cefadroxil	sef-a-DROX-il	capsule, oral liquid	Duricef	Rx
cefazolin	sef-AZ-oe-lin	injection, IV	Ancef	Rx
cephalexin	sef-a-LEX-in	capsule, oral liquid, tablet	Keflex	Rx
Second-Generation Cephalosporins				
cefaclor	SEF-a-klor	capsule, oral liquid	Ceclor	Rx
cefprozil	sef-PROE-zil	oral liquid, tablet	Cefzil	Rx
cefuroxime	se-fyoor-OX-eem	injection, IV, oral liquid, tablet	Ceftin, Zinacef	Rx
Third-Generation Cephalosporins				
cefdinir	SEF-di-neer	capsule, oral liquid	Omnicef	Rx
cefditoren	sef-de-TOR-en	tablet	Spectracef	Rx
cefixime	sef- IK-seem	liquid	Suprax	Rx
cefotaxime	sef-oh-TAX-eem	injection, IV	Claforan	Rx
cefpodoxime	sef-poe-DOX-eem	oral liquid	Vantin	Rx
ceftazidime	SEF-tay-zi-deem	injection, IV	Fortaz	Rx
ceftibuten	sef-TYE-byoo-ten	capsule, oral liquid	Cedax	Rx
ceftizoxime	sef-ti-ZOX-eem	injection, IV	Cefizox	Rx
ceftriaxone	sef-trye-AX-one	injection, IV	Rocephin	Rx
Fourth-Generation Cephalosporins				
cefepime	SEF-e-pim	injection, IV	Maxipime	Rx

generation cephalosporins are used for otitis media in children and for respiratory and urinary tract infections. They can all be dosed orally; cefuroxime (Ceftin, Zinacef) also has IV and IM forms.

The most recently developed third-generation cephalosporin drugs are active against a wide spectrum of gram-negative organisms and are used in severe infections. They are manufactured in a mixture of dosage forms. Because of their long half-life, the agents are also used in ambulatory patients, especially children, with dosing done before and after school. Orally active third-generation cephalosporins include **ceftibuten (Cedax)**, **cefdinir (Omnicef)**, **cefditoren (Spectracef)**, **cefixime (Suprax)**, and **cefpodoxime (Vantin)**. **Ceftriaxone (Rocephin)** is available only as an injectable form. Injection of ceftriaxone is very painful, so it is usually mixed with lidocaine to diminish the discomfort. It is used frequently in emergency room settings and is used to treat STDs.

Cefepime (Maxipime) is an injectable fourth-generation cephalosporin and is considered to have broad-spectrum coverage. It is used for treating pneumonia, urinary tract infections, and sepsis caused by gram-negative organisms. Cefepime is considered as effective as **ceftazidime (Fortaz)**, but it is more cost-effective because cefepime is given twice daily, whereas ceftazidime is dosed three times daily. Because of their activity against *Pseudomonas*, both are used for hospital-acquired infections.

The IV forms of these drugs can be mixed in either normal saline (**NS**) or a 5% dextrose solution (**D$_5$W**). These solutions are generally placed in either a 50 mL or 100 mL bag and administered over 30 minutes.

Therapeutic Uses of Cephalosporins Cephalosporins are among the drugs of choice for the following conditions.

- dentistry work, oral infections—oral first- and second-generation
- heart and pacemaker procedures (surgical prophylaxis)—cefazolin
- neurosurgical operations (surgical prophylaxis)—cefazolin
- OB/GYN procedures and surgery (surgical prophylaxis)—cefazolin
- orthopedic surgery (surgical prophylaxis)—cefazolin
- upper respiratory and sinus infections—oral second-generation
- urinary tract infections (UTIs)—parenteral third-generation
- meningitis—parenteral third-generation
- intra-abdominal infections—cefoxitin, cefotetan

Warning

All of the cephalosporins look alike when written in the generic form. Watch for dosing and indications for use.

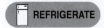

Side Effects and Dispensing Issues of Cephalosporins Cephalosporins share the same side effects as penicillins; a few have also been known to initiate unique toxic reactions. They generally are associated with a lower frequency of toxicity than many other antibiotics. Use of the specific drugs should be gauged by sensitivity testing of the microorganism isolated from the patient.

Several of the cephalosporin drugs have noteworthy dispensing issues. Diabetic patients who are prescribed cefdinir (Omnicef) in oral suspension form must be informed of its high sugar content (2.86 g per teaspoonful). Cefpodoxime (Vantin) is an oral suspension. With the exception of cefdinir (Omnicef) and cefixime (Suprax), which may be stored at room temperature, oral suspensions of cephalosporins must be refrigerated following reconstitution. All liquids should be shaken well immediately before they are administered, because the granules have a tendency to settle to the bottom of the bottle. Shaking will also provide even dosing throughout the regimen. These drugs are reconstituted in the pharmacy. A dropper with milliliter and teaspoon markings should be dispensed with these drugs.

New Drugs Structurally Related to Penicillins and Cephalosporins

Several new beta-lactam drugs, differing slightly from penicillins and the cephalosporins, have been introduced. These are carbapenems, carbacephems, and monobactams, and they are listed in Table 4.6.

One of these drugs, classified as a carbapenem, is **imipenem-cilastatin (Primaxin)**. This drug has excellent in vitro and in vivo activity against gram-positive and gram-negative bacteria. Side effects are similar to those of other beta-lactams except that seizures seem to occur more frequently. A carbapenem, **meropenem (Merrem I.V.)**, has similar coverage, but meropenem is less likely to cause seizures. It is approved for bacterial meningitis and intra-abdominal infections.

Doripenem (Doribax) inhibits cell wall synthesis and kills bacteria. It is indicated for UTIs. 500 mg is reconstituted with 10 mL of normal saline or sterile water for injection and shaken gently. It is then added to 100 mL of normal saline or D_5W and shaken gently again. Doripenem is stable for 8 hours in normal saline and 4 hours in dextrose at room temperature after mixing. It is good for 24 hours if stored in the refrigerator. As with the other carbapenems, patients must be watched for seizures.

Ertapenem (Invanz) is an injectable (once daily) carbapenem approved for severe community-acquired infections.

A monobactam, **aztreonam (Azactam)**, is also being used to treat serious infections, particularly of the urinary tract, with good success and low toxicity. Aztreonam is active only against gram-negative bacilli. The advantage of this drug is an unlikely cross-allergenicity with other beta-lactams. It is used against aerobic gram-negative infections. Patients should notify their physician immediately if skin rash, redness, or itching develops.

Loracarbef (Lorabid), which is in the carbacephem class, is similar to a beta-lactam antibiotic and lyses the bacteria. It is most frequently given to children. The suspension is stable for 14 days at room temperature. The Loracarbef should be taken on an empty stomach.

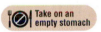 Take on an empty stomach

Tetracyclines and Tigecycline

The **tetracycline** group of drugs is produced by soil organisms. These drugs are broad-spectrum bacteriostatic antibiotics that inhibit protein synthesis in bacteria by binding

TABLE 4.6   Most Commonly Used Carbapenem, Carbacephem, and Monobactam Drugs

Generic Name	Pronunciation	Dosage Form	Brand Name	Dispensing Status
Carbapenems				
ertapenem	er-ta-PEN-em	injection, IV	Invanz	Rx
imipenem-cilastatin	i-mi-PEN-em sye-la-STAT-in	injection, IV	Primaxin	Rx
meropenem	mer-o-PEN-em	IV	Merrem I.V.	Rx
Carbacephem				
doripenem	dore-i-PEN-em	IV	Doribax	Rx
loracarbef	lor-a-KAR-bef	capsule, oral liquid	Lorabid	Rx
Monobactam				
aztreonam	AZ-tree-oh-nam	IV	Azactam	Rx

to ribosomes. The drugs suppress the infection, but they require phagocytes to complete the eradication of the bacteria. Table 4.7 lists the most commonly used tetracycline medications.

Therapeutic Uses of Tetracycline Tetracyclines are among the drugs of choice for the following illnesses.

- acne
- anthrax
- chronic bronchitis
- Lyme disease
- *Mycoplasma pneumoniae* infection (walking pneumonia)
- *Rickettsia* infection (Rocky Mountain spotted fever)
- some sexually transmitted diseases, such as *Chlamydia* infection

Efficacious treatment of STDs requires that all sexual partners be treated at the same time and avoid sexual contact for 3 to 4 days; otherwise reinfection will occur, creating a vicious cycle.

Side Effects and Dispensing Issues of Tetracycline The primary side effects seem to be gastrointestinal upset with nausea and vomiting. Antacids that contain aluminum, calcium, or magnesium and laxatives that contain magnesium, iron, or sodium bicarbonate should not be taken within several hours of taking tetracycline in order to avoid **chelation** (combination of the drug molecule with a metal ion in complexes in which the metal is part of a ring structure of the molecule) with these minerals.

Do not take with ANTACIDS

In recent years, manufacturers have begun to package drugs in the dose quantity. Studies report that this practice seems to promote better compliance but also adds to the cost of the drug. If an insurance company refuses to pay for these drugs, then a generic can be dispensed, and the dosing and strengths described on the package can be used. If an insurance company is resistant to pay for dose packs, then dispense the same drug out of the bottle, with the exact same instructions.

With this drug class, patients should be warned to avoid the sun because the drugs can cause photosensitization. They should also be warned to avoid dairy products with most tetracyclines, with the exception of doxycycline. The tetracyclines must be avoided by pregnant women and young children up to nine years old, because they cause permanent tooth discoloration and may affect bone growth.

Avoid SUN EXPOSURE

When most drugs reach their expiration date, they simply lose effectiveness, but tetracyclines can be toxic and cause a fatal renal syndrome. Therefore, the pharmacy

TABLE 4.7   Most Commonly Used Tetracycline Medications

Generic Name	Pronunciation	Dosage Form	Brand Name	Dispensing Status
demeclocycline	dem-e-kloe-SYE-kleen	tablet	Declomycin	Rx
doxycycline	dox-i-SYE-kleen	capsule, IV, oral liquid, tablet	Vibramycin Oracea Adoxa	Rx
minocycline	mi-noe-SYE-kleen	capsule, IV	Minocin Soladyne	Rx
tetracycline	te-tra-SYE-kleen	capsule, oral liquid, tablet	Sumycin	Rx

technician should always watch the expiration date on these drugs. It is also important to tell patients to take the entire drug regimen, but if any is left, it should be disposed of and not saved for later use.

This class of antibiotics has some delayed-release forms. Care must be taken not to interchange those dosage forms. For example, **Oracea** has a 10 mg dose that is an extended-release doxycycline.

Because of the recent concern over a terrorist attack, government agencies are stock piling tetracycline, which is effective against anthrax. In most situations pharmacy technicians, Homeland Security officials, and fire departments are overseeing this process. Because of their potential toxicity, it is extremely important that these drugs be rotated and, when out of date, that they be destroyed.

Tigecycline Tigecycline (Tygacil) is a new class of drug known as a glycylcycline, which is similar to tetracyclines. Tygacil is used for skin and intra-abdominal infections. It is available only as single-dose 50 mg vial for IV administration. Tigecycline is mixed in D_5W or NS in 100 mL bags and infused over 30 minutes. Tigecycline is listed in Table 4.8.

Macrolides

Macrolide antibiotics are bacteriostatic agents used primarily to treat pulmonary infections caused by *Legionella* and gram-positive organisms. Macrolides inhibit protein synthesis by combining with ribosomes. Clarithromycin (Biaxin), azithromycin (Zithromax, Z Pak), and dirithromycin (Dynabac) cause less gastrointestinal upset than other macrolide antibiotics. Table 4.9 lists the most commonly used macrolides.

Therapeutic Uses of Macrolides Macrolides are among the most commonly prescribed drugs for the following illnesses and other specific bacteria.

- *Chlamydia*
- group A beta-hemolytic streptococcus
- *H. influenzae*
- Legionnaires' disease
- *M. pneumoniae*
- *S. pneumoniae*

An unlabeled but common use of azithromycin is for the treatment of sexually transmitted diseases (STDs). Efficacious treatment of STDs requires that all sexual partners be treated at the same time and avoid sexual contact for 3 to 4 days; otherwise reinfection will occur, creating a vicious cycle.

Side Effects and Dispensing Issues of Macrolides Most antibiotics should be taken on an empty stomach to attain faster absorption; however, some forms of erythromycin can cause severe gastrointestinal distress, and taking them with food can offset some of this distress and improve compliance. Therefore, add a sticker to the

TABLE 4.8 Tigecycline

Generic Name	Pronunciation	Dosage Form	Brand Name	Dispensing Status
tigecycline	Tye-ge-SYE-cleen	IV	Tygacil	Rx

TABLE 4.9 Most Commonly Used Macrolides

Generic Name	Pronunciation	Dosage Form	Brand Name	Dispensing Status
azithromycin	az-ith-roe-MYE-sin	oral liquid, tablet	Zithromax, Z Pak, Zmax	Rx
clarithromycin	kla-rith-roe-MYE-sin	oral liquid, tablet	Biaxin	Rx
dirithromycin	dye-rith-roe-MYE-sin	tablet	Dynabac	Rx
erythromycin base	er-ith-roe-MYE-sin	capsule, tablet, topical	Eryc, Ery-Tab	Rx
erythromycin ethylsuccinate	er-ith-roe-MYE-sin eth-il-SUK-sin-ayt	oral liquid, tablet	E.E.S., EryPed	Rx
erythromycin lactobionate	er-ith-roe-MYE-sin lac-toe-BYE-oh-nayt	injection	Erythrocin	Rx
erythromycin stearate	er-ith-roe-MYE-sin STEER-ate	tablet	Erythrocin	Rx
erythromycin-sulfisoxazole	er-ith-roe-MYE-sin sul-fi-SOX-a-zole	oral liquid	Pediazole	Rx

dispensing container if this is recommended by the accompanying literature or prompted by the computer database. The newer macrolides do not cause as much intestinal distress.

Some of the newer macrolides can be taken with less regard to meals. **Clarithromycin (Biaxin)** may be taken without regard to meals. It is given twice daily. **Biaxin XL**, the extended-release form of clarithromycin, is taken only once a day and is associated with even fewer side effects. It should be taken with food.

Azithromycin (Zithromax) is dispensed in a dose pack **(Z Pak)**. On the first day, the patient takes a loading dose of 500 mg. Maintenance doses of 250 mg once daily are then taken on days 2 through 5, although this regimen can vary depending on the type of infection. There is also a three-pack of 500 mg tablets that should be taken once a day over a 3 day period. **Zmax** is an extended-release powder for oral suspension that delivers a full treatment in one dose. It comes in 1 gram and 2 gram packages and is approved to treat community-acquired pneumonia. Most of the liquids are banana flavored.

The **Z Pak** is an example of a drug that is supplied in a dose pack but can be dispensed from a bottle. The 250 mg and 500 mg tablets can come out of a bottle as well as be dispensed as a package. Just put the same instructions on the label and use the same strength of the drug that is in the package.

Dirithromycin (Dynabac) requires once-daily dosing and should be taken with food.

Ketolides

Ketolide antibiotics block protein synthesis by binding to ribosomal subunits, and they may also inhibit the formation of newly forming ribosomes. Bacteria resistant to macrolides, lincomycin derivatives, and streptogramins are also resistant to ketolides. Ketolides are used to treat bacterial infections in the lungs and sinuses. Metabolism is carried out by the cytochrome P-450 3A4 enzymes, creating a number of drug interactions.

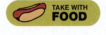

Warning

Erythromycin and azithromycin can be misread, but the dosing should help identify the drug for which the script was written.

An example of a ketolide is presented in Table 4.10. **Telithromycin (Ketek)** is similar to the macrolides. It is approved for mild to moderate community-acquired pneumonia, acute bacterial sinusitis, and acute exacerbation of chronic bronchitis. Patients should not drive while taking this drug, as it can cause blurred vision or difficulty focusing. It also has the very serious side effect of increasing occurrences of **arrhythmia** (irregular heartbeat) and should only be used to treat strep pneumonia that is resistant to penicillin and macrolides.

Warning

Cipro can be easily read as Ceftin (cefuroxime).

Warning

"Ciprofloxacin" and "cephalexin" can look very much alike, depending on the handwriting.

Warning

"Norfloxacin" and "Norflex" (orphenadrine) can easily be misread as each other.

Quinolones

Quinolone antibiotics have strong, rapid bactericidal action against most gram-negative and many gram-positive bacteria. They antagonize the enzyme responsible for coiling and replicating bacterial DNA during growth, causing DNA breakage and cell death. Humans do not have this enzyme, so their cells are unaffected. Table 4.11 lists the most commonly used quinolone drugs.

Therapeutic Uses of Quinolones Quinolones are among the drugs of choice for the following conditions.

- bone and joint infections caused by gram-negative organisms
- infectious diarrhea
- ophthalmic infections (topically)
- some sexually transmitted diseases (STDs)
- upper respiratory infections
- urinary tract infections (UTIs)

Efficacious treatment of STDs requires that all sexual partners be treated at the same time and avoid sexual contact for 3 to 4 days; otherwise reinfection will occur, creating a vicious cycle.

TABLE 4.10   Most Commonly Used Ketolide

Generic Name	Pronunciation	Dosage Form	Brand Name	Dispensing Status
telithromycin	tel-lith-roe-MYE-sin	tablet	Ketek	Rx

TABLE 4.11   Most Commonly Used Quinolone Antibiotics

Generic Name	Pronunciation	Dosage Form	Brand Name	Dispensing Status
ciprofloxacin	sip-roe-FLOX-a-sin	IV, oral liquid, otic, tablet, topical	Cipro	Rx
gatifloxacin	gat-i-FLOX-a-sin	IV, tablet	Tequin	Rx
gemifloxacin	je-mi-FLOX-a-sin	tablet	Factive	Rx
levofloxacin	lee-voe-FLOX-a-sin	IV, oral liquid, tablet	Levaquin	Rx
moxifloxacin	mox-i-FLOX-a-sin	tablet	Avelox	Rx
norfloxacin	nor-FLOX-a-sin	tablet	Noroxin	Rx
ofloxacin	oh-FLOX-a-sin	IV, otic, tablet	Floxin	Rx

Side Effects and Dispensing Issues of Quinolones The side effects are primarily gastrointestinal, with nausea and vomiting. Some joint swelling, dizziness, and an unpleasant taste can also occur. Antacids will interfere with the absorption of quinolones. Quinolones should not be given with theophylline because of the increased risk of theophylline toxicity. These drugs are phototoxic, so patients taking these drugs should be warned to avoid exposure to the sun. Quinolones can cause joint problems and malformations. Patients on quinolones have a tendency to injure tendons. Most quinolone medications are not recommended for use by children or pregnant women.

Streptogramins

Streptogramins inhibit protein synthesis within the bacterial ribosomes. Streptogramins are used to treat gram-positive infections, *Enterococcus faecium*, and vancomycin- and methicillin-resistant infections. This class of antibiotics is an important addition to antimicrobial drug therapy because they provide an alternative to vancomycin. Streptogramins were granted accelerated approval by the Food and Drug Administration (FDA) because of their ability to treat these life-threatening conditions. As shown in Table 4.12, the streptogramins include quinupristin and dalfopristin.

Synercid is a brand-name drug that combines quinupristin and dalfopristin (two streptogramins) at a ratio of 30 parts quinupristin to 70 parts dalfopristin. It is used primarily to treat life-threatening infections associated with vancomycin-resistant *Enterococcus faecium* (VRE).

The side effects of streptogramins are similar to those associated with the quinolones and include nausea, vomiting, joint swelling, and dizziness. Synercid is administered intravenously, and most patients experience an adverse reaction at the infusion site. Prior to administration, IV lines must be flushed with D_5W (5% dextrose) to ensure that the drug does not come into contact with saline or any other medications. Synercid inhibits cytochrome P-450 3A4; as a result, there are some potentially serious drug interactions. Synercid must be stored in a refrigerator.

Aminoglycosides

Aminoglycoside drugs are commonly used to treat serious infections. They exert their bactericidal action by binding to ribosomal subunits, inhibiting bacterial protein synthesis. After the first dose, the dosage should be adjusted according to plasma concentrations of the drug in the individual patient.

Aminoglycoside medications, listed in Table 4.13, are among the most commonly prescribed drugs for treating life-threatening infections due to gram-negative aerobes, **sepsis** (a systemic inflammatory response to infection resulting from blood-borne infections), immunocompromised patients, and peritonitis.

The major side effects of these drugs are **nephrotoxicity** (that is, they are destructive to the kidney) and **ototoxicity** (they damage the organs of hearing). Neuromuscular blockade can also be a problem. Aminoglycosides may cause dose-related changes in

TABLE 4.12   Most Commonly Used Streptogramins

Generic Name	Pronunciation	Dosage Form	Brand Name	Dispensing Status
quinupristin-dalfopristin	qui-NYOO-pris-tin dal-FOE-pris-tin	IV	Synercid	Rx

vestibular and auditory function, ranging from equilibrium problems and hearing problems such as tinnitus to permanent deafness.

New evidence suggests that these drugs can be dosed once a day instead of two to three times daily. Bacterial growth remains suppressed for a while, even after serum levels have declined. Less frequent dosing may help to reduce the toxicity of these drugs, as less of the drug may accumulate in the kidney and ear when there is a brief, high peak and very low trough rather than steady concentrations. Once-daily dosing also reduces costs and simplifies drug monitoring. When dosing once daily, there is usually no need to measure peak drug levels; however, trough levels should be checked before the second dose to make sure the patient is eliminating the drug quickly enough.

Cyclic Lipopeptides

The **cyclic lipopeptide** drugs bind to bacterial membranes and cause the cell membrane to depolarize, thus leading to an inhibition of DNA and RNA (ribonucleic acid) synthesis. Bacterial death follows.

Daptomycin (Cubicin) belongs to this class of drugs and is the most commonly used cyclic lipopeptide (see Table 4.14). It is used for complicated skin infections and is active in treating aerobic gram-positive bacteria. It is also active against antibiotic-resistant gram-positive bacteria. It should not be taken with statins, a class of drugs that lower cholesterol. It comes in an IV dosage form. Lines should be flushed before and after the drug is administered. Side effects include **hypotension** (low blood pressure), headache, insomnia, rash, constipation, nausea, diarrhea, and injection site reactions. It may take up to 30 minutes for this drug to dissolve before it can be mixed as an IV.

TABLE 4.13   Most Commonly Used Aminoglycosides

Generic Name	Pronunciation	Dosage Form	Brand Name	Dispensing Status
amikacin	am-i-KAY-sin	injection, IV	Amikin	Rx
gentamicin	jen-ta-MYE-sin	injection, IV, ophthalmic	Garamycin	Rx
kanamycin	kan-a-MYE-sin	injection, IV	Kantrex	Rx
neomycin	nee-oh-MYE-sin	oral liquid	Mycifradin, Neo-Fradin, Neo Rx	Rx
		topical		
streptomycin	strep-toe-MYE-sin	injection, IV	(none)	Rx
tobramycin	toe-bra-MYE-sin	injection, IV	Nebcin	Rx

TABLE 4.14   Most Commonly Used Cyclic Lipopeptide

Generic Name	Pronunciation	Dosage Form	Brand Name	Dispensing Status
daptomycin	DAP-to-mye-sin	IV	Cubicin	Rx

Other Antibiotics

A number of important antibiotics do not fit into any of the previously discussed groups and are collectively discussed here. These antibiotics, listed in Table 4.15, are structurally distinct from those in other classes and from each other.

Vancomycin (Vancocin)

Vancomycin (Vancocin) is a bactericidal drug that interferes with bacterial wall synthesis. It is especially useful for methicillin-resistant *Staphylococcus aureus* (MRSA) and pseudomembranous enterocolitis (caused by *Clostridium difficile*). However, because vancomycin has been overused, bacterial resistance to this drug is increasing.

Vancomycin is among the most commonly prescribed drugs for the following conditions.

- dialysis patients
- endocarditis
- staph infections (methicillin-resistant *S. aureus*, MRSA)

As a consequence of overuse of vancomycin, the Centers for Disease Control (CDC) has strict guidelines for handling and use of this drug.

Vancomycin can be ototoxic and nephrotoxic. Neutropenia (reduction in white blood cells called neutrophils) can also be a problem. After the first dose, dosing should be based on the individual patient's plasma concentrations.

When dispensed intravenously, 1 gram of vancomycin is usually mixed with at least 250 mL of fluid. Even though the drug diluent ratio is 1 g per 200 mL, it is always best to mix this drug in a larger amount of fluid than the minimum required. This tactic will also prevent the drug from being infused too quickly and prevent the patient from experiencing the flushing known as red man syndrome. The rate of infusion should be no faster than 1 gram per hour. It can also be given orally for *C. difficile*, an infection of the gastrointestinal tract. Metronidazole is also used for this purpose.

Clindamycin (Cleocin)

A derivative of lincomycin, clindamycin (Cleocin) is a broad-spectrum antibiotic that inhibits protein synthesis. It is used for serious gram-positive infections and as a prophylaxis preceding abdominal surgery. It is also frequently dispensed in a topical form for the treatment of acne. It is effective against *Bacteroides fragilis*.

TABLE 4.15   Most Commonly Used Antibiotics Independent of Class

Generic Name	Pronunciation	Dosage Form	Brand Name	Dispensing Status
clindamycin	klin-da-MYE-sin	capsule, injection, IV, oral liquid topical	Cleocin	Rx
linezolid	li-NE-zoh-lid	IV, oral liquid, tablet	Zyvox	Rx
metronidazole	me-troe-NYE-da-zole	capsule, IV, tablet, topical	Flagyl	Rx
pentamidine	pen-TAM-i-deen	inhalant, injection, IV	NebuPent, Pentam	Rx
vancomycin	van-koe-MYE-sin	capsule, IV	Vancocin	Rx

Clindamycin is among the drugs of choice for the following conditions.

- acne
- alternative in dental prophylaxis for patients allergic to penicillin
- anaerobic pneumonia
- bone infections (high concentrations in bone)
- bowel infections
- female genital infections
- intra-abdominal infections

The most serious side effect of clindamycin is pseudomembranous colitis (bloody diarrhea caused when toxin forms in the gut and the innermost layer of the colon is sloughed off). If the patient develops diarrhea, the drug must be discontinued.

Metronidazole (Flagyl)

Metronidazole (Flagyl) is an antibiotic that is effective against fungi and protozoa as well as bacteria. Such capability is unusual because the cells of fungi and protozoa are much more similar to those of humans than to those of bacteria. Metronidazole is used primarily to treat *Trichomonas* infections of the vaginal canal and cervix and of the male urethra. It is also used to treat amebic dysentery, *Giardia* infections of the intestine, and serious infections caused by certain strains of anaerobic bacteria. It disrupts the DNA structure of the microorganism.

Metronidazole is among the drugs of choice for the following bacteria and conditions.

- amebic dysentery
- *Clostridium difficile*
- intestinal infections
- sexually transmitted diseases, *Trichomonas*

Efficacious treatment of STDs requires that all sexual partners be treated at the same time and avoid sexual contact for 3 to 4 days; otherwise reinfection will occur, creating a vicious cycle.

Some side effects include a metallic taste, diarrhea, intolerance to alcohol, and rash. Metronidazole may also discolor the urine. It may be taken with food to decrease gastrointestinal upset.

Do not drink alcoholic beverages when taking this medication

A "Do not drink alcohol" sticker must be attached to this drug. The warning against alcohol consumption is very important with metronidazole as it interacts with alcohol in the same way as disulfiram (Antabuse), a drug that will be discussed in Chapter 7. If the patient consumes alcohol while taking metronidazole, the patient will become nauseated, causing vomiting. In addition, the patient's blood vessels dilate, causing a flushed reaction and headache.

The dosage forms of this drug are capsules, IV, tablets, topical, and vaginal. The topical and vaginal forms are easily confused. The vaginal form has an applicator. Check to be sure which form the prescriber wants if there is any doubt.

Pentamidine (NebuPent, Pentam)

Pentamidine (NebuPent, Pentam) is used as a second-line agent for *Pneumocystis carinii*. Its mechanism of action is unknown. It can be administered intravenously or intramuscularly once daily and by inhalation (drawn into the lungs through the air), once every four weeks. The patient may develop sudden hypotension. Thus, it is important to have emergency drugs and equipment on hand when administering this drug intravenously or intramuscularly.

To administer by inhalation, the dose should be diluted in 6 mL of sterile water and delivered at 6 mL per minute by a jet nebulizer, a device that creates and throws an aerosol spray. Patients who develop wheezing or coughing during therapy may benefit by pretreatment (5 minutes before) with a bronchodilator.

Linezolid (Zyvox)

Linezolid (Zyvox), the first oxazolidinone to be approved by the FDA, inhibits bacterial protein synthesis. It is used to treat MRSA (methicillin-resistant *S. aureus*), VRE (vancomycin-resistant *E. faecium*), and other gram-positive infections. The drug must be protected from light. The dosage forms are IV, oral liquid, and tablet. The IV form comes in an IV bag. It should be administered alone and not given through a line that is administering other drugs. Linezolid is not suitable for simultaneous administration because it has many physical incompatibilities and might precipitate in the line.

Storage of Liquid Antibiotics

Storage of liquid antibiotics is always a problem, because so many of them have to be refrigerated. After the lyophilized (powdered) antibiotics are mixed, some need refrigeration and some may be stored at room temperature. This is very important information the technician may pass onto the patient. It is *not* counseling. No professional judgment is required. Drug storage does not require one to make a decision—the drug is either refrigerated or stored at room temperature—and is a valuable and necessary piece of information. The pharmacy technician may pass this on to the patient or caregiver. Since there are many now that do not require refrigeration and an equal amount that do, patients are often confused. Manufacturers have made an effort to minimize the number of these drugs that do need refrigeration. Table 4.16 is provided to simplify this issue for the pharmacy technician.

Ophthalmic Antibiotics

Some of the antibiotics discussed in this chapter have an **ophthalmic** (eye) dosage form. In contrast, there are very few antibiotics that have an **otic** (ear) form, because the ophthalmic forms are also often used for ear conditions. However, putting an otic medicine in the eye would be extremely painful for the patient. This is because otic medicines are not manufactured with the same **pH** (acidity/alkalinity) as the eye. Ophthalmic (eye) medications are often used in the ear, but otic (ear) medications are *never* used in the eye. Table 4.17 lists antibiotic ophthalmic medications.

Because of the fact that the medication must have the same pH as the eye and because of the extreme sterility demanded in the manufacturing process of ophthalmics, eye drops are very expensive, especially the newer ones. They are often rejected by insurance companies, and a less expensive one must be used. The technician will need to let the prescriber know what is available and which ones the insurance will most likely cover.

Treating Complications of Infections

Drotrecogin alfa (Xigris), presented in Table 4.18, is not an antibiotic (i.e., it does not kill or inhibit the infecting microorganism), yet it is important in treating some patients with complications of sepsis, a life-threatening result of serious infections. It is a recombinant form of Activated Protein C, which is a natural anticoagulant (it prevents blood clotting) and anti-inflammatory. Its anticoagulant properties are very important, and this is the only drug approved for that specific indication. Because of the high cost of this drug, strict guidelines limit its use.

TABLE 4.16 Storage of Liquid Antibiotics

Drug	Brand Name	Refrigerate?
amoxicillin		Yes
amoxicillin-clavulanate	Augmentin	Yes
ampicillin		Yes
azithromycin	Zithromax	No
cefadroxil	Duricef	Yes
cefaclor	Ceclor	Yes
cefpodoxim	Vantin	Yes
cefprozil	Cefzil	Yes
ceftibutin	Cedox	Yes
cephalexin	Keflex	Yes
cefdinir	Omnicef	No
cefixim	Suprax	No
ciprofloxacin	Cipro	No
clarithromycin	Biaxin	No
clindamycin	Cleocin	No
doxycycline	Vibramycin	No
erythromycin		No
erythromycin-sulfasoxazole	Pediazole	No
linezolid	Zyvox	No
levofloxacin	Levaquin	No
loracarbef	Lorabid	Yes
neomycin	Mycifradin	No
nitrofurantoin	Macrobid	No
penicillin		Yes
sulfamethoxazole-trimethoprim	Bactrim, Septra	No
tetracycline	Sumycin	No

TABLE 4.17   Ophthalmic Dosage Forms

Generic Name	Pronunciation	Dosage Form	Brand Name	Dispensing Status
azithromycin	az-ith-roe-MYE-sin	drops	AzaSite	Rx
bacitracin	bas-I-TRAY-cin	ointment	AKtracin	Rx
ciprofloxacin	sip-roe-FLOX-a-sin	drops	Occuflox, Ciprodex	Rx
erythromycin	e-rith-roe-MYE-sin	ointment	Ilotycin	Rx
gatifloxacin	gat-i-floks-a sin	drops	Zymar	Rx
gentamicin	jen-ta-MYE-sin	drops, ointment	Gentak, Genoptic	Rx
moxifloxacin	moks-i-FLOKS-a-sin	drops	Vigamox	Rx
ofloxacin	oh-FLOKS-a sin	drops	Ocuflox	Rx
sodium sulfacetamide	SOE-dee-um-sul-fa-SEE-ta-mide	drops	Bleph 10	Rx
tobramycin	toe-bra-MYE-sin	drops	Tobrex	Rx

TABLE 4.18   Most Commonly Used Adjunct in Treating Sepsis

Generic Name	Pronunciation	Dosage Form	Brand Name	Dispensing Status
drotrecogin alfa	droe-tre-KOE-jin AL-fa	IV	Xigris	Rx

Chapter Terms

aerobic needing oxygen to survive

aminoglycoside a class of antibiotics that inhibit bacterial protein synthesis by binding to ribosomal subunits; commonly used to treat serious infections

anaerobic capable of surviving in the absence of oxygen

antibiotic a chemical substance with the ability to kill or inhibit the growth of bacteria by interfering with bacteria life processes

antiseptic a substance that kills or inhibits the growth of microorganisms on the outside of the body

bacteria small, single-celled microorganisms that exist in three main forms: spherical (i.e., cocci), rod shaped (i.e., bacilli), and spiral (i.e., spirilla)

bactericidal agent a drug that kills bacteria

bacteriostatic agent a drug that inhibits the growth or multiplication of bacteria

broad-spectrum antibiotic an antibiotic that is effective against multiple organisms

cephalosporin a class of antibiotics with a mechanism of action similar to that of penicillins, but with a different antibacterial spectrum, resistance to beta-lactamase, and pharmacokinetics; divided into first-, second-, third-, and fourth-generation agents

chelation combination of an organic molecule such as a drug with a metal in complexes in which the metal ion is part of a ring

community-acquired contracted outside of the hospital

cyclic lipopeptide a new class of antibiotics that bind to bacterial membranes and cause the cell membrane to depolarize, thus leading to an inhibition of DNA and RNA synthesis

disinfectant an agent that frees inanimate objects from infection

D^{5}W dextrose 5% in water

empirical treatment treatment begun before a definite diagnosis can be obtained

Gram staining a staining technique that divides bacteria into gram-positive (purple) or gram-negative (red) based on the properties of their cell walls

hypotension low blood pressure

infection a condition in which bacteria grow in body tissues and cause tissue damage to the host either by their presence or by toxins they produce

ketolide a class of antibiotics that block protein synthesis by binding to ribosomal subunits and may also inhibit the formation of new ribosomes; used primarily to treat bacterial infections in the lungs and sinuses

macrolide a class of bacteriostatic antibiotics that inhibit protein synthesis by combining with ribosomes; used primarily to treat pulmonary infections caused by *Legionella* and gram-positive organisms

nephrotoxicity ability to damage the kidneys

nosocomial acquired by patients in the hospital

NS normal saline

ophthalmic to be used in the eye

otic to be used in the ear

ototoxicity ability to damage the organs of hearing

penicillin a class of antibiotics obtained from *Penicillium chrysogenum*; kill bacteria by preventing them from forming a rigid cell wall, thereby allowing an excessive amount of water to enter through osmosis and cause lysis of the bacterium cell

pH a measurement of acidity or alkalinity. pH 7 is neutral; a solution with a pH above 7 is alkaline; a solution with a pH below 7 is acidic

quinolone a class of antibiotics with rapid bactericidal action against most gram-negative and many gram-positive bacteria; work by causing DNA breakage and cell death; cross the blood-brain barrier

sepsis a systemic inflammatory response to infection resulting from blood-borne infections

Stevens-Johnson syndrome a sometimes fatal form of erythema multiforme (an allergic reaction marked by red blotches on the skin)

streptogramin one of a class of antibiotics that inhibit protein synthesis within the bacterial ribosomes; useful in the treatment of vancomycin- and methicillin-resistant infections

sulfonamides sulfa drugs; a class of bacteriostatic antibiotics that work by blocking a specific step in the biosynthetic pathway of folic acid in bacteria

superinfection a new infection complicating the course of therapy of an existing infection

tetracyclines a class of broad-spectrum bacteriostatic antibiotics that are produced by soil organisms and inhibit protein synthesis by binding to bacterial ribosomes

Chapter Summary

Fighting Bacterial Infections

- Bacteria are single-celled organisms that occur in almost all environments. They can penetrate body tissues and set up areas of infection.
- Gram-negative bacteria predominate in the hospital environment and are often found in hospital-acquired (nosocomial) infections.
- Gram-positive bacteria are most commonly isolated in community-acquired infections.
- General signs of infection that suggest a bacterial origin are fever (101°F or greater) and an increased number (>12,000/mm³) of white blood cells. The onset of fever alone is not diagnostic of bacterial infection.
- The outcome of antibiotic treatment is measured in two ways: (1) the clinical response, meaning the signs and symptoms disappear, or (2) the microbiologic response, meaning the organism is completely eradicated.
- An antibiotic works in one of six ways: (1) preventing folic acid synthesis, (2) inhibiting cell wall formation, (3) blocking protein formation, (4) interfering with DNA formation, or (5) disrupting the cell membrane, or (6) disrupting DNA structure.

- An infection is an invasion of the body by pathogens, resulting in tissue response to organisms and toxins.
- Bacterial infections are contagious until antibiotics have been taken for 24 to 48 hours.
- A bactericidal agent kills bacteria.
- A bacteriostatic agent inhibits growth or multiplication of bacteria.
- A superinfection is a new infection that complicates the course of therapy of an existing infection. It is due to invasion by bacteria or fungi resistant to the drugs in use.
- Antibiotics may interfere with the effectiveness of birth control pills.

Major Classes of Antibiotic Drugs

Sulfonamides

- The sulfa drugs are the oldest antibiotics on the market, so the technician needs to know both the brand names and generic names of these drugs.
- If a patient is allergic to sulfa, the alternative drug is usually nitrofurantoin (Macrobid, Macrodantin). *It is very important that this drug be taken with food to improve absorption.* Ingestion with food also helps to avoid the GI upset that accompanies this drug.

Nitrofurantoin can color urine brown. It is also important to drink plenty of water with this drug and to avoid alcohol.

- Sulfas are used in the treatment of UTIs, otitis media, GI infections, lower respiratory infections, and general infections.
- Patients taking sulfonamides should be told to drink six to eight glasses of water a day to keep the urine dilute and avoid crystallization of the drug in the urine. They should be told to avoid exposure to sunlight and to notify the physician if a rash appears (the most common side effect of the sulfas).

Penicillins

- Penicillin has many therapeutic uses. Ampicillin and amoxicillin have broader antimicrobial spectrums than penicillin G and V. Amoxicillin is used more often because it is dosed only three times a day; ampicillin should be dosed four times a day. Many prescribers are unaware of this difference, so to get better coverage for the patient, they should be called when the drug is dosed inappropriately.
- Penicillin is the drug of choice for streptococcal infections. It is used in gram-positive infections.
- Penicillin is bactericidal in that it kills bacteria by preventing them from forming the rigid wall needed for survival. Human cells do not have cell walls and are, therefore, uninjured by penicillin.
- Penicillin should be taken on an empty stomach with water because food slows its absorption. The acids in fruit juices or colas could deactivate the drug. The most common side effect of the penicillins is diarrhea.
- Antibiotic prophylaxis is recommended for patients with a heart prosthesis, congenital heart disease, idiopathic hypertrophic subaortic stenosis, a heart murmur, mitral valve prolapse, or a history of rheumatic heart disease.
- Patients should be medicated 30 to 60 minutes before a surgical procedure, and then a dose or doses should be given afterward. This varies with the procedure. Dental prophylaxis recommends only a single 2 g dose before dental procedures with no follow-up.
- A patient allergic to penicillin has a 1% possibility of also being allergic to cephalosporins, and vice versa. The pharmacy technician will find both allergies in the computer because most systems enter the drugs under penicillin-cephalosporin allergy.

Cephalosporins

- Cephalosporins have a mechanism of action similar to penicillins but a broader spectrum of coverage.
- The first-generation cephalosporins are similar to the penicillinase-resistant penicillins, with modest gram-negative coverage. The second-generation ones have broader coverage especially against *H. influenzae*. The third generation is active against a wide spectrum of gram-negative organisms. The new fourth-generation cephalosporin is considered "broad spectrum" with both gram-negative and somewhat less gram-positive coverage.
- Cephalosporins are probably the most commonly used antibiotics because they cover a very wide range of organisms and have lower toxicity than other antibiotics with the same coverage.
- Carbapenems, carbacephems, and monobactams are beta-lactams differing slightly from penicillins and cephalosporins.

Tetracyclines and Tigecycline

- Tetracyclines are bacteriostatic. They are the drugs of choice for Rocky Mountain spotted fever and Lyme disease, which are both transmitted by ticks.
- Patients taking tetracycline should be warned to avoid the sun, dairy products, and antacids and to take the drug on an empty stomach. The exception to these effects is doxycycline, which accounts for its popularity. Children and pregnant women should not take tetracyclines.
- Always watch the expiration date on tetracyclines. It can be very dangerous to dispense one of these drugs if it is out of date. When most drugs reach their expiration date, they simply lose effectiveness. That is not true

with tetracyclines; they can cause a fatal renal syndrome. This is especially important with the drugs the government is stocking in case of an anthrax attack.

- Manufacturers are packaging drugs to promote compliance, but this increases the cost. The same drug can be dispensed with the same instructions in less expensive packaging.
- A drug class related to the tetracyclines is glycylcycline. There is only one drug in that class: tigecycline (Tygacil). It is used for skin and intraabdominal infections.

Macrolides

- The macrolides are used primarily to treat pulmonary infections caused by *Legionella* and gram-positive organisms.
- As a rule of thumb, antibiotics are to be taken on an empty stomach to allow faster absorption into the bloodstream. A few, especially the older macrolides, are exceptions to this rule because they cause GI upset. In most cases, food will not lessen the effect of the antibiotic, but will just slow down the absorption rate. A sticker is placed on such antibiotics telling the patient to take the medication with food because their primary side effect is GI upset, and food intake can minimize this.
- Azithromycin (Zithromax, Z Pak) has had extremely good results. When using the Z Pak, the patient takes a loading dose of 500 mg the first day, then 250 mg on each of the next four days. Perhaps this loading regimen and short course, which create very good compliance, accounts for the success of this drug.

Ketolides

- Telithromycin (Ketek) is the only drug in the ketolide class and is similar to the macrolides. It is approved for community-acquired pneumonia exacerbations.

Quinolones

- Quinolones are among the drugs that penetrate bone and thus are good for bone and joint infections. They have many other uses and are especially good for UTIs and upper respiratory infections. Quinolones should not be used in children or pregnant women.

A short course of some of the quinolones can knock out a UTI.

- The primary side effect of the quinolones is GI upset. Antacids should not be taken with these drugs. They are phototoxic and increase the risk of theophylline toxicity.

Streptogramins

- Streptogramins are a drug class with side effects similar to those of the quinolones. They are the alternative for gram-positive bacteria resistant to vancomycin. Since the drugs are such an important advance in antimicrobial therapy, they were approved under the accelerated approval regulations of the FDA. Synercid is a combination of two streptogramins.

Aminoglycosides

- Aminoglycosides are used to treat very serious infections. They are ototoxic and nephrotoxic and may cause neuromuscular blockade. After initial dosing, they should be adjusted according to plasma concentration in the individual patient. Some current evidence supports once-daily dosing; it can be as effective as multiple daily dosing and with fewer side effects.

Cyclic Lipopeptides

- Cyclic lipopeptides are a new class of drugs that bind to bacterial membranes and cause the membrane to depolarize, leading to an inhibition of DNA and RNA synthesis. Daptomycin (Cubicin) belongs to this class of drugs and is used for complicated skin infections.

Other Antibiotics

- Vancomycin (Vancocin) can be ototoxic and nephrotoxic and can cause neutropenia. It is one of the few drugs effective against *Clostridium difficile*, as well as methicillin-resistant *Staphylococcus aureus* (MRSA).
- Clindamycin (Cleocin) has a very broad spectrum, with especially high concentrations in bone. The most serious side effect is pseudomembranous colitis. If diarrhea develops, the drug must be discontinued.

- Metronidazole (Flagyl) is used primarily to treat *Trichomonas* infections of the vaginal canal, cervix, and male urethra. It may discolor the urine. The warning against alcohol consumption is very important with this drug.
- Pentamidine (NebuPent, Pentam) is used as a second-line drug for pneumonia caused by *Pneumocystis carinii.*
- Linezolid (Zyvox), an oxazolidinone, is used to treat MRSA and VRE (vancomycin-resistant enterococcus).

Storage of Liquid Antibiotics

- After reconstitution, some antibiotics need to be stored in the refrigerator, whereas others may be kept at room temperature.
- The pharmacy technician may give the patient the information as to whether the drug needs to be refrigerated—it is not counseling.

Ophthalmic Antibiotics

- Ophthalmic dosage forms may be used in the ear, but otic dosage forms should never be put in the eye.
- Ophthalmic antibiotics are very expensive because of stringent manufacturing requirements. The technician often needs to know which antibiotic is less expensive in order to advise the prescriber.

Treating Complications of Infections

- Drotrecogin alfa (Xigris), which is not truly an antibiotic, is a powerful drug used to treat complications of severe sepsis. It is a recombinant form of Activated Protein C. Its anticoagulant properties are very important.

Drug List

The following drugs were discussed in this chapter. Each generic drug name is followed in parentheses by one or more brand names. If a drug is among the top 200 selling drugs, it will have an asterisk behind it, in this chapter and all the others.

Sulfonamides and Related Drugs
nitrofurantoin (Macrobid*, Macrodantin)
sulfamethoxazole-trimethoprim (Bactrim*, Bactrim DS, Cotrim, Cotrim DS, Septra, Septra DS)*
sulfisoxazole (Gantrisin)

Penicillins
amoxicillin* (Amoxil)*
amoxicillin-clavulanate* (Augmentin)*
ampicillin (Principen)
ampicillin-sulbactam (Unasyn)
carbenicillin (Geocillin)
dicloxacillin (Dycil)
nafcillin (Unipen)
oxacillin
penicillin G (various)
penicillin V (Veetids)*

piperacillin
piperacillin-tazobactam (Zosyn)
ticarcillin (Ticar)
ticarcillin-clavulanate (Timentin)

Cephalosporins
cefaclor (Ceclor)
cefadroxil (Duricef)
cefazolin (Ancef)
cefdinir (Omnicef)*
cefditoren (Spectracef)
cefixime (Suprax)
cefepime (Maxipime)
cefotaxime (Claforan)
cefpodoxime (Vantin)
cefprozil (Cefzil)*
ceftazidime (Fortaz)
ceftibuten (Cedax)

ceftizoxime (Cefizox)
ceftriaxone (Rocephin)
cefuroxime (Ceftin, Zinacef)
cephalexin (Keflex)*

Carbapenems
ertapenem (Invanz)
imipenem-cilastatin (Primaxin)
meropenem (Merrem I.V.)

Carbacephem
doripenem (Doribax)
loracarbef (Lorabid)

Monobactam
aztreonam (Azactam)

Tetracyclines
demeclocycline (Declomycin)
doxycycline (Vibramycin, Oracea, Adoxa)*
minocycline (Minocin, Soladyne)*
tetracycline (Sumycin)

Glycylcycline
tigecycline (Tygacil)

Macrolides
azithromycin (Zithromax, Z Pak, Zmax,
    AzaSite)*
clarithromycin (Biaxin)*
dirithromycin (Dynabac)
erythromycin base (Eryc, Ery-Tab, Ilotycin)
erythromycin ethylsuccinate (E.E.S., EryPed)
erythromycin lactobionate (Erythrocin)
erythromycin stearate (Erythrocin)
erythromycin-sulfisoxazole (Pediazole)

Ketolide
telithromycin (Ketek)

Quinolones
ciprofloxacin (Cipro)*
gatifloxacin (Tequin, Zymar)

gemifloxacin (Factive)
levofloxacin (Levaquin)*
moxifloxacin (Avelox)*
norfloxacin (Noroxin)
ofloxacin (Floxin)

Streptogramin
quinupristin-dalfopristin (Synercid)

Aminoglycosides
Amikacin (Amikin)
gentamicin (Garamycin)
kanamycin (Kantrex)
neomycin (Neo-Fradin)
streptomycin
tobramycin (Nebcin)

Cyclic Lipopeptide
daptomycin (Cubicin)

Antibiotics Independent of Classes
clindamycin (Cleocin)*
linezolid (Zyvox)
metronidazole (Flagyl)*
pentamidine (NebuPent, Pentam)
vancomycin (Vancocin)

Adjunct in Treating Sepsis
drotrecogin alfa (Xigris)

Ophthalmics
azithromycin (AzaSite)
bacitracin (Aktracin)
ciprofloxacin (Occuflox, Ciloxan, Ciprodex)
erythromycin (Ilotycin)
gatifloxacin (Zymar)
gentamicin (Gentak, Genoptic)
moxifloxacin (Vigamox)
ofloxacin (Ocuflox)
sodium sulfacetamide (Bleph 10)
tobramycin (Tobrex)

Chapter Review

Pharmaceuticals and Body Functions

Select the best answer from the choices given.

1. It is especially important that a person taking sulfonamides
   a. avoid the sun and drink lots of water.
   b. avoid drinking alcohol.
   c. get sufficient rest and avoid the sun.
   d. take the medication with food.

2. The primary side effect of Augmentin is
   a. drowsiness.
   b. rash.
   c. dry mouth.
   d. diarrhea.

3. Penicillin should be taken with
   a. colas.
   b. water.
   c. fruit juices.
   d. all of the above.

4. The drug of choice (DOC) for "strep throat" is
   a. clindamycin.
   b. tetracycline.
   c. penicillin.
   d. ceftazidime.

5. Which drug is effective against anthrax?
   a. gentamicin
   b. azithromycin
   c. penicillin
   d. doxycycline

6. The DOC for Rocky Mountain spotted fever is
   a. penicillin.
   b. sulfamethoxazole.
   c. gentamicin.
   d. doxycycline.

7. Which drug is it very important to take with food?
   a. methenamine
   b. nitrofurantoin
   c. sulfasalazine
   d. cefpodoxime

8. You can drink milk with all of the listed drugs except
   a. Macrodantin.
   b. Sumycin.
   c. Vibramycin.
   d. Augmentin.

9. Which drug has a large amount of sugar in the oral liquid dosage form?
   a. Vantin
   b. Omnicef
   c. Ceclor
   d. Lorabid

10. Clindamycin has a special affinity for
    a. bone.
    b. eyes.
    c. brain.
    d. heart.

The following statements are true or false. If the an item false, rewrite the statement so that it is true.

_____ 1. Alcohol has no effect on the patient taking Flagyl.

_____ 2. Quinolones can be used safely with theophylline and antacids.

_____ 3. It could be very dangerous to dispense an out-of-date tetracycline.

_____ 4. Ceclor is the drug of choice for strep throat.

_____ 5. Someone who is allergic to penicillin will also be allergic to cephalosporins.

_____ 6. A nosocomial infection is community-acquired.

_____ 7. The onset of fever is always diagnostic of bacterial infection.

_____ 8. Sulfonamide drugs may be used for UTIs and GI upset.

_____ 9. The major side effects of an amino-glycoside are ototoxicity and neph-rotoxicity.

_____ 10. The most common side effect of sulfonamides is a rash.

Diseases and Drug Therapies

1. List the six ways antibiotics work.

2. Give three penicillin and beta-lactamase inhibitor combinations that are frequently used. Provide generic and brand names.

3. List three infections the sulfonamides are used to treat.

4. How do a bactericidal antibiotic and a bacteriostatic antibiotic differ?

5. How do a nosocomial and community-acquired infection differ?

6. Define superinfection.

7. Which auxiliary labels would you put on a sulfa prescription if there is only room for two? (Make a list of all the labels you might need to put on a sulfa drug. Choose the two you think are most important. Defend your choices.)

8. Specifically describe how penicillin kills bacteria.

9. Why is the liquid dosage form of Omnicef rarely prescribed to diabetics?

10. Being a prudent technician, which antibiotics would you put a "Do not drink alcoholic beverages when taking this medication" auxiliary label on?

11. What is dose loading?

12. When would Xigris be used, and what is the most important property of this drug?

13. If someone picks up a prescription for metronidazole (Flagyl) and is on the way to a New Year's Eve party, what medication label should be pointed out to him or her?

14. Why is resistance developing to antibiotics?

15. Describe empirical treatment and when it would be used.

Dispensing Medications

1. You live in a state that allows a CPhT (certified pharmacy technician) to take a prescription over the phone. You take a prescription from the dentist for a patient with mitral valve prolapse. The patient is to have dental work done. The patient is allergic to penicillin, but the dentist does not know this. What do you suggest the dentist substitute for amoxicillin? (Hint: dental prophylaxis)

2. Amoxicillin comes in 500 mg capsules. The next patient the dentist writes for does not have a penicillin allergy. What do the latest guidelines recommend? How many capsules will you dispense?

3. You receive a prescription for a Z Pak. You have azithromycin, but not in the pack. How will you dose the drug?

4. It is hard to remember which labels go on certain drugs. Create a chart listing the antibiotics covered in this chapter that cause photosensitivity. Keep it with you in the pharmacy for reference.

Internet Research

Use the Internet to complete the following assignments.

1. Antibiotic resistance is of serious concern to the medical community as well as society at large. Use Internet resources to write a brief report outlining the current thinking related to antibiotic resistance. Include the popular media as well as more scientific perspectives in your report. Address the following questions: What are the primary concerns about antibiotic resistance? What measures are being taken to address this problem? Is there any difference of opinion between the popular media and the medical community?

2. Research one of the disease states mentioned in this chapter (e.g., Lyme disease, walking pneumonia, or meningitis). Write a short report that describes the disease, its etiology (i.e., causes and origin), signs, symptoms, and treatments (including drug therapies). List your Internet source(s).

What Would You Do?

1. A mother picks up amoxicillin for her son. It is dosed three times a day. She asks whether he can take the drug to school for the middle-of-the-day dose. Can a technician answer this question?

Therapy for Fungal and Viral Infections

5

Learning Objectives

- Understand the differences between fungi and viruses and why the drugs to treat them must have very different mechanisms of action.

- Differentiate antifungal, antiviral, and antiretroviral drugs by their indications, therapeutic effects, side effects, dosages, and administration.

- Use antifungal, antiviral, and antiretroviral terminology correctly in written and oral communication.

- Identify drugs used for HIV and understand their synergism.

Preview chapter terms and definitions.

Fungi and viruses are often confused with each other and with bacteria, but they are vastly different entities. This is why it takes drugs with very different mechanisms of action to treat them. These infections are often related because patients with debilitating viral infections often contract an equally debilitating fungal infection. When the body's natural defenses or natural bacteria are wiped out by an antibiotic, a fungus can take over and reproduce in these same areas of the body. Both viral and fungal infections can be deadly if left untreated.

Fungi and Fungal Diseases

A **fungus** is a single-cell organism that is similar to a human (i.e., animal) cell and to a green plant cell in that all three are **eukaryotic** (having a defined nucleus), in contrast to bacteria, which are **prokaryotic** (lacking a defined nucleus). Fungi (plural of fungus, pronounced FUN-jye) include mushrooms, yeasts, and molds. They are distinguished from green plants by the absence of chlorophyll and reproduction by spores. They are distinguished from animal cells by the presence of a rigid cell wall that is unlike that of bacteria.

All eukaryotic cells have similar molecular machinery for performing life functions such as making proteins, replicating DNA, and storing and releasing energy, different from the corresponding machinery in prokaryotic cells. Therefore, the antibiotics discussed in Chapter 4 that work so well against bacteria do not work against a fungus, and a drug that kills a fungus is likely to be toxic to a human as well. Still, there are some differences between human and fungal cells that can be used as the basis for antifungal drugs. For example, human cell membranes contain **cholesterol** (a eukaryotic sterol that in higher animals is the precursor of bile acids and steroid hormones and a key constituent of cell membranes); the cell membranes of fungi contain **ergosterol**, another form of lipid.

Fungal Diseases

Systemic fungal diseases are most likely to develop in patients whose immune system is depressed by disease, drug therapy (for example, the use of corticosteroids or antineoplastics), or poor nutrition. Patients at risk for fungal infections include those who have recently received transplants and are receiving immunosuppressive medications, patients with an intravenous catheter, and those with some cancers and human immunodeficiency virus (HIV). Superficially, fungi can cause skin infections, especially in areas that are moist, warm, and dark. The nails are a common target of fungal infection. Fungi can also cause systemic infections of the body organs and tissues such as the lungs, brain, and blood. Examples of fungal organisms and the diseases they cause are included in Table 5.1.

The use of antibiotics may cause certain fungal infections by wiping out the body's natural bacterial flora, allowing the fungus to grow and causing a fungal infection. For example, a woman who has been taking an antibiotic may develop a vaginal yeast infection that has to be treated with an antifungal agent.

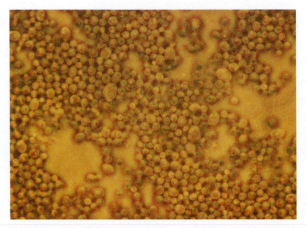

Fungi are unicellular organisms.

TABLE 5.1 Examples of Fungal Organisms and the Resulting Infections

Organism	Fungal Infection	Description of Infection
Aspergillus	aspergillosis	Inflammation in the skin, lungs, or bones
Blastomyces	blastomycosis	Infection through the lungs, producing tumors in the skin and other body tissues
Candida (yeast)	candidiasis	Usually a superficial infection of the mucous membranes, but sometimes systemic
Coccidioides	coccidioidomycosis	Known as Valley fever and endemic to the western United States, Mexico, and South America; an acute but benign self-limiting respiratory infection in its primary form, but a virulent, severe disease of the viscera, CNS, and lungs in its secondary form; sometimes misdiagnosed as lung cancer
Cryptococcus	cryptococcosis	Invasion of CNS most commonly seen in immuno-compromised patients
Histoplasma	histoplasmosis	Usually asymptomatic infection resulting from inhalation of spores, but can cause acute pneumonia

Antifungal Medications

Some antifungal agents prevent the synthesis of ergosterol, a building block for fungal cell membranes. Because human cell membranes use cholesterol instead of ergosterol, they are affected minimally by antifungals. Other antifungal agents act by inhibiting fungal cytochrome P-450, which is different from human cytochrome P-450, so these medications have little effect on human cells, but destroy the cells of the fungi. Some antifungals are available in topical dosage forms and are now available OTC. These topical agents will be discussed in Chapter 15.

Pulse dosing for fungal nail infections is becoming increasingly common. Each pulse dose is usually 1 week per month. Because the drug persists in the nail for several months, this regimen works as well as continuous daily dosing. Since patients take much less drug, treatment is safer and costs less.

Antifungal drugs are dispensed as topical, IV, and systemic agents. Even though the topical agents seem relatively mild compared to other antifungal agents, serious side effects have been reported. Close attention to the dosing regimen is needed to avoid overdosing. Table 5.2 lists the most commonly used antifungals.

TABLE 5.2   Most Commonly Used Antifungals

Generic Name	Pronunciation	Dosage Form	Brand Name	Dispensing Status
amphotericin B	am-foe-TER-i-sin B	IV, topical	Abelcet (ABLC), AmBisome, Amphocin, Amphotec, Fungizone	Rx
clotrimazole	kloe-TRIM-a-zole	lozenge (for oral infection)	Mycelex	Rx
flucytosine	floo-SYE-toe-seen	capsule	Ancobon	Rx
griseofulvin	gri-see-oh-FUL-vin	capsule, tablet	Fulvicin P/G, Gris-PEG	Rx
ketoconazole	kee-toe-KON-a-zole	tablet	Nizoral	Rx
nystatin	nye-STAT-in	oral liquid, tablet, topical, vaginal	Mycostatin	Rx
terbinafine	TER-bin-a-feen	tablet	Lamisil	Rx
terconazole	ter-KON-a-zole	vaginal	Terazol	Rx
Echinocandin				
anidulafungin	ay-nid-yoo-la-FUN-jin	IV	Eraxis	Rx
caspofungin	kas-poe-FUN-jin	IV	Cancidas	Rx
micafungin	mye-ka-FUN-gin	IV	Mycamine	Rx
Triazole				
fluconazole	floo-KON-a-zole	IV, oral liquid, tablet	Diflucan	Rx
itraconazole	i-tra-KON-a-zole	capsule, IV, oral liquid	Sporanox	Rx
posaconazole	poe-sa-KON-azole	oral liquid	Noxafil	Rx
voriconazole	vor-i-KON-a-zohl	IV, oral liquid, tablet	VFEND	Rx

Many of these drug names end in "zole," so if the generic form of the drug ends in "zole" (especially "conazole"), there is a good chance it is an antifungal.

Amphotericin B (Fungizone) is used for blood-borne, life-threatening fungal infections. Amphotericin B interferes with cell wall **permeability** (the ability of a material to allow molecules or ions to pass through it), allowing electrolytes and other substances to leak out. Certain infections may necessitate 4 to 6 weeks of therapy. Cumulative blood levels of the drug should be monitored. The drug must be infused slowly, not mixed or "piggybacked" with other drugs. To avoid precipitation, it should not be mixed with normal saline. It is usually mixed in dextrose and stored in the refrigerator and must be infused within 6 hours of being mixed. Vital signs should be checked periodically during infusion. The following should be monitored closely during therapy: electrolytes; blood urea nitrogen (BUN); serum creatinine; temperature; complete blood count (CBC); and fluid input and output. Antiemetic substances (agents that prevent or eliminate nausea and vomiting; covered in Chapter 10), can reduce the severity of nausea and vomiting. If the patient does not have a central venous catheter, the IV site should be changed frequently, as phlebitis (inflammation of a vein) is common with administration of this drug.

Side effects are fever, chills, shaking, and headache. Prophylaxis with acetaminophen and/or an antihistamine such as diphenhydramine is often necessary to alleviate or prevent infusion-related side effects. A common, serious side effect is renal toxicity. Potassium, calcium, and magnesium stores are often depleted. Anemia (a below-normal concentration of erythrocytes or hemoglobin in the blood) is also common.

Abelcet, AmBisome, and **Amphotec** are lipid complex injectable forms of amphotericin B with less kidney toxicity. These drugs are administered by IV infusion. They are indicated for treating aspergillosis or any type of progressive fungal infection in patients unresponsive to or intolerant of Fungizone. A wide range of side effects similar to those of amphotericin B have been reported.

Clotrimazole (Mycelex), supplied as a **troche** (a small lozenge), is especially effective against oral candidiasis.

Flucytosine (Ancobon) is synergistic with amphotericin B for *Candida* and *Cryptococcus* infections. It is usually given in combination with amphotericin B. The most common side effects are rash and GI upset.

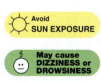

Griseofulvin (Fulvicin P/G, Gris-PEG) is indicated for fungal infections of the hair, skin, and nails. It can be used safely in children. The drug binds to human keratin, making it resistant to infection. The dose is taken with a fatty meal. The patient should avoid exposure to sunlight. If headache occurs, it usually goes away. Dizziness and drowsiness may be side effects.

Ketoconazole (Nizoral) has the same side effect profile as most of the other antifungal agents. Side effects are dose dependent and include nausea, anorexia, and vomiting. Orally it comes in tablet dosage form.

Nystatin (Mycostatin) is most often used in liquid form to swish and swallow, for patients with oral candidiasis, yeastlike fungi causing infection in the mouth.

Terbinafine (Lamisil) kills the fungus instead of just inhibiting its growth. It also persists longer than other antifungals in the nail after drug therapy has been stopped. The oral form is taken once daily for 6 weeks for fingernails and 12 weeks for toenails. For topical applications, terbinafine is the drug of choice for ringworm.

Terconazole (Terazol) is a prescription drug. If a patient has a vaginal fungal infection as a result of antibiotic use, it would be prudent to get the doctor to write a prescription for this drug. It works the same as the OTC vaginal antifungal agents, and often insurance companies will pay for this and not the OTC drugs.

Echinocandins Members of the echinocandin group of antifungal drugs inhibit the synthesis of D-glucan, which is an important cell wall component of the fungus.

Anidulafungin (Eraxis) is an IV antifungal for intra-abdominal, peritoneal, and esophageal *Candida* infections. It must be reconstituted with the provided diluent (an agent that dissolves the substance) and then mixed with D_5W or NS to a specified concentration. The appropriate concentration chart is provided with the drug. Anidulafungin has a loading dose of 200 mg and is followed by 100 mg for a period of 14 days of total therapy.

Caspofungin (Cancidas) was the first drug of this class of antifungal drugs to hit the market, the glucan synthesis inhibitors, that inhibit the synthesis of beta(1,3)-D-glucan, an integral component of the fungal cell wall. It is only available in IV form for the treatment of invasive aspergillosis in patients who are unresponsive to other therapies such as amphotericin B and itraconazole. It seems to have fewer hypersensitivity reactions than the other drugs in this class.

Micafungin (Mycamine) is used to prevent the esophageal *Candida* infection in patients undergoing bone marrow transplants. It is reconstituted and mixed with either NS or D_5W. After the diluent is injected into the vial, it should be gently swirled but not shaken. Once reconstituted, the micafungin preparation is good for 24 hours at room temperature and must be protected from light.

Protect medication from exposure to light

Triazoles Members of the triazole group interfere with cytochrome P-450 and inhibit the formation of the fungal cell wall.

Fluconazole (Diflucan) is metabolized through the cytochrome P-450 system. The oral form is used for vaginal or oral candidiasis, whereas the IV form should be reserved for patients unable to tolerate oral therapy. The most common side effects are headache, rash, and GI upset.

Itraconazole (Sporanox) is especially useful for fungal infections of the nails. The capsule should be taken twice a day with a fatty meal, but should not be taken within 2 hours of taking antacids or H_2 blockers. Because itraconazole can be toxic to the liver, patients should report any unusual nausea, vomiting, jaundice (yellow appearance caused by a deposit of bile pigment in the skin), or changes in the stool to the physician immediately. Capsules should not be substituted for the oral solution, because the solution is more readily absorbed. Patients should drink a cola when taking the capsule, as absorption is improved by increasing stomach acidity.

Posaconazole (Noxafil) is used to prevent invasive *Candida* and *Aspergillus* infections for **immunocompromised** patients (patients who have a deficiency in the immune response system) who are unresponsive to other drugs. It should be administered with a full meal. Because it is an oral suspension, it must be shaken well before the dose is administered. Posaconazole has a broader spectrum of activity than other triazoles. The suspension is cherry flavored.

Voriconazole (VFEND) is an alternative to amphotericin B for life-threatening fungal infections. It can be started intravenously and switched to an oral dose. Voriconazole has serious side effects such as liver toxicity and blurred vision. Patients taking this drug should not drive at night. Voriconazole must be infused over 1 to 2 hours and should not be infused simultaneously with any other products. Voriconazole must be reconstituted and used immediately. If not used within 2 hours, it must be destroyed.

May cause **BLURRED VISION**

Viruses and Viral Infections

A **virus** is a minute infectious agent that is much smaller than a bacterium. Unlike a bacterium, a virus does not have all the components of a cell and thus cannot reproduce on its own. Viruses replicate only within a living host cell by using the host cell's metabolic processes. A virus can infect a spectrum of cells including animal, plant, or bacterial cells. In humans, viruses are among the most common infectious agents. Most common viruses, like other infectious agents, are spread by one of the following routes.

- direct contact
- ingestion of contaminated food and water
- inhalation of airborne particles
- exposure to contaminated body fluids and/or contaminated equipment

The individual virus particle, a **virion**, consists of a core of genetic material, either the deoxyribonucleic acid (DNA) or ribonucleic acid (RNA), and a protein shell, known as a **capsid**, that surrounds and protects the nucleic acid. Depending on the virus, the capsid may be covered with a membrane called an **envelope**, carrying surface proteins that attach to the host cell receptors. A virus without an envelope covering the capsid is called a **naked virus**.

Stages of Viral Infection

Within the body, viral infection takes place at the cellular level in the following stages.

1. The virus attaches to a cell receptor.
2. The virus penetrates the cell as the cell membrane indents and closes around the virus (endocytosis).
3. The virus escapes into cytoplasm.
4. The virus sheds its covering (a process called uncoating) and presents its DNA or RNA to the cell nucleus.
5. This allows the virus to convert the nuclear activity in the cell to viral activity and rapidly reproduce new viral particles. (It uses the energy of the host cell to infect the cell and make more virus.)

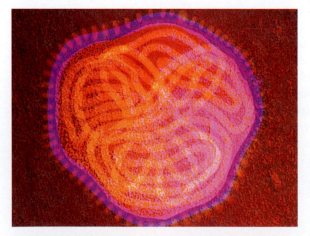

A virus infecting a bacterium (a bacteriophage). A virus does not have all the components of a cell and requires the metabolic and genetic resources of a living cell to replicate itself.

When viruses take over host cell nuclear activity, they synthesize viral nucleic acid and protein, which leads to production of more virus particles. The infected host cell may be so damaged that it disintegrates, releasing bursts of mature virions. If the host cell is not destroyed, the virions are released slowly. If the virus is not a naked virus, the virion acquires its envelope from the nuclear or cell membrane of the host during the release process. All virus-infected cells have some cellular characteristics that differ from those of uninfected cells. These differences provide opportunities to target and block viral division with medications without affecting normal cells.

Influenza, hepatitis B, and HIV are common and significant illnesses caused by viral infections. Influenza (commonly referred to as the **flu**) is an example of a common viral infection; it is due to the influenza virus. Symptoms are usually more severe than those of the common cold and include a rapid onset of malaise (vague discomfort and tiredness), myalgia (muscle pain), headache, chills, and fever. Patients with shortness of breath, wheezing, purulent (consisting of pus) or bloody sputum, fever persisting for more than seven days, or severe muscle pain should be advised to seek medical attention. Patients at high risk for complications secondary to influenza include elderly persons; patients with cardiovascular disease, renal disease, diabetes, or asthma; and immunocompromised patients, such as those with human immunodeficiency virus (HIV) or those who recently received transplants. Annual vaccinations for these patient populations are recommended.

Hepatitis, an inflammation of the liver, has various forms referred to as A through G. It can range from a very benign disease to a serious illness leading to death. It is a viral infection and will be discussed in Chapter 10. However, some of the drugs in this chapter are also used to treat Hepatitis B.

The treatment of **HIV (human immunodeficiency virus)** has been impacted tremendously by new drugs. Today, a diagnosis of HIV is no longer an early death sentence; rather, the patient has a chronic disease that has to be managed. The big issue for the pharmacy team is to be alert for drug interactions. Most regimens include at least three drugs and a complicated dosing schedule. Manufacturers have combined some of these drugs in order to decrease the pill load.

Classification of Viral Infections

Viral infections are classified in several ways. One classification scheme uses the duration or length of time the viral particles have been present in a body and the severity of the symptoms or illness that they cause. Another classification measures the extent of the infection within the body or the parts of the body that are affected. Viral infections can also be classified by the size and shape of the viral particles, genetic makeup (DNA or RNA), host, and induced pathogenic characteristics.

Viral Duration and Severity Within the classification of duration and severity, there are three categories: acute, chronic, and slow. An **acute viral infection** quickly resolves with no latent infection. Examples include the common cold, influenza, and various other respiratory tract viruses. A **chronic viral infection** has a protracted course with long periods of remission interspersed with reappearance; a herpes virus infection is an example. A **slow viral infection** maintains a progressive course over months or years, with cumulative damage to body tissues, ultimately ending in the host's death. HIV (AIDS) is an example of a slow viral infection.

Viral Infection When evaluating the extent of a viral infection, it must be determined whether the infection is local or generalized. A **local viral infection** affects tissues of a single system, such as the respiratory tract, eye, or skin. A **generalized viral infection** has spread or is spreading to other tissues by way of the bloodstream or tissues of the CNS.

Latent Viruses

Latency is a problem with some viruses. After the symptoms of the acute stage of the infection has ceased, these viruses may not have been eradicated but may be lying dormant in the cell in a latent, undetectable form. Later, under certain conditions, possibly years after the initial breakout or transmission of infection, they may reproduce and again behave like an infective agent, causing cell damage. Herpes and HIV can both behave in this manner. Some viruses of this kind can transform normal animal cells into cancer cells.

Virus and Cell Interaction

A virus can have several damaging effects on a host cell. It can alter the cell; incorporate itself into the genetic material of the host cell, thus becoming part of its nucleic acid pool; divide when the host cell divides; or it can kill the host cell.

Most viruses possess several antigens on their surface that stimulate the host to produce immunoglobulins. An **immunoglobulin** is a type of antibody, a molecule produced mostly by white blood cells called B-lymphocytes (as well as by other mechanisms) that matches a specific antigen, as discussed in Chapter 3. An immunoglobulin that matches a viral protein may prevent the virus from attaching to a cell receptor and may also destroy the virus. T-lymphocytes may also become sensitive to viral antigens, at which time they release chemicals to kill the virus or stimulate other cells, such as macrophages, to destroy the virus or virus-infected cells.

A very significant response of some virus-infected cells is the production of **interferon**, a substance that exerts virus-nonspecific but host-specific antiviral activity by inducing genes coding for antiviral proteins that inhibit the synthesis of viral RNA. Although interferon is produced in response to the viral infection, it is coded by the host cell's DNA. Interferon protects neighboring uninfected cells from viral infection and interferes with viral multiplication. Interferon is host cell–specific; that is, interferon molecules made by human cells will work only in human cells.

Vaccination

Prevention of viral infections by providing immunity is the principle of **vaccination**, which was mentioned in Chapter 3 in the context of child immunizations. Vaccination exposes the patient to a component of a virus or an altered viral strain that does not produce infection. The exposure of the body to these foreign (though harmless) materials promotes the growth of B-lymphocytes that produce antibodies that react to the designated virus. Later, if the vaccinated patient encounters the actual virus, the infection cannot develop because the patient's natural defenses are already primed from the vaccine. Because the discovery, testing, production, and implementation of vaccines are very complicated, vaccines are available for only a small number of viruses.

Adding to the difficulty of producing vaccines, some viruses undergo frequent mutations that cause their surface proteins to change, rendering previously effective vaccines useless. Influenza virus is such a virus. Every year a new influenza vaccine is developed according to the genetic changes that are predicted to occur the following year. Because the viruses that cause influenza change from year to year, annual revaccination is needed. The vaccine is only as good as the match it makes with a particular infecting strain of influenza. The vaccine usually becomes available in September and is given throughout the flu season. It is recommended for high-risk populations such as healthcare workers, people in contact with patients with influenza, nursing home residents, public safety workers, individuals 65 years old or older, and **immunocompromised** patients. The vaccine is made from viral particles that are raised in poultry eggs and then inactivated or killed. This is why it is important to confirm that a patient is not allergic to eggs before the vaccine is given. In certain situations, an antiviral medication may be prescribed to patients who cannot take the vaccine or have been exposed to influenza.

Antiviral Agents

There are fewer medications to treat viral infections than there are for bacterial infections. Because antibiotics often disrupt a cellular process that is unique to the bacterium being treated, the medication can be administered without causing toxicity to the patient. In contrast, because viruses use the host's own cellular processes to function and replicate, medications that block the life cycle of a virus are often toxic to the patient, much more so than antifungals and in much the same way as chemotherapy agents for cancer. Thus, **antiviral** drugs have been formulated to seek and prevent the virus cell replication in body fluids or in host cells without interfering with the host cell's normal function. Table 5.3 gives an overview of the most commonly used antiviral agents.

Many of the antiviral agents are potent drugs used to treat difficult diseases, such as HIV. A significant number of antiviral agents have emerged in recent years as a result of the tremendous amount of drug research dedicated to finding treatments for HIV.

Antiviral agents are the drugs of choice for treating viral infections such as:

- cytomegalovirus (CMV) retinitis
- herpes simplex
- herpes simplex keratitis
- herpes zoster (shingles)
- influenza prophylaxis

TABLE 5.3   Most Commonly Used Antiviral Drugs

Generic Name	Pronunciation	Dosage Form	Brand Name	Dispensing Status
Systemic Agents				
acyclovir	ay-SYE-kloe-veer	capsule, IV, ointment, oral liquid, tablet, topical	Zovirax	Rx
amantadine	a-MAN-ta-deen	capsule, oral liquid	Symmetrel	Rx
cidofovir	si-DOF-o-veer	IV	Vistide	Rx
famciclovir	fam-SYE-kloe-veer	tablet	Famvir	Rx
foscarnet	foss-KAR-net	IV	Foscavir	Rx
ganciclovir	gan-SYE-kloe-vir	capsule, IV	Cytovene	Rx
oseltamivir	oh-sel-TAM-i-veer	capsule, oral liquid	Tamiflu	Rx
ribavirin	rye-ba-VYE-rin	aerosol inhalant, capsule, tablet	Copegus, Rebetol, Virazole	Rx
rimantadine	ri-MAN-ta-deen	oral liquid, tablet	Flumadine	Rx
valacyclovir	val-ay-SYE-kloe-veer	capsule	Valtrex	Rx
valganciclovir	val-gan-SYE-kloh-veer	tablet	Valcyte	Rx
zanamivir	zan-AM-e-veer	inhalant	Relenza	Rx
Ocular Agent				
ganciclovir	gan-SYE-kloe-vir	ocular implant	Vitrasert	Rx

Note that the names of many of these drugs end in "vir." If a drug name does end in "vir," most likely it is an anti*viral* drug.

- varicella (chickenpox, shingles)
- hepatitis B

Antiviral side effects can range from mild (headache) to severe (renal disorders). Side effects related to specific agents are outlined in the following section.

Systemic Agents **Acyclovir (Zovirax)** acts by interfering with viral DNA synthesis. It is used to treat genital herpes in certain patients, herpes zoster (shingles), and varicella (chickenpox). The IV form is considered the drug of choice for herpes encephalitis. The dosage regimen changes depending on the type of infection being treated and the patient's status. A range of short- and long-term side effects have been reported. Acyclovir can be used for suppression of herpes in patients with multiple outbreaks.

Amantadine (Symmetrel) prevents absorption of viral particles into the host cell by inhibiting uncoating, which is the removal of the virus capsid proteins to expose the nucleic acid. Amantadine is used in the prophylaxis and treatment of influenza A. Sufficient blood levels of the drug are necessary to prevent infection. If administered after infection has begun, amantadine still may reduce the severity of symptoms. Side effects are rare and relate primarily to the central nervous system, because of these effects, amantadine also has some therapeutic effect on Parkinson disease. Concomitant ingestion of antihistamine or caffeine increases neurotoxicity.

Cidofovir (Vistide) is used for the treatment of cytomegalovirus (CMV) infection. Its advantage is that it can be dosed every two weeks. Cidofovir must be administered intravenously with normal saline and probenecid to reduce the incidence of nephrotoxicity.

Famciclovir (Famvir) is used to manage acute herpes zoster (shingles), to treat recurrent herpes simplex in immunocompromised patients, and to treat genital herpes. The primary side effects are nausea and headache. The advantage of this drug is that it can be dosed less frequently than acyclovir. It is a **prodrug**, a compound that on administration and chemical conversion by metabolic processes becomes an active pharmacological agent. The active compound after biotransformation is penciclovir.

Foscarnet (Foscavir) is used in treating CMV infections in immunocompromised patients. It should be delivered as an IV infusion, rather than as a rapid or bolus injection. Patients must be hydrated, and a prescription for a hydration product should accompany the prescription for foscarnet.

Ganciclovir (Cytovene) is used in treating CMV infections in immunocompromised patients. The pharmacist must follow chemotherapy preparation and dispensing guidelines (see Chapter 16) when mixing, labeling, and packaging this drug. It is available in both IV and an oral form. The IV form should not be used for rapid or bolus injection. Pregnant women should not handle this drug because of its mutagenic (change in genetic material) properties.

Oseltamivir (Tamiflu) is an oral inhibitor of the enzyme neuraminidase, which is carried on the surface of the influenza virus, and this drug is indicated for the treatment or prevention of influenza A and B. As with zanamivir, therapy must be initiated within 48 hours of symptom onset. Food generally improves tolerance, so oseltamivir is generally recommended to be taken orally at breakfast and dinner. (Do not confuse Tamiflu with Flumist, the nasal vaccine.) Oseltamivir has been shown to decrease the duration of the flu by up to three days.

Ribavirin (Virazole) is useful in treating viral infections and is especially useful in treating pediatric patients with respiratory syncytial virus (RSV). It is absorbed systemically from the respiratory tract following nasal and oral inhalation. Absorption depends on respiratory factors and the drug delivery system. Maximal absorption occurs with use of the aerosol generator via an endotracheal tube. This allows the drug to be atomized into a fine mist for inhalation therapy. The highest drug concentrations

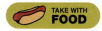
TAKE WITH FOOD

CHEMO PRECAUTIONS

of ribavirin are found in the respiratory tract and erythrocytes. The most common side effects are fatigue, headache, and insomnia. Nausea and anorexia can also occur. Patients who are pregnant or who are planning to become pregnant should not use or administer this drug.

Rimantadine (Flumadine) is indicated for prophylaxis and treatment of infections caused by influenza A virus strains. The most frequent side effects involve the GI and nervous systems. It also has fewer CNS-related side effects than amantadine.

Valacyclovir (Valtrex) is used to treat herpes zoster in immunocompetent adults and to treat genital herpes. It should be taken with plenty of water and within 48 hours of the onset of the zoster rash. It shortens the duration of postherpetic neuralgia. Side effects include nausea, vomiting, diarrhea, and constipation. It is better absorbed than acyclovir, and once absorbed, it is converted to acyclovir in the liver and gut. The end result is higher levels of acyclovir in the blood. It is also given less frequently than acyclovir.

Valganciclovir (Valcyte) is an oral prodrug for ganciclovir. As with ganciclovir, when working with this drug, it is important to follow precautions appropriate for chemotherapy drugs (see Chapter 16). Do not handle broken or crushed tablets. As with chemotherapy drugs, they should be disposed of in special containers. The drug has a Black Box warning regarding its mutagenic properties. Pregnant women should *not* handle this drug.

Zanamivir (Relenza) is indicated for the treatment and prophylaxis of influenza A and B. Therapy with zanamivir must be initiated within 48 hours of the onset of symptoms. The drug is inhaled using a breath-activated plastic device called a diskhaler. The recommended dosage is two inhalations daily, administered at 12 hour intervals, for 5 days. If the patient is also using a bronchodilator, the patient should be instructed to use the bronchodilator immediately prior to the administration of zanamivir. Zanamivir is sometimes prescribed as a prophylactic, especially in nursing homes and other group settings. However, because of the complexities associated with administering the drug, it is prescribed only when there is no other alternative.

Ocular Agent **Ganciclovir (Vitrasert)** is an ocular implant that seems to work better than systemic therapy for CMV retinitis. It does not treat any systemic manifestations.

Warning

Patients who are given Cytovene or Foscavir IV must be well hydrated. If hydration orders are not provided, the physician should be contacted. Some institutions have "standing orders" for hydration when these drugs are prescribed.

HIV-AIDS and Antiretroviral Agents

Human immunodeficiency virus (HIV) causes acquired immunodeficiency syndrome (AIDS), a dysfunction of the immune system associated with a very high mortality rate. Because of the severity of the disease, FDA approval of AIDS-related drugs has been subject to special accelerated processes.

HIV is a **retrovirus**, meaning that it can copy its genetic information, which it carries in the form of RNA, onto the host cell's DNA using an enzyme called **reverse transcriptase**. The host cell's own transcription system then produces new infectious viral RNA from this DNA copy. The DNA copy of the virus can also remain hidden in the host cells and replicate with them after the initial acute infection. **Antiretroviral** agents have been developed specifically to limit the progression of this retrovirus.

There are currently seven classes of antiretroviral drugs.

- nucleoside reverse transcriptase inhibitors (NRTIs)
- non-nucleoside reverse transcriptase inhibitors (NNRTIs)
- nucleotide reverse transcriptase inhibitors (NtRTIs)
- protease inhibitors (PIs)

Warning

One of the biggest problems when treating HIV is noncompliance with the drug regimen due to problematic side effects and complex dosing.

- fusion inhibitors
- chemokine receptors
- integrase inhibitors

Nucleoside Reverse Transcriptase Inhibitors (NRTIs)

A **nucleoside reverse transcriptase inhibitor (NRTI)** prevents the formation of a DNA copy of viral RNA, thus preventing the virus from multiplying or hiding itself. The NRTI molecule resembles a building block for DNA but lacks the attachment site for the next building block, thus terminating the chain being formed. Table 5.4 provides an overview of the NRTIs in current use. As a class these drugs commonly cause GI distress (nausea, diarrhea, abdominal pain). These side effects usually improve within the first two weeks of therapy. More permanent side effects include lactic acidosis with hepatic steatosis (degeneration of the liver).

The NRTIs, with the exception of didanosine, can be taken with or without food and generally do not interfere with other drugs. These agents are usually administered in two to three doses per day.

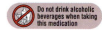

Abacavir (Ziagen) is one of the few HIV drugs that penetrate the CNS. This characteristic makes abacavir an invaluable therapeutic weapon, since HIV itself is able to penetrate and proliferate within the CNS. Although abacavir has few reactions with other drugs, the use of alcohol will increase the drug's toxicity, and patients must be instructed to avoid alcohol completely. Patients should also be cautioned to be on the alert for any of a number of side effects that could signal an adverse and potentially life-threatening reaction to the drug. Fifty percent of patients experience hypersensitivity, a state of altered reaction, to abacavir that generally occurs in the first 6 weeks. These side effects include rash, nausea, abdominal pain, malaise, or respiratory symptoms. The patient must be instructed to contact the prescriber, who will usually stop the medication.

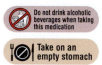

Didanosine (Videx) is always combined with two other antiretroviral agents. However it should not be combined with stavudine (Zerit). Didanosine is indicated in the treatment of advanced HIV in patients who cannot tolerate zidovudine. The patient should allow for an interval of at least 2 hours between the administration of didanosine and any drug that requires gastric acidity for digestion. Alcohol consumption will increase the risk of pancreatitis. For optimal tolerability and absorption, didanosine should be taken on an empty stomach 60 minutes before or 2 hours after meals.

Emtricitabine (Emtriva) simplifies the drug regimen because it is taken once daily. This drug is well tolerated. It is similar to lamivudine. The fact that this drug is

TABLE 5.4   Most Commonly Used Nucleoside Reverse Transcriptase Inhibitors (NRTIs)

Generic Name	Pronunciation	Dosage Form	Brand Name	Dispensing Status
abacavir	a-BAK-a-veer	oral liquid, tablet	Ziagen	Rx
didanosine	di-DAN-oe-seen	capsule, powder	Videx	Rx
emtricitabine	em-trye-SYE-ta-been	capsule	Emtriva	Rx
lamivudine	la-MIV-yoo-deen	oral liquid, tablet	Epivir	Rx
stavudine	STAV-yoo-deen	capsule, oral liquid	Zerit	Rx
zidovudine, AZT	zye-DOE-vyoo-deen	capsule, IV, oral liquid	Retrovir	Rx

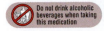

taken once daily and has fewer side effects makes it a major advance in the treatment of HIV. A warning label telling patients taking this medication not to drink alcohol should be attached to the prescription container when dispensing.

Lamivudine (Epivir) is indicated in the treatment of HIV and chronic hepatitis B. Lamivudine must be taken exactly as prescribed. It has the fewest side effects of any of the NRTIs.

Stavudine (Zerit) is typically well tolerated. However, it is associated with an increased risk of peripheral neuropathy. It should also not be prescribed with didanosine or zidovudine because pancreatitis is a side effect when the drugs are combined.

Zidovudine or **AZT (Retrovir)** was one of the first drugs developed specifically for the treatment of HIV. With the exception of stavudine, zidovudine can be combined with any of the other NRTIs. The combination of zidovudine with lamivudine, with or without a protease inhibitor, is recommended for the prevention of HIV after a needlestick or sexual exposure. The most common side effects of zidovudine are headache, anorexia, diarrhea, GI pain, nausea, rash, and anemia.

Non-Nucleoside Reverse Transcriptase Inhibitors (NNRTIs)

A **non-nucleoside reverse transcriptase inhibitor (NNRTI)** inhibits the action of HIV reverse transcriptase but by obstructing the enzyme's mechanical action, not by mimicking a DNA building block. Table 5.5 gives an overview of the most commonly used NNRTIs.

Delavirdine (Rescriptor) is a cytochrome P-450 inhibitor, so it, in contrast to nevirapine and many other NNRTIs, can increase the serum levels of some protease inhibitors. This drug is associated with a lower frequency of rash than nevirapine. Delavirdine should not be taken in tandem with any antacid. Patients should be instructed to avoid the ingestion of antacids for 1 hour before and 1 hour after the administration of delavirdine.

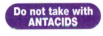

Efavirenz (Sustiva) has a long duration of action relative to other NNRTIs and is dosed only once a day, preferably at bedtime. Patients taking efavirenz should be instructed to avoid high-fat meals. Common side effects include dizziness and headache. The drug may also induce vivid dreams, nightmares, and hallucinations. These typically occur between 1 and 3 hours after administration and will generally subside after 2 to 4 weeks on the drug. Efavirenz is a cytochrome P-450 mixed inhibitor/inducer. It can cause a false cannabinoid (marijuana) test. Efavirenz should not be used in pregnant women.

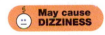

Nevirapine (Viramune) is associated with a high incidence of rash, especially during the early phase of treatment. To mitigate this effect, the drug is typically given at a lower dose during the first 2 weeks of treatment and then increased to the appropriate therapeutic level. Nevirapine is a cytochrome P-450 inducer. The antibiotic rifampin (a drug used to treat tuberculosis) interferes with the efficacy of nevirapine

TABLE 5.5   Most Commonly Used Non-Nucleoside Reverse Transcriptase Inhibitors (NNRTIs)

Generic Name	Pronunciation	Dosage Form	Brand Name	Dispensing Status
delavirdine	de-la-VIR-deen	tablet	Rescriptor	Rx
efavirenz	e-FAV-er-enz	capsule, tablet	Sustiva	Rx
nevirapine	ne-VYE-ra-peen	oral liquid, tablet	Viramune	Rx

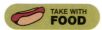
This drug interferes with the effectiveness of oral contraceptives

by reducing its serum concentrations in the body. In turn, nevirapine decreases the serum concentration of the protease inhibitor class of antiretrovirals. As a result, these drugs generally are not prescribed in combination. Nevirapine also decreases the effectiveness of birth control pills. Hepatotoxicity has been reported after one dose. Monitoring liver function tests is imperative.

Nucleotide Reverse Transcriptase Inhibitor (NtRTI)

Like an NRTI, a **nucleotide reverse transcriptase inhibitor (NtRTI)** inhibits the activity of HIV-1 reverse transcriptase by competing with natural nucleic acid building block substrates. When the NtRTI is then incorporated in viral nucleic acid, it terminates the chain formation. The NtRTI is more nearly in the form needed for use by the body than NRTIs are, leading to less toxicity. Table 5.6 lists the only NtRTI available at this time.

Tenofovir (Viread) is similar in structure to the NRTIs. It appears to have fewer drug interactions and side effects than other drugs used to treat HIV. Tenofovir is taken once daily with a meal. It can increase didanosine levels. If used with didanosine, it should be taken 2 hours before or 1 hour after didanosine is taken.

TAKE WITH FOOD

Protease Inhibitors (PIs)

A **protease inhibitor (PI)** inhibits formation of the protease enzyme, which cleaves certain HIV protein precursors that are necessary for the replication of new infectious virions. This mechanism results in the production of immature, noninfectious virions. With the exception of nelfinivir, the PI drugs are typically combined with other antiretroviral drugs, and their use has led to marked clinical improvement and prolonged survival among HIV-infected patients. Because PIs are metabolized through cytochrome P-450, drug interactions are common and can be severe. Table 5.7 provides an overview of the most commonly prescribed PIs. Statins should not be given with these drugs.

Side effects associated with all PIs include redistribution of body fat, referred to as "protease paunch" and characterized by a humped back; facial atrophy (a wasting away); breast enlargement; hyperglycemia (increased level of glucose in the blood); hyperlipidemia (elevated concentration of lipids in the plasma); and possible increase in bleeding episodes in patients with hemophilia, a deficiency of coagulation factor causing a hemorrhagic condition.

Amprenavir (Agenerase) contains much more vitamin E than the recommended daily allowance (RDA). This is because vitamin E enhances absorption of amprenavir. Therefore, patients who are taking this drug should be instructed to avoid the use of any other vitamin E supplements. Amprenavir is contraindicated in patients with sulfa allergies. One side effect peculiar to this drug is numbness around the mouth. The most common side effect associated with amprenavir is nausea.

Atazanavir (Reyataz) is dosed once daily and does not appear to increase cholesterol or triglycerides as most HIV drugs do, but it has other similar side effects. The patient on this drug will turn a little yellow if it is given properly.

TABLE 5.6	Nucleotide Reverse Transcriptase Inhibitor (NtRTI)			
Generic Name	**Pronunciation**	**Dosage Form**	**Brand Name**	**Dispensing Status**
tenofovir	te-NOE-fo-veer	tablet	Viread	Rx

TABLE 5.7   Most Commonly Prescribed Protease Inhibitors (PIs)

Generic Name	Pronunciation	Dosage Form	Brand Name	Dispensing Status
amprenavir	am-PREN-a-veer	capsule, oral liquid	Agenerase	Rx
atazanavir	at-a-ZAN-a-veer	capsule	Reyataz	Rx
darunavir	da-ROON-a-veer	tablet	Prezista	Rx
fosamprenavir	FOS-am-pren-a-veer	tablet	Lexiva	Rx
indinavir	in-DIN-a-veer	capsule	Crixivan	Rx
nelfinavir	nel-FIN-a-veer	oral liquid, tablet	Viracept	Rx
ritonavir	rye-TON-a-veer	capsule, oral liquid	Norvir	Rx
saquinavir	sa-KWIN-a-veer	capsule	Fortovase, Invirase	Rx
tipranavir	tip-RAN-a-veer	capsule	Aptivus	Rx

Darunavir (Prezista) is used in combination with low dose ritonavir and other anti-retroviral agents. The most common side effects are headache, nausea, and diarrhea. Darunavir should be taken with food. This drug received accelerated approval from the FDA so that it could be used in patients resistant to other therapies.

Fosamprenavir (Lexiva) is a prodrug of amprenavir. It is better absorbed and tolerated than amprenavir with less nausea and diarrhea; therefore, it can be taken without regard for meals.

Indinavir (Crixivan) has been shown to be less effective when taken in combination with St. John's wort. Thus, patients who are taking indinavir should be instructed to avoid this herbal remedy. Indinavir is very sensitive to moisture and is therefore always packaged with a desiccant. Patients should be instructed to store the drug in its original container. Indinavir should not be taken with high-fat meals or grapefruit juice. It should be taken on an empty stomach or with a low-fat meal. To lower the incidence of kidney stones, the patient should consume 48 ounces of water daily.

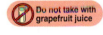

Nelfinavir (Viracept) is well tolerated with the exception of diarrhea, which generally resolves itself with continued use. Loperamide and calcium carbonate can help control the diarrhea. Nelfinavir should be taken with food. Nelfinavir is the only PI, with the exception of high-dose Fortovase, that does not require a **boost** (one drug given to increase the serum levels of another drug).

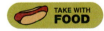

Ritonavir (Norvir) is prescribed primarily for its ability to increase the serum concentrations and decrease dosage frequency of other PIs (this is known as a boost). As such, ritonavir is generally given at a low dose. Ritonavir should be taken with food. This drug has many side effects including an unusual one—an altered sense of taste. Ritonavir, whether in capsule or solution form, should be stored in the refrigerator. It is the most potent inhibitor of cytochrome P-450 and has many drug interactions. This drug is used in combination with many other drugs.

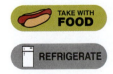

Patients on **saquinavir (Invirase)** should be instructed to avoid sunlight. **Fortovase**, a soft gel preparation, has largely replaced the older formulation Invirase because of its improved bioavailability. Invirase and Fortovase cannot be substituted for one another. Invirase must be taken with Norvir (retonavir) as a boost, but the dosage of Fortovase can be increased and it can be taken without retonavir.

Tipranavir (Aptivus) may have some advantages over other PIs. Its structure is more adaptable to protease binding sites than other PIs. Also, it also has a self

Avoid
SUN EXPOSURE

emulsifying drug delivery system (SEDDS) in the form of a soft gelatin capsule. This improves dissolution and the bioavailability of the drug, which increases systemic circulation and reduces the pill burden. It is given with ritonavir (Norvir) as a boost. Tipranavir is produced as a pink, oblong, and soft gelatin capsule and should be taken with food. The most common side effects are diarrhea, nausea, vomiting, headache, and fatigue. Tipranavir has a Black Box warning because intracranial hemorrhages were produced in clinical studies. It is stored in the refrigerator, but is stable for up to 60 days when not refrigerated.

Fusion Inhibitors

A **fusion inhibitor** prevents HIV from entering the immune cells. This mechanism is a big advance in HIV treatment, because older HIV drugs block replication of the virus only after it has entered the cell. Table 5.8 lists the only fusion inhibitor available at this time.

Enfuvirtide (Fuzeon) is given subcutaneously. It will be administered to HIV patients resistant to older drugs. It is a pregnancy category B drug. It is distributed as a powder, and sterile water is the diluent. It takes 30 to 45 minutes to dissolve. It is very common to have an injection site reaction.

Chemokine Coreceptor

Maraviroc (Selzentry) is the first drug from the **chemokine coreceptor** class to be approved for the R5 Virus, which is a form of HIV; the drug prevents this strain of the virus from attaching to an immune system cell. Maraviroc is to be given with other antiretroviral drugs. It is taken without regard to food. The most common side effect is a cough. While on this drug, patients must be monitored closely for infection. Maraviroc is summarized in Table 5.9.

Integrase Inhibitor

Raltegravir (Isentress) is an **integrase inhibitor**, a seventh class of drugs used to treat HIV. Like reverse transcriptase (blocked by NRTIs, NtRTIs, and NNRTIs) and protease (blocked by PIs), integrase is an enzyme needed for HIV to reproduce. Raltegravir is summarized in Table 5.10. Integrase inserts DNA, produced from viral

TABLE 5.8   Fusion Inhibitor

Generic Name	Pronunciation	Dosage Form	Brand Name	Dispensing Status
enfuvirtide	en-FOO-vir-tide	injection	Fuzeon	Rx

TABLE 5.9   Chemokine Coreceptor

Generic Name	Pronunciation	Dosage Form	Brand Name	Dispensing Status
maraviroc	mah-RAV-er-rock	tablet	Selzentry	Rx

RNA by reverse transcriptase, into the DNA of the host cell. Raltegravir, which blocks the action of integrase, received a priority review and was approved to be used only in combination with other HIV drugs. It reduces the amount of HIV in blood and increases white blood cell count, which helps fight infection. Because HIV patients are immunocompromised, the infection-fighting property of raltegravir is very important.

The most commonly used HIV drugs are listed by group in Table 5.11.

Responding to Exposure to HIV

The Centers for Disease Control (CDC) has developed guidelines for the management of healthcare worker exposures to HIV. These guidelines include recommendations for the administration of antiretroviral drugs as **post-exposure prophylaxis (PEP)**. Healthcare worker risks include exposure to the blood and other body fluids of an HIV-positive patient and needle-stick injuries. Following such an exposure, the administration of an appropriate antiretroviral regimen should begin within 2 hours. Research has shown that prompt treatment can decrease the risk of infection by 80%. Clearly, preventing exposure to HIV through appropriate precautions is the primary means of protection against HIV infection for healthcare workers as well as the public at large. People accidentally exposed to blood with a high virus titer or to deep needle injury should start PEP immediately (within 1 to 2 hours) because they are at high risk of infection.

TABLE 5.10   Integrase Inhibitor

Generic Name	Pronunciation	Dosage Form	Brand Name	Dispensing Status
raltegravir	ral-TEG-ra-veer	tablet	Isentress	Rx

TABLE 5.11   Summary List of HIV Drugs by Class

HIV Drug Classes	HIV Drugs
NRTI, nucleoside reverse transcriptase inhibitor	Ziagen (abacavir), Videx (didanosine), Emtriva (emtricitabine), Epivir (lamivudine), Zerit (stavudine), Retrovir (zidovudine)
NNRTI, non-nucleoside reverse transcriptase inhibitor	Rescriptor (delavirdine), Sustiva (efavirenz), Viramune (nevirapine)
NtRTI, nucleotide reverse transcriptase inhibitor	Viread (tenofovir)
PI, protease inhibitor	Agenerase (amprenavir), Reyataz (atazanavir), Prezista (darunavir), Lexiva (fosamprenavir), Crixivan (indinavir), Viracept (nelfinavir), Norvir (ritonavir), Fortovase, Invirase (saquinavir), Aptivus (tipranavir)
fusion inhibitor	Fuzeon (enfuvirtide)
chemokine coreceptor	Selzentry (maraviroc)
integrase inhibitor	Isentress (raltegravir)

Combining Antiretroviral Medications

None of the antiretroviral medications currently available can eradicate AIDS, but when used appropriately they can decrease viral replication, improve immunological status, and prolong life. The standard care for the treatment of AIDS is to administer three or more drugs in combination. The regimens are difficult to follow because the drugs must be taken around the clock. Consequently, patient compliance is frequently poor. Clear, written instructions for taking the medications, as well as adequate warnings about the potential for drug interactions, may encourage better compliance. Drugs that are dosed once a day show a tremendous improvement in compliance.

Table 5.12 gives an overview of current recommendations for HIV therapy dosing regimens. The following antiretroviral drug combinations should be avoided.

- didanosine with stavudine and **zalcitabine**
- zidovudine with stavudine

In order to simplify the drug regimen and decrease pill load, manufacturers have increasingly moved to drug combinations. There are specific advantages and disadvantages to various combinations. The most obvious advantage is improved compliance. A principal disadvantage is that in these combinations the drugs are in fixed doses; some of these cannot be used in unstable patients who require frequent dose changes to decrease the viral load. Most of the drugs approved by the FDA in the last few years are combination drugs.

Atripla (efavirenz, emtricitabine, and tenofovir) is a combination of three different classes of antiretrovirals—an NNRTI (Sustiva), an NRTI (Emtriva), and an NtRTI (Viread)—in one pill. This is an unusual combination. The virus can be attacked in three different ways by the same pill. The side effects are the same as those of the three individual drugs. The big advantage is that Atripla is dosed once a day and improves compliance. It is recommended as first-line therapy unless the patient is in the first trimester of pregnancy. It was approved through an accelerated process. It has a Black Box warning for lactic acidosis. Atripla must be dispensed in the original unopened container.

Combivir (zidovudine and lamivudine) comes as a capsule and as a syrup for those who have trouble swallowing a capsule. Its ingredients (Retrovir and Epivir) are both NRTIs. The drugs are synergistic and the pill load is decreased. Because Combivir is a fixed dose, it cannot be used in patients requiring dosage adjustments. It cannot be used in children under 12 years.

Warning

Combivir is easily confused with Combivent, a medication for chronic obstructive pulmonary disease.

TABLE 5.12   Antiretroviral Dosing Regimen

Regimen Type	Recommendation	Indications
standard therapy	NNRTI: efavirenz + lamivudine + (zidovudine or tenofovir or stavudine)	HIV positive
	PI: lopinavir-ritonavir + lamivudine + (zidovudine or stavudine)	HIV positive
alternative therapy	3-NRTI: abacavir + lamivudine + (zidovudine or stavudine)	Resistant to usual regimens
post-exposure prophylaxis (PEP)	zidovudine + lamivudine + (indinavir or nelfinavir)	needle sticks and exposure to body fluids or blood of an HIV-positive patient

Epzicom (abacavir and lamivudine) contains two NRTIs (Ziagen and Epivir) in a fixed combination and a single strength. Epzicom can be taken without regard to food, which improves compliance and this is very important because partial compliance can lead to resistance. A card packaged with Epzicom states that if the patient has any two of the following symptoms the prescriber must be contacted immediately and the drug must be discontinued.

- fever
- rash
- nausea and vomiting or diarrhea and cramping
- extreme tiredness or achiness
- shortness of breath, cough, or sore throat

It is very important that the technician remembers to make sure the patient gets this card. Patients are instructed (and warned) to carry the card with them at all times. Always check a second time when dispensing this drug to make sure the patient receives the card, and tell the patient to be sure to read the card. This is *not* counseling.

Kaletra (lopinavir-ritonavir) is a combination of two protease inhibitors. Lopinavir is not supplied alone but only with ritonavir as a boost. Kaletra can cause nausea and vomiting, diarrhea, and pancreatitis. The solution contains alcohol. Ritonavir inhibits the metabolism of lopinavir, allowing increased plasma levels of lopinavir.

Trizivir (lamivudine, abacavir, and zidovudine) consists of three NRTIs (Epivir, Ziagen, and Retrovir) combined into one pill. Note that this combination is the same as Epzicom with Retrovir. Patients can take one tablet twice a day with this drug. It can be taken without regard to food, but if flu-like symptoms or a cough develops, the prescriber will most likely discontinue the drug.

Truvada (emtricitabine and tenofovir) has the same drugs as Atripla without Sustiva (efavirenz); that is, this drug is a combination of Emtriva and Viread. It may be an agent to prevent HIV in the future, but not at this time. Currently it is a drug recommended for occupational exposure to HIV and an option for initial treatment. It is well tolerated and long-acting.

The most commonly employed combinations of antiviral drugs are summarized in Table 5.13.

TABLE 5.13   Summary of Combinations of Antiviral Medications

Generic Name	Pronunciation	Dosage Form	Brand Name	Dispensing Status
abacavir and lamivudine	a-BAK-aveer and la-MIV-yoo-deen	tablet	Epzicom	Rx
abacavir, lamivudine, and zidovudine	a-BAK-a-veer, la-MIVyoo-deen and zye-DOE-vyoo-deen	tablet	Trizivir	Rx
efavirenz, emtricitabine, and tenofovir	e-FAV-e-renz, em-trye-SVE-ta-been & te-NOE-foe-veer	tablet	Atripla	Rx
emtricitabine and tenofovir	em-trye-SVE-ta-been and te-NOE-foe-veer	tablet	Trizivir	Rx
lamivudine and zidovudine	zye-DOE-vyoo-deen and la-MIV-yoo-deen	capsule, syrup	Combivir	Rx
lopinavir and ritonavir	loe-PIN-a-veer and rye-TON-a-veer	capsule, liquid	Kaletra	Rx

The pharmacy technician must understand that when dispensing these drugs that the patient is HIV positive. Discretion and sensitivity are paramount in dealing with these patients.

Chapter Terms

acute viral infection an infection that quickly resolves with no latent infection

antiretroviral a drug that limits the progression of HIV or other retrovirus infections

antiviral an agent that prevents virus replication in a host cell without interfering with the host's normal function

boost one drug given to increase the serum concentration of another drug

capsid a protein shell that surrounds and protects the nucleic acid within a virus particle

chemokine coreceptor a drug that prevents a strain of HIV from attaching to an immune system cell

cholesterol a eukaryotic sterol that in higher animals is the precursor of bile acids and steroid hormones and is a key constituent of cell membranes

chronic viral infection an infection that has a protracted course with long periods of remission interspersed with recurrence

envelope membrane surrounding the capsid in some viruses and carrying surface proteins that attach to cell surface receptors

ergosterol a form of lipid found in the cell membrane of fungi where higher animals have cholesterol

eukaryotic having a defined nucleus, such as an animal or fungal cell

flu influenza, a common viral infection

fungus a single-cell eukaryotic organism (similar to a human cell rather than to bacteria); marked by a rigid cell wall, the absence of chlorophyll, and reproduction by spores

fusion inhibitor a drug that prevents HIV from entering the immune cells

generalized viral infection an infection that has spread to other tissues by way of the bloodstream or the central nervous system

hepatitis viral inflammation of the liver

human immunodeficiency virus (HIV) a retrovirus transmitted in body fluids that causes acquired immune deficiency syndrome (AIDS) by attacking T lymphocytes

immunocompromised having a deficiency in the immune response system

immunoglobulin an antibody that reacts to a specific foreign substance or organism and may prevent its antigen from attaching to a cell receptor or may destroy the organism

interferon a substance that exerts virus-non-specific but host-specific antiviral activity by inducing genes coding for antiviral proteins that inhibit the synthesis of viral RNA

integrase inhibitor a drug that prevents DNA produced by the reverse transcriptase of HIV from becoming incorporated into the patient's DNA

latency the ability of a virus to lie dormant and then, under certain conditions, reproduce and again behave like an infective agent, causing cell damage

local viral infection a viral infection affecting tissues of a single system such as the respiratory tract, eye, or skin

naked virus a virus without an envelope covering the capsid

non-nucleoside reverse transcriptase inhibitor (NNRTI) a drug that inhibits HIV reverse transcriptase by preventing the enzyme from working mechanically

nucleoside reverse transcriptase inhibitor (NRTI) a drug that inhibits HIV reverse transcriptase by competing with natural nucleic acid building block substrates, causing termination of the DNA chain

nucleotide reverse transcriptase inhibitor (NtRTI) a drug that inhibits HIV reverse transcriptase by competing with natural nucleic acid building block substrates, causing termination of chain formation, and is more nearly in the form used by the body than an NRTI

permeability the ability of a material to allow molecules or ions to pass through it

post-exposure prophylaxis (PEP) the administration of antiretrovirals after exposure to HIV

prodrug a compound that, on administration and chemical conversion by metabolic processes, becomes an active pharmacological agent

prokaryotic not having a defined nucleus, like bacteria

protease inhibitor (PI) a drug that prevents the cleavage of certain HIV protein precursors needed for the replication of new infectious virions

pulse dosing a regimen of dosing one week per month; commonly used for treating fungal nail infections

retrovirus a virus that can copy its RNA genetic information into the host's DNA

reverse transcriptase a retroviral enzyme that makes a DNA copy from an RNA original

slow viral infection an infection that maintains a progressive course over months or years with cumulative damage to body tissues, ultimately ending in the host's death

troche a small lozenge

vaccination the introduction of a vaccine, a component of an infectious agent, into the body to produce immunity to the actual agent

virion an individual viral particle capable of infecting a living cell; consists of nucleic acid surrounded by a capsid (protein shell)

virus a minute infectious agent that does not have all the components of a cell and thus can replicate only within a living host cell

Chapter Summary

Fungi and Fungal Diseases

- A fungus is a microscopic, eukaryotic organism, such as mushrooms, yeasts, and molds, that reproduces by spores and does not contain chlorophyll. A difference between human and fungal cells is that human cells contain cholesterol, whereas fungi contain ergosterol. This difference is the basis for some antifungal drugs.
- Systemic fungus diseases are most likely to develop in patients whose immune system is depressed by disease or drug therapy such as the use of corticosteroids or antineoplastics.
- Women who take antibiotics frequently need an OTC antifungal medication to treat vaginitis, which occurs in response to the antibiotic activity.
- Antifungal agents prevent the synthesis of ergosterol, a building block for fungal cell

membranes; or inhibit fungal cytochrome P-450, which is different from human cytochrome P-450; or interfere with the production of the fungal cell wall, which human cells do not have. Therefore, antifungal drugs have little effect on human cells.
- Pulse dosing for fungal nail infections appears to be very effective, with fewer side effects and less costly than continuous daily dosing.
- Amphotericin B causes fever, headaches, shaking, and chills. Intravenous administration of amphotericin B necessitates prophylaxis with an antihistamine, aspirin, or acetaminophen. If there are no accompanying orders, be sure to contact the prescriber. This drug must be infused slowly and cannot be piggybacked or mixed with other drugs.
- Fluconazole (Diflucan) is used primarily for candidiasis.

- Itraconazole (Sporanox) is especially useful for treating fungus under the nails. The capsule dosage form should be taken with a fatty meal, and antacids should be avoided. Itraconazole is especially toxic to the liver, so signs of liver damage such as jaundice (yellowing of the skin) should be monitored.
- Terbinafine (Lamisil) is an antifungal that works in less time and may be even better than itraconazole for fungus under nails. It kills the fungus instead of just inhibiting its growth. The drug persists in the nails even after therapy is completed.
- Flucytosine (Ancobon) is usually given in conjunction with amphotericin B.
- Griseofulvin can be used for fungal infections of the hair, skin, and nails. It is often used in children. It is taken with a fatty meal, and sunlight should be avoided.
- Clotrimazole (Mycelex-7) comes in a troche, especially effective for oral candidiasis.
- Caspofungin (Cancidas) is an antifungal drug approved for use in patients with invasive aspergillosis that is unresponsive to other therapies.

Viruses and Viral Infections

- Viruses are highly specialized infectious agents that replicate within a cell by using the host cell's metabolic process.
- A virus has a spectrum of cells it can infect, and only in these can it multiply. These host cells can be animal, plant, or bacteria.
- All virus-infected cells have some characteristics that are different from those of uninfected cells. These differences offer ways to block viral division without affecting normal cells.
- Latency is a problem with viruses. They can lie dormant and then, under certain conditions, reproduce and behave once more like an infective agent, causing cell damage. Herpes virus and HIV both have this characteristic.
- Some virus-infected cells produce interferon, which protects neighboring uninfected cells from viral infection.

- Even though the body has defense mechanisms, such as producing interferons, some viruses can cause normal animal cells to be transformed into cancer cells.
- A major problem in the development of antivirals is the intimate relationship between host and virus. The search for selective inhibitors of viral activity that are not too toxic to the human host is a major area of research. The use of interferons from outside the body is leading the way.
- Hepatitis B is a viral infection.
- When someone is diagnosed with HIV, it is no longer an early death sentence, but a chronic disease.
- The IV form of acyclovir is the drug of choice for a form of herpes encephalitis and for severe herpes in immunocompromised persons.
- Famciclovir (Famvir), acyclovir (Zovirax), and valacyclovir (Valtrex) are used to manage acute herpes zoster.
- Amantadine (Symmetrel) and rimantadine (Flumadine) can be prescribed for influenza prophylaxis or treatment. Flumadine has fewer side effects. Symmetrel is also used for Parkinson's disease.
- Ganciclovir (Cytovene) is used primarily in treating cytomegalovirus (CMV) infections in immunocompromised patients. When mixing this drug, technicians must use chemotherapy agent precautions, and the drug must be labeled appropriately. It is also very important that hydration (IV fluids) orders accompany an order for this drug. If these orders are missing, contact the prescriber.
- An inhalation antiviral is ribavirin (Virazole). Maximum absorption occurs with the use of the aerosol generator via an endotracheal tube. Side effects are fatigue, headache, and insomnia. Virazole is especially useful in patients with respiratory syncytial virus (RSV), which usually occurs in children. Pregnant women *must* avoid exposure to ribavirin.
- Ganciclovir (Vitrasert) is an ophthalmic antiviral.

HIV-AIDS and Antiretroviral Agents

- Human immunodeficiency virus (HIV) is a retrovirus. It copies its RNA onto DNA using the reverse transcriptase enzyme and inserts the copy into the DNA of the host cell.
- Nucleoside reverse transcriptase inhibitors (NRTIs) mimic a DNA building block to inhibit the actions of reverse transcriptase, preventing the multiplication of the virus.
- Zidovudine or AZT (Retrovir) was one of the first drugs available specifically for treatment of HIV. (Even though you need to know what AZT means, do not use this abbreviation for this drug, it could lead to medication errors.)
- Non-nucleoside reverse transcriptase inhibitors (NNRTIs) inhibit the action of reverse transcriptase, preventing the formation of the DNA copy of viral RNA.
- Nucleotide reverse transcriptase inhibitors (NtRTIs) mimic a DNA building block to stop the formation of the DNA copy with less toxicity than with NRTIs.

- Protease inhibitors (PIs) inhibit the protease enzyme, which cleaves certain HIV protein precursors that are necessary for replication of the virus.
- Fusion inhibitors and chemokine coreceptors prevent HIV from entering the immune cells.
- An integrase inhibitor blocks the enzyme integrase, which inserts DNA produced by reverse transcriptase into the patient's DNA.
- The standard of care for HIV patients involves the combination of three or more antiretroviral drugs. Since these regimens are often complex and difficult to follow, compliance is an issue. None of the current drugs can eradicate the disease, but they can improve immunological status and prolong life. Some drug combinations should be avoided; didanosine with stavudine and zalcatabine, zidovudine with stavudine.
- More and more manufacturers are combining these drugs into one tablet in order to decrease the pill load and improve compliance. This is very important because partial compliance in these patients can lead to drug resistance.

Drug List

The following drugs were discussed in this chapter. Each generic drug name is followed in parentheses by one or more brand names. (Only two drugs in this list are among the top 200 selling drugs.)

Antifungals

amphotericin B (Abelcet, AmBisome, Amphocin, Amphotec, Fungizone)
anidulafungin (Eraxis)
butenafine (Mentax)
caspofungin (Cancidas)
clotrimazole (Mycelex)
fluconazole* (Diflucan)
flucytosine (Ancobon)
griseofulvin (Fulvicin P/G, Gris-PEG)
itraconazole (Sporanox)
ketoconazole (Nizoral)
micafungin (Mycamine)
nystatin (Mycostatin)
posaconazole (Noxafil)

terbinafine (Lamisil)
terconazole (Terazol)
voriconazole (VFEND)

Antivirals

Systemic Agents

acyclovir (Zovirax)*
amantadine (Symmetrel)
cidofovir (Vistide)
famciclovir (Famvir)
foscarnet (Foscavir)
ganciclovir (Cytovene)
oseltamivir (Tamiflu)
ribavirin (Copegus, Rebetol, Virazole)
rimantadine (Flumadine)

valacyclovir (Valtrex)*
valganciclovir (Valcyte)
zanamivir (Relenza)

Ocular Agent
ganciclovir (Vitrasert)

Antiretrovirals

NRTIs
abacavir (Ziagen)
didanosine (Videx)
emtricitabine (Emtriva)
lamivudine (Epivir)
stavudine (Zerit)
zidovudine, AZT (Retrovir)

NNRTIs
delavirdine (Rescriptor)
efavirenz (Sustiva)
nevirapine (Viramune)

NtRTIs
tenofovir (Viread)

PIs
amprenavir (Agenerase)
atazanavir (Reyataz)

darunavir (Prezista)
fosamprenavir (Lexiva)
indinavir (Crixivan)
nelfinavir (Viracept)
ritonavir (Norvir)
saquinavir (Fortovase, Invirase)
tipranavir (Aptivus)

Fusion Inhibitors
enfuvirtide (Fuzeon)

Chemokine Coreceptor
maraviroc (Selzentry)

Integrase Inhibitor
raltegravir (Isentress)

Combinations
abacavir and lamivudine (Epzicom)
abacavir, lamivudine and zidovudine
   (Trizivir)
efavirenz, emtricitabine, and tenofovir
   (Atripla)
emtricitabine and tenofovir (Truvada)
lamivudine and zidovudine (Combivir)
lopinavir and ritonavir (Kaletra)

Chapter Review

Pharmaceuticals and Body Functions

Select the best answer from the choices given.

1. Which listed drug is used as prophylaxis for influenza and also in treating Parkinson's disease?
   a. zidovudine
   b. rimantadine
   c. amantadine
   d. ganciclovir

2. Which listed drug requires the pharmacy technician to use chemotherapy agent precautions when mixing?
   a. Zovirax
   b. Cytovene
   c. Famvir
   d. Videx

3. Which listed drug is a lipid complex and less toxic than the older IV form of the drug?
   a. Zovirax
   b. Cytovene
   c. Abelcet
   d. Videx

4. Which listed drug should not be taken in combination with didanosine?
   a. stavudine
   b. ritonavir
   c. zidovudine
   d. indinavir

5. Which of the following drugs should be stored in its original container with a desiccant?
    a. saquinavir
    b. indinavir
    c. zanamivir
    d. oseltamivir

6. Which drug listed below must have a card dispensed with it?
    a. Epzicom
    b. Fortovase
    c. Atripla
    d. Retrovir

7. Which drug is the most used to boost another drug?
    a. Norvir (ritonavir)
    b. Selzentry (maraviroc)
    c. Viread (tenofovir)
    d. Fuzon (enfuvirtide)

8. Which two antifungals come in an IV dosage form?
    a. fluconazole and amphotericin B
    b. fluconazole and griseofulvin
    c. griseofulvin and amphotericin B
    d. clotrimazole and ketoconazole

9. Which antifungal is especially useful for treating fungal infection in the nails because of the shorter time span needed for treatment?
    a. Gris-PEG
    b. Sporanox
    c. Mycostatin
    d. Mycelex-7

10. Which vaginal antifungal requires a prescription?
    a. Monistat 3
    b. Gyne-Lotrimin
    c. Mycelex-7
    d. Terazol

The following statements are true or false. If an item is false, rewrite the question so it is true.

_____ 1. Gris-PEG is used for fungal infections of the hair, skin, and nails.

_____ 2. The patient taking Fulvicin P/G should be told to take the dose on an empty stomach and get plenty of sun.

_____ 3. The most common side effects of fluconazole (Diflucan) are headache, rash, and GI upset.

_____ 4. A virus cannot reproduce outside the cell.

_____ 5. Virus host cells can be animal, plant, or bacterial.

_____ 6. A virus cannot lie dormant and then under certain conditions reproduce and again behave like an infective agent.

_____ 7. The elderly, patients with cardiovascular or renal disease, and patients with diabetes or asthma are *not* at risk for influenza.

_____ 8. Acyclovir (Zovirax) is available in the following dosage forms: IV, oral, suppository, and topical.

_____ 9. Most antiviral and antifungal agents are very expensive.

_____ 10. The largest group of antiretrovirals is the PIs.

Diseases and Drug Therapies

1. Identify two classifications for a virus.

2. Explain why you would not mix amphotericin B with normal saline.

3. Explain how pulse dosing works.

4. What are the most common side effects of Nizoral?

5. Why is latency a problem with some viruses?

Dispensing Medications

1. You receive the following prescription. This is the only one given for this patient.

   Joe Brown
   Amphotericin B one (1) mg/kg over six (6) hr every other day. Mix in D_5W.

   a. If Mr. Brown weighs 150 pounds, how much will you mix?

   b. Give at least two reasons for calling the doctor.

2. You receive the following prescription:

   Joe Lee
   Foscarnet sixty (60) mg/kg IV over one (1) hr q8h for two (2) weeks.

   a. If Mr. Lee weighs 180 pounds, how much will you mix?

   b. This is the only prescription you receive. What has the doctor forgotten?

3. You receive the following prescription:

   Jim Tucker
   Dispense four (4) weeks' supply.
   lamivudine one hundred fifty
     (150) mg bid # ____
   zidovudine three hundred (300)
     mg bid # ____

   a. How many of each will you dispense?

   b. What might be the patient's diagnosis?

Internet Research

Use the Internet to complete the following assignments.

1. Create a table listing four to six drugs for HIV treatment; include their generic and brand names and their side effects. List your Web sources.

2. Find current HIV/AIDS statistics. How many individuals in the United States are HIV-positive? At what rate (individuals per year) is the virus spreading? Make sure to include the date and source of the information in your report. Do you think it is difficult to get an accurate figure? Why or why not? List your Internet sources.

What Would You Do?

1. The drug being dispensed to the patient is Kaletra. The other technician working with you does not want to wait on the patient for fear of contacting the disease. How will you respond to the technician and the patient?

Anesthetics and Narcotics

6

Learning Objectives

- Understand the central and peripheral nervous systems, their functions, and their relationship to drugs.
- Recognize different dosage forms and understand how the drug delivery system works.
- Learn how drugs affect body systems and where they work in the body.
- Understand the concepts of general and local anesthesia, and know the functions of these agents.
- Define the action of neuromuscular blocking agents in reducing muscle activity.

- Distinguish between narcotic and nonnarcotic analgesia.
- Understand the different classes of narcotics and the role of the technician in monitoring these drugs.
- Become familiar with the various types of agents for migraine headaches.

Preview chapter terms and definitions.

The nervous system coordinates the other body systems and is the body's link with the outside world. It works continuously to preserve homeostasis, keeping the other physiologic systems of the body in a normal state. The neurotransmitters, chemical messengers that are an integral part of this system, control the behavior of most drugs in the body. Their activity determines the reactions of anesthetics, analgesics (pain relievers), and narcotics as well as their interactions with each other and with the other body chemicals and systems. This chapter will concentrate on anesthesia agents and narcotic analgesics.

The Nervous System

The nervous system is responsible for transmitting information over a vast network throughout the body. The type of cells of which this network is made is a **neuron**, and the way it transmits information is by releasing a chemical substance known as a **neurotransmitter.** Neurotransmitters stimulate or inhibit activity in their target cells, especially other neurons. Neurons and neurotransmitters are important in the study of drugs and drug actions, and the relationships between them are illustrated in Figure 6.1.

The Central Nervous System

The **central nervous system (CNS)** consists of the brain and the spinal cord, the two organs that evaluate incoming information and determine responses. The CNS coordinates and controls the activity of other body systems as well. Sense organs throughout the body detect heat, cold, pain, and the presence of chemicals and convert that information into a chemical/electrical message. The message is transmitted to the spinal cord, the brain stem, and the cerebral cortex. As the impulses pass through the memory and emotional areas of the lower brain, they are compared with previous experiences on the basis of "like, dislike, or do not care." The thought process is based on a series of chemical reactions from the sense organs. The process involves the neurotransmitters released at each connection; some are stimulatory and others are inhibitory. When the balance between the two is disturbed, the person may experience any of a number of physical, mental, or emotional disorders. The primary CNS transmitters are acetylcholine, norepinephrine, dopamine, gamma-aminobutyric acid (GABA), glutamate and serotonin (also known as 5-hydroxytryptamine). Glutamate is the most common neurotransmitter in the brain and it is always excitatory.

The Peripheral Nervous System

The **peripheral nervous system (PNS)** consists of the **afferent system**, nerves and sense organs that bring information to the CNS, and the **efferent system**, nerves that dispatch information out from the CNS. The efferent system has two parts: the autonomic nervous system and the somatic nervous system. The primary PNS transmitters are acetylcholine and norepinephrine.

FIGURE 6.1   Neurotransmitters Being Released from a Neuron

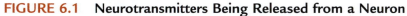
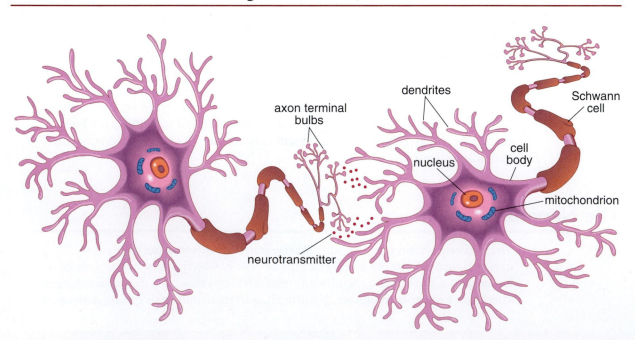

The Autonomic Nervous System The **autonomic nervous system (ANS)** regulates activities of structures that are not under voluntary control and thus are (usually) below the level of consciousness. The ANS controls respiration, circulation, digestion, body temperature, metabolism, blood glucose, pupil dilation, GI motility, sweating, and certain glandular functions. By making these unconscious adjustments, the ANS maintains internal balance. In the ANS, there are two neurons between the CNS and the muscle or glandular tissue it innervates. The ANS has two major components: the sympathetic nervous system and the parasympathetic nervous system as described in Figure 6.2. The major transmitters of the sympathetic system are acetylcholine, norepinephrine, dopamine, glutamate, and epinephrine. The only neurotransmitter of the parasympathetic system is acetylcholine.

The Somatic Nervous System The second part of the PNS, the **somatic nervous system**, is concerned with skeletal muscles, which perform voluntary actions. There is only one neuron between the CNS and the skeletal muscles. Acetylcholine is the only neurotransmitter.

Major Neurotransmitters

The major neurotransmitters have the following actions.

- Acetylcholine (ACh) acts on receptors in smooth muscle, cardiac muscle, and exocrine glands; anticholinergics block these receptors.
- GABA (gamma-aminobutyric acid), a major CNS neurotransmitter, acts on GABA receptors to regulate the message delivery system of the brain. GABA is present in many nerve endings in the brain.

FIGURE 6.2
The Autonomic Nervous System

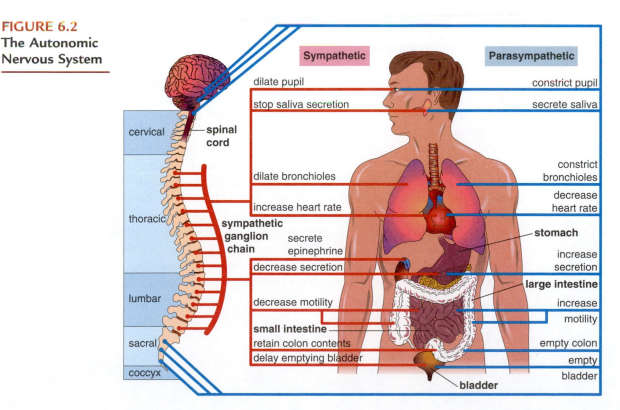

- Dopamine acts on receptors in the CNS and kidneys. Dopamine receptors are blocked by specific dopamine-blocking drugs.
- Epinephrine acts on cardiac receptors and bronchodilator adrenergic receptors. It is also referred to as adrenaline, the fight-or-flight chemical.
- Norepinephrine acts on alpha and beta receptors and is blocked by drugs classified as alpha- and beta-adrenergic blockers.
- Serotonin acts on receptors in smooth muscle and gastric mucosa. It produces vasoconstriction (constriction or drawing together of blood vessels, thus decreasing blood flow). Serotonin is a major CNS neurotransmitter implicated in emotional responses to certain stimuli and in conditions of depression and anxiety.
- Glutamate may be crucial to some forms of learning and memory.

Drug Effects on the Nervous System

Numerous drugs mimic or influence the action of chemical mediators that affect neurotransmitter release and reception. Transmitters bind to receptors, which in most instances are proteins within the cell membrane of the cell receiving the message. When a transmitter binds to a receptor, a molecular change occurs in the receptor compound, triggering further changes. For many receptors, neurotransmitter binding causes the cell membrane to be more permeable to various ions, which then directly affect the receptor cell either to create or suppress an electrical signal. Other receptors activate enzyme systems that promote chemical reactions within the cell.

The following important receptors all respond to the neurotransmitters epinephrine and norepinephrine, produced by the sympathetic nervous system. The primary function of the following receptors are:

- **Alpha receptors** constrict blood vessels (vasoconstriction, raising blood pressure), but they also cause decongestion.
- **Beta-1 receptors** (β_1) increase the heart rate and contractive force of the heart.
- **Beta-2 receptors** (β_2) influence bronchodilation.

The most important actions of the beta-adrenergic receptors are bronchodilation and heart stimulation. Notice that alpha and beta-2 receptors have opposite effects on blood vessels. Which effect occurs depends on the concentration of epinephrine. Beta-2 receptors widen the vessels in response to moderate levels, while higher levels of transmitter stimulate the alpha receptors to narrow the vessels.

Drugs may act by blocking receptors, thereby preventing the transmitters from binding to them. For example, anticholinergic drugs block the acetylcholine receptors, and the physiologic result is just the opposite of that produced by ACh. In the cardiovascular system, ACh reduces heart rate and contraction and lowers arterial pressure through vasodilation. In the smooth muscles, ACh increases motility (the ability to move spontaneously) in the gastrointestinal and urogenital systems, bronchial constriction in the respiratory system, and pupil constriction (miosis) of the eyes. In the glands, it increases secretions.

The anticholinergic drugs can have important side effects in certain groups of patients. Some reactions to watch for include

- decreased GI motility (constipation)
- decreased sweating

- decreased urination (urinary retention)
- dilated pupil (mydriasis) and blurred vision
- dry eyes
- dry mouth

Anesthesia

Before 1846, surgical procedures were uncommon. Practitioners had only a simplistic understanding of the pathophysiology of disease and its surgical treatment. Aseptic technique and prevention of wound infection were almost unknown. The lack of satisfactory anesthesia was also a major deterrent to surgery. Typically, an operation was done only in emergency situations (e.g., amputating a limb).

Some pain relief methods were available. Drugs like alcohol, hashish, and opium derivatives were taken by mouth. Physical methods were sometimes used, such as packing the limb in ice or inducing ischemia (deficiency of blood) with a tourniquet before amputation. Unconsciousness was achieved by a blow to the head or strangulation. Most commonly, though, the patient was simply restrained by force. No wonder surgery was a last resort!

Drugs that enable painless and controlled surgical, obstetric, and diagnostic procedures form the cornerstone of modern pharmacologic therapy. These drugs, known as anesthetics, are classified as general or local, according to the type of anesthesia they induce. They are provided in a variety of dosage forms and strengths. The hallmark of anesthetic drugs is controllability. For this reason, most potent anesthetics are gases or vapors, which can be quickly introduced into the patient's air supply and quickly removed. One anesthetic may be superior to another, depending on the clinical circumstances. Final selection is based on the drugs and anesthetic techniques judged safest for the patient. A physician who oversees administration of anesthesia during surgery is known as an **anesthesiologist**.

The physiologic effects of anesthesia involve many systems.

- **Nervous System** All nerve tissue function in the peripheral system is depressed.
- **Respiratory System** Function is depressed, and the anesthesiologist controls oxygen concentration and ventilation (exchange of air between the lungs and the ambient air). Inhalant anesthetics, which are drawn into the lungs, generally irritate the respiratory tract and salivary glands, causing increased mucus secretion, coughing, and spasm.
- **Endocrine System** Some anesthetics cause pituitary secretion of antidiuretic hormone (ADH), which may cause postoperative urinary retention. The adrenal medulla may release epinephrine and norepinephrine, which can counter depression caused by inhibited nerves.
- **Cardiovascular System** The activity of cardiac muscle in the myocardium is reduced, and the resultant loss of tone reduces blood pressure. Vagus nerve inhibition increases the heart rate. Some drugs make the heart sensitive, which may cause arrhythmias (variations from the normal rhythm of the heart).
- **Skeletal Muscular System** Anesthesia depresses systems within the brain and spinal reflexes, causing some muscle relaxation.
- **GI System** Common GI effects are nausea and vomiting.
- **Hepatic System** Some medications are suspected of causing liver changes.

The goals of balanced anesthesia are

- amnesia—to eliminate the patient's memory of the procedure
- adequate muscle relaxation—to keep the patient still and the patient's muscles from contracting
- adequate ventilation—to maintain adequate oxygen concentration
- pain control—to eliminate or greatly reduce the patient's pain

General Anesthetics

General anesthesia is the unique condition of reversible unconsciousness and absence of response to otherwise painful stimuli. It is characterized by four reversible actions:

- unconsciousness (unawareness)
- analgesia (relieving pain)
- skeletal muscle relaxation
- amnesia on recovery

The indicators used to assess the degree of general anesthesia are

- blood pressure
- hypervolemia (abnormal increase in the volume of circulating fluid, i.e., plasma, in the body) and hypovolemia (abnormal decrease in the plasma volume)
- oxygen level
- pulse
- respiratory rate
- tissue perfusion (the passage of a fluid through the vessels of a specific organ)
- urinary output (reduction in urine volume sends more blood to the brain)

General anesthetics are administered in several different ways, and several factors must be considered before, during, and after their administration. Some of these considerations are briefly discussed in this section.

Preanesthetic Medications Medication is sometimes used preoperatively to help control the effects of anesthesia. The purpose is to control sedation, reduce postoperative pain, provide amnesia, and decrease anxiety. Review of the individual patient's medication history is important in determining which anesthetic to use.

Several classes of drugs offer agents to be used before anesthesia.

- Narcotics alleviate pain and depress the respiratory center. (As will be explained later in this chapter, morphine is the most important narcotic analgesic. It is the standard against which all others are measured.)
- Drugs such as benzodiazepines are the most used preoperative sedatives. They can cause amnesia, which is a desirable quality in a drug when anesthetizing a patient. They relieve anxiety as well as act as an anticonvulsant. Phenothiazines are often prescribed for their antiemetic properties as well as their sedative effects.

Malignant Hyperthermia **Malignant hyperthermia** is a rare, but serious, side effect of anesthesia associated with a marked increase in intracellular calcium levels. This syndrome, which involves a sudden and rapid rise in body temperature with accompanying irregularities in heart rhythms and breathing, must be treated immediately. Other symptoms include a greatly increased body metabolism, muscle rigidity (inflexibility or stiffness), and fever of 110 °F or more. Malignant hyperthermia is potentially life-threatening. Death may result from cardiac arrest, brain damage, internal hemorrhaging, or failure of other body systems. This syndrome must be identified and treated early for a good outcome.

Treatment involves the intravenous (IV) infusion of the drug **dantrolene (Dantrium)**. It is a skeletal muscle relaxant used to treat multiple sclerosis (MS), stroke, cerebral palsy, and spinal cord injury and will be discussed in Chapter 13. Dantrolene is thought to reduce muscle tone and metabolism by either preventing the ongoing release of calcium from the storage sites in the muscle or by enhancing the reuptake of calcium. All hospitals require that a drug kit for the treatment of malignant hyperthermia be immediately accessible wherever anesthesia is administered.

It is usually the responsibility of the pharmacy technician to maintain these malignant hyperthermia kits and to make sure that the drugs are always in date.

Dantrolene, in particular, has a very short shelf life and must be replenished frequently. A malignant hyperthermia kit generally contains the following components.

- dantrolene
- sterile water
- procainamide
- furosemide
- glucose
- sodium bicarbonate, 7.5%

Inhalant Anesthetics All inhalant anesthetics reduce blood pressure. Fluids are often given before surgery to help counter this drop in blood pressure. These agents also make the patient hypervolemic. The respiratory system excretes 80% to 90% of inhalant anesthetics. A reduction in renal function, caused by a decreased renal blood flow with reduced glomerular filtration, is common after anesthesia. Nausea and vomiting may also occur. Table 6.1 lists the most commonly used inhalant anesthetics. These anesthetics are stored under high pressure and are provided by the manufacturer in steel cylinders. Though informally referred to as "compressed gas," some of these chemicals are actually in liquid form in the cylinders, but they transform into a gas when released.

Nitrous oxide is not a potent anesthetic, and it usually is used with other agents. It will reduce blood pressure. Activity includes analgesia only, with no amnesia or skeletal muscle relaxation. It may be used alone, as in dental procedures, which is the most common use of this drug. It has the tremendous advantage of being rapidly eliminated; its disadvantage is that it may cause hypoxia, or a reduction in the oxygen supplied to a tissue, despite adequate perfusion by blood. In balanced anesthesia, it is supplemented with hypnotics (barbiturates or benzodiazepines), analgesics (intravenous narcotics), and muscle relaxants. It is administered with more powerful anesthetics, such as halothane, to hasten the uptake of the more powerful agent.

Enflurane (Ethrane) has the advantages of rapid induction and recovery. A short-acting barbiturate is usually infused first to render the patient unconscious. Enflurane is a mild stimulant of bronchial and salivary secretions. The disadvantages are excessive depression of the respiratory and circulatory systems. High concentrations may stimulate seizures in susceptible patients, and

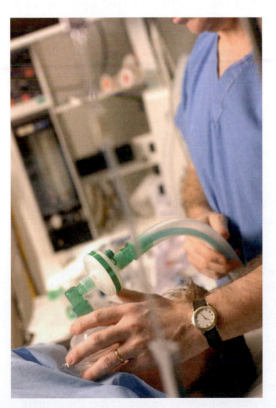

Anesthesiologist applying inhalant anesthetics during surgery.

TABLE 6.1   Most Commonly Used Inhalant Anesthetics

Generic Name	Pronunciation	Dosage Form	Brand Name	Dispensing Status
desflurane	des-FLOO-rayn	gas	Suprane	Rx
enflurane	EN-floo-rayn	gas	Ethrane	Rx
halothane	HA-loe-thayn	gas	(none)	Rx
isoflurane	eye-soe-FLOO-rayn	gas	Forane	Rx
nitrous oxide (N_2O)	NYE-trus OX-ide	gas	(none)	Rx

malignant hyperthermia is a possibility. It causes uterine relaxation, which prohibits its use during labor.

Isoflurane (Forane) produces rapid induction and recovery, with no excessive tracheal or salivary secretions. The disadvantages are progressive respiratory and blood pressure depression, with possible malignant hyperthermia. It may cause less renal and hepatic toxicity than any other commonly employed anesthetic.

Desflurane (Suprane) is an easily controllable anesthetic with rapid onset and rapid recovery. It is often used in ambulatory surgery. It reduces the required dose of neuromuscular blocking agents. It produces a high incidence of moderate to severe upper respiratory irritation for children and is therefore not recommended for use in the pediatric population for induction of anesthesia. It can be used for maintenance.

Sevoflurane (Ultane) is an ether (gas) used for induction and maintenance of general anesthesia. It is usually used with desflurane. It is the preferred agent for mask induction due to its lesser irritation to mucous membranes.

Injectable Anesthetics   The injectable anesthetics include the ultrashort-acting barbiturates and benzodiazepines. The IV products are very lipid soluble. They are distributed initially to the brain, liver (where they are metabolized), kidneys, and other organs with high-volume blood flow and later to fat and muscle. Body distribution lowers concentrations that maintain anesthesia. Most of the injectable anesthetics are administered by an IV drip, but some do have other dosage forms. Table 6.2 lists the most commonly used injectable anesthesia agents. Note that some of these agents can be administered in ways other than by injection. Almost all of the injectible anesthetics are controlled substances.

Etomidate (Amidate) is used to supplement a weak anesthetic (e.g., nitrous oxide) or for short procedures such as gynecologic ones (e.g., dilation and curettage). It may cause transient involuntary muscle contractions. Nausea and vomiting are common during the recovery period.

Fentanyl (Sublimaze) can be used as a preoperative medication and a narcotic-analgesic. It is used extensively for open-heart surgery procedures because it lacks some of the cardiac depressant (diminishing heart function) actions of other anesthetics. It is used as a supplement in balanced anesthesia. The lozenge, which is raspberry flavored, is used extensively with children and is often used as a preoperative medication for a child. The IV form of this drug is used most often in the operating room. The potency of Fentanyl is much greater than that of morphine. It has several analogs that are used exclusively in the operating room. **Alfentanil (Alfenta)** is an ultrashort-acting (5–10 minutes) analgesic. **Sufentanil (Sufenta)** is five to ten times more potent than fentanyl. **Remifentanil (Ultiva)** is the shortest-acting opioid. It has the benefit of rapid offset, even after prolonged infusions during surgeries. Anesthesiologists like

Warning

Diprivan and Diflucan might be confused. This could be life-threatening if an ICU patient who needs Diflucan for an infection receives Diprivan instead.

TABLE 6.2   Most Commonly Used Injectable Anesthesia Agents

Generic Name	Pronunciation	Dosage Form	Brand Name	Dispensing Status	Control Schedule
alfentanil	al-FEN-ta-nil	IV	Alfenta	Rx	C-II
etomidate	e-TOM-i-date	IV	Amidate	Rx	NA
fentanyl	FEN-ta-nil	IV	Sublimaze	Rx	C-II
fentanyl-droperidol	FEN-ta-nil droe-PER-i-dole	injection	(none)	Rx	C-II
ketamine	KEET-a-meen	injection, IV	Ketalar	Rx	C-III
morphine	MOR-feen	injection, IV	(various)	Rx	C-II
propofol	PROE-po-fole	IV	Diprivan	Rx	NA
remifentanyl	rem-i-FEN-a-nil	IV	Ultiva	Rx	C-II
sufentanil	soo-FEN-ta-nil	IV	Sufenta	Rx	C-II
Barbiturates					
methohexital	meth-oh-HEX-i-tal	IV	Brevital	Rx	C-IV
thiopental	thye-oh-PEN-tal	IV	Pentothal	Rx	C-III
Benzodiazepines					
diazepam	dye-AZ-e-pam	injection, IV, oral liquid, tablet	Valium	Rx	C-IV
lorazepam	lor-AZ-e-pam	injection, IV, tablet	Ativan	Rx	C-IV
midazolam	mid-AZ-oe-lam	injection, IV, syrup	Versed	Rx	C-IV

the fact that patients regain consciousness quickly. Fentanyl is frequently administered intrathecally as part of spinal anesthesia.

Ketamine (Ketalar) produces a sort of anesthesia known as dissociative amnesia, in which the patient appears to be awake but neither responds to pain nor remembers the procedure. This agent enhances muscle tone and increases blood pressure, heart rate, and respiratory secretions. Onset is quick (within 30 seconds), and effects last five to ten minutes.

Propofol (Diprivan) is used for maintenance of anesthesia, sedation, or treatment of agitation of patients in the intensive care unit. It has demonstrated antiemetic properties. The side effects are drowsiness, respiratory depression, motor restlessness, and increased blood pressure. Propofol changes urine color to green, pink, or rust. Any unused drug must be discarded after 12 hours. Propofol should be administered by slow infusion and mixed only with 5% dextrose. It is a white emulsion, stable in glass containers, and should be stored at room temperature. Because propofol is the only white emulsion in use in anesthesia, some healthcare workers think it does not need to be labeled, which is incorrect. When drawn up, propofol must be labeled immediately.

The barbiturates **thiopental (Pentothal)** and **methohexital (Brevital)** are used primarily for induction in short procedures. Respiratory depression, yawning, coughing, or laryngospasm may occur. In the patients that are awake, these agents may cause excitement or delirium in the presence of pain. Methohexital is the shorter-acting of the two. Both agents can be used to induce anesthesia prior to administration of another agent or alone for short procedures. The big advantages of the barbiturates are rapid induction, fast recovery, and little postanesthetic excitement or vomiting.

The benzodiazepines, **diazepam (Valium)**, **lorazepam (Ativan)**, and **midazolam (Versed)**, are used for induction, short procedures, and dental procedures. They are metabolized to active products, so they work longer than the barbiturates. Midazolam has the fastest onset of action, greatest potency, and most rapid elimination and is thus the preferred agent. It obliterates any memory of what has occurred during the procedure, even though the patient can carry on a conversation during the procedure. Some of these conversations can be quite interesting. Benzodiazepines are also useful for controlling and preventing seizures induced by local anesthetics.

Antagonists Antagonists (listed in Table 6.3) are used to reverse benzodiazepine and narcotic overdoses, whether administered during surgery or under some other condition. All operating rooms and emergency rooms maintain an adequate, quickly accessible supply of these drugs. Wherever narcotics are used, a supply of antagonists must be available.

Flumazenil (Romazicon) antagonizes benzodiazepines by competing at receptor sites. It blocks sedation, recall, and psychomotor impairment. It is used for complete or partial reversal of sedative effects of the benzodiazepines used as general anesthesia or to reverse the effects of a benzodiazepine overdose. Adverse reactions are headache, nausea, vomiting, dizziness, and agitation.

Naloxone (Narcan) is an antagonist that competes for the opiate receptor sites. Although this drug has a greater affinity for the receptor, its action is much shorter than that of the competing narcotic. Thus, when the naloxone wears off, the opioid will reattach to the receptor. Consequently, naloxone must be given repeatedly until the opioid is cleared from the patient's system. Naloxone must be stored in a dark compartment.

Nalmefene (Revex) partially or completely reverses the effects of opiate, including respiratory depression. The half-life is about 10 hours compared with 1 hour for Narcan. (The half-life of heroin and morphine is approximately 2 hours, whereas that of meperidine is approximately 4 hours.)

Neuromuscular Blocking Agents

Muscle movements during surgery can be very dangerous for the patient. **Neuromuscular blocking** agents paralyze the patient's skeletal muscles, which enables a surgeon to operate with greater accuracy and safety. Neuromuscular blocking is often used as an adjunct to general anesthesia to enable **endotracheal intubation**, or the insertion of a tube into the trachea to maintain an open airway and deliver general anesthesia directly to the lung. The administration of neuromuscular blocking agents results in immediate skeletal muscle paralysis. When stocking neuromuscular blocking agents, the technician should always flag this type of drug with a sticker to alert everyone explicitly that the drug will paralyze whoever receives it.

TABLE 6.3	Most Commonly Used Antagonists to Reverse Overdoses			
Generic Name	Pronunciation	Dosage Form	Brand Name	Dispensing Status
flumazenil	floo-MAZ-eh-nil	injection	Romazicon	Rx
nalmefene	NAL-me-feen	injection	Revex	Rx
naloxone	nal-OX-one	injection	Narcan	Rx

Every effort should be made to make sure these agents are not stored close to a look-alike drug. Neuromuscular blocking agents are some of the most dangerous drugs.

Table 6.4 gives an overview of the most commonly used neuromuscular blocking agents. As noted in the table, many of these agents must be stored in a refrigerator.

There are two mechanisms for achieving neuromuscular blockade. **Succinylcholine (Quelicin)**, often referred to as "sux," is the only agent that works via a depolarizing (neutralizing) mechanism. All other neuromuscular blocking agents are considered to be nondepolarizing agents. Succinylcholine works as an agonist of the nicotinic cholinergic receptors. These receptors briefly allow ions to pass through when acetylcholine binds to them, producing a pulse of electrical current that causes the muscle to contract. Succinylcholine holds the ion channels open, causing a persistent depolarization at the motor endplate—that is, it shorts out the electrical signal. The result is a sustained brief period of flaccid (weak, lax, and soft) skeletal muscle paralysis. Bradyarrhythmias (irregular and slow heartbeats) may occur; if they do, they are reversed with atropine.

The nonpolarizing agents work as competitive antagonists to acetylcholine at the nicotinic cholinergic receptors; that is, they prevent acetylcholine from binding to the receptors to start the electrical signal, but the signal is not shorted out. Many of them have the syllable "cur" in their names, indicating that they act like curare, a South American arrow poison.

Agents to Reverse Neuromuscular Blocking Agents

To reverse the effects of a nondepolarizing blocking drug requires the administration of one of several **anticholinesterase** agents, including neostigmine (Prostigmin), edrophonium (Enlon), and pyridostigmine (Mestinon). These drugs potentiate the action of acetylcholine by inhibiting its destruction by the enzyme acetylcholinesterase and thereby restore the transmission of impulses across the neuromuscular junctions. Many of the anticholinesterase agents are also used in the treatment of myasthenia gravis.

Table 6.5 gives an overview of the pharmacologic agents most commonly used to reverse neuromuscular blockers.

TABLE 6.4   Most Commonly Used Neuromuscular Blocking Agents

Generic Name	Pronunciation	Dosage Form	Storage	Brand Name	Dispensing Status
Short Duration					
succinylcholine	sux-in-il-KOE-leen	injection, IV	refrigerate	Quelicin	Rx
Intermediate Duration					
atracurium	a-tra-KYOO-ree-um	IV	refrigerate	Tracrium	Rx
cisatracurium	sis-a-tra-KYOO-ree-um	IV	refrigerate	Nimbex	Rx
rocuronium	roe-kyoor-OH-nee-um	IV	refrigerate	Zemuron	Rx
vecuronium	ve-kyoo-ROE-nee-um	IV	room temperature	Norcuron	Rx
Extended Duration					
mivacurium	mye-va-KYOO-ree-um	IV	room temperature	Mivacron	Rx
pancuronium	pan-kyoo-ROE-nee-um	IV	refrigerate	(none)	Rx

Local Anesthetics

Local anesthesia produces a transient and reversible loss of sensation in a defined area of the body. It relieves pain without altering alertness or mental function. The introduction of cocaine as a topical ophthalmologic anesthetic in 1884 opened the first era of local anesthesia, and cocaine is still used today for procedures on the eye and nasal passages. The second era began in 1904 with the introduction of procaine, the first local anesthetic suitable for injection. Lidocaine, introduced in the 1940s, is the most widely used local anesthetic. Local anesthetics, especially topical agents, are commonly combined with other drugs, so a variety of combinations are currently available on the market.

Local anesthetics are available in a variety of dosage forms for use in a range of conditions. These dosage forms and applications are

- topical (drops, sprays, lotions, ointments)—to treat sunburn, insect bites, hemorrhoids
- infiltration (superficial injection)—to suture (stitch) cuts, perform dental procedures, and block small nerves
- nerve block (injection)—to prevent transmission of the pain impulse
- IV—for reasons other than anesthesia
- epidural (injection into the space outside the dura mater membrane of the vertebral canal)—to block afferent pain nerve impulses to provide regional anesthesia
- spinal (subarachnoid or intrathecal injection into the innermost space of the spinal cord)—to block afferent pain nerve impulses from the lower part of the body

Local anesthetics decrease the neuronal membrane's permeability to sodium ions. This results in inhibition of depolarization with resultant blockade of conduction.

Local anesthesia is advantageous because all types of nervous tissue are affected—sensory and motor. The action is reversible, with recovery and no residual nerve damage. Nerve fibers (cells) determine the degree and speed with which a local anesthetic acts. In response to the activity of the anesthetic, function is lost in the following order.

1. pain perception
2. temperature sensation
3. touch sensation
4. proprioception (recognition of body position/posture and joint positions)
5. skeletal muscle tone

Local anesthetics depress the small, unmyelinated fibers first and the larger, myelinated fibers (fibers surrounded by a myelin sheath of Schwann cells) last. The time of onset of action is shorter for smaller fibers, and the concentration of drug required is smaller. Systemic action depends on the time the drug is in contact with nerve tissue. Inflammation reduces tissue pH, thereby reducing drug activity. Vasodilation caused

TABLE 6.5	Most Commonly Used Anticholinesterase Agents to Reverse Neuromuscular Blocking			
Generic Name	Pronunciation	Dosage Form	Brand Name	Dispensing Status
edrophonium	ed-roe-FOE-nee-um	IV	Enlon	Rx
neostigmine	nee-oh-STIG-meen	IV	Prostigmin	Rx
pyridostigmine	peer-id-oh-STIG-meen	IV, syrup, tablet	Mestinon	Rx

by the agent itself affects the duration of action. Many local anesthetics cause vasodilation, resulting in the drug being absorbed more rapidly into the bloodstream and diluted. Addition of a vasoconstrictor (epinephrine), even at a concentration of 5 parts per million, slows absorption of a drug into the bloodstream. Dentists commonly employ epinephrine to keep the local anesthetic drug at the injection site so that numbness will last longer. Epinephrine should *not* be used as a vasoconstrictor in areas of fingers, toes, ears, nose, or external genitals, because cutting blood flow at these extremities may result in ischemia and subsequent gangrene. Alkalization enhances drug penetration and onset of activity.

Local anesthetics are classified by their chemistry into two classes: esters and amides. An **ester** contains a –COO– group, which is relatively easily broken down, so ester local anesthetics are short-acting and are metabolized mainly by pseudocholinesterase of the plasma and tissue fluids. An **amide** contains a –CONH– group, which is more difficult to break down, so amide local anesthetics are longer-acting and are metabolized by liver enzymes. Metabolites of both classes are excreted in urine. Table 6.6 lists the most commonly used local anesthetics in these two classes.

Local anesthetics are given to produce a pharmacologic response in a well-defined area of the body. Occasionally, the anesthetic is absorbed into the blood from the

TABLE 6.6   Most Commonly Used Local Anesthetics

Generic Name	Pronunciation	Dosage Form	Brand Name	Dispensing Status
Esters				
benzocaine	BEN-zoe-kayn	cream, ear drops, gel, lozenge, ointment, oral liquid, oral paste, spray	Americaine	OTC
chloroprocaine	klor-oh-PROE-kayn	epidural	Nesacaine	Rx
dyclonine	DYE-kloe-neen	liquid	Cepacol Maximum Strength	OTC
procaine	PROE-kayn	injection, IV	Novocain	Rx
tetracaine	TET-ra-kayn	gel, injection, ointment, oral liquid	Cepacol Viractin	OTC
		IV	Pontocaine	Rx
Amides				
bupivacaine	byoo-PIV-a-kayn	injection	Marcaine	Rx
levobupivacaine	lee-voe-byoo-PIV-a-kayn	injection, IV	Chirocaine	Rx
lidocaine	LYE-doe-kayn	cream, gel, injection, oral, patch solution, topical	L-M-X, Solarcaine Aloe Extra Burn Relief	OTC
		IV	Xylocaine, Lidoderm	Rx
lidocaine-epinephrine	LYE-doe-kayn ep-i-NEF-rin	injection	Xylocaine with Epinephrine	Rx
lidocaine-prilocaine	LYE-doe-kayn PRIL-oh-kayn	cream	EMLA	Rx
mepivacaine	me-PIV-a-kayn	injection, IV, single- and multi-dose vial	Carbocaine	Rx

administration site. It can then affect organs along the way, with the most serious effects on the blood vessels, heart, and brain.

All local anesthetics, except cocaine (which is used for eye and nose surgery), cause relaxation of vascular smooth muscles and can lead to vascular collapse. Hypersensitivity or an allergy to a particular local agent can cause histamine release at the injection site. The most common reactions to the ester class of local anesthetics are skin rashes, edema (an abnormal accumulation of fluid in intercellular spaces of the body), and asthma. This hypersensitivity usually develops when the agent is used frequently or for prolonged periods. An amide can generally be substituted for an ester to avoid these hypersensitivity reactions.

Lidocaine (Lidoderm) can also be administered as a patch, an adhesive strip that should be placed directly onto dry, clean skin at the site of pain. The patch should be applied only to intact skin and may be cut with scissors to fit a smaller area. As many as three patches may be applied in one area if the patch is too small to cover the painful area. The patch is worn for 12 hours and then removed for 12 hours. Hands should be washed immediately after applying the patch. A patch is especially useful for shingles.

Pain Management

Pain is the activation of electrical activity in afferent neurons with sensory endings in peripheral tissue that have a higher firing threshold than those of temperature or touch. These neurons are activated by stimulation sufficient to cause tissue damage. Pain is primarily a protective signal to warn of damage or the presence of disease. It is also part of the normal healing process. This process involves inflammation, in which protective cells move into the injured area and release chemical mediators that cause fluids and plasma proteins to leak into the surrounding tissue. The result is repair and healing, but also stimulation of pain nerve endings. Pain perception arises from the transmission of nerve impulses.

The challenges in pain management are to assess the patient properly and to select the most successful and cost-effective therapy for the patient and the patient's family. Goals of management include enhancing functionality and productivity to improve the patient's quality of life. It has been shown that pain is often under-treated, and this deficiency can in some cases delay recovery from the condition causing the pain. To achieve adequate pain control, pain medication must sometimes be administered around the clock.

In January 2001, the Joint Commission on the Accreditation of Healthcare Organizations (JCAHO) issued its pain management standards, which are used to evaluate the performance of healthcare providers. The new standards emphasize the right of patients to receive appropriate pain management and education. The standards define pain as the "fifth" vital sign, along with temperature, pulse, respiration, and blood pressure. Healthcare providers must make regular pain intensity assessments. Inadequate pain control can increase the need for opioids.

Pain is classified as acute, chronic nonmalignant, and chronic malignant.

- **Acute** This type of pain is associated with trauma or surgery. Acute pain is usually easier to manage by identifying and treating the cause, and it disappears when the body heals.
- **Chronic Nonmalignant** This type of pain may have a diagnosed or an undiagnosed cause, such as a nonmalignant disease. The pain lasts for more than three months and may respond poorly to treatment. Chronic nonmalignant pain

may have signs and symptoms of depression in patients with a high tolerance of pain. The neurotransmitters involved in pain transmission are the same as those involved with depression (norepinephrine, dopamine, serotonin). Chronic pain syndrome is a form of this type of pain. In this syndrome, pain lasts longer than three months, may or may not have an identifiable physical or chemical basis, creates an overwhelming lifestyle burden for the patient, and does not respond to medication.

- **Chronic Malignant** This type of pain accompanies malignant disease and often increases in severity as the disease progresses.

Acute and chronic pain differ in one important way. Whereas acute pain has a beginning and an end and warns of a problem, chronic pain does not cease when an illness or injury is cured or healed. With chronic pain the suffering includes a sense of helplessness and hopelessness. Total pain has physical, psychological, social, and spiritual components. Adequate sleep, mood elevation, diversion, sympathy, and understanding all can raise an individual's pain threshold. Alternatively, fatigue, anxiety, fear, anger, sadness, depression, and isolation can lower the pain threshold. Uncontrolled pain is a potent factor in lowering the pain threshold.

Physiologic responses to pain are as varied as the patients themselves. These responses include

- catabolism (tissues, such as muscle, break down)
- delayed stomach and bowel function
- impaired immune response
- increased autonomic activity (heart rate and blood pressure)
- increased metabolism
- muscle rigidity
- negative emotional response (depression)
- shallow breathing
- water retention

Inadequate treatment of pain can have adverse physiological, psychological, and immunological effects. Good clinical care must be based on the optimization of risk/benefit considerations. The major sources of pain, its characteristics, and their treatment are listed in Table 6.7.

Sympathetically mediated pain occurs from oversensitivity to a pain stimulus; that is, pain occurs when no pain should be felt. Nerve damage usually occurs as a result of

TABLE 6.7 Major Sources of Pain

Source	Areas Involved	Characteristics	Treatment
somatic	body framework (bones, muscles, ligaments)	throbbing, stabbing, well localized	narcotics, NSAIDs, nerve blockers
visceral	kidneys, intestines, liver	aching, throbbing, sharp, gnawing, crampy, deep squeezing; associated with sweating, nausea, vomiting	narcotics, NSAIDs, nerve blockers, antiemetics
neuropathic	nerves (destruction)	burning, aching, numbing, tingling, viselike, knifelike, constant	antidepressants, anticonvulsants
sympathetically mediated	overactivity in sympathetic system	occurring when no pain should be felt	nerve blockers

trauma to the area. Hair, nail, and skin changes result (e.g., color, overgrowth of hair); swelling and changes in skin temperature are common.

Narcotics

A **narcotic** is a pain-modulating chemical that tends to cause insensibility or stupor, such as morphine or codeine. Generally, a narcotic is an **opiate**: a substance that either is derived from opium (juice from the unripe seed capsule of the opium poppy, *Papaver somniferum*) or chemically resembles the opium derivatives.

Opiates work because they are agonists of **opioid** receptor sites having their main effects on the CNS, GI tract, and, to a lesser extent, peripheral tissues. The body (specifically, the brain) produces three distinct types of natural opioids—endorphins, enkephalins, and dynorphins—in response to pain stimuli. As pain increases, the levels of these chemicals also increase. When opioid receptors are activated, nerve transmission to CNS centers for pain processing is decreased, so the sensation of pain is diminished. Narcotics bind to the same receptors as these natural substances, causing activation. The pain receptors in the CNS are in the limbic system, thalamus, hypothalamus, midbrain, and spinal cord. Additional receptors are found in the adrenal medulla and nerve plexus. The primary opioid receptors associated with analgesia are denoted as mu, delta, and kappa.

Narcotics have the following effects.

- **Analgesia** Narcotics reduce pain from most sources (organs, trauma, myocardial infarction, terminal illness, and surgical wounds). Some pain is unresponsive to opiates.
- **Sedation** Narcotics allay anxiety and cause drowsiness.
- **Euphoria and Dysphoria** Narcotics produce feelings of well-being or feelings of disquiet, restlessness, or malaise, respectively. In addition, all narcotics have the potential to induce tolerance and dependence.

Narcotics also reduce the cough reflex and respiratory drive; increase mental clouding; and can cause nausea, vomiting, and constipation.

Patients can develop tolerance to pain therapy within days or weeks. As a result, dosages may need to be titrated every day or two. A good rule of thumb is to increase the current dose by 50% when needed, based on evaluation of pain control. After long-term treatment and disease regression, dosage may often be reduced without signs of withdrawal or recurrence of pain. Patients in pain have activated endorphin systems and are pharmacologically, physiologically, and biochemically different from drug abusers. Patients with medical reasons for their pain who are treated with appropriate opiates rarely become addicted.

Although opioids frequently impair judgment and psychomotor function for a period following the onset or acceleration of therapy, after a few days these adverse effects usually diminish markedly.

Opioids are associated with a high incidence of constipation. Thus, an opioid regimen often requires a clinically prescribed bowel program, such as stimulant laxatives, to produce an adequate

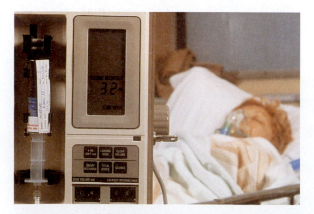

A patient-controlled analgesia pump can allow the patient to regulate the amount of pain medication she receives. This results in better pain control with less drug used.

response if constipation develops. Nausea is also a side effect of narcotics. An anti-emetic (nausea drug) should be available to these patients.

An effective means of controlling pain in hospitalized patients is the **patient-controlled analgesia (PCA) pump**. The patient regulates, within certain limits, the amount of drug received by pushing a button controlled only by the patient. Better pain control can be achieved with lower doses when patients administer the drug on pain onset. Once pain has been ongoing for a long time, it is much more difficult to control. Another remarkable development in pain control is the transdermal patch. By providing stable blood levels of drug, the patch seems to control pain more effectively than other forms of delivery while allowing the patient to remain more alert.

Persistent pain should be treated in a stepwise fashion: first acetaminophen, then **nonsteroidal anti-inflammatory drugs** (**NSAIDs**), and then the opioids. A simple scheme for analgesic selection is known as the **analgesic ladder**, which is illustrated in Figure 6.3.

FIGURE 6.3   Analgesic Ladder

The World Health Organization analgesic ladder for pain relief. Source: World Health Organization

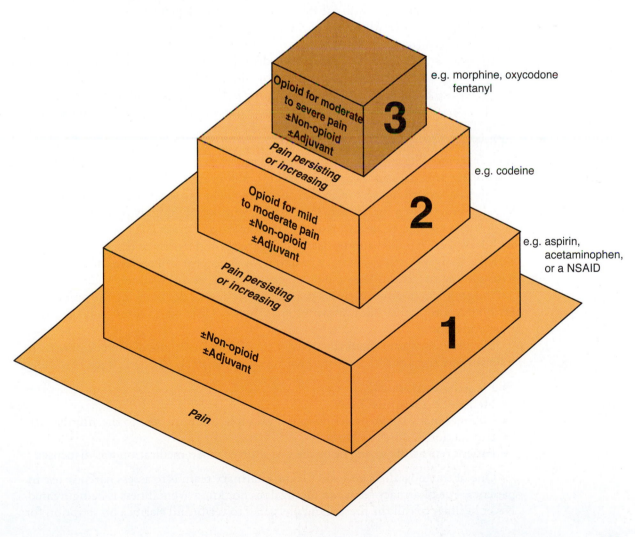

1. Mild-to-moderate pain is treated with acetaminophen or an NSAID (prototype: aspirin) and an adjuvant (enhancement) analgesic.
2. If adequate relief is not achieved, a nonnarcotic analgesic (e.g., an NSAID) is given with a "weak" opioid (prototype: codeine).
3. If this fails, the patient is given a strong opioid (prototype: morphine), with an adjuvant analgesic if indicated.

Symptoms of narcotic overdose are respiratory depression, decreased body temperature, decreased blood pressure, tachycardia (abnormally rapid heart rate), and coma. The treatment is assisted ventilation and a narcotic antagonist.

Addiction and Dependence

Underprescribing of opioids for nonmalignant pain is not uncommon because these are controlled substances that may cause addiction, and physicians are concerned with regulatory authorities as well as the risk that the patient may become addicted. Now, however, healthcare providers are increasingly aware that chronic pain is not being adequately treated and that opioids are appropriate when other treatments fail or are not tolerated. Chronic opioid therapy has a low risk of addiction when used appropriately for pain.

Although patients undergoing chronic opioid therapy do become physically dependent, addiction must not be confused with dependence. **Dependence** is a physical and emotional reliance on a drug. Patients who are dependent will experience an abstinence syndrome (withdrawal) when drug therapy is discontinued or when the dose is reduced substantially.

In contrast, **addiction** is a compulsive disorder that leads to continued use of the drug despite harm to the user. Symptoms of addiction include preoccupation with drugs, refusal to taper medication off, a strong preference for a specific opioid (usually for short-acting over long-acting drugs), and a general decrease in ability to function. An addicted patient generally does not take the medication as prescribed. Opioid addicts have a tendency to rely on multiple prescribers and pharmacies to conceal their behavior. Pharmacy technicians must be alert to these signs of addiction when dispensing opioids, as it is their legal and moral responsibility to notify the pharmacist and/or prescribing physician if drug-seeking behavior is suspected. The technician should always watch for abuse of these drugs, without prejudging patients.

A patient will be more successful at overcoming addiction if the symptoms of withdrawal are handled appropriately. Drugs that bind tightly to the opioid receptors do this. An agent with a stronger attraction for a receptor will replace another agent with a lesser attraction. The opioid antagonists work in this manner because they have a stronger attraction for receptors than analgesic agents do. Blocking the opioid action may prevent withdrawal symptoms. Table 6.8 lists drugs commonly used to treat addiction.

The pharmacy team should be aware of the potential of abuse of narcotic drugs. The following are signs of addiction; the pharmacy technician should be alert to these things:

- Forged prescriptions
- Frequent prescription loss
- Changes made to the prescription; for example, adding a zero to the number 10
- Unsanctioned dose escalation
- Patient repeatedly saying he or she was shorted when medication was dispensed

One of the most difficult tasks for the pharmacy team is to assess narcotic use in patients. The pharmacy team commonly does not know what illness is being treated. Never hesitate to call the prescribing physician to verify and clarify a prescription for

TABLE 6.8   Most Commonly Used Drugs to Treat Addiction

Generic Name	Pronunciation	Dosage Form	Brand Name	Dispensing Status	Control Schedule
buprenorphine	byoo-pre-NOR-feen	injection, sublingual tablet	Buprenex, Subutex	Rx	C-III
buprenorphine-naloxone	byoo-pre-NOR-feen nal-OX-oan	sublingual tablet	Suboxone	Rx	C-III
methadone	METH-a-doan	injection, tablet	Dolophine	Rx	C-II

pain. Although the intention is certainly not to cause patients to feel uncomfortable or embarrassed, the pharmacy team must always be on the alert for those who abuse these medications, because addiction itself is an illness.

It is very important that the pharmacy team acknowledge the value of opioids in the treatment of pain as well as the potential for drug diversion. The federal regulation pertinent to controlled substances states that prescriptions can be "issued for a legitimate medical purpose by an individual practitioner acting in the usual course of his or her professional practice." It is imperative that documentation be in the medical records. The pharmacy team must serve both as gatekeeper and as advocate for patients who are in pain.

Buprenorphine (Buprenex, Subutex) is used for the management of moderate to severe pain and to prevent opioid withdrawal. This drug attaches to the opioid receptors and acts both as an agonist and as an antagonist. The patient should start with Subutex. The tablet should be placed under the tongue until it dissolves. It should not be swallowed.

Buprenorphine-naloxone (Suboxone) is given after the patient has completed a course of buprenorphine, which takes 3 to 4 days. The patient is then maintained on this drug. It is only approved to treat opioid dependence. Prescribers must have two DEA numbers to write for this drug, and the second number is issued when the prescriber has met the appropriate requirements. The pharmacy technician must always check for this second DEA number on all prescriptions for Suboxone. It is a C-III drug and is limited to qualifying prescribers. Like buprenorphine, it too is administered sublingually.

Methadone (Dolophine) is used as a pain reliever and to prevent withdrawal symptoms in patients addicted to opiate drugs who are enrolled in a treatment program. Alcohol, when added to methadone, can slow breathing and cause death. The concentrated form of methadone is packaged as a dispersible tablet and as a concentrated solution. Both must be mixed with 4 ounces of liquid. Patients should ingest the prepared solution immediately after it is mixed. Methadone is a C-II controlled substance.

Narcotic Analgesics

Warning

The words Codeine and Lodine (an NSAID) can look alike if written with poor handwriting.

A drug that alleviates pain is known as an **analgesic.** An analgesic medication that consists of, or is derived from, an opioid is a **narcotic analgesic.** Table 6.9 describes the most commonly used single narcotic analgesics. Table 6.10 gives an overview of pharmacotherapeutic options for moderate-to-severe pain.

Narcotics have no set or optimal dose. Dose requirements vary with the severity of pain, the individual response to pain, the patient's age and weight, and the presence of concomitant disease. Morphine is the standard against which all other narcotics are

TABLE 6.9 Most Commonly Used Narcotic Analgesics

Generic Name	Pronunciation	Dosage Form	Brand Name	Dispensing Status	Control Schedule
butorphanol	byoo-TOR-fa-nawl	IM, IV, nasal spray	Stadol	Rx	C-IV
codeine	KOE-deen	IM, tablet	Codeine Contin	Rx	C-II
fentanyl	FEN-ta-nil	IM, IV, buccal, patch, transmucosal	Actiq, Duragesic, Fentora, Ionsys	Rx	C-II
hydromorphone	hye-droe-MOR-foan	IM, IV, oral liquid, tablet	Dilaudid	Rx	C-II
meperidine	me-PER-i-deen	IM, IV, syrup, tablet	Demerol	Rx	C-II
morphine	MOR-feen	capsule, IM, IV, suppository, tablet	Astramorph/PF, Avinza, Duramorph, Kadian, MS Contin, MSIR	Rx	C-II
oxycodone	ok-see-KOE-doan	capsule, oral liquid, tablet	OxyContin	Rx	C-II
oxymorphone	ok-see-MOR-foan	IM, IV, suppository	Numorphan, Opana, Opana ER	Rx	C-II
pentazocine	pen-TAZ-oh-seen	IM, IV, tablet	Talwin	Rx	C-IV
propoxyphene	proe-POX-i-feen	capsule	Darvon	Rx	C-IV

TABLE 6.10 Pharmacotherapeutic Options for Moderate-to-Severe Pain

Indication	Pharmacotherapeutic Options for Treatment
bone pain	NSAIDs
	calcitonin
	dexamethasone
	prednisone
cancer pain	opioids
fibromyalgia	antidepressants
	opioids
lower back pain	muscle relaxants
	opioids
neuropathic pain	antidepressants
	anticonvulsants
osteoarthritis	NSAIDs
	glucocorticoid injections

TABLE 6.11   Comparative Doses of Narcotic Analgesics

Generic Name	Brand Name	Dose Equivalent to 10 mg IM Morphine
morphine	(many)	10 mg
codeine	(many)	130 mg, injection
fentanyl	Sublimaze	0.1 mg, IV
hydromorphone	Dilaudid	1.5 mg, injection
meperidine	Demerol	300 mg, oral
methadone	Dolophine	10–20 mg, oral
oxycodone-acetaminophen	Percocet	30 mg, oral
oxycodone-aspirin	Percodan	30 mg, oral
oxymorphone	Numorphan	1.5 mg, IV

Note: These equivalents will vary slightly depending on reference.

measured. Some drugs are more potent than morphine, but none are more effective when given in equianalgesic doses. Table 6.11 lists common narcotic analgesics and provides dosage equivalents to 10 mg of morphine.

Warning

Percocet is packaged in different strengths. Technicians must be careful to fill the prescription in the correct strength.

Narcotics can be delivered by several routes. Oral doses of most drugs are essentially equivalent to rectal suppository doses, and intramuscular doses are essentially equivalent to subcutaneous doses. A subcutaneous dose of morphine is two to three times as potent as an oral dose. When patients cannot tolerate oral medications (e.g., because they suffer from nausea or vomiting), the rectal suppository route should be considered. Another alternative is subcutaneous or IV infusion. Intravenous doses are usually more potent than intramuscular or subcutaneous doses. The route and administration affect both the onset and duration of action. Long-acting opioids are usually better choices because there is less euphoria potential for addiction and sleep disturbance. The quality of life is improved because, even though it is dependent on taking pills, there are fewer pills to take.

Warning

Avinza (morphine) and Invanz (ertapenem; see Chapter 4) can easily be confused when one is reading a prescription.

Whatever the route, patient comfort is the goal, and the response of the patient should be the basis for dosage adjustments. The key to effective pain management is constant reassessment. Doses should be titrated, and the dose should be repeated at a time *before* the pain recurs (adjusted to each individual). The right dose is the dose that controls pain without excessive or intolerable adverse effects.

Narcotics may produce a range of side effects in individual patients. Side effects should be anticipated and minimized so that pain relief is not offset by creating other distressing symptoms. Some common effects are mental confusion, reduced alertness, nausea, vomiting, dry mouth, constipation, urinary retention, histamine release (flush, wheal, and flare), vessel dilation, inflammatory process, and bronchial constriction (especially in persons with asthma).

Narcotics inhibit normal peristalsis (waves of contractions that pass along tubular organs to propel their contents), causing local spasms and reduced linear movement. All patients taking regular doses of a narcotic become constipated and should be maintained on some form of stimulant laxative from the outset of narcotic therapy. Stool softeners and increased fluid intake may be of benefit. Urinary retention can result because of spasmodic activity of the urethra (the tubular organ through which urine passes from the bladder) and major sphincter (ringlike muscle that closes a natural orifice) of the bladder. This can last from 24 to 48 hours and is most pronounced in patients over 55 years of age. The patient can also experience postural hypotension.

Respiratory depression is dose related. Appropriately prescribed narcotics rarely cause clinically significant respiratory depression. Any narcotic should be used with caution in patients with chronic obstructive pulmonary disorder (COPD) or asthma; for these patients, reduction of the dosage is necessary.

Narcotics act on an area identified as the chemotrigger zone (CTZ), which in turn acts on the vomiting center to produce emesis (the act of vomiting). This can be very dangerous in a patient heavily sedated with narcotics, because it can result in aspiration of vomitus into the airway. Morphine is especially likely to cause nausea because of the drug's stimulatory effect on the CTZ and inhibitory effect on GI motility. Antiemetics may be given to prevent or offset this reaction.

Narcotics can also stimulate seizures in patients with convulsive disorders. Most narcotics are metabolized by the liver; thus, serious liver disease may cause the patient to become comatose (a state of profound unconsciousness). Reduced doses must be used in these patients.

Consumption of alcohol with any of these drugs can cause immediate death. It can result in the absorption and rapid release of the opioid, which will lead to breathing depression.

When these drugs are dispensed, *they must always be counted twice*. The number is then circled on either the label of the bottle or the label attached to the back of the prescription. It is not unusual for abusers to call back and say they were shorted. These circles will show that whoever dispensed the drug did count it twice and it is not likely to be short.

Butorphanol (Stadol) is a more potent analgesic than morphine, yet it has less cardiovascular effects and respiratory sensitivity. It is a synthetic opiate that is a partial agonist. It is especially used to manage pain during labor. It binds to opiate receptors in the CNS. It is also used intranasally for migraine headaches.

Codeine is an opioid analgesic primarily used as an antitussive (coughing) or antidiarrheal medicine, but it can also be used as an analgesic. It is an alkaloid derived from opium. Codeine is converted to morphine in the liver, is not approved for IV administration, and is most frequently marketed with acetaminophen. Combinations of codeine with another drug used for mild to moderate pain or diarrhea are C-III, C-IV, or C-V controlled substances. Even in those locales where dilute codeine preparations are available OTC, very few pharmacists will sell it without a prescription. To do so, they must maintain a log. Many states have their own laws regarding these products. Codeine is considered less addictive than other opiates.

Fentanyl can be administered as a patch **(Duragesic)** and as a lozenge **(Actiq).** Before these dosage forms came out, fentanyl was rarely prescribed outside of the operating room (OR) or intensive care unit (ICU). The transdermal patches are used for chronic pain management. They should not be used for acute pain, such as that experienced immediately after surgery. Prescribers are not always aware of this limitation; if the prescriber is unaware, it is the pharmacy technician who has to catch this inappropriate prescribing for fentanyl. The patch is applied to a dry area on the body and remains there for 72 hours. The patch works by releasing fentanyl into body fats. The fatty tissue stores the drug and slowly releases it into the bloodstream. These patches must not be cut. Body temperature, skin type, and placement of the patch have major effects on how effective the pain control is. Fentanyl lozenges are berry-flavored and should be swabbed on the mucosal surfaces inside the mouth and under the tongue. They are most effective when consumed over a period of 10 to 15 minutes and absorbed through the mucosal surface of the mouth and cheeks. The lozenge is less effective if swallowed. A disadvantage of this dosage form is that it is very hard for nurses to docu-

Warning

Morphine sulfate and magnesium sulfate are often confused, especially when the prescriber uses the abbreviation MSO_4 or $MgSO_4$.

ment how much of the lozenge has been consumed. **Fentora,** the buccal pellet, is effervescent and absorbed through the buccal mucosa. An advantage of this dosage form is quicker absorption into the blood stream at lower dosage levels. **Ionsys** is a system that transports the drug into the body through a 3-volt lithium battery.

Hydrocodone (Vicodin, Lortab, etc.) was the top-selling drug in the United States in 2006. It is sold only in combination with other drugs, such as acetaminophen or aspirin. It is very popular as an antitussive in cough syrups, many of which were removed from the market by the FDA in 2008. (See information in Table 6-12, which lists combinations of opioids and an analgesic used for pain control.) Hydrocodone is a semisynthetic opioid derived from two naturally occurring opiates (codeine and thebaine). It relieves pain by binding to opioid receptors in the brain and spinal cord. Hydrocodone is the most abused prescription drug, which could help account for the sales, which have increased significantly in recent years, as have diversion and illicit use. Hydrocodone is habit-forming and can lead to physical and psychological addiction. It is a very popular drug and one the pharmacy technician will need to watch very carefully.

Hydromorphone (Dilaudid) is becoming more popular in the treatment of chronic pain. It is preferred over morphine in many cases because of its superior solubility and speed of onset. Hydromorphone has a less troublesome side effect profile. Furthermore, patients experience less nausea and vomiting with hydromorphone than with alternatives, and it has no troublesome metabolites.

Meperidine (Demerol) changes the way the body senses pain. It is used to control mild to moderate pain. Meperidine produces less nausea than most of the other opioids. However, it produces a metabolite that can cause serious problems when used for a long time. For that reason, it should never be used long term. The syrup should be diluted in order to prevent numbing of the mouth. It can be used as an adjunct to anesthesia.

Morphine (MS Contin, MSIR, Kadian, Avinza) is the principal alkaloid obtained from opium. It is a very versatile drug used in many different settings. Morphine is a strong analgesic used for the relief of severe and chronic pain, for preoperative sedation, and as a supplement to anesthesia. It is the drug of choice for the pain of myocardial infarction (heart attack). As with other opiate agonists, clinical effects other than pain relief include cough suppression, hypotension, nausea, and vomiting. Morphine is also very dangerous. An overdose causes the patient to stop breathing.

Morphine is administered orally, parenterally, intrathecally, epidurally, and rectally. When administered via the intravenous route it is three to six times more potent than when it is administered orally. Morphine has significant first-pass metabolism and is readily absorbed from the gut and is absorbed even faster rectally. **Avinza** is long-acting form that should be taken once a day. **Kadian** is also a slow release form of this drug.

Some confusion arises with the morphine sulfate forms of morphine. There are two types of morphine sulfate: MSIR and MS Contin. **MSIR (morphine sulfate immediate release)** is immediately available and is used for breakthrough pain. The other sulfate form of morphine, **MS Contin,** is used for pain control over a longer period of time (*contin*uous release). MS Contin is usually dosed for 12 hour periods, whereas MSIR is usually dosed for 4 hours. The minimum effective plasma concentration varies widely from patient to patient. Many factors affect the minimum concentration, including age, prior opiate therapy, medical condition, and emotions. Yet another morphine sulfate product, **DepoDur,** is an extended-release epidural injection that works for up to 48 hours.

Nalbuphine (Nubain) is injected into a large muscle and inhibits pain pathways by changing the perception of pain. It is used to control pain primarily in labor. CNS depression is a side effect.

Warning

Lortab and Lorabid (a cephalosporin antibiotic; see Chapter 4) can be confused. The dosing should help identify the prescribed drug.

Oxycodone (OxyContin, OxyIR, Roxicodone,) is used to relieve mild to severe pain. It is provided in either liquid and or tablet form. The most commonly used forms of this drug are combined with other analgesics such as acetaminophen or aspirin. Oxycodone causes CNS depression, which impedes mental abilities. It is a much abused drug and has a high street value. Oxycodone is one of the drugs the pharmacy technician must watch carefully for abuse, not only by patients but also by fellow workers. When a prescriber writes for Oxycotin, the extended release (ER) form must be used.

Oxymorphone (Opana, Opana ER) is a morphine-like opioid agonist. It is a semi-synthetic compound that stimulates opioid receptors in the CNS, producing analgesia. Oxymorphone is approximately three times as potent as oral morphine. It is indicated for the management of moderate to severe pain when an opioid analgesic is needed around the clock for an extended period of time. Oxymorphone doses must not be broken, chewed, or dissolved, as doing so would lead to rapid release and a fatal dose. Unlike other opioids, oxymorphone should be taken on an empty stomach, because taking it with food can lead to excessive peak levels.

Pentazozine (Talwin) is a synthetically prepared narcotic used to treat mild to moderate pain. It is sold only in combination with other drugs. It is more likely to cause hallucinations than other opioids.

Propoxyphene (Darvon) is used to relieve mild to moderate pain. The most popular dosage form is combined with acetaminophen.

Combination Drugs for Managing Pain

The combination of a narcotic and a nonnarcotic oral analgesic often results in analgesia superior to that produced by either agent alone. Relieving pain on two fronts (peripherally and centrally) enhances relief and facilitates use of lower doses of each agent. This produces a more favorable side effect profile. The purpose of combining drugs is twofold: (1) increasing pain relief through drug synergy and (2) limiting the intake of addictive substances. The most commonly used combination of drugs for controlling pain are listed in Table 6.12.

Many of these drugs come in varying strengths. Oxycodone and hydrocodone both come in several different combinations of doses of both the analgesic and the narcotic. It is very important to make sure that both strengths agree with the prescription.

One serious risk that is commonly overlooked with the combination drugs is aspirin or acetaminophen toxicity. When a prescription is filled, the pharmacy technician should check to make sure the patient is not getting more than 4 grams of aspirin or acetaminophen per day. Often, prescribers are concerned only with the addiction potential of the narcotic and overlook this important toxicity. The technician who checks this possibility performs a valuable service for the patient. The different dosage combinations of oxycodone and hydrocodone were developed to address this very issue.

Pharmacy technicians must also constantly be on the alert regarding C-III, C-IV, and C-V drugs. Prescriptions for those substances may be refilled for no more than five times and are good for no more than 6 months. After this time, the patient must get a new prescription. C-II substances have absolutely no refills.

Meperidine and promethazine make an interesting combination. This drug combination produces less nausea than other similar agents, because the promethazine helps to control the nausea. This combination is very useful for patients who develop nausea as a result of opioids. Also, because both drugs produce sedation, the combination likewise is very sedating.

TABLE 6.12   Most Commonly Used Combination Drugs for Control of Pain

Generic Name	Pronunciation	Dosage Form	Brand Name	Dispensing Status	Control Schedule
acetaminophen-codeine	a-seat-a-MIN-oh-fen KOE-deen	capsule, elixir, tablet	Phenaphen with Codeine, Tylenol with Codeine	Rx	C-III, C-V
hydrocodone-acetaminophen	hye-droe-KOE-done a-seat-a-MIN-oh-fen	capsule, elixir, tablet	Lortab, Vicodin, Lorcet	Rx	C-III
meperidine-promethazine	me-PER-i-deen-proe-METH-a-zeen	capsule	Mepergan	Rx	C-II
oxycodone-acetaminophen	ox-i-KOE-done a-seat-a-MIN-oh-fen	capsule, tablet	Endocet, Percocet, Tylox	Rx	C-II
oxycodone-aspirin	ox-i-KOE-done AS-pir-in	capsule	Endodan, Percodan	Rx	C-II
oxycodone-ibuprofen	ox-i-KOE-done-eye-byoo-PROE-fen	tablet	Combunox	Rx	C-II
pentazocine-naloxone	pen-TAZ-oh-seen-nal-OX-one	tablet	Talwin NX	Rx	C-IV
propoxyphene-acetaminophen	proe-POX-i-feen a-seat-a-MIN-oh-fen	tablet	Darvocet-N 100	Rx	C-IV

Migraine Headaches

A **migraine headache** is a severe, throbbing, unilateral headache accompanied by neurologic and GI disturbances that can severely affect quality of life and daily function. The headache is caused by dilation of cerebral surface vessels. Nausea, vomiting, and anorexia are common. Approximately 90% of all migraine sufferers report nausea. Photophobia (sensitivity to light), phonophobia (sensitivity to sound), and hyperesthesia (increased sensitivity to stimulation) are also common. Oral contraceptives can exacerbate migraine, partly because of their estrogen component.

Classic migraine has five components: prodrome (a symptom indicating the onset), aura, headache, headache relief, and postdrome (knowing it is gone). About 30% of migraine attacks are preceded by a subjective sensation or motor phenomenon known as an **aura,** which entails visual or sensory disturbances, or both: flashing lights; shimmering heat waves; bright lights; dark holes in the visual field; blurred, cloudy vision; or even a transient loss of vision. The headache generally dissipates in 6 hours but sometimes lasts 1 to 2 days.

The pathogenesis of the migraine is not completely understood. One well-known theory, referred to as the **vascular theory,** proposes that migraines are caused by vasodilation and the concomitant mechanical stimulation of sensory nerve endings. Researchers now suspect that the mechanism is more complicated than this.

The neurotransmitter serotonin (also known as 5-hydroxytryptamine or 5-HT) appears to be involved in the pathogenesis of migraine. Serotonin is a potent vasoconstrictor, and its concentration in platelets increases just before migraine attacks and decreases afterward. Thus, changes in serotonin level parallel the migraine symptoms. It has been theorized that stimulating certain subclasses of serotonin receptors in the cerebral and temporal arteries will cause vasoconstriction, which inhibits neural transmission, thereby alleviating migraine caused by excessive dilation of cranial arteries. As a result of this theory, several serotonin receptor agonists have come into use.

Diet, stress, sleep habits, certain medications, hormonal fluctuations, depression, atmospheric changes, and environmental irritants have all been implicated as causative factors that lower the threshold for neural transmission in the trigeminal nerve system, which is implicated in migraine.

The initial treatment for migraine should focus primarily on nondrug interventions. Identifying and eliminating trigger factors may be effective in many patients. For example, a quiet environment and sleep may help as many as 25% of patients during an acute attack. Lying down in a dark room often helps. When symptoms are severe or debilitating and attacks are frequent, drug therapy may be indicated. Sedative, antiemetic, and narcotic agents are helpful.

The medications used in migraine therapy can be divided into two classes: prophylactic therapy and abortive therapy, each of which is discussed briefly in the following paragraphs.

Prophylactic therapy attempts to prevent or reduce recurrence. Prophylaxis is indicated if migraines occur more than twice a month, occur in predictable patterns, or become refractory (stop responding) to acute therapy. Propranolol (Inderal) is the drug of choice for prophylaxis for migraines. Prophylactic therapies for migraines include the following classes of drugs:

- anticonvulsants
- beta blockers
- calcium channel blockers
- estrogen (can also be a causative factor)
- feverfew (an herb frequently used but without scientific data to support its use)
- NSAIDs
- selective serotonin reuptake inhibitors (SSRIs)
- tricyclic antidepressants

Abortive therapy for migraine headaches treats acute migraine headaches after they occur. The abortive drugs should be taken at the first sign of a headache. Patients must be educated to understand the importance of treating the attack as soon as possible—long before it develops into a full migraine, when the treatment is much less effective. Abortive therapy treatment is most effective when it begins at the first sign of aura or headache. The traditional therapies for acute migraine include simple analgesics, NSAIDs, and ergotamine-containing medications. These have been joined more recently by the serotonin receptor agonists.

Research has shown that combination regimens are more effective at treating migraine headaches and have lower recurrence rates than monotherapy. These advantages are especially true for combinations of a triptan and an NSAID.

Table 6.13 gives an overview of the most commonly used agents for migraine headaches. Several groups of drugs used to treat migraine headaches are discussed in the sections that follow.

Triptans—Selective Serotonin Receptor Agonists

These migraine-specific products offer good efficacy and rapid onset of action. They bind to serotonin receptors, causing dilated blood vessels in the dura mater to constrict. They are available in various dosage forms. If a patient does not respond to one, he or she may respond well to another.

TABLE 6.13   Most Commonly Used Agents for Migraine Headaches

Generic Name	Pronunciation	Dosage Form	Brand Name	Dispensing Status	Control Schedule
Triptans—Selective 5-HT Receptor Agonists					
almotriptan	al-moe-TRIP-tan	tablet	Axert	Rx	
eletriptan	el-ih-TRIP-tan	tablet	Relpax	Rx	
frovatriptan	froe-va-TRIP-tan	tablet	Frova	Rx	
naratriptan	NAR-a-trip-tan	tablet	Amerge	Rx	
rizatriptan	rye-za-TRIP-tan	sublingual tablet, tablet	Maxalt, Maxalt-MLT	Rx	
sumatriptan	soo-ma-TRIP-tan	injection, nasal spray, tablet	Imitrex	Rx	
zolmitriptan	zohl-mi-TRIP-tan	nasal spray, tablet	Zomig	Rx	
Ergot Preparations					
dihydroergotamine	dye-hye-droe-er-GOT-a-meen	injection, nasal spray	D.H.E. 45, Migranal	Rx	
ergotamine	er-GOT-a-meen	sublingual tablet	Ergomar	Rx	
ergotamine-caffeine	er-GOT-a-meen KAF-een	rectal suppository	Cafergot	Rx	
Antiemetic Agents					
chlorpromazine	klor-PROE-ma-zeen	capsule, injection, oral liquid, rectal suppository, syrup, tablet	Thorazine	Rx	
metoclopramide	met-oh-KLOE-pra-mide	injection, oral liquid, tablet	Reglan	Rx	
prochlorperazine	proe-klor-PER-a-zeen	capsule, injection, oral liquid, rectal suppository, tablet	Compazine	Rx	
Opioid Analgesic					
butorphanol	byoo-TOR-fa-nawl	injection, IV, nasal spray	Stadol, Stadol NS	Rx	C-IV
Beta Blocker					
propranolol	proe-PRAN-oh-lawl	capsule, injection, oral liquid, tablet	Inderal	Rx	
Other					
acetaminophen, aspirin, caffeine	a-seet-a-MIN-oh-fen-AS-pi-rin-KAF-een	tablet	Excedrin Migraine	OTC	
butalbital-acetaminophen-caffeine	byoo-TAL-bi-tal a-seet-a-MIN-oh-fen KAF-een	capsule, tablet	Fioricet	Rx	
butalbital-aspirin-caffeine	byoo-TAL-bi-tal AS-pir-in KAF-een	capsule	Fiorinal	Rx	C-III
isometheptene-dichloralphenazone-acetaminophen	eye-soe-meth-EP-teen dye-klor-al-FEN-a-zone a-seet-a-MIN-oh-fen	capsule	Midrin	Rx	C-IV
tramadol	TRA-ma-dawl	tablet	Ultram	Rx	

Almotriptan (Axert) has one of the highest oral bioavailabilities. It is also better tolerated than some of the other migraine medications.

Eletriptan (Relpax) has quite a few interactions, so the technician should be sure to check the computer system before dispensing. The maximum is two doses in 24 hours, but it does seem to last longer than most migraine treatments.

Frovatriptan (Frova) has a slow onset but a relatively long half-life.

Naratriptan (Amerge) is the gentlest triptan because it has slow onset and a favorable safety profile. It has a long half-life, which is generally associated with a low likelihood of migraine recurrence.

Rizatriptan (Maxalt and Maxalt-MLT) oral tablets are quickly absorbed and have the most rapid onset of action of all the oral migraine therapies. Many patients experience relief as soon as 30 minutes after taking this drug. The tablet is dissolved under the tongue. **Maxalt** is not absorbed as rapidly as **Maxalt-MLT.**

Sumatriptan (Imitrex) first entered the market as a subcutaneous injection and now is also available in tablet form and as a nasal spray. When injected, sumatriptan is effective in approximately 15 minutes. Sumatriptan may cause tingling, warm sensation, chest discomfort, dizziness, vertigo, and discomfort at the injection site. It has little or no activity on dopamine, beta-adrenergic, and alpha-adrenergic receptors. Side effects, including nausea, vomiting, and peripheral vasoconstriction, are relatively uncommon. The use of alcohol, of course, should be avoided because alcohol is a major contributor to migraines. The maximum recommended adult dose (subcutaneous route) is two 6 mg doses in 24 hours. A second dose may be administered at least 1 hour after the first dose if some improvement occurs but the migraine is still not relieved. The subcutaneous administration route is especially beneficial to patients with diminished gastric absorption or nausea and vomiting. The autoinjector is very easy to use. The patient should receive an injection at the first sign of a headache.

Zolmitriptan (Zomig) is similar to sumatriptan. It constricts cerebral blood vessels and reduces inflammation of sensory nerves. The dose can be repeated in 2 hours, but the patient should never take more than 10 mg in 24 hours.

Ergot Derivatives

Ergotamine, an alkaloid derived from the ergot group of fungi, which live parasitically on grasses such as rye, is used in the treatment of migraine headaches. The ergotamine molecule is similar to several neurotransmitters; its effectiveness in migraine is due to its activity as a vasoconstrictor. To be effective, ergotamine therapy should be initiated early in the attack. Ergotamine has significant adverse effects that limit its usefulness. The most common, regardless of the administration route, are nausea and vomiting. These effects may be exacerbated if a rectal suppository is used, because absorption is enhanced. Ergotism (a syndrome of progressive vasoconstriction and ischemia of vital organs) and ergot headache (a medication–headache cycle occurring with daily use of ergotamine) have been reported. To avoid these adverse effects, patients should be instructed regarding the maximum daily and weekly dosages and the importance of avoiding ergotamine use on consecutive days or more than twice a week.

Dihydroergotamine (Migranal) is a nasal spray that constricts peripheral and cranial blood vessels. This drug does not work as quickly as sumatriptan (Imitrex), but the effect lasts longer. Patients should administer one spray in each nostril, repeating in 15 minutes for a total of 4 sprays. The head should not be tilted while spraying so that the drug remains in the nostril for absorption. Any drug not used within 24 hours should be discarded. Once the ampule is broken, the drug becomes less potent.

Ergotamine-caffeine (Cafergot) is a direct vasoconstrictor of smooth muscle in cranial blood vessels and is used to treat migraines. The dose should be titrated to each patient. The patient should be told to initiate treatment at the first sign of an attack and not to exceed the recommended dose.

Antiemetic Agents

Metoclopramide (Reglan) can be used to reduce nausea and vomiting and enhance the absorption of other antimigraine products by reducing gastritis (inflammation of the stomach). Currently, many physicians are prescribing aspirin and metoclopramide in place of oral sumatriptan. The combination seems to have fewer side effects. Metoclopramide tends to cause drowsiness, but sumatriptan is more likely to cause nausea, fatigue, and weakness. Physicians are prescribing 1000 mg of aspirin with 10 mg of metoclopramide.

Chlorpromazine (Thorazine) is effective in some migraines unresponsive to ergotamines. It has antiemetic properties. The side effects include drowsiness, extrapyramidal effects, and orthostatic hypotension. This is also the only drug approved by the FDA for the treatment of hiccups.

Opioid Analgesic

Butorphanol (Stadol, Stadol NS) is a mixed narcotic agonist-antagonist. The nasal spray form is an inhalant with central analgesic actions. It is used to manage moderate to severe pain. It can be addictive and is a C-IV controlled substance. Each bottle of the nasal spray delivers only fourteen doses—fewer if it is primed before each use. The nasal spray is most commonly used, but the drug also comes as an injection that can be given either by IV or intramuscularly.

Other Antimigraine Agents

Tramadol (Ultram), when given in combination with an NSAID such as ibuprofen, has a high success rate in treating migraines. Because the drug has a slow onset, it was being promoted as a nonaddictive substance. However, recent evidence suggests that there is, in fact, some potential for addiction with this drug.

Warning

Tramadol and Toradol (an NSAID) could be confused.

Isometheptene-dichloralphenazone-acetaminophen (Midrin) has fewer side effects than ergotamine, but it is less effective for some people. The patient should take two capsules at the beginning of an attack and then one every 1 to 2 hours until cessation of headache, up to five capsules in 12 hours. It is a combination analgesic (acetaminophen), sedative (dichloralphenazone), and vasoconstrictor (isometheptene). It has been effective for mild-to-moderate migraine attacks. Sedation and gastrointestinal distress occur frequently, but rebound headache is not common. The most frequent side effects are dizziness, insomnia, nausea, vomiting, and transient numbness.

Acetaminophen, aspirin, and caffeine in combination **(Excedrin Migraine)** were reported in one study to give very good results in migraine pain. Many common headaches, including migraines, respond to this combination.

Chapter Terms

addiction a compulsive disorder that leads to continued use of a drug despite harm to the user

afferent system the nerves and sense organs that bring information to the CNS; part of the peripheral nervous system

alpha receptors (alpha-adrenergic receptors) nerve receptors that control vasoconstriction, pupil dilation, and relaxation of the GI smooth muscle in response to epinephrine

amide a compound containing a –CONH– group; a longer-acting local anesthetic that is metabolized by liver enzymes

analgesic a drug that alleviates pain

analgesic ladder a guideline for selecting pain-relieving medications according to the severity of the pain and whether agents lower on the ladder have been able to control the pain

anesthesiologist a physician who oversees administration of anesthesia during surgery

antagonists drugs used to reverse the effects of other drugs, such as in treatment of benzodiazepine or narcotic overdoses

anticholinesterase a drug that potentiates the action of acetylcholine by inhibiting the enzyme acetylcholinesterase, which breaks acetylcholine down

aura a subjective sensation or motor phenomenon that precedes and marks the onset of a migraine headache

autonomic nervous system (ANS) the part of the efferent system of the PNS that regulates activities of body structures not under voluntary control

beta-1 receptors nerve receptors on the heart that control the rate and strength of the heartbeat in response to epinephrine

beta-2 receptors nerve receptors that control vasodilation and relaxation of the smooth muscle of the airways in response to epinephrine

central nervous system (CNS) the brain and spinal cord

dependence a physical and emotional reliance on a drug

efferent system the nerves that dispatch information out from the CNS; part of the peripheral nervous system

endotracheal intubation insertion of a tube into the trachea to keep it open

ester a compound containing a –COO– group; a short-acting local anesthetic, metabolized by pseudocholinesterase of the plasma and tissue fluids

general anesthesia a condition characterized by reversible unconsciousness, analgesia, skeletal muscle relaxation, and amnesia on recovery

local anesthesia the production of transient and reversible loss of sensation in a defined area of the body

malignant hyperthermia a rare, but serious, side effect of anesthesia associated with an increase in intracellular calcium and a rapid rise in body temperature

migraine headache a severe, throbbing, unilateral headache, usually accompanied by nausea, photophobia, phonophobia, and hyperesthesia

narcotic analgesic pain medication containing an opioid

neuromuscular blocking skeletal muscle paralysis

neuron a nerve cell that transmits information

neurotransmitter a chemical substance that is selectively released from a neuron and stimulates or inhibits activity in the neuron's target cell

nonsteroidal anti-inflammatory drug (NSAID) a drug such as aspirin or ibuprofen that reduces pain and inflammation

opiate a narcotic that is either derived from opium or synthetically produced to resemble opium derivatives chemically

opioid a substance, whether a drug or a chemical naturally produced by the body, that acts on opioid receptors to reduce the sensation of pain

pain the activation of electrical activity in afferent neurons with sensory endings in peripheral tissue with a higher firing threshold than those of temperature or touch; a protective signal to warn of damage or presence of disease; the fifth vital sign; classified as acute, chronic nonmalignant, and chronic malignant

patient-controlled analgesia (PCA) pump a means of pain control whereby the patient can regulate, within certain limits, the administration of pain medication

peripheral nervous system (PNS) the nerves and sense organs outside the CNS

somatic nervous system the part of the efferent system of the PNS that regulates the skeletal muscles

vascular theory a theory that proposes that migraine headaches are caused by vasodilation and the concomitant mechanical stimulation of sensory nerve endings

Chapter Summary

The Nervous System

- The primary CNS transmitters are acetylcholine, norepinephrine, dopamine, GABA, glutamate, and serotonin.
- The primary PNS transmitters are acetylcholine and norepinephrine.
- The major transmitters of the sympathetic system are acetylcholine, norepinephrine, dopamine, and epinephrine.
- The only transmitter of the parasympathetic system is acetylcholine.
- If a drug is classified as an anticholinergic, the following side effects may occur: decreased GI motility, decreased urination, pupil dilation, decreased sweating, dry eyes, and dry mouth.

Anesthesia

- Drugs that allow painless, controlled surgical, obstetric, and diagnostic procedures constitute the cornerstone of modern pharmacologic therapy. The hallmark of anesthetic drugs is controllability. For this reason, most potent anesthetics are gases or vapors.

- One anesthetic may be superior to another, depending on the clinical circumstances. Final selection is based on those drugs and anesthetic techniques judged safest for the patient.
- General anesthesia is the unique condition of reversible unconsciousness and absence of response to stimulation. It is characterized by four reversible actions: unconsciousness, analgesia, skeletal muscle relaxation, and amnesia on recovery.
- The purposes of premedication are sedation, helping with postoperative pain relief, and reducing anxiety.
- Dantrolene (Dantrium) is a skeletal muscle relaxant; it is the drug of choice to treat malignant hyperthermia.
- The advantage of nitrous oxide is that it is rapidly eliminated.
- Fentanyl is used extensively for open-heart procedures because it lacks some of the cardiac depressant actions of other anesthetics.
- Naloxone (Narcan), nalmefene (Revex), and flumazenil (Romazicon) are given to reverse overdoses of specific drugs.

- Neuromuscular blocking is important as an adjunct to general anesthesia to facilitate endotracheal intubation and to ensure that the patient does not move during surgery.
- Blocking agents act via a depolarizing mechanism or as antagonists to acetylcholine at receptor sites on the muscle cell.
- Anticholinesterase agents reverse neuromuscular blockers.
- Local anesthetics are advantageous because they affect all types of nervous tissue. They relieve pain without altering alertness or mental function.

Pain Management

- Pain itself can be a disease; it is classified as acute, chronic nonmalignant, or chronic malignant.
- Pain is now considered to be the "fifth" vital sign.
- All narcotics have the potential to induce tolerance and dependence.
- The effects of narcotics differ on different individuals.
- The patient-controlled analgesia (PCA) pump is an effective means of controlling pain; the pump allows the patient to regulate, within certain limits, the amount of drug received. Better pain control is achieved with less drug.
- The transdermal patch provides pain control and allows the patient to remain more alert than with most other methods.
- Methadone (Dolophine), buprenorphine (Buprenex, Subutex), and buprenorphine-naloxone (Suboxone) are drugs used to treat opioid addiction.
- Morphine is the standard against which all other narcotic analgesics are measured.

- Fentanyl is manufactured as a lozenge and a patch. The patch is approved for chronic use, not acute pain following surgery.
- Narcotics act on an area of the brain identified as the chemotrigger zone, which in turn stimulates the vomiting center.
- It is as important to watch the aspirin or acetaminophen dose in narcotic combination analgesics as it is to watch the narcotic dose.
- The pharmacy team must serve as the advocate and gatekeeper when dispensing narcotics.

Migraine Headaches

- Patients with migraine headaches should be taught to initiate therapy immediately at the first hint of an episode.
- Treatments for migraine headaches are divided into two groups: abortive and prophylactic therapies.
- Prophylactic drugs include anticonvulsants, beta blockers, calcium channel blockers, estrogen, feverfew, NSAIDs, SSRIs, and tricyclic antidepressants.
- Sumatriptan (Imitrex) is used for the relief of migraine headaches. It should be used at the first sign of headache. If it brings partial, but not total, relief, the patient may receive a second dose at least 1 hour after the first dose.
- Midrin is a combination drug with fewer side effects than ergotamine. The patient should take two capsules at the onset of headache and then one every 1 to 2 hours until the pain stops, up to 5 capsules in 12 hours.

Drug List

The following drugs were discussed in this chapter. Each generic drug name is followed in parentheses by one or more brand names.

Inhalant Anesthetics
desflurane (Suprane)
enflurane (Ethrane)
halothane
isoflurane (Forane)
nitrous oxide
sevoflurane (Ultane)

Injectable Anesthetics
alfentanil (Alfenta)
etomidate (Amidate)
fentanyl* (Sublimaze)
fentanyl-droperidol
ketamine (Ketalar)
morphine
propofol (Diprivan)
remifentanyl (Ultiva)
sufentanil (Sufenta)

Barbiturates
methohexital (Brevital)
thiopental (Pentothal)

Benzodiazepines
diazepam (Valium) *
lorazepam (Ativan)*
midazolam (Versed)

Antagonist to Reverse Malignant Hyperthermia
dantrium (Dantrolene)

Antagonists to Reverse Overdoses
flumazenil (Romazicon)
nalmefene (Revex)
naloxone (Narcan)

Neuromuscular Blocking Agents
atracurium (Tracrium)
cisatracurium (Nimbex)
mivacurium (Mivacron)
pancuronium
rocuronium (Zemuron)
succinylcholine (Quelicin)
vecuronium (Norcuron)

Agents to Reverse Neuromuscular Blocking
edrophonium (Enlon)
neostigmine (Prostigmin)
pyridostigmine (Mestinon)

Local Anesthetics

Esters
benzocaine (Americaine)
chloroprocaine (Nesacaine)
dyclonine (Cēpacol Maximum Strength)
procaine (Novocain)
tetracaine (Cēpacol Viractin, Pontocaine)

Amides
bupivacaine (Marcaine)
levobupivacaine (Chirocaine)
lidocaine (L-M-X, Solarcaine Aloe Extra Burn Relief, Xylocaine)
lidocaine-epinephrine (Xylocaine with Epinephrine)
lidocaine-prilocaine (EMLA)
mepivacaine (Carbocaine)

Drugs Used to Treat Addiction
buprenorphine (Buprenex, Subutex)
buprenorphine-naloxone (Suboxone)
methadone (Dolophine)

Narcotic Analgesics
butorphanol (Stadol)
codeine (Codeine Contin)
fentanyl (Actiq, Duragesic, Fentora, Ionsys)
hydromorphone (Dilaudid)
meperidine (Demerol)
morphine (Astramorph/PF, Avinza, Duramorph, Kadian, MS Contin, MSIR)
oxycodone (OxyContin, OxyIR, Roxicodone)*
oxymorphone (Numorphan, Opana, Opana ER)
pentazocine (Talwin)
propoxyphene (Darvon)

Combination Drugs

acetaminophen-codeine (Phenaphen with
  Codeine, Tylenol with Codeine)*
hydrocodone-acetaminophen (Lortab,
  Vicodin, Lorcet)*
meperidine-promethazine (Mepergan)
oxycodone-acetaminophen (Endocet,
  Percocet, Tylox)*
oxycodone-aspirin (Endodan, Percodan)
oxycodone-ibuprofen (Combunox)
pentazocine-naloxone (Talwin NX)
propoxyphene-acetaminophen (Darvocet-N
  100)*

Migraine Headaches

Triptans—Selective 5-HT Receptor Agonists

almotriptan (Axert)
eletriptan (Relpax)
frovatriptan (Frova)
naratriptan (Amerge)
rizatriptan (Maxalt, Maxalt-MLT)
sumatriptan (Imitrex)*
zolmitriptan (Zomig)

Ergot Derivatives

dihydroergotamine (D.H.E. 45, Migranal)
ergotamine (Ergomar)
ergotamine-caffeine (Cafergot)

Antiemetic Agents

chlorpromazine (Thorazine)
metoclopramide (Reglan)*
prochlorperazine (Compazine)

Opioid Analgesic

butorphanol (Stadol, Stadol NS)

Beta Blocker

propranolol (Inderal)

Other

acetaminophen-aspirin-caffeine (Excedrin
  Migraine)
butalbital-acetaminophen-caffeine (Fioricet)
butalbital-aspirin-caffeine (Fiorinal)
isometheptene-dichloralphenazone-
  acetaminophen (Midrin)
tramadol (Ultram)*

Chapter Review

Pharmaceuticals and Body Functions

Select the best answer from the choices given.

1. If a drug is classified as an anticholinergic,
   it would have all the following effects
   except
   a. decreased urination.
   b. watery eyes.
   c. pupil dilation.
   d. decreased sweating.

2. The purpose of preanesthetic medications is
   a. sedation.
   b. to help with pain relief.
   c. anxiety reduction.
   d. all of the above
   e. none of the above

3. Someone has been given too much Versed
   (midazolam) in the operating room.
   The surgical resident cannot recall the
   name of the drug that should be given
   but sends a stat order to the pharmacy
   for an antagonist. You should notify the
   pharmacist and prepare
   a. diazepam.
   b. dantrolene.
   c. flumazenil.
   d. thiopental.
   e. nitrous oxide.

4. Which narcotic has a dangerous metabolite
   if used long term?
   a. meperidine
   b. oxycodone
   c. morphine
   d. oxymorphone
   e. pentazocine

5. A patient who had outpatient surgery the previous day awakens in the morning and urinates. The urine is green. The patient's caretaker calls, wanting to know whether any drugs dispensed to the patient would cause this. Which drug did the patient receive?
   a. ketamine
   b. Amidate
   c. Diprivan
   d. fentanyl
   e. Dantrium

6. The pharmacy technician is stocking the OR suite that is used for open-heart surgery. Which of the following anesthetics would definitely need to be stocked?
   a. Ketalar
   b. etomidate
   c. Diprivan
   d. fentanyl
   e. Dantrium

7. Which is the most widely used local anesthetic?
   a. cocaine
   b. lidocaine
   c. chloroprocaine
   d. tetracaine
   e. dyclonine

8. Which inhalant anesthetic causes no amnesia or skeletal muscle relaxation and is frequently used in dental procedures?
   a. methoxyflurane
   b. nitrous oxide
   c. halothane
   d. Ethrane
   e. isoflurane

9. Which OTC drug has been shown to give good control for headaches?
   a. Excedrin Migraine
   b. Fentora
   c. Mepergan
   d. sumatriptan
   e. Metoclopromide

10. Which drug is a combination drug?
    a. Sufenta
    b. Midrin
    c. Narcan
    d. Diprivan
    e. none of the above

The following statements are true or false. If the answer is false, rewrite the statement so it is true.

_____ 1. The pharmacy team must serve both as gatekeeper and advocate when dispensing narcotics.

_____ 2. One reason for the many doses of combination drugs is to reduce the amount of the non-narcotic analgesic.

_____ 3. Nausea and constipation are both side effects of narcotics.

_____ 4. Even though literature indicates that pain is undertreated, pain medications are among the top selling drugs in this country.

_____ 5. Alpha-adrenergic receptors cause vasodilation.

_____ 6. The hallmark of anesthetic drugs is controllability.

_____ 7. Nitrous oxide has a tremendous advantage of being rapidly eliminated.

_____ 8. Local anesthetics depress the small, unmyelinated fibers last and the larger, myelinated fibers first.

_____ 9. Pain itself can be a disease.

_____ 10. All narcotics have the potential to produce tolerance and dependence.

Match the following brand names with their generic names.

1. Inderal _____   a. zolmitriptan

2. Zomig _____   b. pentazocine

3. Reglan _____   c. metoclopramide

4. Talwin _____   d. propranolol

Classify the following drugs as (a) schedule II, (b) schedule III, (c) schedule IV, (d) not controlled.

5. Demerol	_____	21. Americaine	_____
6. succinylcholine	_____	22. acetaminophen-codeine	_____
7. fentanyl	_____	23. Reglan	_____
8. naloxone	_____	24. Percocet	_____
9. ergotamine	_____	25. Percodan	_____
10. propoxyphene	_____	26. Dilaudid	_____
11. MS Contin	_____	27. Midrin	_____
12. edrophonium	_____	28. Imitrex	_____
13. Revex	_____	29. Darvocet-N 100	_____
14. Lortab	_____	30. dantrolene	_____
15. Tylenol III	_____	31. hydrocodone-acetaminophen	_____
16. Vicodin	_____	32. propoxyphene-acetaminophen	_____
17. nitrous oxide	_____	33. morphine	_____
18. diazepam	_____		
19. Duragesic	_____		
20. Xylocaine	_____		

Diseases and Drug Therapies

1. List (a) the goals of balanced anesthesia and (b) indices to assess the degree of general anesthesia.

2. Discuss local anesthetics. Include (a) advantages and (b) order of function loss.

3. Discuss pain. Include (a) classification and (b) major sources and areas involved.

4. Discuss narcotics. Include (a) reactions and (b) analgesic ladder.

Dispensing Medications

1. Outline a stepwise approach to treating migraines. Include the drug of choice for prophylaxis of migraines.

2. Why must dantrolene always be stored near an OR?

3. You are the patient and are going to have the following operations. Choose the appropriate anesthetic.
   a. tooth extraction
   b. open-heart surgery

Internet Research

Use the Internet to complete the following assignments.

1. Research current news stories related to the Controlled Substances Act. Find two articles related to pharmaceuticals and summarize each in two or three sentences. List your Internet sources.

2. Research the use of narcotics in the management of chronic pain. Look up the JCAHO pain management standards and compare JCAHO's treatment of the subject to that of two or three other sites. Describe the main controversies surrounding this issue. Why do you think it is important to have standards and guidelines in place? List your Internet sources and comment on the usefulness of each site.

What Would You Do?

1. One of your favorite patients, an elderly lady, comes in and hands you a prescription for her lorazepam. She usually gets #30 but often runs out and tries to get refills early. She frequently looses her medication. This prescription says "#80"; however, a part of the 8 is in a different ink color. How would you handle this situation?

Psychiatric and Related Drugs

7

Learning Objectives

- Differentiate antidepressant, antipsychotic, and antianxiety agents.
- Be prepared to discuss the antidepressant classes, their uses, and their side effects.
- Know why and how lithium and other drugs are used in treating bipolar disorders.
- Be familiar with antipsychotics and the drugs that prevent their side effects.

- Define anxiety, learn its symptoms, and know the drugs used in its treatment.
- Recognize the course and treatment of panic disorders, insomnia, and alcoholism.

 Preview chapter terms and definitions.

Mental disorders are among the most disabling conditions that healthcare professionals see. Many have their cause in the interaction of central nervous system (CNS) chemicals. For the patient and the patient's family, these diseases can be overwhelming and frightening. Often, control of symptoms is the only treatment that can be offered. These states include depression, posttraumatic stress disorder, seasonal affective disorder, bipolar disorder, psychotic disorders, anxiety, panic attacks, sleep disorders, and alcoholism.

Depression and Mood Disorders

Clinical **depression** is the most common severe psychiatric disorder. Depression is characterized by feelings of pessimism, worry, intense sadness, loss of concentration, slowing of mental processes, and problems with eating and sleeping. Its symptoms may include dysphoric mood or loss of interest in almost all usual activities, low self-esteem, pessimism, self-pity, significant weight loss or gain, insomnia or hypersomnia, extreme restlessness, loss of energy, feelings of worthlessness, diminished ability to think, feelings of guilt, recurrent thoughts of death, and suicide attempts. The patient feels life has no meaning. Women are more likely than men to have depression, with the peak years usually from ages 35 to 45. Depression occurs later in life in men.

In addition to depression, there are several different recognized types of mood disorders. **Mania** is a mood of extreme excitement, excessive elation, hyperactivity, agitation, and increased psychomotor activity. **Bipolar disorder** patients have mood swings that alternate between periods of major depression and periods of mild to severe chronic agitation (mania). **Unipolar depression** is major depression with no previous occurrence of mania. **Post-traumatic stress disorder (PTSD)** was first recognized in World War I combat veterans, in whom it was called "shell shock," but it has emerged as a major civilian illness since the September 11, 2001, terrorist attacks, the Iraq war, and Hurricane Katrina. PTSD is now the fourth most common psychiatric illness. Most people involved in a traumatic event have a brief period of difficulty, but if persistent anxiety or recurrent fear lasts more than a month after the end of the traumatic event or disturbs work or personal life, it needs to be treated. Finally, **seasonal affective disorder (SAD)** is a form of major depression that occurs in the fall and winter and remits in the spring and summer.

A **neurotransmitter** is a chemical produced by a nerve cell and involved in transmitting information in the body, as was discussed in Chapter 6. Neurotransmitters are important in mood disorders and other mental disorders. Drug therapy for depression is aimed at changing the levels of neurotransmitters, specifically serotonin and norepinephrine. Antidepressants are classified based on which neurotransmitter they affect and how. A **selective serotonin reuptake inhibitor (SSRI)** blocks the reuptake (i.e., reabsorption) of serotonin, thus increasing the concentration of that neurotransmitter with little effect on another important neurotransmitter, norepinephrine. SSRIs have the benefit of producing fewer side effects than older antidepressants. A **serotonin norepinephrine reuptake inhibitor (SNRI)** increases both serotonin and norepinephrine. It is believed that the earlier **tricyclic antidepressant (TCA)** class of medications acts similarly by preventing neuron reuptake of norepinephrine and/or serotonin. Antidepressants of the **monoamine oxidase inhibitor (MAOI)** class inhibit enzymes that break down norepinephrine and serotonin, therefore allowing these neurotransmitters to build up in the synapse, as with the SSRIs and TCAs.

Unlike most other drugs, antidepressants generally have a delay of onset of 10 to 21 days. They should never be used on an "as needed" basis to treat depression.

Antidepressants *as a class* are required by the FDA to include a Medication Guide. These guides must be given to all patients of all ages with every dispensing of an antidepressant. Medication Guides are "required for drug products that present a serious and significant" concern. Technicians should make sure that every antidepressant has this Medication Guide attached. This is just one reason it is important to know which drugs are antidepressants. It is also important to remember that antidepressants are *not* controlled substances.

SSRIs and SNRIs are much safer than the tricyclic antidepressants. However, combined with certain other drugs, they can be fatal. This effect is known as **serotonin syndrome,** and it occurs when drugs that increase serotonin levels are combined with drugs that themselves stimulate the serotonin receptors, causing the receptors to be overstimulated. The FDA has a warning that discusses the dangers of combining triptans (serotonin receptor agonists used to treat migraine, discussed in Chapter 6) with antidepressants, a combination that can occur frequently because many people who suffer from migraine headaches are also depressed. Although serotonin syndrome is rare, it can be fatal, partly because it is difficult to diagnose. It causes mental state changes and neuromuscular abnormalities, as well as other symptoms. Many prescribers are unaware of these dangerous interactions. Pharmacy technicians should be aware of these, and will see warnings for these on their computer screen (from pharmacy database information) and from insurance companies. If a patient is prescribed drugs that could cause such interactions, the pharmacy technician should notify both pharmacist and prescriber.

Selective Serotonin Reuptake Inhibitors

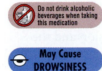
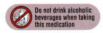
The most commonly used SSRIs for the treatment of depression are listed in Table 7.1.

Fluoxetine (Prozac) is the most established agent in this drug class. It is indicated for major depression and **obsessive-compulsive disorder (OCD)** (recurrent, persistent urges to perform repetitive acts such as hand washing). Adverse effects include nervousness, insomnia, drowsiness, **anorexia** (loss of appetite), nausea, and diarrhea. Most patients lose weight, but a few may gain weight. Patients should avoid alcohol. Pharmacists should be alert for possible interaction with phenytoin (Dilantin). This interaction can raise the serum phenytoin to toxic levels. Patients should take the drug in the morning to avoid insomnia. Fluoxetine plus light treatment (exposure to white light for a specific time period early in the morning, upon awakening) has shown good results for SAD.

Citalopram (Celexa) is considered to be an SSRI, although it is structurally different from the other drugs in this class. This drug has relatively few drug interactions because it is metabolized through an alternative pathway. It is ideal for patients who are required to take a number of different prescriptions concurrently. Citalopram is approved for obsessive-compulsive disorder as well as depression.

Sarafem is a brand of fluoxetine specifically targeted for women suffering from premenstrual dysphoric disorder (PMDD), which is a severe form of premenstrual syndrome (PMS). Serotonin levels are thought to influence the hormonal fluctuation that occurs just prior to the onset of menstruation. Although some women will benefit by taking the drug only during the week prior to menses, most will need to take it daily to achieve the desired effect. It comes in a seven-day pack containing 10 mg or 20 mg capsules.

Escitalopram (Lexapro) is the s-isomer of citalopram (isomers are chemical compounds of identical composition but with different arrangements of atoms). It is more potent with fewer side effects.

Fluvoxamine is effective for major depression and may be useful in managing anxiety; it is also approved for treatment of obsessive-compulsive disorders. The primary side effect is nausea. Alcohol should be avoided, as should administration with phenytoin (Dilantin). Hard candy can relieve the side effect of dry mouth. Fluvox, the brand form of this drug, has been voluntarily removed from the market, but many prescribers still write for Fluvox, and fluvoxamine is to be dispensed.

TABLE 7.1	Most Commonly Used SSRIs and Related Drugs for Depression			
Generic Name	Pronunciation	Dosage Form	Brand Name	Dispensing Status
citalopram	sye-TAL-oh-pram	oral liquid, tablet	Celexa	Rx
escitalopram	es-sye-TAL-oh-pram	oral liquid, tablet	Lexapro	Rx
fluoxetine	floo-OX-e-teen	capsule, oral liquid, tablet	Prozac, Sarafem	Rx
fluvoxamine	floo-VOX-a-meen	tablet	(none)	Rx
paroxetine	pa-ROX-e-teen	oral liquid, tablet	Paxil	Rx
sertraline	SER-tra-leen	oral liquid, tablet	Zoloft	Rx

The indications for **paroxetine (Paxil)** are depression, obsessive-compulsive disorder, and panic disorder. Side effects are nausea, headache, ejaculatory disturbances, and sweating.

Sertraline (Zoloft) is indicated for depression and obsessive-compulsive disorder. The primary side effect reported by patients is nausea when they first begin to take the drug; it may also cause drowsiness. It should be taken once daily without regard for food. Patients should respond in the first 8 weeks of therapy.

Serotonin and Norepinephrine Reuptake Inhibitors

For patients for whom SSRIs are not effective, serotonin and norepinephrine reuptake inhibitors (SNRIs) offer potential relief. SNRIs affect both serotonin and norepinephrine reuptake, which makes them more effective for treating pain than drugs that affect only one neurotransmitter. These drugs will commonly be prescribed for pain alone. The most commonly used SNRIs in the treatment of depression are listed in Table 7.2.

Duloxetine (Cymbalta) is approved for treatment of major depression and the management of pain associated with diabetic neuropathy. It is a potent inhibitor of serotonin and norepinephrine and a weak inhibitor of dopamine reuptake, providing a more balanced reuptake inhibition. It cannot be discontinued abruptly, but rather its dosage must be tapered. It has more interactions than the other drugs in this class.

Venlafaxine (Effexor) blocks reuptake of both serotonin and norepinephrine and is prescribed for depression. It is sometimes refered to informally as "Prozac with a punch." A sustained increase in blood pressure may result from its use, and it may produce manic episodes. Side effects include sweating, headache, somnolence, nausea, vomiting, dry mouth, blurred vision, and abnormal ejaculation or orgasm. At lower doses it primarily affects serotonin, whereas at higher doses it also affects norepinephrine.

Desvenlafaxine (Pristiq), the major metabolite of venlafaxine, is approved for depression and hot flashes. Pharmacokinetically, it works in the same way as venlafaxine, but it does not produce all of the unpleasant side effects. Additionally, desvenlafaxine is currently the only nonestrogenic drug available for hot flashes. This is significant, because many of the estrogens previously used for hot flashes have been taken off the market. It is anticipated that many women who cannot tolerate estrogen will be prescribed desvenlafaxine. Finally, desvenlafaxine is also used for fibromyalgia and neuropathic pain.

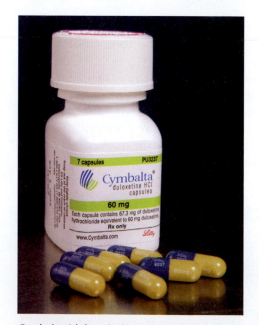

Cymbalta (duloxetine), a serotonin and norepinephrine reuptake inhibitor, has recently been approved by the FDA for treatment of major depression.

Cyclic Antidepressants

The cyclic antidepressants include varieties that contain three fused rings of carbon atoms (tricyclic) and four fused rings (tetracyclic). Tricyclic antidepressants (TCAs) produce a response in greater than 50% of patients. Usually, a therapeutic course of 10 to 20 days is needed before improvements are apparent. Once the acute phase has subsided, the patient should continue to take the drug for 6 to 12 months to reduce risk of relapse. TCAs have anticholinergic (blocking the neurotransmitter acetylcholine) side effects, which can decrease urinary urgency; therefore TCAs may be used in children with bed-wetting problems. Table 7.3 lists the most commonly used cyclic antidepressants. Table 7.4 lists the anticholinergic and sedative properties of antidepressants.

The TCAs can be cardiotoxic in high doses, and this primary side effect needs to be monitored. Patients (particularly the elderly) may experience postural hypotension (a blood pressure decrease) of 20 mm Hg; arrhythmias and central nervous system (CNS) toxicity (in overdose) may also occur. Deaths have occurred from these cardiac arrhythmias. Treatment should begin with a low dose, increased as needed to attain a response. Sedation (calming or causing drowsiness), another side effect, occurs especially in the first few days and may last several weeks; however, most patients become tolerant to this effect. It is usually prudent to advise the patient to take these drugs at bedtime. Dry mouth, blurred vision, constipation, and urinary retention (an anticholinergic effect) may all resolve within a few weeks. Patients also need to avoid prolonged sun exposure.

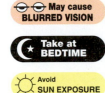

TABLE 7.2 Most Commonly Used Serotonin and Norepinephrine Reuptake Inhibitors

Generic Name	Pronunciation	Dosage Form	Brand Name	Dispensing Status
desvenlafaxine	des-ven-la-FAX-een	tablet	Pristiq	Rx
duloxetine	doo-LOX-a-teen	capsule	Cymbalta	Rx
venlafaxine	ven-la-FAX-een	capsule, tablet	Effexor	Rx

TABLE 7.3 Most Commonly Used Cyclic Antidepressants

Generic Name	Pronunciation	Dosage Form	Brand Name	Dispensing Status
Tricyclic Antidepressants (TCAs)				
amitriptyline	a-mee-TRIP-ti-leen	injection, tablet	Elavil	Rx
clomipramine	cloe-MIP-ra-meen	capsule	Anafranil	Rx
desipramine	des-IP-ra-meen	tablet	Norpramin	Rx
doxepin	DOX-e-pin	capsule, cream, oral liquid	Sinequan, Zonalon	Rx
imipramine	im-IP-ra-meen	capsule	Tofranil	Rx
nortriptyline	nor-TRIP-ti-leen	capsule, oral liquid	Aventyl, Pamelor	Rx
protriptyline	proe-TRIP-ti-leen	tablet	Vivactil	Rx
trimipramine	trye-MIP-ra-meen	capsule	Surmontil	Rx
Tetracyclic Antidepressants				
maprotiline	ma-PROE-ti-leen	tablet	Ludiomil	Rx
mirtazapine	meer-TAZ-a-peen	tablet	Remeron	Rx

TABLE 7.4   Anticholinergic and Sedative Properties of Common Antidepressants

Generic Name	Properties	
	Anticholinergic	Sedative
amitriptyline	+ + + + +	+ + + +
bupropion	–	–
citalopram	–	–
clomipramine	+ + + +	+ + + +
desipramine	+ +	+ +
doxepin	+ + +	+ + + +
duloxetine	–	+
escitalopram	–	–

Note: The greater the number of + signs, the stronger the property.

Tricyclic Antidepressants **Doxepin (Sinequan, Zonalon)** has some unusual dosage forms. As a cream (Zonalon) it is used for pruritus (itching) in adults and the elderly. It is applied three or four times a day. The topical form should not be used for more than 8 days. The oral liquid is used by dentists as a topical for "burning mouth syndrome." The oral form is best taken at bedtime, because it does cause drowsiness. It should not be taken with carbonated beverages or grape juice because these drinks can reduce its effectiveness. Overall, doxepin is a very versatile drug.

Imipramine (Tofranil) is used primarily for nocturnal enuresis (bed wetting) in children.

Tetracyclic Antidepressants **Maprotiline** is indicated for treating depression accompanied by anxiety. Side effects are similar to those of the TCAs, and it has a high seizure potential. It may cause seizures in patients without a history of these disorders. The effects may not be felt for 3 to 6 weeks after initiation of therapy. The drug should not be discontinued abruptly.

Mirtazapine (Remeron) is used to treat mild to severe depression and is especially useful for patients who suffer from nausea. It is an alpha-2 agonist. Like other antidepressants, mirtazapine increases active levels of serotonin and norepinephrine in the synapse, but rather than blocking the reuptake of these neurotransmitters, it is thought to work by blocking receptors that normally inhibit the release of the neurotransmitters. Mirtazapine seems to have some antianxiety effects and should be taken at bedtime.

Monoamine Oxidase Inhibitors

Monoamine oxidase inhibitors (MAOIs) inhibit the activity of the enzymes that break down catecholamines (a group of neurotransmitters used by the sympathetic nervous system, including epinephrine, dopamine, and norepinephrine), thus allowing these transmitters to build up in the synapse. MAOIs are a second-line treatment because of their many interactions with foods and other drugs, but they may be effective for certain patients. These drugs are most beneficial in atypical depression. They are similar in efficacy and adverse effects to TCAs, but they are not as cardiotoxic and may offer some advantages to patients with angina and cardiac conduction defects. At present they are primarily used to treat conditions other than depression. Table 7.5 lists the most commonly used MAOIs.

When dispensing any of these drugs, the pharmacist should check the patient profile for interactions with other drugs. If a patient is taking an MAOI and the physician changes to another class of antidepressant, the patient must wait at least 2 weeks for the MAOI to clear the system (washout period) before starting the second drug. MAOIs generally cause weight gain and edema.

Severe hypertensive reactions have occurred when an MAOI has been taken with food containing a high level of tyramine (a compound that occurs in aged cheese and many meats and vegetables). The clinical result is sudden onset of a painful, throbbing, occipital headache; if severe, the condition may progress to severe hypertension, profuse sweating, pallor, palpitation, and occasionally death.

In addition to providing full disclosure on the drug prescribed, the pharmacist should give the patient detailed instructions on foods and other drugs to be avoided. Patients taking these drugs must absolutely *not* ingest aged cheeses, concentrated yeast extracts, pickled fish, sauerkraut, or broad bean pods because of the high levels of tyramine in these foods. Severe interactions may also occur when someone taking an MAOI takes amphetamine, ephedrine, levodopa, meperidine, or methylphenidate.

Selegiline (Eldepryl, Emsam) is primarily used in Parkinson disease as an adjunct in the management of patients in whom levodopa/carbidopa therapy is becoming ineffective. There is some use of selegiline in Alzheimer disease as well. Selegiline can be administered either orally or as a patch. The patch has some distinct advantages over the the oral form. For example, with the patch selegiline bypasses first-pass metabolism, which allows it to reach higher levels in the CNS compared with oral administration. Even though administration as a patch presents less potential for food interactions, patients still need to watch their diet. Patches are available in boxes of 30. A patch should be applied immediately upon removal from the sealed packet; applied to dry, intact skin on the upper body; and worn for 24 hours. Because of serotonin syndrome, this drug should not be given with other antidepressants. The patch should increase compliance.

Other Antidepressant Drugs

Table 7.6 presents the most commonly used antidepressant medications that do not fit into the previously discussed groups.

Bupropion (Wellbutrin, Zyban) is a dopamine-uptake inhibitor with no direct effect on serotonin or monoamine oxidase, and it does not present anticholinergic, antihistaminic, or adrenergic effects. Bupropion has also been approved as an aid to smoking cessation as well as for seasonal affective disorder. The maximum daily dose

TABLE 7.5 Most Commonly Used Monoamine Oxidase Inhibitors (MAOIs)

Generic Name	Pronunciation	Dosage Form	Brand Name	Dispensing Status
phenelzine	FEN-el-zeen	tablet	Nardil	Rx
selegiline	seh-LEDGE-i-leen	capsule, patch, tablet	Eldepryl, Emsam	Rx
tranylcypromine	tran-il-SIP-roe-meen	tablet	Parnate	Rx

TABLE 7.6   Most Commonly Used Miscellaneous Antidepressant Drugs

Generic Name	Pronunciation	Dosage Form	Brand Name	Dispensing Status
bupropion	byoo-PROE-pee-on	tablet	Wellbutrin, Zyban	Rx
nefazodone	nef-AY-zoe-done	tablet		Rx
trazodone	TRAZ-oh-done	tablet	Desyrel	Rx

should not exceed 450 mg. It may take 3 to 4 weeks for the full effects to be realized. The drug should not be discontinued abruptly. It causes less erectile dysfunction than other antidepressants. Bupropion is manufactured in several forms, which can cause confusion for the technician. At times it is difficult to determine which form the prescriber intended. Forms of bupropion, together with daily dosing rates, include the following:

- Wellbutrin, three times a day
- Wellbutrin SR, twice a day
- Wellbutrin XL, once per day

Budepion SR is a sustained version of bupropion, like Wellbutrin SR, so it is dosed twice a day. Zyban for smoking cessation is initiated at once a day for 3 days then twice a day for 7 to 12 weeks.

You may get a prescription for this drug written in any of these forms. The dosing is the clue as to which drug you will need to dispense. When in doubt, always clarify the form and dosage with the prescriber.

Bupropion has negligible anticholinergic and andrenergic effects. It does not cause sedation, blood pressure effects, or electrocardiographic (ECG) changes. Effects that may occur are headache, impairment of cognitive skills, nausea and vomiting, dry mouth, constipation, seizures, and impotence. There is significant interaction between bupropion and haloperidol, MAOIs, or trazodone.

Nefazodone is closely related to trazodone. The brand Serzone was voluntarily removed from the market by the manufacturer because of the possibility of causing severe liver damage. The generic is still being manufactured and has experienced a modest resurgence in sales because it is approved for PTSD, which, as discussed earlier, has received more attention over the last several years.

Trazodone (Desyrel) exerts its effect by preventing the reuptake of serotonin and norepinephrine. It is a serotonin inhibitor/antagonist, which means it works slightly differently from the SNRIs. It has a much better side effect profile than the TCAs. It has no anticholinergic effects and no effects on cardiac conduction. It may cause orthostatic hypertension, which can be offset by taking with food. There is much concern that it might have a serious interaction with ginkgo. The drug should be given at bedtime because it can cause drowsiness. Patients should avoid alcohol and sun exposure.

Cases of abnormal penile erection **(priapism)** have been reported with trazodone; some even require surgical intervention. This makes it a drug to avoid in young males, but it is very effective in older men for the relief of depression.

Warning

Wellbutrin SR is usually dosed two times daily. Wellbutrin XL has a once-a-day dosing. Mistaking these could lead to an overdosing or underdosing.

May Cause DROWSINESS

Do not drink alcoholic beverages when taking this medication

Avoid SUN EXPOSURE

Drugs Used in Bipolar Disorders

Lithium compounds are the most commonly prescribed drugs for bipolar mood disorders; these lithium compounds are generally referred to simply as "lithium." If a patient is experiencing three or more of the following symptoms or signs of increased neurological activity, the diagnosis could be mania.

- decreased need for sleep
- distractibility
- elevated or irritable mood
- excessive involvement in pleasurable activities with a large potential for painful consequences (e.g., financial irresponsibility, sexual indiscretions, alcohol or drug abuse, or reckless driving)
- grandiose ideas
- increase in activity (socially, at work, or sexually)
- pressure to keep talking (emotional lability)
- racing thoughts

Depressive episodes are characterized by

- sadness; excessive crying
- low energy
- loss of pleasure
- difficulty concentrating
- irritability
- thoughts of death or suicide

The first episode of bipolar disorder typically occurs at about age thirty, may last several months, and usually remits spontaneously. Without treatment, however, many patients experience one or more subsequent episodes.

The objective of therapy is to treat acute episodes and prevent subsequent attacks. The specific mechanism of lithium is unknown, but it is believed to alter levels of specific brain chemicals (neurotransmitters) or cause changes in brain receptor sensitivity. Table 7.7 presents the drugs most often used to treat bipolar disorder. Antidepressants are used very carefully when a patient is in the depressive pole because they can trigger a manic episode.

Lithium (Eskalith, Lithobid) may indirectly interfere with sodium transport in nerve and muscle cells. It also affects the synthesis and storage of CNS neurotransmitters. Lithium promotes norepinephrine reuptake and increases the sensitivity of

TABLE 7.7   Most Commonly Used Drugs to Treat Bipolar Disorders

Generic Name	Pronunciation	Dosage Form	Brand Name	Dispensing Status
carbamazepine	kar-ba-MAZ-e-peen	capsule, oral liquid, tablet	Epitol, Tegretol	Rx
divalproex	dye-VAL-pro-ex	capsule, tablet	Depakote	Rx
lithium	LITH-ee-um	capsule, oral liquid, tablet	Eskalith, Lithobid	Rx
olanzapine-fluoxetine	oh-LAN-za-peen floo-OX-e-teen	capsule	Symbyax	Rx
valproic acid	val-PRO-ik AS-id	capsule, IV, oral liquid	Depakene	Rx

serotonin receptors. The usual dosage of lithium is 300 mg, two to three times daily. Therapeutic blood levels are usually attained within 5 to 10 days after the start of therapy. Levels of 0.6 to 0.8 mEq/L are effective for most patients. To avoid toxicity, the patient must have blood tests regularly and take the medication at a specific time. Even if the patient is taking a therapeutic dosage, a slight tremor, especially of the hands, may occur. Salt intake should remain constant during treatment because it can affect lithium blood levels. Alcohol intake increases the potential for toxicity.

Lithium is the drug of choice for treating bipolar (manic-depressive) disorder and acute mania, and for prophylaxis of unipolar and bipolar disorders. An antipsychotic agent may be added initially to the regimen to control the hostility and agitation that sometimes accompany mania. When the blood level of lithium reaches therapeutic levels, the antipsychotic can be discontinued. Lithium is the only mood stabilizer that has consistently been shown to decrease the risk of suicide for bipolar patients.

Carbamazepine (Epitol, Tegretol) affects the sodium channels that regulate nerve cells. This drug is indicated in bipolar disorder and is also used as an anticonvulsant. It is considered a second-line treatment to lithium and is used for patients who do not respond to lithium or cannot tolerate its side effects. It produces a response in a majority of manic patients within 10 days. Side effects, which may be alleviated by briefly decreasing the dose to slow the rate of accumulation in the blood, include dizziness, ataxia (irregularity of muscular action), clumsiness, slurred speech, double vision, and drowsiness.

Divalproex (Depakote) and **valproic acid (Depakene)**, referred to as *valproates*, are particularly effective in patients with rapid changes of mood (rapid cyclers) and the elderly. They also work well as an adjunct to lithium and may replace lithium for some of these patients. They should be taken with food or milk but not with carbonated drinks. Sore throat, fever, fatigue, bleeding, or bruising should be reported to the physician. These are symptoms of thrombocytopenia (decrease in the number of platelets), which can be a side effect of these drugs. Valproates may also cause drowsiness and impair judgment or coordination.

Olanzapine-fluoxetine (Symbyax) is an approved treatment for bipolar disorder. A combination drug, olanzapine-fluoxetine helps with the depression in bipolar disorder and does not seem to increase mania. It is available in different dosage combinations. The drug should be taken at night and may cause drowsiness, sexual dysfunction, hyperglycemia, and orthostatic hypotension.

Psychosis

The primary indication for using **antipsychotic** drugs (or **neuroleptic** drugs, as they are sometimes called) is **schizophrenia**. Schizophrenia is a chronic psychotic disorder manifested by retreat from reality, delusions, hallucinations, ambivalence, withdrawal, and bizarre or regressive behavior.

Dopamine and, to a lesser degree, serotonin are the major neurotransmitters implicated in schizophrenia. Dopamine receptors occur in four pathways: the limbic system (nerve fibers surrounding the upper brain stem), which controls emotions; the frontal cortex, which controls thought, learning, and memory; the basal ganglia, which affect control of voluntary muscle movement; and the pathway for the release of the hormone prolactin, which can cause sexual dysfunction. The first of these four pathways, involving the limbic system, is the one responsible for psychotic experiences when dopamine levels are excessive. The "older" or "typical" antipsychotic drugs antagonize dopamine receptors in all four of the dopamine pathways, leading to negative side effects. In particular, drug action in the pathway involving the basal ganglia causes muscle control problems, referred to as **extrapyramidal symptoms**.

After the turn of the twenty-first century, some important improvements were made in the development of antipsychotic agents to improve efficacy and reduce negative side effects. The "new" or "atypical" antipsychotic medications are designed to limit dopamine-blocking ability to the limbic system pathway rather than all four pathways. The atypical agents are now considered the first-line agents.

Antipsychotic drugs are chosen on the basis of cost, limited adverse effects, and a patient's response history. Drugs do not alter the natural course of schizophrenia. They do reduce symptoms such as thought disorders, hallucinations, and delusions, but rarely eliminate them. Symptoms such as emotional and social withdrawal, ambivalence (conflicting emotional attitudes), and poor self-care usually do not respond to drug treatment. Most therapeutic gains occur in the first 6 weeks, but maximum response may take up to 12 to 18 weeks. Discontinuation of these drugs leads to relapse of symptoms. Evidence shows that drug therapy does not reverse memory impairment, confusion, or intellectual deterioration.

Typical Antipsychotic Medications

Table 7.8 lists the typical antipsychotic medications that are most frequently prescribed. In low doses, **prochlorperazine (Compazine)** is commonly used as an antiemetic. In high doses, however, it can be used as an antipsychotic. It is rarely prescribed this way, but in unusual circumstances it can occur, so the technician needs to be aware of this usage of this drug. The only antipsychotic drug that has a ceiling dose is **thioridazine**, which should not exceed 800 mg per day because abnormal pigment deposits in the retina may result in blindness.

These older agents are identified as "typical" or "first generation" antipsychotics and are effective, but serious long-term side effects limit their use. Prescribers are avoiding these drugs and moving toward the newer "atypical" antipsychotics, described in a later section.

TABLE 7.8   Most Commonly Used Typical Antipsychotic Drugs

Generic Name	Pronunciation	Dosage Form	Brand Name	Dispensing Status
fluphenazine	floo-FEN-a-zeen	injection, tablet	Prolixin	Rx
haloperidol	hal-oe-PAIR-i-dawl	injection, oral liquid, tablet	Haldol	Rx
loxapine	LOX-a-peen	capsule, oral liquid	Loxitane	Rx
molindone	moe-LIN-done	oral liquid, tablet	Moban	Rx
perphenazine	per-FEN-a-zeen	injection, oral liquid, tablet	Trilafon	Rx
prochlorperazine	proe-klor-PAIR-a-zeen	capsule, injection, oral liquid, suppository, tablet	Compazine	Rx
thioridazine	thye-oh-RID-a-zeen	oral liquid, tablet		Rx
thiothixene	thye-oh-THIX-een	capsule, injection, oral liquid	Navane	Rx
trifluoperazine	trye-floo-oh-PAIR-a-zeen	injection, oral liquid, tablet	Stelazine	Rx

Side Effects of Antipsychotic Drugs

Side effects of antipsychotic drugs run the gamut from minor annoyances to serious problems that may not be reversible. Sedation that lasts as long as 2 weeks is a common side effect. Tolerance develops, which is minimized by administering the total daily dose at bedtime. The patient may experience the following side effects.

- **Anticholinergic** Dryness of the mouth, eyes, and throat; blurred vision; and constipation. Problems occur at the beginning of treatment, but tolerance develops.
- **Cardiovascular** Postural hypotension and increase in pulse rate of about 20 bpm (beats per minute) with a change in position. These events may cause fainting or falling, most often in the elderly.
- **Dermatologic** Excessive tanning or burning and a steely gray appearance to the skin after years of therapy, due to drug accumulation in melanocytes. With increased usage of the newer drugs, this effect is becoming rare.
- **Endocrine** Hyperglycemia (high blood sugar), lack of menses, lactation in nonpregnant females, breast enlargement in males, change in sex function and drive (females, increases; males, decreases). Patients on antipsychotics should be monitored closely for weight gain, development of diabetes, and an increase in cholesterol levels.
- **Hematologic** Some reversible or nonreversible bone marrow depression.
- **Ophthalmologic** Deposit of melanin-drug complex in lens and retina, resulting in blindness.
- **Withdrawal** Relapse.
- **Neurologic** Extrapyramidal side effects due to an imbalance of cholinergic and dopaminergic transmitters. Dopaminergic blockade results in excessive cholinergic effects. Coadministration of anticholinergic drugs can balance out some of these. Side effects develop in 40% to 60% of patients, with early-onset symptoms developing within the first 4 weeks.

The following muscle coordination conditions develop from the cholinergic and dopaminergic imbalance as early-onset symptoms.

- **Dystonia** Involuntary tonic contraction of skeletal muscles, mostly of the head, face, and shoulders. The tongue may protrude, and the patient experiences difficulty talking and swallowing.
- **Akathisia** Motor restlessness. Patients complain that they are unable to sit or stand still and that they feel a compulsion to pace. Feelings of apprehension, irritability, and uneasiness may also appear. While standing, the patient may rock to and fro or shift weight from one leg to the other. This occurs most frequently in the middle-aged, especially women.
- **Pseudoparkinsonism** Tremor, rigidity, and slow movement; apathy with little facial expression; difficulty in walking or a shuffling gait; and drooling. The treatment is reducing the dose, changing to an agent less likely to produce extrapyramidal side effects, or giving anticholinergics.

Late-onset neurologic side effects occur after 6 months of treatment. **Tardive dyskinesia** involves involuntary movements of the mouth, lips, and tongue that are sometimes accompanied by involuntary movements of the limbs or trunk. These actions are made worse by emotional upsets but disappear during sleep. Onset can be insidious and often occurs while the patient is taking the drug. The condition is potentially irreversible, even if the drug is discontinued. Drug withdrawal reveals the presence and severity of tardive dyskinesia. Once tardive dyskinesia appears, it is rarely progressive and usually either becomes static or slows, improving gradually over weeks or months. Currently, there is no satisfactory treatment. Anticholinergics make the condition worse.

Table 7.9 lists drugs that are commonly used to minimize the side effects of antipsychotic medications. **Benztropine (Cogentin)** is an anticholinergic that may produce an immediate, but not necessarily complete, response to excess muscle activity resulting from antipsychotic administration. **Meclizine (Antivert)** and **diphenhydramine (Benadryl)** are antihistamines.

Atypical Antipsychotic Drugs

Although atypical antipsychotic agents are much better tolerated than the older agents, they are associated with metabolic side effects such as weight gain, hyperglycemia, new-onset diabetes, and dyslipidemia. The most commonly prescribed atypical antipsychotic medications are listed in Table 7.10 and briefly discussed below.

Aripiprazole (Abilify) is a dopamine system stabilizer. Whereas antipsychotic medications such as haloperidol (Haldol) typically are dopamine receptor antagonists, this atypical antipsychotic blocks both dopamine and serotonin receptors. Unlike typical antipsychotic agents, it has the potential to act differently in different parts of the brain depending on endogenous dopamine activity. Also, unlike some atypical antipsychotics, aripiprazole does not prolong the **QT interval** (the time between depolarization and repolarization of the ventricles of the heart during a heartbeat), and it may cause less weight gain than typical antipsychotic drugs. This could make it

TABLE 7.9 Most Commonly Used Drugs to Minimize the Side Effects of Antipsychotic Drugs

Generic Name	Pronunciation	Dosage Form	Brand Name	Dispensing Status
benztropine	BENZ-troe-peen	injection, IV, tablet	Cogentin	Rx
diphenhydramine	dye-fen-HYE-dra-meen	capsule, injection, IV, oral liquid, tablet	Benadryl	OTC, Rx
meclizine	MEK-li-zeen	tablet	Antivert	OTC

TABLE 7.10 Most Commonly Used Atypical Antipsychotic Drugs

Generic Name	Pronunciation	Dosage Form	Brand Name	Dispensing Status
aripiprazole	air-i-PIP-ra-zole	tablet	Abilify	Rx
clozapine	KLOE-za-peen	tablet	Clozaril	Rx
olanzapine	oh-LAN-za-peen	injection, tablet	Zyprexa	Rx
paliperidone	pal-ee-PAIR-i-done	tablet	Invega	Rx
quetiapine	kwe-TYE-a-peen	tablet	Seroquel	Rx
risperidone	ris-PAIR-i-done	oral liquid, tablet	Risperdal	Rx
ziprasidone	zi-PRAS-i-done	capsule, injection	Geodon	Rx

a significant option for treatment of schizophrenia. It is thought that this drug improves dopamine activity and modulates motor function and prolactin secretion. It has a low risk of motor and other side effects. This drug is used primarily for bipolar disorder but has also received approval for major depressive disorder.

Clozapine (Clozaril), a weak blocker of D_1 and D_2 dopamine receptors, is indicated for managing schizophrenic patients. It also blocks some serotonin, alpha-adrenergic, and histamine CNS receptors. Its most serious side effect is a reduction in white blood cells, for which it carries a Black Box warning. Leukocyte counts should be obtained weekly for the duration of therapy. Frequent blood samples *must* be taken and the results documented by the pharmacy. Before the drug is dispensed, the pharmacy must receive blood work reports, and the technician must document that the white blood count (WBC) is greater than 3500/mm³ and that the absolute neutrophil count (ANC) is greater than 2000/mm³. The patient should report any lethargy, fever, sore throat, flulike symptoms, or indications of infection. However, medication should not be stopped abruptly.

Olanzapine (Zyprexa) is used for schizophrenia. Like clozapine and risperidone, olanzapine blocks dopamine and serotonin receptors, but it causes fewer movement disorders and is more effective than either drug. It does not affect white blood cells as clozapine does, so frequent blood monitoring is not necessary with olanzapine. Side effects are dizziness, drowsiness, constipation, dry mouth, and weight gain. Patients *must* avoid alcohol. This drug appears to help patients by decreasing distorted thinking or obsessive-compulsive behavior concerning food. It helps patients respond better to behavioral therapy. It can be used for either anorexia nervosa or weight gain.

Paliperidone (Invega) is an active metabolite of risperidone. It is used in the treatment of schizophrenia. Paliperidone works as well as risperidone, but with fewer side effects. It is a sustained release tablet and is dosed once a day. There are few interactions with other drugs, because it is not extensively metabolized in the liver. Advantages of paliperidone include low weight gain, fewer extrapyramidal symptoms, and significant efficacy in the treatment of schizophrenia. Invega uses an extended release technology called **OROS** (osmotic-controlled release oral delivery system), in which the drug dissolves through pores in the tablet shell; when empty, the tablet shell, known as a **ghost,** is excreted in the stool. These tablets must not be crushed or broken. It is recommended the drug be taken in the morning. One side effect of paliperidone that needs to be monitored is orthostatic hypotension.

Quetiapine (Seroquel) is structurally related to clozapine but has a lower incidence of the hematologic toxicities associated with clozapine.

Risperidone (Risperdal) is a mixed serotonin-dopamine antagonist. It binds to serotonin receptors in the CNS and the peripheral nervous system with a very high affinity and binds to dopamine receptors with less affinity. The binding of serotonin receptors and dopamine receptors is thought to improve negative symptoms of psychosis and reduce the incidence of extrapyramidal side effects. Risperidone is indicated for the management of psychotic disorders (e.g., schizophrenia) and dementia in the elderly. Furthermore, it is the first drug that has been approved for **autism,** a disorder, first exhibited in childhood, characterized by repetitive behavior and lack of ability for social interaction and communication; when combined with mental retardation, autism can be expressed through mood swings, irritability, tantrums, aggression, and self-injury, and the medication can be used to treat these symptoms. The primary side effects of risperidone are hypotension, sedation, and anxiety. There is a significant interaction with paroxetine (Paxil).

Ziprasidone (Geodon), which is used for schizophrenia, causes less weight gain than other antipsychotic agents. This is an important advantage, because for most

Warning

Clozaril and Clinoril (sulindac, a medication for rheumatoid arthritis pain) can be confused.

Warning

Zyprexa looks and sounds like Zyrtec (antiallergy medication); be careful in dispensing.

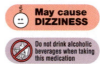

antipsychotics, weight gain is often the reason that patients quit taking their medication. The major problem with ziprasidone is that it prolongs the QT interval, which may lead to arrhythmia and death. Ziprasidone can be given intramuscularly.

Anxiety

Anxiety is a state of uneasiness characterized by apprehension and worry about possible events. Anxiety is a common complaint made to physicians. It is a collection of unpleasant feelings identical to the fearful feelings experienced under conditions of actual danger. The patient feels generalized tension and apprehension and startles easily. Other symptoms include uneasiness and nervousness at work or with people or vague, nagging uncertainty about the future, which may lead to chronic fatigue, headaches, and insomnia.

Exogenous anxiety (anxiety caused by factors outside the organism) develops in response to external stresses. The response may be appropriate if conditions warrant apprehension and fear.

Endogenous anxiety (anxiety caused by factors within the organism) is not related to any identifiable external factors but occurs spontaneously as a result of a defined abnormality in cellular function in the CNS. The most common way that people deal with anxiety is by consumption of alcohol. Excessive use of alcohol is common in patients with anxiety.

Antianxiety Agents

Antianxiety agents (also called sedatives) include both noncontrolled and controlled substances (see Table 7.11). The most commonly used antianxiety drugs are the benzodiazepines, which are also effective in insomnia, panic disorders, alcohol withdrawal syndrome, convulsive disorders, and muscle spasms. When used short term, they can be effective in controlling anxiety. They are used in the lowest possible doses that control the symptoms while minimizing side effects.

Patients taking antianxiety drugs should be monitored closely for onset of depression, which occurs in about one-third of cases. Patients who discontinue medication have a high rate of relapse. The drug must be tapered to avoid withdrawal reactions.

Benzodiazepines may cause physical or psychological dependence, or both. **Alprazolam (Xanax)**, **lorazepam (Ativan)**, and **oxazepam (Serax)** produce no active metabolites and thus do not have prolonged effects. Patients should understand that continued dosing may cause physical dependence and that stopping the drug abruptly may result in withdrawal side effects. The onset of withdrawal usually occurs 1 to 2 days after discontinuing the drug.

Among the side effects of the benzodiazepines are

- dependence if duration of therapy exceeds 3 months (in general, a patient should not remain on the drug more than 6 months)
- drug accumulation during multiple dosing (fat-soluble)
- link to birth defects if taken early in pregnancy
- muscle relaxation, reduced muscle coordination, impaired reflexes
- paradoxical (at variance with the normal rule) excitement (hostility, rage, destructive behavior)
- sedation

TABLE 7.11   Most Commonly Used Antianxiety Agents

Generic Name	Pronunciation	Dosage Form	Brand Name	Dispensing Status	Control Schedule
amoxapine (TCA)	a-MOX-a-peen	tablet	(none)	Rx	
buspirone (azapirone)	byoo-SPYE-rone	tablet	BuSpar	Rx	
hydroxyzine (antihistamine)	hye-DROX-i-zeen	capsule, injection, oral liquid	Vistaril	Rx	
meprobamate	me-proe-BAM-ate	tablet	Miltown	Rx	C-IV
paroxetine (SSRI)	pa-ROX-e-teen	oral liquid, tablet	Paxil	Rx	
propranolol (beta blocker)	proe-PRAN-oh-lawl	capsule, IV, oral liquid, tablet	Inderal	Rx	
trifluoperazine (antipsychotic)	trye-floo-oh-PAIR-a-zeen	injection, oral liquid, tablet	Stelazine	Rx	
venlafaxine (azapirone SNRI)	ven-la-FAX-een	capsule, tablet	Effexor	Rx	
Benzodiazepines					
alprazolam	al-PRAZ-oh-lam	oral liquid, tablet	Xanax	Rx	C-IV
chlordiazepoxide	klor-dye-az-e-POX-ide	capsule	Librium	Rx	C-IV
clorazepate	klor-AZ-e-pate	tablet	Tranxene	Rx	C-IV
diazepam	dye-AZ-e-pam	injection, IV, oral liquid, tablet	Valium	Rx	C-IV
lorazepam	lor-AZ-e-pam	injection, IV, oral liquid, tablet	Ativan	Rx	C-IV
oxazepam	ox-AZ-e-pam	capsule, tablet	Serax	Rx	C-IV

Propranolol (Inderal) is a nonspecific beta blocker widely used to treat the physical symptoms of anxiety but currently is not approved for that indication. It reduces heart rate and thereby decreases nervousness due to stage fright or test anxiety. It is useful for tremors in these situations.

Hydroxyzine Pamoate (Vistaril), used for some anxious patients, has sedating qualities and is widely used as a preoperative sedative and sleeping pill. This drug is thought to depress subcortical areas of the CNS. (Hydroxyzine chloride – Atarax is used for itching.)

Warning

Vistaril and Zestril (lisinopril, antihypertensive) are easily mistaken for each other.

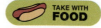
TAKE WITH FOOD

Buspirone (BuSpar) acts by selectively antagonizing serotonin receptors without affecting the receptors for benzodiazepine and gamma-aminobutyric acid (GABA). Buspirone should be taken with food, and the patient should report any changes in the senses (hearing, smell, or taste). It takes about 2 weeks to see the full effect of this drug. It has few side effects; nausea and headache are the most common. Buspirone has shown little potential for abuse. It is also used for depression.

Venlafaxine (Effexor), described earlier as a serotonin and norepinephrine reuptake inhibitor, is also considered a first-line treatment for anxiety. It is structurally related to buspirone (BuSpar). When used as an antidepressant, it has been shown to decrease anxiety. It is not sedating and has minimal if any impact on psychomotor

Warning

Buspirone and bupropion are frequently confused when not clearly written out.

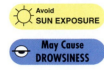

Avoid SUN EXPOSURE

May Cause DROWSINESS

function and is not associated with tolerance or dependence. It does take several weeks to become fully effective.

Trifluoperazine (Stelazine) has been effective in treating nonpsychotic anxiety. It has a high potential for pseudoparkinsonism, dystonias (impairment of muscular tonus), and tardive dyskinesia, so it is usually given with an antihistamine or benztropine. It blocks dopaminergic receptors. Therapy requires several weeks before the full effects can be seen. The patient should avoid sunlight.

Meprobamate (Miltown), when used as an anxiety agent, acts primarily on the hypothalamus, thalamus, limbic system, and spinal cord. Meprobamate also has value in treating muscle rigidity and contractions. Sedation is the primary side effect.

Panic Disorders

Panic is a form of intense, overwhelming, and uncontrollable anxiety. It is neither a voluntary, controllable emotion nor a condition that can be avoided by ignoring it or wishing it away.

Panic attacks have a definite onset and end spontaneously. They occur in public or at home, sometimes interrupting sleep. They are characterized by a sense of fear, apprehension, a premonition of serious illness, and fear of a life-threatening attack. The criteria for diagnosis are three attacks in a three-week period, not stimulated by physical exertion, life-threatening situations, or exposure to phobic stimulus, and at least four of the following symptoms: dyspnea (labored breathing), palpitations, chest pain or discomfort, choking sensation, dizziness, feelings of unreality, tingling in hands or feet, hot or cold flashes, sweating, numbness, and trembling.

Pathophysiology of Panic Disorders Panic disorders appear to result from a neurochemical defect in part of the brain. In some persons, the brain stem functions abnormally. This abnormality, often characterized by progressive oversensitivity, can develop at any age and occurs in the *locus caeruleus*, a group of synapses in the brain stem at the level of the pons and medulla. The locus coeruleus determines the organism's level of arousal. Sensory information that arrives from all parts of the body passes through this major neurologic junction before being distributed to other parts of the brain. If an abnormality occurs in the locus coeruleus, incoming signals are affected, depending on both the current state of the organism and the nature of the arriving messages. If incoming messages are inappropriately amplified to signal a life-threatening stress, the organism is aroused to defense or flight. Excessive amplification of incoming messages gives rise to a state of excessive arousal, excessive autonomic discharges, and increased respiratory drive. If the incoming message is calm and nonthreatening, the stimuli are toned down, and the locus does not overreact.

Panic patients are unusually sensitive to the stimulant effects of low doses of caffeine and sodium lactate that, when infused, alter intracellular pH and increase impulse transmission through the brain, causing panic symptoms.

Treatment of Panic Disorders A panic attack is postulated to be of neurochemical origin and has both emotional and physical components. Antianxiety and psychotherapeutic measures have proved inadequate because neither type of drug restores normal neurochemical function to the locus coeruleus. The most successful treatment combines antipanic medication and behavioral therapy.

Psychotherapy is the preferred treatment in panic disorders for patients whose symptoms cause significant discomfort or impairment. Panic disorders have a true biochemical basis and can be effectively treated. These disorders should be viewed with the same objectivity as other chronic, incurable, but drug-controllable diseases.

Short-term administration of an antianxiety agent may be indicated. Drug therapy blocks the autonomic expression of the panic. The benzodiazepines, buspirone, and, to a lesser extent, the beta-adrenergic blocking agents are the most appropriate pharmacologic alternatives. Diphenhydramine, hydroxyzine, and other antihistamines are sometimes prescribed, especially for elderly patients. The TCA imipramine (Tofranil) has also proved effective.

Sleep and Sleep Disorders

Sleep is fundamental to human health (as well as for all mammals and many other vertebrates). Sleep research has recognized four stages of sleep:

- Stage I involves nonrapid eye movements (NREM). The subject is somewhat aware of his or her surroundings and is relaxed (4% to 5% of sleep time).
- Stage II also involves NREM. The subject is unaware of surroundings but can be easily awakened (50% of sleep time).
- Stages III and IV involve rapid eye movements (REM). The subject's sleep is characterized by increased autonomic activity and by episodes of REM sleep with dreaming, if possible. This deep sleep (20 to 25% of sleep time), which occurs four to five times per night (for a total of >90 minutes), is important to physical rest.

Many adults have trouble sleeping. Approximately 6% seek a physician's help. **Insomnia** is characterized by difficulty falling or staying asleep, or not feeling refreshed on awakening. The symptoms of insomnia are indications for using a **hypnotic** (a drug that induces sleep).

Insomnia may be a chronic condition or an occasional or short-term problem. Transient insomnia is not really a sleep disorder. It is usually a response to an acute stressful event and can normally be expected to improve with time as the person adapts to the stress. Chronic insomnia is most often of multifaceted origin. The first evaluation of patients should include sleep, drug, medical, and psychiatric histories.

Some types of sleep disorders can be caused by various events or conditions. The causes can be

- situational: job stress, hospitalization, or travel
- medical: pain, respiratory problems, or GI problems
- psychiatric: schizophrenia, depression, or mania
- drug induced: alcohol, caffeine, or sympathomimetic agents

In these cases, diagnosis and effective treatment of the cause can usually eliminate the need for using hypnotic drugs. Treating only the symptoms of insomnia can make it difficult to recognize and treat the underlying illness. Furthermore, it can subject patients to potentially habitual or physical dependence on the drugs.

Narcolepsy

Narcolepsy is a sleep disorder involving recurring inappropriate episodes of sleep during the daytime hours. There is no known cause. Onset usually occurs in adolescents or young adults, and this disorder continues throughout life. It occurs four times more frequently in men than women. Narcolepsy exhibits four characteristic symptoms. First, the patient feels sleepy during the daytime, proceeding almost immediately into REM sleep without first entering NREM. The desire to sleep can be resisted only briefly. Second, the patient experiences **cataplexy**, or short periods of muscle weakness or loss of muscle tone, associated with sudden emotions such as joy, fear, or anger. Third, sleep paralysis occurs as the patient falls asleep or immediately upon awakening. The patient wishes to move but finds that, for a brief period, he or she cannot. Fourth, the patient has very vivid hallucinations at the onset of sleep.

Therapeutic approaches include drug and nondrug therapy. Nondrug therapy includes lifestyle changes to establish a consistent sleep schedule, avoidance of shift work, and especially avoidance of alcohol. Stimulants such as methylphenidate and dextroamphetamine have been the drug therapy mainstay for sleepiness. (These drugs will be discussed in Chapter 8.) Tricyclic antidepressants and SSRIs work well with cataplexy. Two drugs specifically approved for narcolepsy are listed in Table 7.12.

One drug approved for narcolepsy is **modafinil (Provigil).** It is a nonamphetamine stimulant, but it is a Schedule IV controlled substance. Modafinil is also approved for shift-work disorder, which is a disturbance in the circadian rhythm (bodily cycles that occur within a 24 hour period at about the same time each day) and is a response to changes in exposure to light and dark. These problems affect people who work at night. Modafinil is currently being evaluated for attention-deficit hyperactivity disorder (ADHD) and situations where extended alertness is critical, such as for flight crews. The mechanism of action is unclear, but it does increase mental alertness.

Armodafinil (Nuvigil) is structurally related to modafinil. It is approved for excessive sleepiness caused by sleep apnea, narcolepsy, or shift-work sleep disorder. The mechanism of action is unknown. Armodafinil should be taken in the morning or 1 hour before going to work if taken for shift-work sleep disorder. It will not cure sleep apnea, but it will help diminish the symptoms. Armodafinil should not be taken close to the time of sleep and should not be taken for longer than 12 weeks. When prescribed to treat sleep apnea, armodafinil is commonly combined with a continuous positive airway pressure (CPAP) machine. This CPAP machine consists of an air pump, connected to a mask, that blows pressurized air into the nose while sleeping. It does not interrupt normal sleep patterns. The most serious side effect of armodafinil is a skin rash. If a rash appears, the patient should immediately stop taking armodafinil. Since the drug works on the central nervous system, alcohol should be avoided while taking this drug. Armodafinil should never be used in place of getting enough sleep, and it may decrease the effectiveness of birth control pills.

Treatment of Sleep Disorders

Effective treatment of sleep disorders necessitates both pharmacologic and nonpharmacologic measures. For patients with clearly defined insomnia, pharmacologic treatment consists primarily of the adjunctive use of hypnotics. Table 7.13 lists the most

TABLE 7.12	Drugs Used to Treat Narcolepsy					
Generic Name	Pronunciation	Dosage Form	Brand Name	Dispensing Status	Control Schedule
armodafinil	ar-moe-DAF-i-nil	tablet	Nuvigil	Rx	C-IV
modafinil	moe-DAF-i-nil	tablet	Provigil	Rx	C-IV

TABLE 7.13 Most Commonly Used Sleep Agents

Generic Name	Pronunciation	Dosage Form	Brand Name	Dispensing Status	Control Schedule
Benzodiazepines					
alprazolam	al-PRAZ-oh-lam	oral liquid, tablet	Xanax	Rx	C-IV
chlordiazepoxide	klor-dye-az-e-POX-ide	capsule	Librium	Rx	C-IV
clorazepate	klor-AZ-e-pate	tablet	Tranxene	Rx	C-IV
diazepam	dye-AZ-e-pam	injection, IV, oral liquid, tablet	Valium	Rx	C-IV
estazolam	es-TAZ-oe-lam	tablet	ProSom	Rx	C-IV
flurazepam	floo-RAZ-e-pam	capsule	Dalmane	Rx	C-IV
lorazepam	lor-AZ-e-pam	injection, IV, oral liquid, tablet	Ativan	Rx	C-IV
oxazepam	ox-AZ-e-pam	capsule, tablet	Serax	Rx	C-IV
quazepam	KWA-ze-pam	tablet	Doral	Rx	C-IV
temazepam	tem-AZ-e-pam	capsule	Restoril	Rx	C-IV
triazolam	trye-AY-zoe-lam	tablet	Halcion	Rx	C-IV
Barbiturates					
amobarbital	am-oh-BAR-bi-tal	capsule, injection, IV, tablet	Amytal	Rx	C-II
butabarbital	byoo-ta-BAR-bi-tal	oral liquid, tablet	Butisol	Rx	C-III
secobarbital	see-koe-BAR-bi-tal	capsule	Seconal	Rx	C-II
Antihistamines					
diphenhydramine	dye-fen-HYE-dra-meen	capsule, cream, injection, IV, oral liquid, tablet	Benadryl	OTC, Rx	
hydroxyzine	hye-DROX-i-zeen	capsule, injection, oral liquid, tablet	Atarax, Vistaril	Rx	
Hypnotics					
chloral hydrate	KLOR-al HYE-drate	capsule, oral liquid, suppository		Rx	C-IV
ramelteon	ra-MEL-tee-on	tablet	Rozerem	Rx	
Z hypnotics					
eszopiclone	es-zo-PIK-lone	tablet	Lunesta	Rx	C-IV
zaleplon	ZAL-e-plon	capsule	Sonata	Rx	C-IV
zolpidem	ZOLE-pi-dem	tablet	Ambien	Rx	C-IV

commonly used agents for sleep disorders, several of which are among the antianxiety medications listed in Table 7.11. Nonpharmacologic treatment includes supportive counseling and behavioral treatment. The components of this therapy are

- normalizing the sleep schedule as to bedtime and waking time
- increasing physical exercise during the daytime
- discontinuing use of alcohol as a sedative
- sleeping a total of only 7 to 8 hours in a 24 hour period
- reducing caffeine and nicotine intake
- eliminating any drug (e.g., decongestant) that could lead to insomnia

A person facing a clearly identified external stress (i.e., grief reaction) may become anxious and have difficulty sleeping. A 1 to 3 week course of treatment with a hypnotic agent may be justified in such instances. Hypnotic drugs should be used only as an adjunct to medical therapeutic measures.

Therapy with hypnotic agents decreases the time it takes to fall asleep, reduces early morning awakenings, increases total sleep, and improves quality of sleep. Three specific criteria guide the choice when prescribing a hypnotic drug.

- The agent must have low addiction and suicide potential.
- The agent must minimally alter electroencephalographic patterns (brain imaging) and not depress REM sleep.
- The agent must have minimum interaction with other drugs.

These criteria suggest use of the benzodiazepine class of drugs. The FDA has specifically approved five benzodiazepines for hypnotic use: estazolam, flurazepam, quazepam, temazepam, and triazolam.

A new class of drug called the Z hypnotics has emerged and is replacing the benzodiazepines as the preferred treatment for sleep disorders. The big advantage that these newer drugs have over benzodiazepines is that seizures do not occur if the drug therapy is abruptly discontinued, as can happen with benzodiazepines. Furthermore, Z hypnotics have relatively short half-lives and do not significantly impact REM sleep, as the other hypnotics do.

Patients should be informed of the limitations of drugs used to induce sleep. To reduce the risk of habituation and increase the duration of effectiveness, they should be taken as needed, rather than every night. It is easy to slip into the habit of taking these drugs every day, and the patient may not be able to sleep without them. Therapy should be started with a small dose, to be increased only if the initial dose is ineffective. Sleep agents are best administered 1 hour before bedtime.

The primary side effect of sleep medications (seen more often with high doses) is CNS depression, which results in dizziness, confusion, next-day drowsiness, and impaired reflexes. Some patients, particularly the elderly, may exhibit paradoxical reactions (excitation, irritability, and, occasionally, aggressive behavior). Anterograde amnesia (impaired memory for the event) may also occur after taking a hypnotic.

Below are additional comments on some of the sleep agents listed in Table 7.11.

Some barbiturates are hypnotics, including **amobarbital (Amytal)**, a Schedule II controlled substance; **butabarbital (Butisol)**, Schedule III; and **secobarbital (Seconal)**, Schedule II. Barbiturates work by depressing the sensory cortex, decreasing motor activity, altering cellular function, and producing drowsiness, sedation, and hypnosis. The Schedule IIs and Schedule IIIs are used only for short-term therapy. Use is rare because the side effect profile includes significant abuse potential, tremors, confusion, high suicide potential, and hangover.

Hydroxyzine (Atarax, Vistaril) and **diphenhydramine (Benadryl)** are both antihistamines used for sleep. The antihistamines are the safest drugs for treating insomnia. They can be given to children and the elderly, and there is no addiction. Even if patients become accustomed to taking a dose at night to help them fall asleep, they can still sleep without one if they are sufficiently tired.

Chloral hydrate, a hypnotic, has quick onset with no rebound. Dependence is a problem. It also interacts with warfarin.

Ramelteon (Rozerem) is approved for sleep onset insomnia. It is a melatonin receptor agonist, so there is no potential for abuse, and it is not a controlled substance. It is more potent than melatonin. It has not been shown to be effective in sleep maintenance disorders but just for initiating sleep. It has rapid onset and no next-day hangover.

Side effects of the Z hypnotics may include sleepwalking or eating with no recall of the events. There have also been reports of people driving (sleepdriving) with no recall of the event. The FDA is looking at these side effects and encouraging manufacturers to include these side effects in their labeling.

Patients using a hypnotic should use it only a limited number of times each week, and that use should be restricted to a 4 to 6 week period.

Eszopiclone (Lunesta) is similar to zolpidem, however the FDA has approved it for chronic insomnia. It causes an unpleasant taste, which usually disappears after a couple of weeks. The medication should be taken immediately before bedtime.

Zaleplon (Sonata), the shortest-acting hypnotic, has a duration of action of 4 hours. It can be taken in the middle of the night. Depending on when the drug is taken, there should be little leftover morning grogginess. Use should be limited to 7 to 10 days. Zaleplon has the advantage of having the lowest risk of next-day cognitive function impairment. Patients should be warned to take this drug right before going to bed and to make sure they have enough time to sleep before the drug wears off.

Zolpidem (Ambien) has the hypnotic and many of the anxiolytic properties of the benzodiazepines, but it is structurally dissimilar. It has a high affinity for the benzodiazepine receptors, especially the omega$_1$ receptors, but has reduced effects on skeletal muscle and seizure threshold. Rarely is mechanical ventilation required for an overdose. Zolpidem is used for short-term treatment of insomnia. The side effects are dizziness, headache, nausea, diarrhea, and next-day drowsiness. Like zaleplon, this drug also should not be taken for more than 10 days. The pharmacy technician should watch the prescriptions and alert the pharmacist if it is prescribed for a longer period of time. Of course, there may be exceptions. **Ambien CR** is approved for long-term use. It is a controlled release form that contains 12.5 mg, of which 10 mg is released immediately, then 2.5 mg later in the night to help maintain sleep. It prevents early awakening.

Alcoholism

The American Medical Association recognizes alcoholism as a disease that can be arrested but not cured. Alcoholism is a lifetime disease and is potentially fatal. Alcoholics are in emotional pain and use alcohol to kill that pain. Part of the nature of the disease is that alcoholics do not believe they are ill (denial). Hope for recovery lies in their ability to recognize a need for help, their desire to stop drinking, and their willingness to admit that they cannot cope with the problems by themselves.

Alcoholism is a complex genetic disease. The abuser has a different level of brain chemicals, different levels of enzymes, or altogether different enzymes that metabolize the alcohol at different rates and quantities than in nonalcoholics. Thus, genetic makeup may affect a person's chance of becoming an alcoholic.

Effects of Alcohol on Metabolism

Ethanol (alcohol) is an anesthetic. As with any anesthesia, intake of a large quantity of ethanol causes loss of consciousness. However, the margin between loss of consciousness and medullary paralysis is smaller than with general anesthesia. The emetic (vomit-inducing) action usually prevents death by preventing absorption of lethal concentrations. Most deaths from alcohol are due to aspiration of vomitus during unconsciousness.

The habitual drinker has an increased ability to metabolize ethanol rapidly, which increases tolerance. Neurons in the CNS adapt to the presence of ethanol, and the drinker learns to compensate to some extent for the depressant action.

Abuse of alcohol takes a heavy toll on many aspects of health. Heavy beer drinking may lead to the serious complication of obesity coupled with vitamin deficiency. In the later stages of alcoholism, gastritis and loss of appetite, organic brain damage, alcoholic psychosis, and dementia occur. Cirrhosis (irreversible damage) of the liver results from fatty synthesis and excessive buildup of lipid compounds.

Dependence and Withdrawal from Alcohol

Chemical dependence is the inability to control the use of some physical substance; the person is unable to stop the use or limit the amount taken. Dependence is often a physical condition that cannot be cured by willpower. A person can be chemically dependent without showing obvious signs. Symptoms of dependence are listed in Table 7.14. To resolve their problem, alcoholics must take four steps toward recovery.

1. Acknowledge the problem.
2. Limit the time spent with substance users.
3. Seek professional help.
4. Seek support from recovering alcoholics.

Abrupt withdrawal of alcohol can precipitate a variety of symptoms, some of which are serious and even life-threatening. Table 7.15 lists withdrawal symptoms. The first signs of withdrawal appear within a few hours. In mild withdrawal, symptoms may disappear in 1 to 2 days; in severe withdrawal, symptoms may last 1 to 2 weeks.

Benzodiazepines are considered the standard of care for detoxification. Their dosage must be adjusted to the needs of individual patients. Benzodiazepines will also prevent detoxification-related seizures and **delirium tremens ("DTs")**, a condition,

TABLE 7.14   Symptoms of Dependence on Alcohol
Blackouts or lapses of memory
Concerns of family, friends, and employers about the drinking
Doing things that cause regret afterwards while under the influence of alcohol
Financial or legal problems from drinking
Loss of pleasure without alcohol
Neglecting responsibilities
Trying to cut down or quit drinking but failing
Drinking alone; hiding evidence
Drinking to forget about problems
Willingness to do almost anything to get alcohol

TABLE 7.15	Alcohol Withdrawal Symptoms	
Agitation	Mental disturbances
Circulatory disturbances	Nausea and vomiting
Convulsions	Restlessness
Delirium tremens (DTs)	Sweating
Digestive disorders	Temporary suppression of REM sleep
Disorientation	Tremor
Extreme fear	Weakness
Hallucinations	

caused by cessation of alcohol consumption, in which coarse, irregular tremors are accompanied by vivid hallucinations.

Therapy may also necessitate administering a sedative, anticonvulsant, beta blocker, antipsychotic drug, or a combination of these. In addition, when an alcoholic enters a treatment program, comes to an emergency room, or is admitted into the hospital, the patient is usually given folic acid (Folvite), thiamine (B$_1$), and a multipurpose vitamin. This treatment is given because liver damage, imbalanced fluid intake, and imbalanced nutrition cause alcoholics to be deficient in vitamins, particularly the water-soluble ones.

Alcohol Antagonists

There are four drugs approved for treating alcohol dependence (see Table 7.16). Any drug regimen must be accompanied by psychosocial support.

Acamprosate (Campral), which has been shown to be moderately effective in clinical trials, is thought to work by restoring balance between neuronal excitation and neuronal inhibition. This reestablishment of balance reduces the negative effects of abstinence from alcohol and ideally diminishes the chances that a relapse of alcohol consumption is triggered. A combination of disulfiram and acamprosate may work better than either drug alone. The most common adverse effects include headache, diarrhea, flatulence, and nausea. Drug therapy should be combined with a comprehensive management program that includes psychosocial support. Acamprosate is taken three times a day, with meals—because food increases absorption. This regimen may also improve compliance and may help prevent alcohol cravings and prevents relapse. Acamprosate, however, will not treat delirium tremens.

Disulfiram (Antabuse) stops the metabolism of alcohol at the acetaldehyde stage, allowing the latter to accumulate in body tissues. When a patient on disulfiram consumes alcohol, the acetaldehyde causes violent side effects almost instantaneously. These include

- blurred vision
- confusion
- difficulty breathing
- face becoming hot and scarlet
- intense throbbing in head and neck
- chest pain
- nausea

TABLE 7.16   Most Commonly Used Alcohol Antagonists

Generic Name	Pronunciation	Dosage Form	Brand Name	Dispensing Status
acamprosate	a-kam-PROE-sate	tablet	Campral	Rx
disulfiram	dye-SUL-fi-ram	tablet	Antabuse	Rx
naltrexone	nal-TREX-one	tablet, injectable	ReVia, Vivitrol	Rx
topiramate	toe-PYRE-a-mate	capsule, tablet	Topamax	Rx

- severe headache
- severe vomiting
- thirst
- uneasiness

These side effects are known as Antabuse-like reactions. The patient usually becomes exhausted and sleeps for several hours after symptoms have worn off. Patients who are taking disulfiram must examine food labels to be sure they do not inadvertently ingest alcohol in an everyday product (e.g., cough medicines, mouthwashes, flavorings, salad dressings, and wine vinegars). Several other prescription drugs can produce an antabuse-like reaction when combined with alcohol. These include metronidazole, some cephalosporins, and certain oral hypoglycemic drugs. Warning labels that instruct patients not to consume alcohol while taking these drugs should be placed on the containers.

Naltrexone (ReVia) is a pure opiate antagonist that blocks the effects of endogenous opioids released as a result of alcohol consumption, making alcohol consumption less pleasurable. It is used to treat alcohol dependence. Naltrexone can cause an acute withdrawal syndrome in opiate-dependent patients, including nausea, dizziness, headache, and weight loss. The patient should be stable after alcohol withdrawal before starting this drug. To prevent withdrawal symptoms, those with a history of opiate intake must be opiate-free before starting the drug. **Vivitrol** is the injectable extended-release form of this drug. It decreases the effectiveness of opiates for pain, cough, and diarrhea. Patients on this drug should wear a medical alert pendant or bracelet so that, if they end up in the emergency room, the staff will know not to provide opiates. The drug must be refrigerated, except for the week just before injection. It is a single-use carton that contains the drug in powdered form, diluent and syringe. It is administered IM, monthly in alternating buttocks.

REFRIGERATE

The anticonvulsant **topiramate (Topamax)** seems to reduce cravings for alcohol. It takes about 6 weeks to be effective. The dosage must be slowly increased. Phamacological research suggests that topiramate inhibits alcohol-induced release of dopamine in the midbrain. The use of topiramate combined with behavioral therapy looks promising. Topiramate has poor compliance because it must be taken on a daily basis.

Chapter Terms

anorexia loss of appetite for food

antipsychotics drugs that are used to treat schizophrenia; reduce symptoms of hallucinations, delusions, and thought disorders; also called neuroleptics

anxiety a state of uneasiness characterized by apprehension and worry about possible events

autism a disorder that first appears in childhood, characterized by repetitive behavior and impairment in social interaction and communication; it can be expressed through mood swings, irritability, tantrums, aggression, and self-injury

bipolar disorder a condition in which a patient presents with mood swings that alternate between periods of major depression and periods of mild to severe chronic agitation

cataplexy short periods of muscle weakness and loss of muscle tone associated with sudden emotions such as joy, fear, or anger; a symptom of narcolepsy

delirium tremens (DTs) a condition caused by cessation of alcohol consumption in which coarse, irregular tremors are accompanied by vivid hallucinations

depression a condition characterized by the feeling that life has no meaning, pessimism, intense sadness, loss of concentration, and problems with eating and sleeping

endogenous anxiety anxiety caused by factors within the organism

exogenous anxiety anxiety caused by factors outside the organism

extrapyramidal symptoms disorders of muscle movement control caused by blocking dopamine receptors in the basal ganglia

ghost empty shell of an OROS tablet, excreted in the stool after the drug has dissolved

hypnotic a drug that induces sleep

insomnia difficulty falling asleep or staying asleep or not feeling refreshed on awakening

mania a mood of extreme excitement, excessive elation, hyperactivity, agitation, and increased psychomotor activity

monoamine oxidase inhibitor (MAOIs) an antidepressant drug that inhibits the activity of the enzymes that break down catecholamines (such as norepinephrine) and serotonin

narcolepsy a sleep disorder in which inappropriate attacks of sleep occur during the daytime hours

neuroleptics see antipsychotics

neurotransmitter a chemical produced by a nerve cell and involved in transmitting information in the body

obsessive-compulsive disorder (OCD) a mental disorder characterized by recurrent, persistent urges to perform repetitive acts such as hand washing

osmotic-controlled release oral delivery system (OROS) a drug delivery system that allows the drug to dissolve through pores in the tablet shell; the empty shell, called a ghost, is passed in the stool

panic intense, overwhelming, and uncontrollable anxiety

priapism abnormal penile erection

posttraumatic stress disorder (PTSD) a disorder characterized by persistent agitation or persistent, recurrent fear after the end of a traumatic event and lasting for over a month or impairing work or relationships

QT interval the time between depolarization and repolarization of the ventricles of the heart during a heartbeat, as shown on the electrocardiogram

seasonal affective disorder (SAD) a form of depression that recurs in the fall and winter and remits in the spring and summer

schizophrenia a chronic psychotic disorder manifested by retreat from reality, delusions, hallucinations, ambivalence, withdrawal, and bizarre or regressive behavior

selective serotonin reuptake inhibitor (SSRI) an antidepressant drug that blocks the reuptake of serotonin, with little effect on norepinephrine and fewer side effects than other antidepressant drugs

serotonin and norepinephrine reuptake inhibitor (SNRI) an antidepressant drug that blocks the reabsorption of both serotonin and norepinephrine, increasing the levels of both neurotransmitters

serotonin syndrome a possibly fatal condition caused by combining antidepressants that increase serotonin levels with other medications that also stimulate serotonin receptors

tardive dyskinesia involuntary movements of the mouth, lips, and tongue

tricyclic antidepressant (TCA) one of a class of antidepressant drug, developed earlier than the SSRIs and SNRIs, that also prevent neuron reuptake of norepinephrine and/or serotonin

unipolar depression major depression with no mania

Chapter Summary

Depression and Mood Disorders

- Antidepressants are not controlled substances.
- Antidepressants are classified as SSRIs (selective serotonin reuptake inhibitors), TCAs (tricyclic and tetracyclic antidepressants), SNRIs (serotonin and norepinephrine reuptake inhibitors), and MAOIs (monamine oxidase inhibitors).
- SSRIs block the reuptake of serotonin, with little effect on norepinephrine. They have fewer side effects than the older antidepressant medications.
- TCAs can be cardiotoxic in high doses.
- MAOIs are a second-line treatment because of their many interactions with drugs and foods.
- The maximum daily dose of bupropion (Wellbutrin, Zyban) should not exceed 450 mg.
- It may take at least 2 weeks for some of the antidepressants to be effective.
- Lithium is the drug of choice for treating bipolar (manic-depressive) disorder and acute mania and for prophylaxis of unipolar and bipolar disorders.

- A patient taking lithium *must* have frequent blood tests to assess lithium levels and maintain a therapeutic range.
- Carbamazepine (Tegretol) or divalproex (Depakote) may be substituted if patients cannot tolerate lithium.

Psychosis

- An antipsychotic that has a ceiling dose is thioridazine, which should not exceed 800 mg/day.
- The older agents are identified as "typical" or first-generation antipsychotics and are effective, but serious long-term side effects limit their use. Prescribers are steering away from these drugs and moving toward the newer "atypical" antipsychotics such as aripiprazole (Abilify), clozapine (Clozaril), olanzapine (Zyprexa), paliperidone (Invega), quetiapine (Seroquel), risperidone (Risperdal), and ziprasidone (Geodon).
- Anticholinergics can minimize some of the side effects of typical antipsychotic drugs.

Anxiety

- Anxiety is a state of uneasiness characterized by apprehension and worry about possible events.
- The most common self- prescribed and/or administered remedy for anxiety is alcohol.
- The benzodiazepines, buspirone, and, to a lesser extent, the beta blockers are the most appropriate pharmacologic treatments for panic attacks.
- A sedative is an antianxiety drug; a hypnotic drug induces sleep. Some drugs fit both descriptions.

Sleep and Sleep Disorders

- All hypnotic agents except the benzodiazepines and chloral hydrate reduce REM sleep.
- Benzodiazepines that are FDA-approved for hypnotic use are estazolam (ProSom), flurazepam (Dalmane), quazepam (Doral), temazepam (Restoril), and triazolam (Halcion).
- Hypnotic medications should be administered 1 hour before bedtime.
- Patients should take hypnotic drugs only a limited number of times each week, and the duration of use should be restricted to a 4 to 6 week period.

- Rozerem is not a controlled substance because it works in a different way from other hypnotics.
- The Z hypnotics are the preferred treatment of sleep disorder.
- Zaleplon (Sonata) is the shortest-acting hypnotic, with a duration of action of 4 hours. Therefore it may be taken in the middle of the night.
- Zolpidem (Ambien), a Schedule IV drug, has many of the same properties as the benzodiazepines, but it is structurally dissimilar.
- Eszopiclone (Lunesta) is approved for long-term use.
- Antihistamines are the safest drugs to use in treating insomnia.

Alcoholism

- Alcoholism is an incurable and potentially fatal disease. It can be controlled through behavioral changes.
- Alcoholism is linked to genetics.
- Alcoholics have an increased ability to metabolize ethanol rapidly, and neurons in the CNS adapt to the presence of ethanol.
- Four drugs have been approved for treatment of alcoholism; they are disulfiram (Antabuse), acamprosate (Campral), topiramate (Topamax), and naltrexone (ReVia).

Drug List

The following drugs were discussed in this chapter. Each generic drug name is followed in parentheses by one or more brand names.

Antidepressants

SSRIs and SNRIs
citalopram (Celexa)*
escitalopram (Lexapro)*
desvenlafaxine (Pristiq)
duloxetine (Cymbalta)
fluoxetine (Prozac*, Sarafem)
fluvoxamine
paroxetine (Paxil)

sertraline (Zoloft)*
venlafaxine (Effexor)*

Tricyclic Antidepressants (TCAs)
amitriptyline (Elavil)*
clomipramine (Anafranil)
desipramine (Norpramin)
doxepin (Sinequan, Zonalon)
imipramine (Tofranil)
nortriptyline (Aventyl, Pamelor)

protriptyline (Vivactil)
trimipramine (Surmontil)

Tetracyclic Antidepressant
maprotiline (Ludiomil)
mirtazapine (Remeron)*

Monoamine Oxidase Inhibitors (MAOIs)
phenelzine (Nardil)
selegiline (Eldepryl)
tranylcypromine (Parnate)

Miscellaneous Antidepressants
bupropion (Wellbutrin, Zyban)*
nefazodone
trazodone (Desyrel)*

Drugs for Bipolar Disorders
carbamazepine (Epitol, Tegretol)
divalproex (Depakote)
lithium (Eskalith, Lithobid)
olanzapine-fluoxetine (Symbyax)
valproic acid (Depakene)

Antipsychotics

Typical Antipsychotics
fluphenazine (Prolixin)
haloperidol (Haldol)
loxapine (Loxitane)
molindone (Moban)
perphenazine (Trilafon)
prochlorperazine (Compazine)
thioridazine
thiothixene (Navane)
trifluoperazine (Stelazine)

Atypical Antipsychotics
aripiprazole (Abilify)
clozapine (Clozaril)
olanzapine (Zyprexa)*
paliperidone (Invega)
quetiapine (Seroquel)*
risperidone (Risperdal)*
ziprasidone (Geodon)

Drugs Used to Minimize the Effects of Antipsychotics
benztropine (Cogentin)
diphenhydramine (Benadryl)
meclizine (Antivert)

Antianxiety Agents
amoxapine
buspirone (BuSpar)*
hydroxyzine (Vistaril)
meprobamate (Miltown)
paroxetine (Paxil)*
propranolol (Inderal)
trifluoperazine (Stelazine)
venlafaxine (Effexor)

Benzodiazepines
alprazolam (Xanax)*
chlordiazepoxide (Librium)
clorazepate (Tranxene)
diazepam (Valium)*
estazolam (ProSom)
flurazepam (Dalmane)
lorazepam (Ativan)*
oxazepam (Serax)
quazepam (Doral)
temazepam (Restoril)*
triazolam (Halcion)

Stimulant
modafinil (Provigil)
armodafinil (Nuvigil)

Sleep Agents

Barbiturates
amobarbital (Amytal)
butabarbital (Butisol)
secobarbital (Seconal)

Antihistamines
diphenhydramine (Benadryl)
hydroxyzine (Atarax, Vistaril)

Hypnotic
chloral hydrate
ramelteon (Rozerem)

Others
eszopiclone (Lunesta)
zaleplon (Sonata)
zolpidem (Ambien)*

Alcohol Antagonists
acamprosate (Campral)
disulfiram (Antabuse)
naltrexone (ReVia)
topiramate (Topamax)*

Chapter Review

Pharmaceuticals and Body Functions

Select the best answer from the choices given.

1. Antidepressants are classified as all of the following except:
   a. SSRIs
   b. cyclic
   c. NSAIDs
   d. SNRIs

2. If the patient is taking a therapeutic dose of lithium, there will be a slight tremor of the
   a. hand.
   b. foot.
   c. eyes.
   d. head.

3. Which drug can be safely taken with alcohol?
   a. lithium
   b. Valium
   c. Ativan
   d. none of the above

4. Advances made in antipsychotic medications are
   a. improved efficacy
   b. reduced negative side efects
   c. drugs are better tolerated
   d. all of the above

5. Which drug must have blood work faxed to the pharmacy before it can be dispensed?
   a. Tegretol
   b. clozaril
   c. carbamazepine
   d. none of the above

6. Antipsychotic drugs are chosen on the basis of
   a. cost.
   b. side effects.
   c. the patient's history of response.
   d. all of the above.

7. The antipsychotic with a ceiling dose is
   a. molindone.
   b. loxapine.
   c. thioridazine.
   d. trifluoperazine.

8. An adverse effect of the antipsychotics is
   a. dry mouth.
   b. constipation.
   c. blurred vision.
   d. all of the above.

9. Which drug class is used to treat anxiety, panic disorder, sleep disorder?
   a. SSRIs
   b. MAOIs
   c. SNRIs
   d. benzodiazepines

10. Which drug is recommended to treat tardive dyskinesia?
    a. Benadryl
    b. hydroxyzine
    c. Antivert
    d. none of the above

The following statements are true or false. If the answer is false, rewrite the statement so it is true.

_____ 1. The most-used drugs to treat anxiety are the SSRIs.

_____ 2. The only drug approved by the FDA for panic disorder is Valium.

_____ 3. The most successful treatment of panic attacks is behavioral therapy and antipanic medication.

_____ 4. Withdrawal symptoms in alcoholics may be treated by anticonvulsants, sedatives, and beta blockers.

_____ 5. A side effect of the hypnotics could be sleep driving.

_____ 6. Two drugs specifically used to treat alcoholism are topiramate and Antabuse.

_____ 7. Sometimes alcohol addiction has no physical signs.

_____ 8. Benzodiazepines are the best hypnotics, and they should be used routinely as the first-line treatment for sleeplessness.

_____ 9. An MAOI might be a good choice for an antidepressant in a patient with Parkinson disease.

_____ 10. Desyrel is a good antidepressant in a young male, but a poor choice in an elderly man.

Diseases and Drug Therapies

1. List at least five symptoms of depression.

2. List five symptoms of bipolar disorders.

3. List four noncontrolled medications for anxiety.

4. Which three benzodiazepines used to treat anxiety clear the body most quickly?

5. Which five benzodiazepines are approved for hypnotic use?

6. List the four steps toward recovery for an alcoholic.

7. List the effects of alcohol when combined with Antabuse.

8. List some practical methods of inducing sleep other than drug use.

9. List the side effects of antipsychotics.

10. List three types of depression.

Dispensing Medications

You receive the following incorrect prescriptions. Identify the error in each.

1. Ativan 2 mg
   tid #90
   refills 12

2. thioridazine 400 mg
   tid #90
   refills 12

3. Ambien 5 mg #30
   every day at bedtime
   refills 12

Internet Research

Use the Internet to complete the following assignments.

1. Find Internet sources listing potential drug and food interactions for three of the antidepressants discussed in this chapter. Do you think the information provided on these sites is reliable? Why or why not? Create a table listing the drugs you researched along with their corresponding drug and food interactions.

2. Research bipolar mood disorder. What are the modes of treatment for this disease (including drug treatment)? What are the most common signs and symptoms of this disorder? List your Internet sources.

What Would You Do?

1. The person at the counter reeks of alcohol and begins to berate you because you are not filling the prescription fast enough. How would you handle this situation?

Drugs for Central Nervous System Disorders

8

Learning Objectives

- Develop an understanding of the physiologic processes that occur in epilepsy.
- Classify seizures and the goals of therapy.
- Understand that specific drugs are used in different classes of seizures.
- Be familiar with Parkinson disease and the drugs used in its treatment.
- Identify the drugs and goals of therapy for attention-deficit disorders.

- Realize that some drugs may be used for several disease states.
- Recognize drugs used to treat Alzheimer disease.

STUDY PARTNER

Preview chapter terms and definitions.

The central nervous system (CNS) disorders cause a range of complex, distressing, and life-threatening symptoms, some of which are nonresponsive to treatment. They often leave the patient unable to function normally. The chemicals involved in the thought process and motor activity form the basis of some of these diseases and the rationale for their treatment. These diseases include epilepsy in its various forms, Parkinson disease, myasthenia gravis, attention-deficit disorders, amyotrophic lateral sclerosis, multiple sclerosis, and Alzheimer disease. For some of these diseases, medical science is still searching for definitive treatment.

Epilepsy

Epilepsy is a fairly common neurologic disorder characterized by paroxysmal (sudden and recurring) seizures. It involves disturbances of neuronal electrical activity that interfere with normal brain function. These abnormal discharges may occur only in a specific area of the brain or may spread extensively throughout the brain. These discharges may not provoke obvious clinical symptoms, yet seizures may nevertheless be taking place.

Epilepsy is a symptom of brain dysfunction. All epilepsy patients have seizures, but not all patients with seizures have epilepsy. Some have a single unprovoked seizure in their lifetime; 1% to 2% have chronic epilepsy.

Seizures

A **seizure** is caused by disordered abnormal electrical discharges in the cerebral cortex (the main portion of the brain), resulting in a change in behavior of which the patient is not aware. Conscious periods may or may not be accompanied by loss of control over movements or distortion of the senses. When body movement is lost, it may be in only one area of the body or in the entire body.

Seizures result from the sudden, excessive firing of a small number of neurons, often without an exogenous (outside the organism) trigger, and the spread of the electrical activity to adjacent neurons. These firings can result in a **convulsion**, an involuntary contraction or series of contractions of the voluntary muscles.

Each neuron is in one of three states: resting, firing, and returning to rest. The balance between excitatory and inhibitory impulses determines whether a neuron fires. Neurons operate through the movement of ions across the cell membrane. Negative ions, such as chloride, entering a neuron inhibit it from firing, whereas positive ions such as sodium or calcium entering the cell excite it and make it more likely to fire. The ion flows are controlled by molecules in the cell membrane known as ion channels, which in turn are controlled by neurotransmitters binding to them. Some neurotransmitters bind to receptors that let positive ions in and excite the cell, whereas others bind to receptors that let negative ions in and inhibit firing. Healthy persons have a balance between excitation and inhibition. In persons with epilepsy, there is an imbalance between excitation and inhibition among the neurotransmitters. When excitation is excessive relative to inhibition, neurons can fire uncontrollably, leading to a seizure. Glutamate, an excitatory amino acid neurotransmitter, and gamma-aminobutyric acid (GABA), an inhibitory neurotransmitter, play the greatest role in seizures. Other contributors are the CNS chemicals involved in the thought process and motor activity. These CNS chemicals are

- acetylcholine (ACh)
- aspartate
- dopamine
- glutamate
- glycine
- norepinephrine
- serotonin

The levels of neurotransmitters are determined in part by the levels of the enzymes that produce them. Upsetting the enzymes disrupts the balance and leads to seizures, especially if the disruption results in a high ratio of glutamate to GABA. The majority of seizures are caused by the following event or condition:

- alcohol or drug withdrawal
- epilepsy
- high fever
- hypoglycemia, hyperglycemia (low and high sugar in serum, as from diabetes)
- infection (meningitis)
- neoplasm (brain tumor)
- trauma or injury (head, hematoma)

The two major types of seizures are partial and generalized. Each is further subdivided into additional types, according to their manifestations.

Partial Seizures A **partial seizure** is localized in a specific area of the brain and almost always results from injury to the cerebral cortex. Approximately 65% of people with epilepsy suffer from partial seizures. Partial seizures occur in two distinct types, each of which can progress to generalized seizures. In a simple partial seizure, the patient does not lose consciousness, may have some muscular activity manifested in twitching, and may have sensory hallucinations (visual or auditory phenomena). In the other type of partial seizure, the complex partial seizure, the patient experiences impaired consciousness, often with confusion, blank stare, and postseizure amnesia.

Generalized Seizures A **generalized seizure** involves simultaneous malfunction in both hemispheres of the brain and has no local origin. This type of seizure sometimes occurs in the absence of injury or known structural abnormality. Generalized seizures are classified by type and include tonic-clonic, absence, myoclonic, and atonic seizures.

- The **tonic-clonic seizure** (formerly often called a **grand mal seizure**) occurs in two phases. The tonic portion of the seizure begins with the body becoming rigid, and the patient may fall. This lasts for a minute or less. The clonic portion usually is initiated with muscle jerks, and may be accompanied by shallow breathing, loss of bladder control, and excess salivation (foaming at the mouth). Jerking continues for a few minutes. After the attack, the patient is drowsy and confused for moments or hours.
- The **absence seizure** (formerly often called a **petit mal seizure**) begins with interruption of the patient's activities by some or all of the following signs: blank stare, rotating eyes, uncontrolled facial movements, chewing, rapid eye blinking, twitching or jerking of an arm or leg, but no generalized convulsions. Seizures last from 10 seconds to 2 minutes but are rarely longer than 30 seconds. The patient may experience up to 100 attacks a day. Often, the person has a premonition of the attack through unusual sensations of light, sound, and taste, known as an aura. After the attack, the patient continues normal activities. Seizures are most prevalent during the first 10 years of life; 50% of children with absence seizures have tonic-clonic activity as they grow older.
- A **myoclonic seizure** occurs with sudden, massive, brief muscle jerks, which may throw the patient down, or nonmassive, quick jerks of the arm, hand, leg, or foot. Consciousness is not lost, and this seizure type can occur during sleep.
- An **atonic seizure** begins with sudden loss of both muscle tone and consciousness. The patient may collapse, the head may drop, and the jaw may slacken. An arm or leg may go limp. The seizure lasts a few seconds to a minute, and then the patient can stand and walk again.

Status epilepticus is a serious disorder involving continuous tonic-clonic convulsions, with or without a return to consciousness, that last at least 30 minutes. It is characterized by high fever and lack of oxygen severe enough to cause brain damage or death. Of the patients who have convulsive status epilepticus, 10% die regardless of treatment, often as a complication of sudden drug withdrawal. Therapy is aimed at stopping the convulsions and preventing brain damage.

Antiepileptic Drug Therapy

Epilepsy can have a profound effect on one's health, quality of life, and ability to function. The optimum antiepileptic therapy would be complete seizure control without compromising the patient's quality of life. Thus, therapy with anticonvulsant drugs has two goals: (1) to control seizures or reduce their frequency so that the patient can live an essentially normal life and (2) to prevent emotional and behavioral changes that may result from the seizures.

Approximately 30% of epilepsy patients are poorly controlled with medication, and 30% do not comply with therapy because some of the side effects of the drugs are unpleasant. The most common side effects are sedation and loss of cognitive processes (i.e., mental perception, memory, judgment).

As described previously, seizures occur when the effect of excitatory neurotransmitters is excessive relative to the effect of inhibitory neurotransmitters. Drugs to control seizures work by reducing the excitation or increasing the inhibition so that neurons do not fire out of control. Not surprisingly, many drugs used to control seizures are used, or have been used in the past, to treat other conditions characterized by excessive excitation, such as mania, anxiety, or panic.

The most important concept in treating epilepsy is to begin with monotherapy (using a single drug). Except in life-threatening situations, single-drug therapy should be initiated at one-fourth to one-third of the usual daily dosage. The dosage is then increased gradually over 3 to 4 weeks until seizures are controlled or adverse side effects occur. Once an optimal dosage has been determined, it is essential that the plasma concentration of the drug remain stable to ensure seizure control and minimize the risk of side effects.

For patients who do not respond positively to antiepileptic monotherapy, the use of more than one drug (polytherapy) should be considered. Monotherapy is preferred to polytherapy, however, because it costs less and has potential for fewer adverse effects, drug interactions, and compliance problems.

One possible reason for nonresponsiveness to antiepileptic drug therapy is that the agent is inappropriate for the seizure type. In the past, most patients with epilepsy were treated with phenytoin, phenobarbital, or both. Clinicians now recognize that different seizure types require different antiepileptic agents. A drug that controls one seizure type may exacerbate another type. The newer drugs are seizure-specific; that is, their pharmacologic action is directed toward controlling a certain type of seizure activity.

The need for therapy should be evaluated periodically. Some patients can discontinue therapy if they have been seizure-free for several years. To discontinue an antiepileptic drug, the dosage should be decreased gradually over 2 to 6 months. Abrupt discontinuation should be avoided because of the risk of triggering status epilepticus or other withdrawal seizures.

The potential for drug interactions during antiepileptic therapy is high. Antiepileptic drugs interact with each other and with other drugs through two major mechanisms. They can induce or inhibit the liver enzymes responsible for drug metabolism. They can also cause drug displacement from plasma protein.

Table 8.1 presents the most commonly used **anticonvulsant** drugs (drugs to control seizures). These drugs all have relatively narrow therapeutic ranges. In some patients, *even minor changes in bioavailability can compromise control or result in toxicity.* Maintaining a consistent rate and extent of absorption, and thus stable plasma concentrations, is important. Factors that can alter either the rate or the extent of absorption include storage conditions, the drug's physical and chemical characteristics, the dosage form, and the patient's physical condition. Pharmacokinetic interactions result from some alteration of absorption, protein binding, metabolism, or elimination. Because of the narrow therapeutic ranges of this class of drugs, even the very small allowable differences in manufacturing can have an effect on the ability of the drug to control episodes. For this reason, prescribers often will not allow generic

TABLE 8.1   Most Commonly Used Anticonvulsant Drugs

Generic Name	Pronunciation	Dosage Form	Brand Name	Dispensing Status	Control Schedule
carbamazepine	kar-ba-MAZ-e-peen	oral liquid, tablet	Epitol, Tegretol	Rx	
clonazepam	kloe-NAZ-e-pam	tablet	Klonopin	Rx	C-IV
diazepam	dye-AZ-e-pam	injection, IV, oral liquid, tablet	Valium	Rx	C-IV
divalproex	dye-VAL-pro-ex	capsule, tablet	Depakote	Rx	
ethosuximide	eth-oh-SUX-i-mide	capsule, oral liquid	Zarontin	Rx	
fosphenytoin	fos-FEN-i-toyn	IV	Cerebyx	Rx	
gabapentin	gab-a-PEN-tin	capsule, oral liquid, tablet	Neurontin	Rx	
lamotrigine	la-MOE-tri-jeen	tablet	Lamictal	Rx	
levetiracetam	lev-a-tur-AS-a-tam	tablet	Keppra	Rx	
lorazepam	lor-AZ-e-pam	injection, IV, oral liquid, tablet	Ativan	Rx	C-IV
oxcarbazepine	ox-kar-BAZ-e-peen	oral liquid, tablet	Trileptal	Rx	
phenobarbital	fee-noe-BAR-bi-tal	capsule, injection, IV, oral liquid, tablet	Luminal Sodium	Rx	C-IV
phenytoin	FEN-i-toyn	capsule, IV, oral liquid, tablet	Dilantin	Rx	
pregabalin	pree-GAB-a-lin	capsule	Lyrica	Rx	C-V
primidone	PRYE-mih-done	tablet	Mysoline	Rx	
tiagabine	te-AG-a-been	tablet	Gabitril	Rx	
topiramate	toe-PYRE-a-mate	tablet	Topamax	Rx	
valproic acid	val-PRO-ik AS-id	capsule, injection, oral liquid	Depakene	Rx	
zonisamide	zoh-NIS-a-mide	capsule	Zonegran	Rx	

drugs to be used, so pharmacy technicians should watch for these drugs to be written DAW (dispense as written), or "brand only." If the computer automatically changes the drug to the generic, the technician will often have to change it back to the brand.

Carbamazepine, phenytoin, divalproex, and valproic acid act to stabilize the neuronal membrane and may decrease the release of excitatory neurotransmitters. Barbiturates and benzodiazepines enhance the inhibitory effect of GABA. The mechanism of gabapentin is unknown, but it does not interact with GABA receptors (despite its name).

For status epilepticus, **diazepam (Valium)** is the drug of choice; given in IV dosage form, it takes 30 to 60 seconds for the effects to become apparent. If this does not work, then **phenytoin (Dilantin)**, given in IV form, or barbiturates are administered. If antiepileptic therapy does not work and the seizure continues for more than 60 minutes, intubation and general anesthetics are used as a last resort.

Carbamazepine (Epitol, Tegretol) is used in the prophylaxis of generalized tonic-clonic, partial (especially complex-partial), and mixed partial or generalized seizure disorders. It is also used to treat bipolar disorders, as described in Chapter 7. The antiepileptic effect may be related to its effects on sodium channels to limit sustained, repetitive firing and alter synaptic transmission. Blood monitoring is important, because carbamazepine induces its own metabolism, so the plasma concentration may be lower than expected. The patient should report bleeding, bruising, jaundice, abdominal pain, pale stools, mental disturbances, fever, chills, sore throat, or mouth ulcers. The drug may also cause drowsiness. Patients may need to use carbamazepine produced by only one manufacturer when taking this drug, which requires the pharmacy to dispense the brand, not a generic. As with all the other anticonvulsant medications, carbamazepine has many interactions with other drugs. The side effects of carbamazepine can be serious, the most serious being aplastic anemia, but this is rare. The drug should be taken with food to offset GI disturbances.

The only indication for **clonazepam (Klonopin)**, a Schedule IV benzodiazepine, is prophylaxis of seizures. It suppresses the spike-and-wave discharge in absence seizures by depressing nerve transmission in the motor cortex. The patient should be told to avoid alcohol and other CNS depressants and not to discontinue the drug abruptly. Physical or psychological dependence may result from its use. (Even though this drug is a benzodiazepine, a member of a class discussed in Chapter 7, it is discussed only here and not with the other benzodiazepines.)

Diazepam (Valium) is the drug of choice for status epilepticus, as stated previously. Diazepam can also be administered as a rectal gel (Diastat). It is used in patients who need intermittent treatment to control increased seizure activity, or clusters. Diazepam is supplied in a prefilled unit dose rectal delivery system. The pharmacy team must set the syringe and lock the dose in before it is dispensed. It can be used in the home. It is best to wait until the patient or caregiver picks up the drug to lock in the dose, in case the person decides not to get it. Once the dose is locked in, it cannot be changed.

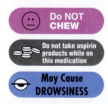

Divalproex (Depakote) and **valproic acid (Depakene),** which are also indicated for treatment of manic episodes in bipolar disorder (Chapter 7), may also increase the availability of GABA and are indicated for managing simple and complex absence seizures, mixed seizure types, and myoclonic and generalized tonic-clonic seizures. They may also be effective in partial seizures and infantile (early childhood) spasms. The patient should take the dose with water (not with a carbonated drink) and should not chew, break, or crush the tablets or capsules. Patients should be warned not to use aspirin or aspirin products, because these could lead to *serious* valproic acid toxicity. Routine hepatic and hematologic tests are indicated during therapy. Patients should report severe or persistent sore throat, fever, fatigue, bleeding, or bruising. Side effects include drowsiness and impaired judgment or coordination.

Ethosuximide (Zarontin) is the drug of choice for absence seizures. It increases the seizure threshold. Because of its long half-life, it can usually be given once daily to achieve therapeutic plasma concentrations, but it is often divided between two daily doses to reduce gastrointestinal side effects. The patient should be told to take the dose with food and not to discontinue it abruptly. The drug may cause drowsiness and impair judgment. Patients should have a complete blood count (CBC) every 4 months during therapy. The side effects are drowsiness, headache, dizziness, nausea, and vomiting.

Fosphenytoin (Cerebyx) can be used instead of IV phenytoin. It is a prodrug (precursor or inactive form) that is rapidly converted to phenytoin after administration. It has the advantage of being water soluble and, therefore, better tolerated. This means fewer infusion reactions (pain, burning, or tissue damage) and more

Warning

Cerebyx looks and sounds like Celexa (citalopram, an antidepressant) and Celebrex (celecoxib, used for treating arthritis pain); be careful in dispensing.

Warning

Neurontin and Noroxin (norfloxacin, an antibiotic) can be confused, but they can be differentiated by dosage. Neurontin is usually 100 mg and Noroxin is 400 mg.

Warning

Lamictal, Lamisil (terbinafine, an antifungal), and Lomotil (diphenoxylate/atropine, used in the treatment of diarrhea) could be easily mistaken for each other.

Warning

Boxed warnings are special warnings about a drug highlighted in a box in the FDA-approved product information. A Black Box warning is the most serious.

reliable treatment. It does have an unusual side effect of brief, intense itching, usually in the groin, which might be a reaction to the phosphate in the injection, but this reaction is not an allergic response.

Gabapentin (Neurontin) is used as an **adjunct** (a drug added to existing therapy) for drug-refractory (not responsive to treatment) partial and generalized seizures, secondary to the initial seizure in adults with epilepsy. It is not effective for absence seizures. Gabapentin was designed to mimic the neurotransmitter GABA, but studies have shown that it must have another mechanism of action. Unlike other anticonvulsant drugs, it does not modify plasma concentrations of standard anticonvulsant medication. Side effects are somnolence (sleepiness or unnatural drowsiness), dizziness, **ataxia** (irregular muscle movements), fatigue, nystagmus (involuntary, rapid movement of the eyeballs), tremors, and double vision. There are no reported significant drug interactions. Renal function should be monitored. Gabapentin is a well-accepted treatment option for patients with neuropathic pain. Other uses not as well documented include bipolar disorder, migraine prevention, hot flashes, multiple sclerosis, attention deficit, and alcohol withdrawal. Because it is generally well tolerated and easy to use, gabapentin is a very popular drug.

Gabapentin is being prescribed for neuropathic pain, a stinging and burning pain resulting from nerve damage, such as the type of pain seen in patients with diabetic neuropathy or post-herpetic neuralgia. This pain is treated first with tricyclic antidepressants. If that does not work, the next step is anticonvulsants. Gabapentin seems to work well for some patients, even those with severe and refractory pain. It is also less sedating than the other agents.

Lamotrigine (Lamictal) provides add-on therapy for adults with partial seizures, with or without generalized secondary seizures. The drug works by blocking sodium channels, thereby reducing neuron excitation. Lamotrigine does not affect serum concentrations of phenobarbital, phenytoin, or primidone, but it may affect the pharmacokinetics or pharmacodynamics of carbamazepine and valproic acid. The drug has a Black Box warning about fatal rashes in the FDA-approved product information. The patient should be advised to call the physician immediately if a rash appears, but the drug should not be discontinued abruptly. Life-threatening rashes with this drug are much more common in children, and lamotrigine is not to be used in patients less than 16 years old.

Lorazepam (Ativan) is often used to treat alcoholic seizures. It must be administered by IV as soon as possible when used for this purpose. Alcoholic seizures can be deadly. Most "recreational" drugs can be stopped abruptly ("cold turkey"), but abrupt withdrawal of alcohol can kill. People who consume very large amounts of alcohol must be weaned off of it by means of a medication such as lorazepam. The benzodiazepines and alcohol drips are used for this purpose. Any time a "stat" order is received for a benzodiazepine, it implies that someone is having a seizure and needs the drug immediately to prevent further damage. The injectable form of this drug is stored in the refrigerator. It is good for 30 days unrefrigerated.

Levetiracetam (Keppra) is an adjunctive therapy for partial seizures. Its mechanism of action is unknown, and it is structurally unrelated to other anticonvulsants. It was initially developed to improve cognition (the ability to perceive, think, and remember). The pharmacokinetics of this drug are simple; there is little potential for drug interactions, and serum level monitoring is not required. It should be a drug that is easily dispensed. However, there is no evidence that doses greater than 300 mg per day are effective, so the pharmacy technician should watch the dosage and alert the pharmacist if a doctor writes a prescription for a dose greater than this. Levetiracetam causes drowsiness.

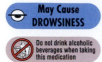

Oxcarbazepine (Trileptal) blocks voltage-sensitive sodium channels and thereby stabilizes hyperexcited neurons. This drug is most frequently used as an adjunct to other therapies, but it can be used as monotherapy for partial seizures. Female patients taking oxcarbazepine must be warned that this drug decreases the effectiveness of birth control pills. Patients should also be warned about the potentially debilitating drowsiness associated with oxcarbazepine therapy.

Phenobarbital (Luminal Sodium) is used for generalized tonic-clonic and partial seizures because it interferes with the transmission of impulses from the thalamus to the cortex of the brain. Use of alcohol and other CNS depressants should be avoided. The drug should not be stopped abruptly. Phenobarbital is a Schedule IV agent because it has abuse potential. It can cause drowsiness and paradoxical hyperexcitability in children and the elderly. Periodic blood tests are required.

When filling a prescription for phenobarbital, the pharmacy technician should always check the patient's profile in the computer for other drugs being prescribed. Phenobarbital has several interactions with other drugs. If the patient has a rash or exhibits excessive drowsiness, ataxia, **dysphagia** (difficulty swallowing), slurred speech, and confusion while taking this drug, the physician should be notified immediately.

Phenytoin (Dilantin) is used to manage generalized tonic-clonic, simple-partial, and complex-partial seizures and to prevent seizures after head trauma and neurosurgery. It works in the motor cortex by promoting sodium ion outflow from cells, thus stabilizing the membrane threshold. It is useful for all types of seizures except absence. In some patients, small changes in dosage result in large changes in serum concentration. Side effects may or may not be related to dosage and may be reversible when the dosage is reduced. Table 8.2 lists phenytoin's dosage-related and non-dosage-related side effects.

Patients should receive routine hepatic and hematologic tests. Phenytoin must be discontinued if even a mild rash appears. The symptoms usually occur within the first 8 weeks of therapy and include hepatitis, lymphadenopathy, and hematologic alterations. The rash can progress to the life-threatening Stevens-Johnson syndrome.

Antacid and phenytoin doses should be spaced 2 to 3 hours apart. Phenytoin is a potent inducer of hepatic microsomal enzymes and binds avidly to plasma proteins. Therefore, it interacts with many other drugs.

TABLE 8.2   Phenytoin Side Effects

Dose-Related	Ataxia (irregularity of muscular action)
	Diplopia (the perception of two images of a single object)
	Dizziness
	Drowsiness
	Encephalopathy (degenerative brain disease)
	Involuntary movements (when concentration is greater than 30 mcg/mL)
Non-Dose-Related	Gingival hyperplasia (abnormal increase in cells that increases the volume of the tissue covering the tooth-bearing border of the jaw)
	Peripheral neuropathy (noninflammatory pathological disturbance or pathological change in areas away from the center of the body, such as arms or legs; pain in the extremities)
	Vitamin deficiencies

Intravenous phenytoin should never be infused faster than 50 mg/minute. For diluting phenytoin to allow for a safe infusion, normal saline is the only suitable vehicle. It is one of the few drugs that might be mixed by a nurse outside the pharmacy because it precipitates so quickly. IV phenytoin should be marked as a "high alert" drug in a hospital setting because of the many problems it presents. This is one of the few drugs that may need to be dispensed as "brand only." If a generic is used, then only one manufacturer should be used. The small allowable manufacturing differences can alter therapeutic levels because the therapeutic index is very narrow for this drug. The FDA allows the **AUC** (**area under the curve,** a measure of drug concentration in the body) of a generic and a brand medication to fall within 3% of each other. For most drugs this is negligible, but for epileptic drugs it can make a difference in efficacy.

Pregabalin (Lyrica) reduces the release of several neurotransmitters, including glutamate, norepinephrine, and **substance P** (a sensory neurotransmitter, mediating pain, touch, and temperature, a potent vasoactive substance). Pregabalin is thought to bind to calcium channels and modulate calcium influx. Pregabalin is structurally similar to gabapentin (and is informally referred to as "son of gabapentin"), but is more potent. Pregabalin produces fewer side effects than gabapentin and other anticonvulsant drugs, probably because it is efficacious at lower doses. Also, pregabalin can be titrated more readily and may have a faster onset. Furthermore, pregabalin has few interactions. It is approved as an adjunct only (added onto another drug) for partial seizures. It is important to remember that pregabalin is a controlled substance (Schedule V), because it can cause euphoria and withdrawal. It is also approved to treat diabetic neuropathy or nerve pain that continues after shingles. It must not be stopped abruptly.

Primidone (Mysoline) is indicated in generalized tonic-clonic and complex-partial seizures. Metabolic reactions in the liver transform primidone into phenobarbital, so the therapeutic and side effects profiles are similar to those of phenobarbital. Because megaloblastic anemia is a rare side effect of primidone, annual CBCs are recommended.

Tiagabine (Gabitril) blocks the reabsorption of GABA, which allows it to bind to nerve cells that may enhance normal brain activity. Tiagabine should be taken with food and not stopped abruptly, but tapered. Tiagabine can actually *cause* seizures, which has occurred in patients taking it for off-label uses who do not have epilepsy. The FDA has issued a warning about taking tiagabine for off-label uses, because prescribers would not expect a drug *for* seizures actually to *cause* seizures.

Topiramate (Topamax) is prescribed for treating partial-onset seizures in adults. Although its mechanism of action is not well understood, the most common theories propose that topiramate blocks sodium channels and subsequently enhances the activity of GABA and antagonizes glutamine receptors. It is add-on therapy to carbamazepine or phenytoin. It works well but causes significant cognitive effects (e.g., slowed thinking, slowed speech, and difficulty concentrating). Therapy should start with a low dose and be titrated slowly over 8 weeks. Topiramate can increase phenytoin levels. It is a weak carbonic anhydrase inhibitor, so it increases the risk of kidney stones. Patients should drink plenty of water.

Zonisamide (Zonegran) is a sulfonamide with anticonvulsant activity. Patients must be warned about the potentially serious sulfonamide reactions, and the pharmacy technician should check for sulfa allergies when dispensing this drug. Patients should also be instructed to report any skin rashes and to drink six to eight glasses of water a day to reduce the risks of kidney stones.

Parkinson Disease

Parkinson disease is characterized by muscular difficulties and postural abnormalities, usually affecting persons over age 60. Three characteristic signs of Parkinson disease are tremor while resting, rigidity, and akinesia (absence of movement). These may manifest by poor posture control, shuffling gait, and loss of overall muscle control (e.g., flexed stance, difficulty in turning, and hurried gait). With the elderly population increasing in number, we can expect to see more cases of this debilitating disease in the upcoming years.

Physiology of Parkinson Disease

Parkinson disease occurs as a result of pathologic alterations in the extrapyramidal system, a complex functional unit of the CNS involved in controlling motor activities. The extrapyramidal system is composed of the **basal nuclei** (also called the basal ganglia); these are symmetric, subcortical masses of gray matter embedded in the lower portions of the cerebral hemisphere. Parkinson disease is the most common of the extrapyramidal diseases. No definitive test exists for this disease, so it is diagnosed almost exclusively by its symptoms.

Voluntary movement requires complex neurochemical messaging in the brain. Nerve impulses travel, by means of electrical impulses and neurotransmitters, from the cerebral cortex to the basal nuclei and back to the cerebral cortex via the thalamus (see Figure 8.1 for the features of the brain). Transmission of information about the initiation of movement, muscle tone, and posture is affected by the balance of neurotransmitters in the basal nuclei. Normal movement requires that the two primary neurotransmitters—dopamine, an inhibitor, and acetylcholine (ACh), a stimulator—be in balance.

FIGURE 8.1
Cutaway View of the Brain

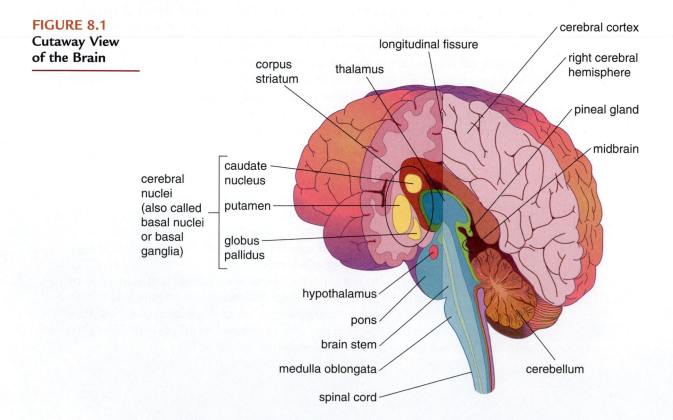

In a healthy person, dopaminergic neurons (neurons that release dopamine when they fire) in the **substantia nigra** (a collection of dark gray substance, found deep within the midbrain and illustrated in Figure 8.2) release an amount of dopamine sufficient to control the stimulating effect of acetylcholine on large motor and fine muscle movements. In Parkinson disease, however, there is progressive destruction of dopaminergic neurons in the nigrostriatal pathway, so an insufficient amount of dopamine is produced to counterbalance acetylcholine production. This results in a predominance of cholinergic neuronal activity, which produces excessive motor nerve stimulation.

Parkinson Disease Drug Therapy

Drug therapy for Parkinson disease has greatly improved the functional ability and clinical status of patients. Nevertheless, drug therapy aims only at symptomatic relief; it does not alter the underlying disease process. Temporary or prolonged remission allows the patient to live a productive life. Currently, there is no cure for Parkinson disease, so the goals of treatment are to minimize disability and help patients maintain the highest possible quality of life. Levodopa is considered to be the gold standard. Meanwhile, the search continues for new agents to prolong the length of effective treatment or reverse the disease. Table 8.3 presents the most commonly used agents for patients with Parkinson disease.

The side effects of the drugs can be a problem in the treatment of Parkinson disease. Drugs with numerous problems may necessitate constant changes in the medication. Often, the patient will need emotional and psychological support as well.

Amantadine (Symmetrel), an antiviral encountered in Chapter 4 as a prophylaxis and treatment for influenza, is also used to treat Parkinson disease. Its anti-Parkinson activity is a result of blocking the reuptake of dopamine into presynaptic neurons and causing direct stimulation of postsynaptic dopamine receptors. The second dose of the day should be taken in the early afternoon to decrease the incidence of insomnia. Abrupt discontinuation of therapy should be avoided.

Benztropine (Cogentin) blocks central cholinergic receptors, helping to balance cholinergic activity in the basal ganglia. Indications for the use of this drug are acute

Warning

Amantadine, ranitidine (gastric acid reducer), and rimantadine (another antiviral) look alike.

FIGURE 8.2
The Substantia Nigra

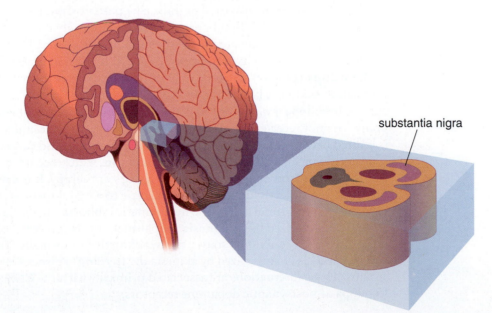

substantia nigra

TABLE 8.3 Most Commonly Used Anti-Parkinson Agents

Generic Name	Pronunciation	Dosage Form	Brand Name	Dispensing Status
amantadine	a-MAN-ta-deen	capsule, oral liquid, tablet	Symmetrel	Rx
benztropine	BENZ-troe-peen	injection, IV, tablet	Cogentin	Rx
bromocriptine	broe-moe-KRIP-teen	capsule, tablet	Parlodel	Rx
entacapone	en-TAK-a-pone	tablet	Comtan	Rx
levodopa	lee-voe-DOE-pa	capsule	Dopar	Rx
levodopa-carbidopa	lee-voe-DOE-pa kar-bi-DOE-pa	tablet	Sinemet	Rx
levodopa-carbidopa-entacapone	lee-voe-DOE-pa kar-bi-DOE-pa en-TAK-a-pone	tablet	Stalevo	Rx
pramipexole	pra-mi-PEX-ole	tablet	Mirapex	Rx
rasagiline	ra-SAJ-i-leen	tablet	Azilect	Rx
ropinirole	ro-PIN-a-role	tablet	ReQuip	Rx
selegiline	seh-LEDGE-ah-leen	capsule	Eldepryl, Zelapar	Rx
tolcapone	TOLE-ka-pone	tablet	Tasmar	Rx

dystonic reactions, Parkinson disease, and drug-induced extrapyramidal reactions (such as those caused by antipsychotics). Benztropine may also prolong dopamine's effects by blocking dopamine reuptake and storage at central receptor sites. This drug should be administered after meals to prevent GI irritation. Constipation is the primary side effect. The drug should not be discontinued abruptly.

Bromocriptine (Parlodel) is an ergot alkaloid with dopaminergic properties. It improves symptoms of Parkinson disease by directly stimulating dopamine receptors in the corpus striatum. It is usually used with levodopa or levodopa-carbidopa. The drug should be taken with food or milk. The patient should limit use of alcohol and avoid exposure to cold. Blood pressure should be closely monitored. Drowsiness, nausea, and hypotension are the most common side effects. It also inhibits prolactin secretion and has been used to dry up milk production in breast-feeding mothers.

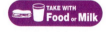

Levodopa (Dopar), a precursor of dopamine, crosses the blood-brain barrier and is metabolized in the brain into dopamine, which does not itself cross the blood-brain barrier. Levodopa is also converted into dopamine by the peripheral tissues, so the brain does not receive the full dose. This drug has very undesirable effects. The dosage is limited because of the potential for nausea, vomiting, and cardiac arrhythmia.

Another problem is the **on-off phenomenon,** which occurs in as many as two-thirds of Parkinson patients after about 5 years of therapy. It is a wide fluctuation of functional states, ranging from a hyperkinetic to a hypokinetic state, potentially occurring several times a day. The hyperkinetic (abnormally increased motor function) state is characterized by **dyskinesia** (impairment of the power of voluntary movement) and good functional status; the hypokinetic (abnormally diminished motor activity) state is characterized by akinesia or "freezing" episodes and painful dystonic spasms. These fluctuations are associated primarily with the CNS availability of levodopa at postsynaptic dopamine receptors.

Patients may be well controlled on levodopa for several years and then, suddenly, assume a state of akinesia, masked facies (a relentless, unblinking stare without emotional expressiveness), and stooped posture. The drug may just as suddenly start working again. It also causes neuropsychiatric disorders, dementia (organic loss of intellectual function), loss of memory, hallucinations, and postural hypotension (reduced blood pressure in certain positions, due to inhibition of neurons responsible for vasoconstriction). Levodopa should be carefully titrated to provide optimal control at minimal doses so that the on-off phenomenon is delayed as long as possible.

Levodopa-carbidopa (Sinemet) is probably the most commonly used drug in Parkinson disease. The carbidopa prevents loss of the drug from the CNS by conversion to dopamine in the peripheral nervous system, and it results in fewer dopaminergic side effects. Carbidopa does not affect the CNS metabolism of levodopa, and lower doses of levodopa can be used as brain concentrations of dopamine increase. There is a smoother, more rapid induction into therapy with this drug.

Levodopa-carbidopa-entacapone (Stalevo) is a combination drug for patients who experience a "wearing off" of the beneficial effects of levodopa. Entacapone, boosts efficacy and helps the effect last longer. The combination is often less costly than buying the drugs separately.

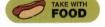

Pramipexole (Mirapex), a dopamine agonist, is more selective for dopamine D_2 receptors but has also been shown to bind to D_3 and D_4 receptors. This drug works as well as other anti-Parkinson drugs but has fewer side effects. Unlike bromocriptine, pramipexole is not an ergot derivative. Pramipexole should be prescribed early in the disease, either as a monotherapy or in combination with levodopa-carbidopa. It should be taken with food to reduce nausea. Pramipexole is approved for **restless leg syndrome** (an overpowering urge to move the legs, especially at rest). It may help with the pain of fibromyalgia but is not yet approved for this disease.

Rasagiline (Azilect) is a monoamine oxidase inhibitor (MAOI), which blocks the breakdown of dopamine. It is similar to selegiline. Rasagiline is used as initial therapy in early stages of Parkinson disease to improve symptoms. It can also be added to levodopa to prolong the effects of this latter drug. Rasagiline should not be taken for 2 weeks prior to surgery. Like other MAOIs, rasagiline can cause a hypertensive crisis, as described in Chapter 7, if the patient ingests foods that contain tyramine, such as matured cheeses, cured meats, fava or broad bean pods, tap or draft beers, sauerkraut, or soy sauce.

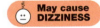

Ropinirole (ReQuip), like pramipexole, is a dopamine agonist, binding with higher affinity at the D_3 receptors. The precise mechanism of action is unknown. It can be taken without regard to food. Hypotension, especially at the beginning of therapy or dose escalation, can cause severe dizziness, especially with a change in position. Ropinirole also is approved for restless leg syndrome.

Selegiline (Eldepryl, Emsam, Zelapar) is a potent MAOI that affects MAO type B, found primarily in the brain. Selegiline plays a major role in the metabolism of dopamine and may increase dopaminergic activity by interfering with dopamine breakdown. The daily dose should not exceed 10 mg. Zelapar is a dosage form that dissolves in the mouth. Because absorption is higher with Zelapar, doses are lower than with related drugs. EmSam is the transdermal form of selegiline and is approved only for depression, not for Parkinson disease; therefore EmSam was discussed in Chapter 7.

Tolcapone (Tasmar) is the first of a new class of anti-Parkinson agents known as **catechol-O-methyl transferase (COMT)** inhibitors. The inhibition of COMT, an enzyme that metabolizes levodopa in the body, allows greater levels of levodopa to reach the brain, thereby extending the drug's beneficial life. The COMT inhibitors have no clinical effect unless they are combined with levodopa. Tolcapone was approved by the FDA in 1998 but has since been linked to three fatal liver injuries. As

Warning

Selegiline and sertraline (an SSRI-type antidepressant) both contain a vertical letter, but if the vertical is crossed, it is probably *t* and the name is probably sertraline. The dosage for selegiline is 5 mg, and the dosages for sertraline are 25 mg, 50 mg, and 100 mg. When a dosage is in doubt, it is always safest to call the prescriber to confirm.

a result, the medication now carries a warning label recommending that its use be limited to people who do not respond to or are not appropriate candidates for other available treatments. Tolcapone has been shown to increase patient "on-time" by an average of 2 to 3 hours per day. The drug should be discontinued if the patient does not demonstrate any improvement within 3 weeks.

Entacapone (Comtan) is the second COMT inhibitor to be approved by the FDA. Whereas tolcapone penetrates the CNS, entacapone acts peripherally. Thus, entacapone is expected to be less toxic than tolcapone. Entacapone is indicated for patients who are experiencing a deteriorating response to levodopa in the earlier stages of motor fluctuations. This drug can be taken without regard to food.

Other Central Nervous System Disorders

Several other neurologic disorders share symptoms and signs with the convulsive disorders and Parkinson disease. They include myasthenia gravis, attention-deficit hyperactivity disorder and attention-deficit disorder, amyotrophic lateral sclerosis (ALS), multiple sclerosis (MS), and Alzheimer disease.

Myasthenia Gravis

Myasthenia gravis is a disorder of the interface between nerves and muscles, resulting from autoimmune damage to acetylcholine (Ach) receptors at the **motor end plate** (connection point between a nerve and a muscle; see Figure 8.3); as a result, the muscles cannot respond to the nerve signal to move them. The disorder is characterized by weakness and fatigability, especially of the skeletal muscles. For some individuals, weakness is relatively constant, but for others, weakness is typically enhanced by exercise and diminishes with rest. The first symptoms may be **ptosis** (paralytic drooping of the upper eyelid), **diplopia** (double vision), or blurred vision; these may be accompanied or followed by **dysarthria** (imperfect articulation of speech), dysphagia, extremity weakness, and respiratory difficulty. The clinical course is variable and includes spontaneous remissions and exacerbations.

FIGURE 8.3
Motor End Plate

The interface between the nervous system and the muscular system is the neuromuscular junction.

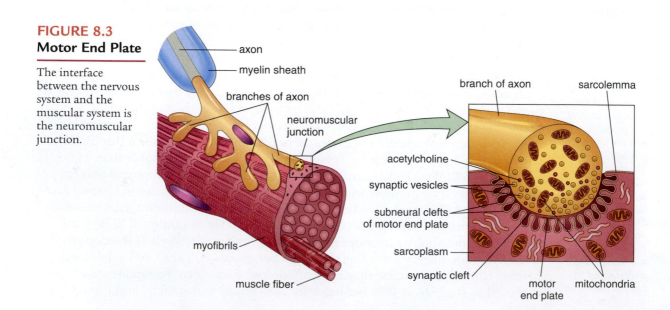

Acetylcholinesterase inhibitors can produce clinical improvement in all forms of myasthenia gravis. They allow ACh to last longer and may be used with corticosteroids. Although drug therapy does not inhibit or reverse the basic immunologic flaw, it does enable the ACh remaining in the junction sites to interact with ACh receptors for longer periods of time. Table 8.4 lists the most commonly used drugs for myasthenia gravis.

Edrophonium (Enlon, Reversol) is used to diagnose myasthenia gravis. It often markedly improves patients' strength. The response lasts 5 minutes.

Neostigmine (Prostigmin) and **pyridostigmine (Mestinon)** are used to treat myasthenia gravis or to reverse the effects of nondepolarizing muscle relaxants. They block ACh hydrolysis by cholinesterase, resulting in ACh accumulation at cholinergic synapses and thereby increasing stimulation of cholinergic receptors at the neuromuscular junction. Neostigmine and pyridostigmine interact with procainamide, quinidine, corticosteroids, succinylcholine, and magnesium. These drugs should be taken with food or milk. It is equally important to take them exactly as directed and at the same time each day.

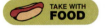

When neostigmine and pyridostigmine are delivered by oral, intramuscular, or IV routes, they facilitate transmission of impulses across the neuromuscular junction. Side effects are generally due to exaggerated pharmacologic effects. The most common side effects are salivation and **muscle fasciculation** (a small, local, involuntary muscular contraction visible under the skin). The prescriber should be notified of any nausea, vomiting, muscle weakness, severe abdominal pain, or difficulty in breathing.

Azathioprine (Imuran) suppresses cell-mediated hypersensitivity, alters antibody production, and reverses neuromuscular blockade. It is taken with food to avoid nausea. The side effects of immunosuppressive drugs are leukopenia (reduction of leukocytes), pancytopenia (abnormal depression of blood cells), infection, GI irritation, and abnormal liver function tests.

Cyclophosphamide (Cytoxan), an alkylating agent, prevents cell division by cross-linking deoxyribonucleic acid (DNA) strands. Guidelines for preparing and disposing of chemotherapeutic agents should be followed. Fluids should be taken liberally (3 L per day). Cystitis is a frequently occurring side effect, even months after therapy has been discontinued. Other urinary tract effects may include urinary bladder fibrosis, hematuria, and renal tubular necrosis. Uric acid, CBCs, and renal and hepatic functions should be monitored. Alopecia (hair loss) is a side effect, as are nausea, vomiting, and bone marrow depression.

TABLE 8.4 Most Commonly Used Agents for Myasthenia Gravis

Generic Name	Pronunciation	Dosage Form	Brand Name	Dispensing Status
azathioprine	ay-za-THYE-oh-preen	IV, tablet	Imuran	Rx
cyclophosphamide	sye-kloe-FOS-fa-mide	IV, tablet	Cytoxan	Rx
edrophonium	ed-roe-FOE-nee-um	injection, IV	Enlon, Reversol	Rx
neostigmine	nee-oh-STIG-meen	injection, IV, tablet	Prostigmin	Rx
pyridostigmine	peer-id-oh-STIG-meen	injection, IV, oral liquid, tablet	Mestinon	Rx

Attention-Deficit Disorders

Several types of attention-deficit disorders are recognized. Chief among these are **attention-deficit hyperactivity disorder (ADHD)** and attention-deficit disorder (ADD). In general, both of these disorders are treated with the same drugs; therefore, in this text they both will be referred to as ADHD. Most of the drugs used to treat ADHD and ADD are amphetamines or amphetamine derivatives; they have a high addictive quality and therefore they are classified as Schedule II. The FDA has determined that drugs used for this purpose as a group must provide a medication guide for the patient or caretaker including the two substances that are not Schedule II drugs. The technician can check for this when the drug is handed to the patient or caregiver. Although ADHD is thought of as a disease of childhood, some symptoms can persist into adult life. Several drugs are used primarily for this disorder, and they are listed in Table 8.5.

Atomoxetine (Strattera) is a nonstimulant, selective inhibitor of the reuptake of norepinephrine, which controls impulsivity and activity. It is the only nonstimulant medication indicated for the treatment of ADHD in patients 6 years and older. Atomoxetine has been shown to be as effective as psychostimulants and therefore can be a reasonable alternative with a lower risk for abuse. It is not a controlled substance, so prescriptions can be refilled and called in. Atomoxetine should be used as a first-line agent. Like other drugs for attention-deficit disorders, atomoxetine can cause weight loss and slow growth.

Methylphenidate (Concerta, Daytrana, Metadate, Metadate ER, Methylin, Ritalin, Ritalin-SR), a Schedule II agent, is the drug of choice to treat attention-deficit disorders; it is also used for narcolepsy. Methylphenidate improves concentration for many patients by increasing levels of neurotransmitters in the brain. It should be used as an adjunct to psychosocial measures. Like amphetamine, it has a paradoxical calming effect in hyperactive children. A CBC with differential (number of types of cells) and platelet count should be monitored during long-term therapy. To help prevent the development of tolerance, the patient can skip methylphenidate doses,

TABLE 8.5　Most Commonly Used Agents for Attention-Deficit Disorders

Generic Name	Pronunciation	Dosage Form	Brand Name	Dispensing Status	Control Schedule
atomoxetine	at-oh-MOX-e-teen	capsule	Strattera	Rx	
dexmethylphenidate	dex-meth-il-FEN-i-date	tablet	Focalin	Rx	C-II
dextroamphetamine-amphetamine	dex-troe-am-FET-a-meen am-FET-a-meen	tablet	Adderall	Rx	C-II
lisdexamfetamine	liss-dex-am-FET-a-meen	capsule	Vyvanse	Rx	C-II
methylphenidate	meth-il-FEN-i-date	tablet	Concerta, Daytrana Metadate, Metadate ER, Methylin, Ritalin, Ritalin-SR	Rx	C-II
modafinil	moe-DAF-i-nil	tablet	Sparlon	Rx	

Note: all of these drugs require a Medication Guide.

especially during times of low-stress, such as during weekends and vacation. When the patient resumes medication, he or she may be able to decrease the necessary dosage. Caffeine may decrease this drug's efficacy, so the patient should avoid coffee, tea, and colas. The patient should get plenty of rest. This drug does have abuse potential.

Concerta is dosed once per day, which allows it to be given only in the morning. The outer layer of Concerta dissolves to release part of the dose immediately. The rest of the tablet is an OROS tablet (described in Chapter 7 in connection with paliperidone), which releases the drug slowly through pores in the tablet, leaving a ghost tablet that passes through the stool. **Daytrana** is the patch form of methylphenidate. It is worn for 9 hours and then removed. The drug is in the adhesive.

Dexmethylphenidate (Focalin) consists of the dextro isomer of methylphenidate. An **isomer** is one of two (or more) compounds that contain the same number and type of atoms but have different molecular structures. Many biologically active substances have isomers whose molecules are mirror images of each other, like a pair of gloves. Such isomers are often distinguished by the terms "dextro" (right) and "levo" (left). Methylphenidate is such a compound, with D (dextro) and L (levo) isomers. Dexmethylphenidate contains only the more active dextro isomer of methylphenidate. Because dexmethylphenidate only contains one isomer, it is expected to have fewer side effects than methylphenidate. Like methylphenidate, it is a Schedule II drug.

Dextroamphetamine-amphetamine (Adderall), a Schedule II agent, is an alternative to other stimulants. Its effects can last about 6 hours, long enough to get some children through the school day. The primary side effect is depression as the drug wears off.

Lisdexamfetamine (Vyvanse) is dextroamphetamine chemically bonded to the amino acid lysine. Enzymes in the GI tract cleave the lysine, leaving dextroamphetamine, an active drug. The attachment to lysine is intended to reduce the abuse potential of the drug, which is a problem with dextroamphetamine. Once the lysine is cleaved, the dextroamphetamine is absorbed rapidly, so this drug is still a Schedule II substance. A Medication Guide must be dispensed with this drug.

Modafinil (Sparlon, Provigil) has a different mechanism of action than other drugs used for treatment of ADHD. The exact mechanism for this drug is unclear, but it does increase mental alertness. Provigil, available as an uncoated tablet, is approved only for narcolepsy, whereas Sparlon, which is available in the slower-releasing coated tablet, is approved only for ADHD.

Amyotrophic Lateral Sclerosis (ALS)

Amyotrophic lateral sclerosis (ALS), also known as **Lou Gehrig disease** after the New York Yankees star who died of this disease in 1941, is a progressive degenerative disease of the nerves that leads to muscle weakness, paralysis, and eventually death. It is thought to be caused by excessive levels of glutamate, an excitatory neurotransmitter that causes nerve damage.

The only drug approved to treat this syndrome is **Riluzole (Rilutek)**. It inhibits the release of glutamate, inactivates sodium channels, and interferes with intracellular events following transmitter binding at excitatory receptors. Riluzole has been shown to improve survival by approximately 3 months in some patients.

Multiple Sclerosis (MS)

Multiple sclerosis (MS) is an autoimmune disease in which the myelin sheaths around nerves, which serve as electrical insulation, degenerate. The patient loses use of the muscles, and often eyesight is affected. In the later stages of the disease, there is severe trembling. Some drugs can slow the progression of the disease, but there is no cure. Table 8.7 lists the agents most commonly used to treat MS.

Baclofen (Lioresal) is a skeletal muscle relaxant used to treat MS, spinal cord lesions, intractable hiccups, and bladder spasticity. It inhibits transmission of reflexes at the spinal cord level with resultant relief of muscle spasticity. Onset requires 3 to 4 days. Baclofen should be taken with food or milk and may cause drowsiness.

Glatiramer acetate (Copaxone) seems to block the autoimmune reaction against myelin that leads to nerve damage. It decreases the frequency of relapses, but it has not been shown to slow disease progress. It is given every day by subcutaneous injection. It may cause local injection-site reactions and brief flushing, chest pain, and shortness of breath; these side effects are bothersome but benign.

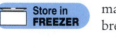

Interferon beta-1a (Avonex, Rebif) is used for ambulatory patients with relapsing-remitting MS. It reduces the frequency of attacks in patients with this form of MS. It also delays disability (the only drug that has been able to do this). It is given every other day. Most patients report flu-like symptoms, and to avoid these, prophylaxis with acetaminophen is indicated. It is also recommended that the drug be taken in the evening to avoid these symptoms. A photosensitivity reaction may occur. The drug should not be exposed to high temperatures or freezing.

Mitoxantrone (Novantrone) is a chemotherapeutic agent. It has been shown to slow the progression of MS and to reduce relapses. It is given intravenously every 3 months.

Tizanidine (Zanaflex) is indicated to reduce muscle spasticity in MS and spinal cord injuries. This drug works via the inhibition of presynaptic motor neurons. It is

TABLE 8.6   Agent to Treat Amyotrophic Lateral Sclerosis

Generic Name	Pronunciation	Dosage Form	Brand Name	Dispensing Status
riluzole	RIL-yoo-zole	tablet	Rilutek	Rx

TABLE 8.7   Most Commonly Used Agents for Multiple Sclerosis

Generic Name	Pronunciation	Dosage Form	Brand Name	Dispensing Status
baclofen	BAK-loe-fen	injection, tablet	Lioresal	Rx
glatiramer acetate	gla-TIR-a-mer AS-a-tate	injection	Copaxone	Rx
interferon beta-1a	in-ter-FEER-on BAY-ta 1A	injection	Avonex, Rebif	Rx
interferon beta-1b	in-ter-FEER-on BAY-ta 1B	injection	Betaseron	Rx
mitoxantrone	mye-toe-ZAN-trone	IV	Novantrone	Rx
tizanidine	tye-ZAN-i-dine	tablet	Zanaflex	Rx

the first oral drug approved for spasticity since baclofen (Lioresal). It is structurally similar to clonidine and has similar side effects (dry mouth, sedation, dizziness, and hypotension).

Alzheimer Disease

Alzheimer disease was first described by Alois Alzheimer, a German psychiatrist, in 1907. It is a degenerative disorder of the brain that leads to progressive dementia (loss of memory, intellect, judgment, orientation, and speech) and changes in personality and behavior. In the early stages of the disease, the patient complains of memory deficit, forgetfulness, and/or misplacement of ordinary items. Depression is a part of the disease profile. As the disease progresses, complex tasks become impossible (for example, managing personal finances), and concentration becomes poor; in the final stages, the patient suffers complete incapacitation, disorientation, and failure to thrive.

Two neurochemical mechanisms for cognitive impairment have been identified. One is that not enough of the neurotransmitter acetylcholine is produced to give a reliable signal. The other is that some of the receptors for the neurotransmitter glutamate are hyperactive and cause the neuron to fire even when there is no glutamate present.

Table 8.8 lists drugs most commonly used to treat Alzheimer disease. These drugs slow the disease but do not cure or reverse it. There are no agents that will reverse the cognitive abnormalities. Four of the medications listed in Table 8.8 (Aricept, Razadyne, Exelon, and Cognex) are cholinesterase inhibitors, which increase the levels of acetylcholine. Namenda, which is used early in the disease, blocks hyperactive glutamate receptors. The other drug listed in Table 8.8 is the OTC herbal remedy ginkgo.

Warning

Aricept and Aciphex (rabeprazole, a drug for gastroesophageal reflux disease) labels are nearly identical.

The depression associated with the disease is often treated with antidepressants, as determined by existing symptoms and adverse drug reaction profiles. Amitriptyline should be avoided in these patients because it blocks acetylcholine receptors. Agitation and sleep disturbances should be treated with short-acting benzodiazepines.

Tacrine (Cognex) is a cholinesterase inhibitor. The most common side effect is an increase in liver function values. It is metabolized through cytochrome P-450, so it interacts with other drugs that are metabolized through that system. It must be taken four times a day on an empty stomach because side effects include nausea and vomiting.

Donepezil (Aricept) is similar to tacrine but causes fewer side effects and is more convenient. Both tacrine and donepezil improve memory and alertness, but donepezil

TABLE 8.8   Most Commonly Used Agents for Alzheimer Disease

Generic Name	Pronunciation	Dosage Form	Brand Name	Dispensing Status
tacrine	TAK-reen	tablet	Cognex	Rx
donepezil	don-EP-a-zil	tablet	Aricept	Rx
galantamine	ga-LAN-ta-meen	oral liquid, tablet	Razadyne	Rx
ginkgo	GING-ko	tablet	(many)	OTC
memantine	MEM-an-teen	tablet	Namenda	Rx
rivastigmine	riv-a-STIG-meen	capsule, oral liquid, patch	Exelon	Rx

is more selective for the cholinesterase that is in the CNS. This means less nausea, vomiting, and diarrhea. Also, liver function tests are not necessary. Unlike tacrine, donepezil is given only once a day at bedtime.

Galantamine (Razadyne) is a cholinesterase inhibitor derived from daffodil bulbs. It is better tolerated than rivastigmine but not as well as donepezil. The oral forms of the drug should be taken with meals. This drug is rarely used because of deaths reported in some of the clinical trials.

The herb **ginkgo** has shown good results in improving cognitive function and social behavior in Alzheimer patients. There are good scientific studies to support the use of this herb in this disease state. The active ingredients have antioxidant and anti-inflammatory effects. Ginkgo improves blood flow and inhibits platelet aggregation. Because it is an OTC drug, it is much less expensive than the other drugs. It takes 6 to 12 weeks to see improvement. The concentrated ginkgo tablets should be used, because they contain the highest concentration of the active ingredients. Teas will not work. Patients on warfarin should not take ginkgo.

Memantine (Namenda) works by blocking the glutamate receptors known as NMDA receptors because they also respond to the chemical N-methyl-D-aspartate (NMDA). These receptors are excessively excitable in Alzheimer disease and can cause neurons to fire even without the neurotransmitter. Memantine may have fewer side effects and is better tolerated than other drugs used to treat this disease. The physician will have starter doses to titrate the patient to the optimal dose. After the patient is stabilized and the optimal dose is established, the pharmacy will get a prescription. The results of clinical trials suggest that memantine slows advancement of Alzheimer disease.

Rivastigmine (Exelon) is similar to donepezil but has fewer interactions. However, it is more difficult to dose and administer. The patch dosage form was specifically designed for Alzheimer patients. It is a matrix formulation. It is thought this drug increases brain acetylcholine levels through inhibition of acetylcholinesterase. It is approved to treat mild or moderate dementia due to either Parkinson disease or Alzheimer disease.

Chapter Terms

absence seizure a type of generalized seizure characterized by a sudden, momentary break in consciousness; formerly often called petit mal seizure

adjunct a drug used with another drug

Alzheimer disease a degenerative disorder of the brain that leads to progressive dementia and changes in personality and behavior

amyotrophic lateral sclerosis (ALS) a degenerative disease of the motor nerves; also called Lou Gehrig's disease

anticonvulsant a drug to control seizures

ataxia irregular muscle movements

atonic seizure a type of generalized seizure characterized by sudden loss of both muscle tone and consciousness

attention-deficit hyperactivity disorder (ADHD) a neurologic disorder characterized by hyperactivity, impulsivity, and distractibility

area under the curve (AUC) a measure of drug concentration in the blood

basal nuclei symmetric, subcortical masses of gray matter embedded in the lower portions of the cerebral hemisphere; part of the extrapyramidal system; also called basal ganglia

catechol-O-methyl transferase (COMT) an enzyme that metabolizes levodopa in the body; inhibited by certain anti-Parkinson agents

convulsion involuntary contraction or series of contractions of the voluntary muscles

diplopia the perception of two images of a single object

dysarthria imperfect articulation of speech

dyskinesia impairment of the power of voluntary movement

dysphagia difficulty in swallowing

epilepsy a neurologic disorder involving sudden and recurring seizures

generalized seizure a seizure that involves both hemispheres of the brain simultaneously and has no local origin; can be a tonic-clonic (grand mal), absence (petit mal), myoclonic, or atonic seizure

grand mal seizure see tonic-clonic seizure

isomer one of two or more compounds that contain the same number and type of atoms but have different molecular structures

Lou Gehrig disease see amyotrophic lateral sclerosis (ALS)

motor end plate the neuromuscular junction, where the nervous system and muscular system meet to produce or stop movement

multiple sclerosis (MS) an autoimmune disease in which the myelin sheaths around nerves degenerate

muscle fasciculation a small, local, involuntary muscular contraction visible under the skin

myasthenia gravis an autoimmune disorder of the neuromuscular junction in which the ACh receptors are destroyed at the motor end plate, preventing muscles from responding to nerve signals to move them

myoclonic seizure a type of generalized seizure characterized by sudden muscle contractions with no loss of consciousness

on-off phenomenon a wide fluctuation between abnormally increased and abnormally diminished motor function, present in many Parkinson patients after about 5 years of levodopa therapy

Parkinson disease a neurologic disorder characterized by akinesia, resting tremor, and muscular rigidity

partial seizure an abnormal electrical discharge centered in a specific area of the brain; usually caused by a trauma

petit mal seizure see absence seizure

ptosis paralytic drooping of the upper eyelid

restless leg syndrome an overpowering urge to move the legs, especially at rest

seizure abnormal electrical discharges in the cerebral cortex caused by sudden, excessive firing of neurons; result in a change in behavior of which the patient is not aware

status epilepticus a serious disorder involving tonic-clonic convulsions that last at least 30 minutes

substance P a potent neurotransmitter mediating sensations of pain, touch, and temperature

substantia nigra a layer of gray substance separating parts of the brain

tonic-clonic seizure a type of generalized seizure characterized by body rigidity followed by muscle jerks; formerly called a grand mal seizure

Chapter Summary

Epilepsy

- Epilepsy is a common neurologic disorder defined as paroxysmal seizures. It involves disturbances of neuronal electrical activity that interfere with normal brain function.
- Two major classifications of seizures are generalized and partial.
- The objective of antiepileptic drug therapy is to eliminate seizures without compromising the patient's quality of life because of adverse effects.
- Different seizure types require different drugs.
- All anticonvulsants have very narrow dose/therapeutic ranges. A slight dosage change can result in loss of seizure control or toxicity; therefore, prescribers often write for the brand name drug.
- Boxed warnings are special warnings about a drug highlighted in a box in the FDA-approved product information. A Black Box warning is the most serious.

Parkinson Disease

- For normal movements to be performed, the two primary neurotransmitters—dopamine (an inhibitor) and acetylcholine (a stimulator)—must be in balance. In Parkinson disease, these transmitters are not in balance.

- Dopamine will not cross the blood-brain barrier.
- Sinemet, a levodopa-carbidopa preparation, is probably the most commonly used drug in Parkinson disease.
- Bromocriptine (Parlodel) is used to treat Parkinson disease; it is also used to dry up breast milk in a nursing mother.
- Selegiline (Eldepryl) is an MAOI used in treating Parkinson disease.

Other Central Nervous System Disorders

- Acetylcholinesterase drugs can produce clinical improvement in all forms of myasthenia gravis.
- Methylphenidate (Concerta, Daytrana, Metadate, Metadate ER, Methylin, Ritalin, Ritalin-SR) is the drug of choice to treat attention-deficit disorders. It is a CNS stimulant and Schedule II controlled substance used primarily for attention-deficit disorders. Improved dosage forms allow the drug to be taken only in the morning, and one form comes as a patch, improving compliance.
- Atomoxetine (Strattera) and modafinil (Sparlon) are the only nonstimulant medications indicated for treatment of ADHD in patients 6 years and older.

- Riluzole (Rilutek) is the first drug approved for amyotrophic lateral sclerosis (Lou Gehrig disease). It inhibits the release of glutamate and seems to improve survival by about 3 months.
- Among the drugs used to treat multiple sclerosis are two chemically different interferons.
- Glatiramer acetate (Copaxone) is an MS drug that must be kept frozen.
- Tizanidine (Zanaflex) is the first oral drug approved for spasticity since baclofen (Lioresal).

- Alzheimer disease is a progressive form of dementia.
- Tacrine (Cognex) and donepezil (Aricept) are used to treat Alzheimer disease; donepezil has fewer side effects.
- There is evidence that memantine (Namenda) slows Alzheimer disease.
- Ginkgo has been shown to have good results in improving cognitive function and social behavior in Alzheimer patients in some studies.

Drug List

The following drugs were discussed in this chapter. Each generic drug name is followed in parentheses by one or more brand names.

Anticonvulsants
carbamazepine (Epitol, Tegretol)
clonazepam (Klonopin)*
diazepam (Valium)
divalproex (Depakote)*
ethosuximide (Zarontin)
fosphenytoin (Cerebyx)
gabapentin (Neurontin)*
lamotrigine (Lamictal)*
levetiracetam (Keppra)
lorazepam (Ativan)
oxcarbazepine (Trileptal)
phenobarbital (Luminal Sodium)
phenytoin (Dilantin)
pregabalin (Lyrica)*
primidone (Mysoline)
tiagabine (Gabitril)
topiramate (Topamax)*
valproic acid (Depakene)*
zonisamide (Zonegran)

Anti-Parkinson Agents
amantadine (Symmetrel)
benztropine (Cogentin)
bromocriptine (Parlodel)
entacapone (Comtan)
levodopa (Dopar)

levodopa-carbidopa (Sinemet)
levodopa-carbidopa-entacapone (Stalevo)
pramipexole (Mirapex)
rasagiline (Azilect)
ropinirole (ReQuip)
selegiline (Eldepryl)
tolcapone (Tasmar)

Myasthenia Gravis
azathioprine (Imuran)
cyclophosphamide (Cytoxan)
edrophonium (Enlon, Reversol)
neostigmine (Prostigmin)
pyridostigmine (Mestinon)

Attention-Deficit Disorders
atomoxetine (Strattera)*
dexmethylphenidate (Focalin)
dextroamphetamine-amphetamine (Adderall)*
lisdexamphetamine (Vyvanse)
methylphenidate (Concerta, Daytrana, Metadate, Metadate ER, Methylin, Ritalin, Ritalin-SR)*
modafinil (Sparlon)

Amyotrophic Lateral Sclerosis (ALS)
riluzole (Rilutek)

Multiple Sclerosis (MS)
baclofen (Lioresal)
glatiramer acetate (Copaxone)
interferon beta-1a (Avonex, Rebif)
interferon beta-1b (Betaseron)
mitoxantrone (Novantrone)
tizanidine (Zanaflex)

Alzheimer Disease
donepezil (Aricept)*
galantamine (Razadyne)
ginkgo
memantine (Namenda)
rivastigmine (Exelon)
tacrine (Cognex)

Chapter Review

Pharmaceuticals and Body Functions

Select the best answer from the choices given.

1. Seizures can be caused by
   a. epilepsy.
   b. alcohol withdrawal.
   c. infection.
   d. all of the above

2. The two major classifications of seizures are
   a. generalized and partial.
   b. simple-partial and complex-partial.
   c. tonic-clonic and atonic.
   d. absence and myoclonic.

3. Goals of epilepsy therapy are
   a. to control seizures or reduce their frequency to the extent that the patient can live essentially a normal life.
   b. to prevent emotional and behavioral changes.
   c. a and b
   d. none of the above

4. Which is the only indication for Klonopin?
   a. MS prophylaxis
   b. ADHD
   c. Alzheimer disease
   d. seizure prophylaxis

5. Which drug has a boxed warning about fatal rashes?
   a. Cerebyx
   b. Klonopin
   c. Lamictal
   d. Neurontin

6. Which oral liquid drug should be well shaken before administering?
   a. phenytoin
   b. primidone
   c. clonazepam
   d. fosphenytoin

7. Which anticonvulsant is a scheduled drug?
   a. phenytoin
   b. primidone
   c. carbamazepine
   d. phenobarbital

8. Which drug is metabolized to phenobarbital?
   a. carbamazepine
   b. primidone
   c. phenytoin
   d. valproic acid

9. Which anticonvulsants are used to treat bipolar disorders?
   a. carbamazepine and valproic acid
   b. phenytoin and ethosuximide
   c. phenobarbital and gabapentin
   d. clonazepam and Klonopin

10. The two noncontrolled substances to treat ADHD are:
    a. ReQuip and Mirapex
    b. Adderall and Ritalin
    c. Strattera and Sparlon
    d. Aricept and Razadyne

The following statements are true or false. If the answer is false, rewrite the statement so it is true.

_____ 1. The drug of choice for convulsive status epilepticus is Klonopin.

_____ 2. Dopamine crosses the blood-brain barrier.

_____ 3. Sinemet is an anti-Parkinson drug that has an "on-off" phenomenon.

_____ 4. The most commonly used drug in Parkinson disease is levodopa.

_____ 5. Amantadine can be used for prophylaxis and treatment of flu.

_____ 6. Parlodel can be used to dry up milk in a nursing mother.

_____ 7. Alzheimer drugs cannot reverse the disease but only slow the progression.

_____ 8. Copaxone must be kept frozen.

_____ 9. Lyrica is a controlled substance.

_____ 10. Vyvanse is the least addictive of the ADHD drugs.

Diseases and Drug Therapies

1. List five causes of seizures.

2. List the three stages of neuron activity.

3. What is the big advantage of Lamictal in the treatment of seizures?

4. What are the uses of Parlodel?

Dispensing Medications

The following prescriptions are brought in. Identify a possible disease state that is being treated.

1. 25-year-old woman: Parlodel

2. 10-year-old boy: Zarontin

3. 50-year-old man: Parlodel

4. 50-year-old man: Sinemet

5. 20-year-old man: Symmetrel

6. 50-year-old man: Emsam

7. 50-year-old man: Provigil

8. 10-year-old boy: Ritalin

9. 35-year-old man: Rilutek

10. 25-year-old woman: Betaseron

Internet Research

Use the Internet to complete the following assignments.

1. Locate information related to ongoing clinical trials aimed at the development of new treatments for Parkinson disease. Create a table listing at least five experimental therapies. Indicate the phase (one through three) of testing currently under way and where (institution and country) the trials are taking place. List your Internet sources.

2. Identify three Internet sites that offer guidance related to the management of epilepsy. Which of these sites would you recommend most highly to a patient and why?

What Would You Do?

1. A patient brings in a prescription for Lyrica. It has 12 refills on it. What is wrong with that prescription and what would you do?

Respiratory Drugs

9

Preview chapter terms and definitions.

Learning Objectives

- Differentiate the pulmonary diseases.
- Understand the pathophysiology and treatment of asthma.
- Define the goals of asthma treatment.
- Discuss the pathophysiology and treatment of emphysema and chronic bronchitis.
- Describe other diseases related to the lungs.
- Be aware of the reemergence of tuberculosis and of treatment for this disease.
- Understand how the antitussives, expectorants, decongestants, and antihistamines differ, and be able to describe their uses.
- Know why some drugs are prescribed for their side effects.
- Outline smoking cessation plans and supportive therapy.

The pulmonary diseases include asthma, chronic obstructive pulmonary disease (COPD), and other related disorders. COPD encompasses two major diseases: emphysema and chronic bronchitis. COPD is irreversible. Asthma, a reversible syndrome, obstructs inspiration, whereas emphysema and chronic bronchitis obstruct expiration. Related diseases, also obstructive, include pneumonia, cystic fibrosis, respiratory distress syndrome, tuberculosis, and histoplasmosis. In addition, the lungs are frequently attacked by less severe upper respiratory tract infections, including the common cold. Four classes of drugs are used to treat symptoms of the common cold, but as yet, no drug can truly cure the common cold. Smoking, which is closely linked to many respiratory diseases, is thus included in this chapter. Several innovative drugs are available to help the smoker quit.

Asthma

Asthma is a disease in which inflammation (irritation in the lungs) causes the patient's airways to tighten. It occurs in intermittent attacks that involve a reversible airway obstruction, and it is precipitated by specific triggering events that vary in severity from patient to patient.

Figure 9.1 shows the upper and lower airways (upper and lower respiratory tracts), through which gases pass in the respiratory system. Oxygen flows through and across membrane surfaces, where it is exchanged with carbon dioxide, as shown in Figure 9.2. In asthma and COPD, as a result of the obstructed airways, less oxygen is available to exchange with carbon dioxide, or the amount of exchange surface area is diminished.

Asthma is most commonly classified as allergic, exercise induced, or nonallergic. An allergic component is present in 35 to 55% of patients. The allergens that provoke asthma are airborne and evoke the response through classic allergic pathways as described in Chapter 3. The asthmatic lung is more sensitive and responds to lower doses of allergen challenge than the normal lung. Studies strongly support the concept of genetic predisposition to developing asthma.

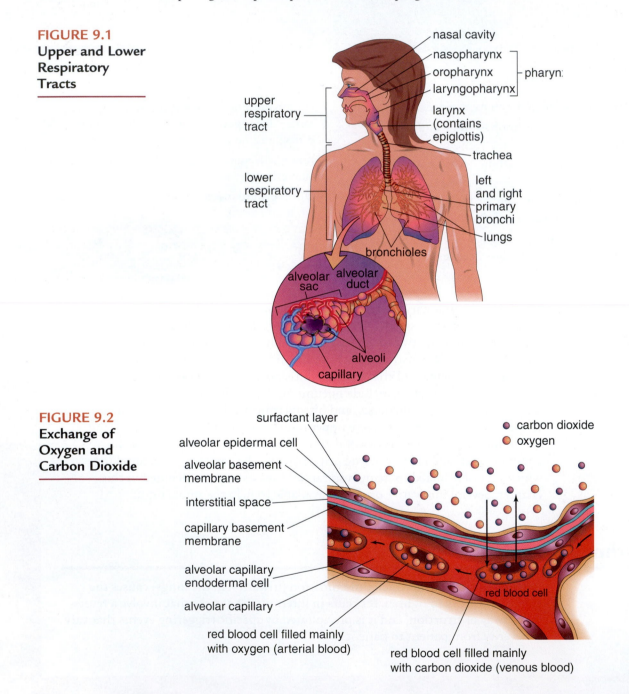

FIGURE 9.1
Upper and Lower Respiratory Tracts

nasal cavity
nasopharynx
oropharynx } pharynx
laryngopharynx
upper respiratory tract
larynx (contains epiglottis)
trachea
lower respiratory tract
left and right primary bronchi
lungs
bronchioles
alveolar sac   alveolar duct
alveoli
capillary

FIGURE 9.2
Exchange of Oxygen and Carbon Dioxide

surfactant layer
alveolar epidermal cell
alveolar basement membrane
interstitial space
capillary basement membrane
alveolar capillary endodermal cell
alveolar capillary
• carbon dioxide
• oxygen
red blood cell
red blood cell filled mainly with oxygen (arterial blood)
red blood cell filled mainly with carbon dioxide (venous blood)

However it is precipitated, asthma has the following characteristics: reversible small-airway obstruction, progressive airway inflammation, and increased airway responsiveness to a variety of endogenous and exogenous stimuli. These characteristics translate into recurrent episodes of wheezing (a whistling respiratory sound), dyspnea (labored or difficult breathing), and cough that have both acute (short, severe course) and chronic (persisting for a long time) manifestations in most patients.

Asthma differs from normal pulmonary defense mechanisms in its severity of **bronchospasm** (spasmodic contraction of the smooth muscles of the bronchioles, or small airways) and apparent failure of normal dilator muscle systems, excessive production of mucus that plugs airways, and the presence of sometimes severe long-term inflammatory reactions that may lead to patchy shedding of the lining of small airways.

The Asthmatic Response

Mast cells mediate a variety of cells and events in the inflammatory process. These cells are activated by immunoglobulin E (IgE), air inhalation during exercise, cold weather, and allergens. Their activation leads to airway obstruction caused by smooth-muscle contractions, increased secretion of mucus, and increased vascular permeability (see Figure 9.3).

An asthma attack consists of two phases or responses. The first response is often triggered by an antigen (any substance capable, under appropriate conditions, of inducing a specific immune response) antibody reaction. This phase is characterized by degranulation of the mast cells, which release histamine and other mediators, resulting in immediate bronchospasm and increased production of mucus, which often forms plugs in the small airways, with plasma leaking into tissue. This results in the release of mediators: histamines, chemotactic factor, platelet-activating factor, bradykinin, prostaglandins, and leukotrienes. The second response is bronchoconstriction with delayed, sustained reactions, including epithelial damage, that make the airway more sensitive to further challenge, even weeks after exposure. The late response causes self-sustaining inflammation.

FIGURE 9.3
The Asthmatic Response

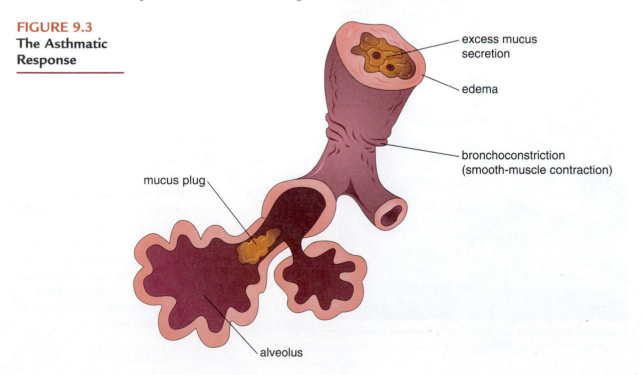

excess mucus
secretion

edema

bronchoconstriction
(smooth-muscle contraction)

mucus plug

alveolus

The most useful means of assessing the severity of asthma is with an instrument known as a **peak flow meter**, which measures **peak expiratory flow rate (PEFR)**. Patients forcefully blow into the peak flow meter, and PEFR is recorded in liters per minute. A measurement below 50% indicates a medical alert; immediate treatment with a bronchodilator and anti-inflammatory agent is needed, and the physician should be notified.

Goals of Asthma Care and Management of the Disease

For the patient, the goals of asthma care are to

- sleep well every night
- be able to go to work or school every day
- be free from wheezing all day
- have good control of coughing
- be able to continue with activities and exercise
- tolerate medicines well

As part of good asthma care, the asthmatic patient must learn to manage the disease and its complications and to limit the amount of exposure to irritants that will cause airway inflammation. The patient needs to learn what can trigger asthma attacks and how to control those trigger factors. For example, the patient with asthma should avoid contact with smoke as much as possible, because smoke is detrimental to patients with asthma. Also, because most people with asthma are allergic to dust mites, patients should follow simple dust mite control steps, including washing sheets and mattress pads at least once a week in hot (130 °F or hotter) water. Asthma patients should obtain a yearly flu vaccination.

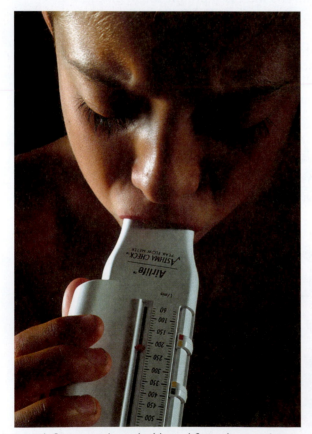

A peak flow meter is a valuable tool for asthma patients to use to measure and manage symptoms.

Symptoms alone are not always the best measure of respiratory status. For this reason, patients must learn to use a peak flow meter to measure peak expiratory flow rate (PEFR). The peak flow meter should be used twice a day and the results recorded in a diary as an aid to better management. Often, simply adjusting the asthma medications on the basis of the peak flow meter readings helps manage asthma effectively.

It is imperative that patients with asthma and their caregivers be aware of the signs and symptoms of **status asthmaticus**, which is a potentially life-threatening condition. An episode of status asthmaticus begins like any other asthma attack, but unlike an ordinary attack, it does not respond to normal management. The patient suffering from such an episode experiences increasing difficulty in breathing and exhibits blue lips and nail beds. The patient may lose consciousness. Status asthmaticus clearly constitutes a medical emergency, and the patient should receive prompt attention. This may require a visit to the emergency room.

Asthma Drug Therapy

Drug therapy is the mainstay of asthma management. The appropriate drug therapy depends on the persistence of the asthma attacks the patient suffers. The disease begins with intermittent attacks and may progress to mild-to-severe, persistent symptoms.

An important method of administering asthma medications is by a **metered dose inhaler (MDI)**—sometimes called a "puffer"—that contains medication and compressed gas. The MDI delivers a specific amount of medication with each actuation. The idea is to suspend the medication in particles or droplets that are fine enough to penetrate to the deepest parts of the lungs.

The prescribing physician usually orders the MDI to be used with a **spacer**. A spacer is recommended to decrease the amount of spray deposited on the back of the throat and swallowed. The spacer chamber holds the drug mist until the patient is ready to breathe. It also allows the patient to breathe the mist in at a slower, more effective rate, which, in turn, provides much better penetration of the drug into the lungs. Side effects are reduced because the drug is delivered to the lower portions of the lungs and fewer particles are left in the mouth and throat to be absorbed. A spacer is extremely useful for children and the elderly who have a hard time coordinating an inhaler. Very strong evidence supports the use of spacers.

Historically, the propellant of MDIs has been chlorofluorocarbons (CFCs). Unfortunately, CFCs migrate into the atmosphere, undergo various chemical reactions, and are depleting and destroying the protective ozone layer. CFCs were banned in the late 1980s. In 2008 the FDA required all MDIs to convert to hydrofluoroalkane (HFA) as the propellant; these are known as HFA inhalers. Studies have shown that HFA propellant produces a finer mist that has a better pulmonary deposit of particles and does not produce serum or tissue accumulation when given at 12 hour intervals. Another alternative to CFC-propelled inhalers is the dry-powder inhaler, which does not use gases. Many manufacturers are incorporating asthma drugs into dry-powder devices. A pellet is placed in the inhaler and crushed, and when the user inhales, the inhaler is activated.

MDIs need to be primed (the inhaler should be shaken for 5 seconds before releasing a spray) before the first use, if dropped, or if not used for several weeks. They should also be shaken well before each use. The following are the steps involved in using an HFA MDI:

1. Remove cap and shake inhaler.
2. Breathe out all the way.
3. Place mouthpiece between lips.
4. Press down on inhaler, hold for a few seconds, then breathe in slowly.
5. Hold breath and count to 10.
6. Breathe out slowly.

Steps for using a dry-powder MDI are as follows:

1. Activate the inhaler, insert disk, etc.
2. Breathe out all the way.
3. Put the mouthpiece to your lips and breathe in *quickly*.
4. Hold breath and count to 10.
5. Breathe out slowly.

If the asthma medication prescription calls for a second puff, wait approximately 1 minute, then go back to step 1. If another inhaler has been prescribed, wait 5 minutes before using it. Always clean the mouthpiece after each use and rinse the mouth if a corticosteroid is used. Treatment should be reviewed every 3 to 6 months.

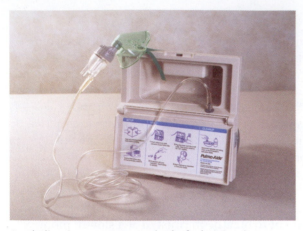

A nebulizer is a common method of administering asthma medication. It is especially effective for children.

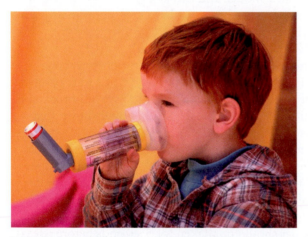

If a spacer is added to a metered dose inhaler, the medication will penetrate deeper into the tissue of the lungs than if the MDI is used without a spacer.

The primary difference between the two inhalers is that with the HFA inhaler, the patient should breathe in *slowly*, whereas with the dry-powder inhaler the patient should breathe in *quickly*. The most common use by far of inhaled medications is for the treatment of asthma.

Because of the complicated series of steps required to use gas-propelled and dry-powder inhalers, they are not recommended for very young children. Asthma medication can be administered to children by a **nebulizer**, a device in which a stream of air flows past a liquid and creates a fine mist, which the patient inhales while breathing normally through a mouthpiece or mask. The drug thus has a higher likelihood of being deposited farther into the lungs. This delivery system is very effective. If not properly cleaned and cared for, a home nebulizer can be a source of bronchitis and infections. Therefore, nebulizers should be cleaned daily.

Table 9.1 lists the most commonly used agents for asthma. Long-term control medications are cromolyn sodium, nedocromil, inhaled steroids, theophylline, long-acting beta$_2$ agonists, and leukotriene antagonists. Quick relief medications for reversal of acute exacerbations include short-acting beta$_2$ agonists, systemic corticosteroids, and ipratropium. Some physicians may begin patients at a higher step to gain control and then reduce therapy to the minimum required for control. There is evidence supporting a more aggressive initial approach.

Because beta blockers can constrict the bronchial tubes, their use is contraindicated in patients with asthma. Asthmatics should not use antihistamines in an acute attack. Many asthmatics are sensitive to aspirin and other drugs such as nonsteroidal anti-inflammatory drugs (NSAIDs), penicillin, cephalosporin, and sulfa drugs.

Bronchodilators A **bronchodilator** is an agent that relaxes smooth-muscle cells of the bronchioles. As a result, airway diameter increases, improving the movement of gases into and out of the lungs. Asthmatics need both a long-term medication and a rescue medication to treat asthma and control exacerbations. For long-term needs, inhaled corticosteroids are the most effective medications. When using different medications the bronchodilators should always be used first. Long-term control should be maintained with leukotriene receptor antagonists, cromolyn, long-acting beta agonists, and corticosteroids. Xolair (omalizumab) should be used only in resistant cases.

In terms of a rescue medication, the drug of choice is **epinephrine (EpiPen, Primatene Mist)**. For acute attacks, it is given subcutaneously immediately. Many asthmatics carry an EpiPen to use in the event of an attack. Epinephrine acts as a bronchodilator through beta$_2$ receptors, relaxing smooth muscles and relieving bronchospasms. The OTC aerosol Primatene Mist should not be used more than eight times per day.

Warning

Epinephrine and ephedrine can be easily confused.

TABLE 9.1   Most Commonly Used Agents for Asthma

Generic Name	Pronunciation	Dosage Form	Brand Name	Dispensing Status
Bronchodilators				
albuterol*	al-BYOO-ter-awl	aerosol, capsule, inhalation, oral liquid	Proventil, Proventil HFA, Ventolin HFA, ProAir HFA	Rx
epinephrine*	ep-i-NEF-rin	inhalation , injection, IV	EpiPen	Rx
			Primatene Mist	OTC
formoterol	for-MOE-ter-awl	inhalation	Foradil, Perforomist	Rx
ipratropium*	i-pra-TROE-pee-um	inhalant, solution	Atrovent	Rx
isoproterenol	eye-soe-proe-TER-e-nole	IV	Isuprel	Rx
levalbuterol	lee-val-BYOO-ter-awl	inhalation	Xopenex	Rx
metaproterenol*	met-a-proe-TER-e-nawl	inhalation, oral liquid, tablet	Alupent	Rx
pirbuterol	peer-BYOO-ter-awl	inhalation	Maxair	Rx
salmeterol	sal-ME-te-rawl	inhalation	Serevent	Rx
terbutaline	ter-BYOO-ta-leen	injection, tablet	Brethine	Rx
tiotropium	tye-oh-TRO-pee-um	inhalation	Spiriva	Rx
Xanthine Derivatives				
aminophylline	am-in-OFF-i-lin	IV, suppository, tablet	Truphylline	Rx
theophylline	thee-OFF-i-lin	capsule, IV, oral liquid, tablet	Theo 24, TheoAir	Rx
Leukotriene Inhibitors				
montelukast	mon-te-LOO-kast	oral liquid, tablet	Singulair	Rx
zafirlukast	za-FEER-loo-kast	tablet	Accolate	Rx
zileuton	zye-LOO-ton	tablet	Zyflo	Rx
Corticosteroids				
beclomethasone	bek-loe-METH-a-sone	inhalation, nasal spray	Beconase AQ, QVAR, Vanceril	Rx
budesonide*	byoo-DES-oh-nide	capsule, inhalation	Entocort EC, Pulmicort Respules, Pulmicort Turbuhaler, Rhinocort	Rx
dexamethasone	dex-a-METH-a-sone	tablet	Decadron	Rx
flunisolide	floo-NIS-oh-lide	inhalation	AeroBid	Rx
fluticasone*	floo-TIK-a-sone	inhalation, nasal spray	Flonase, Flovent	Rx
hydrocortisone	hye-droe-KOR-ti-sone	injection	Solu-Cortef	Rx
methylprednisolone	meth-il-pred-NIS-oh-lone	injection, IV, oral liquid, tablet	Medrol Dose Pack, Solu-Medrol	Rx

TABLE 9.1   Most Commonly Used Agents for Asthma (continued)

Generic Name	Pronunciation	Dosage Form	Brand Name	Dispensing Status
mometasone furoate	moe-MET-a-sone FYOOR-oh-ate	inhalation	Asmanex	Rx
prednisolone	pred-NIS-oh-lone	oral liquid, tablet	Orapred, Pediapred	Rx
prednisone	PRED-ni-sone	oral liquid, tablet	Deltasone	Rx
triamcinolone*	trye-am-SIN-oh-lone	inhalation, injection, nasal spray	Azmacort, Nasacort AQ	Rx
Mast Cell Stabilizers				
cromolyn sodium*	KROE-moe-lin SOE-dee-um	capsule, inhalation, nasal spray, ophthalmic solution, oral liquid	Crolom, Gastrocrom, Intal, Opticrom	Rx
			Nasalcrom	OTC
nedocromil	ne-DOK-roe-mil	inhalation	Tilade	Rx
Monoclonal Antibody				
omalizumab	oh-mah-lye-ZOO-mab	injection	Xolair	Rx
Combination Drugs				
budesonide/formoterol	byoo-DES-oh-nide/for-MOE-ter-awl	inhalation	Symbicort	Rx
fluticasone-salmeterol	floo-TIK-a-sone sal-ME-te-rawl	inhalation	Advair Diskus	Rx

*These products are produced in forms as well as inhalants, such as liquids (for use in nebulizers), syrups, and injections. Pharmacists and pharmacy technicians should always carefully read the prescription and choose the correct dosage form.

Side effects of epinephrine can be serious and thus need to be monitored. The alpha agonist actions of the drug increase blood pressure, which increases risk of angina, aortic rupture, and cerebral hemorrhage due to vasoconstriction. The $beta_1$ agonist action causes palpitation, tachycardia, and arrhythmias. The $beta_2$ agonist action causes central nervous system (CNS) stimulation (nervousness, tremor, anxiety, nausea, vomiting) and relaxation of uterine muscles. The $beta_2$ agonists may also cause dry mouth.

The pharmacy technician should be alert to the potential for patient overdependence on short-acting $beta_2$ agonists. If the patient is using more than one canister per month, the pharmacist should notify the prescribing physician. Such overdependence is generally a sign that the patient's asthma is not being adequately controlled and that the physician needs to consider alternative treatment regimens.

Albuterol (Proventil HFA, Ventolin HFA, ProAir HFA) is a bronchodilator used in cases of airway obstruction, such as asthma or COPD. It relaxes bronchial smooth muscle by acting on pulmonary $beta_2$ receptors with little effect on heart rate. Albuterol is administered by inhalation or orally for relief of bronchospasms. Duration is 3 to 6 hours. Proventil HFA and ProAir HFA (hydrofluoroalkane) are both albuterol inhalers that do not use chlorofluorocarbons (CFCs), but the two *cannot* be interchanged. Side effects include tremor and nervousness. If a prescriber writes a prescription for an albuterol inhaler any of the three brands may be used.

Formoterol (Foradil) is a long-acting bronchodilator approved for the long-term maintenance of asthma, for preventing bronchospasms, and for the prevention of exercise-induced asthma. It is a selective beta$_2$ agonist, which means that it acts locally in the lungs to relax smooth muscle and inhibit the release of mast cells. It has a faster onset than salmeterol, working within minutes. Formoterol is supplied in a capsule that is to be loaded into a dry-powder inhaler, *not* to be taken orally. Formoterol must be refrigerated until dispensed, but it does not need to be refrigerated after dispensing, at which time it is good for 4 months. The technician must mark on the box the date after which the drug should not be used. This date is either the expiration date or 4 months after the drug was dispensed, whichever comes first.

Proper administration of formoterol is important. A capsule is placed in the chamber of the inhaler, and the mouthpiece is closed. The capsule is pierced by pressing and releasing the buttons on the side. *The patient should then inhale quickly and deeply,* which causes the capsule to spin, dispensing the drug. The patient should then hold their breath as long as possible. The capsule should be checked to ensure that all of the powder was released; if it was not, then it should be inhaled again. The most common side effect is tremor. Even though this drug has a quick onset, it should *not be used* to treat acute asthma. If it is being used to prevent exercise-induced asthma, it should be used 15 minutes before exercise. No more than one capsule should be used in 12 hour.

Ipratropium (Atrovent) blocks the action of acetylcholine in bronchial smooth muscle, causing bronchodilation. It is derived from atropine and is used for prevention, not for acute management. It is a short-acting agent and is not absorbed into general circulation when inhaled, so it does not cause arrhythmias. The technician should make sure the patient is not allergic to peanuts before dispensing this drug. Soy lecithin is used as a suspending agent in the inhaler. Because soybeans and peanuts are closely related, a very dangerous cross-reaction can occur if the patient has a peanut allergy. The warning about the possible allergy problem may not show up in the computer when the drug is dispensed.

Isoproterenol (Isuprel) is indicated for treating reversible airway obstruction, as in asthma or COPD. It stimulates beta$_1$ and beta$_2$ receptors, resulting in relaxation of bronchial, GI, and uterine smooth muscle, increased heart rate and contractility, and vasodilation of peripheral vasculature. It may be used up to five times a day with no more than two inhalations at one time and 1 to 5 minutes between inhalations; no more than six inhalations should be administered in 1 hour.

Albuterol, discussed previously, occurs in two isomeric forms, one of which is the active component of the compound. **Levalbuterol (Xopenex)** is the active isomer of albuterol. Levalbuterol can be prescribed at lower doses than albuterol and is thought to have fewer side effects than albuterol.

Metaproterenol (Alupent) is a bronchodilator for airway obstruction, such as asthma or COPD. It has a rapid onset of action within minutes, a peak effect in approximately 1 hour, and prolonged effect (4 hour); it acts primarily on beta$_2$ receptors, with little or no effect on heart rate.

Pirbuterol (Maxair) is a short-acting bronchodilator used to prevent and treat reversible bronchospasm, especially asthma. It is a selective beta$_2$ agonist with a duration of action of 4 to 6 hours. The patient should not exceed the recommended dose of 12 inhalations per day. Allow at least 2 minutes between inhalations and at least 5 minutes before using inhaled steroids.

Salmeterol (Serevent) is indicated for maintenance therapy of asthma. It is a beta$_2$ agonist with a long duration of action and an onset of action in 30 to 60 minutes. Salmeterol is taken twice a day. It should be reserved for patients with more serious asthma or those already receiving anti-inflammatory therapy. Its long duration of action makes it particularly useful for nocturnal symptoms of asthma. Salmeterol should not be used to treat rescue situations. Improper use of this drug has been implicated in deaths. Salmeterol is available as a dry powder inhaler.

Terbutaline (Brethine) is a long-acting bronchodilator for reversible airway obstruction and bronchial asthma. It can be used parenterally for status asthmaticus. Excessive use may lead to paradoxical bronchoconstriction. If this occurs, the patient should discontinue the medication immediately. It is a beta$_2$ agonist. (Terbutaline is also used in obstetrics as a premature labor inhibitor because of its relaxation of uterine muscle.)

Xanthine Derivatives   A **xanthine derivative** is a drug, structurally similar to caffeine, that causes relaxation of airway smooth muscle, thus causing airway dilation and better air movement.

Theophylline is a phosphodiesterase inhibitor that reverses early bronchospasm associated with antigens or irritants. **Aminophylline (Truphylline)** is the more soluble ethylenediamine salt of theophylline. Theophylline improves the contractility of the fatigued diaphragm. It can be used as a bronchodilator in reversible airway obstruction due to asthma, chronic bronchitis, or emphysema. Blood levels are maintained at 10 mcg/mL to 20 mcg/mL. Theophylline has many interactions, however, and blood levels can become elevated quickly. Consequently, it is used only in lung disease unresponsive to other drugs. Theophylline can also be used for neonatal (the first four weeks after birth) apnea and bradycardia.

Leukotriene Inhibitors   Leukotrienes are metabolized from arachidonic acid, which is also responsible for forming prostaglandins. Leukotrienes increase accumulation of fluid in the spaces between cells, mucus, and vascular permeability, permitting substances to pass through the blood vessels; they are 100 to 1,000 times more potent than histamine for these effects. A **leukotriene inhibitor** blocks either the synthesis of, or the body's inflammatory responses to, the leukotrienes. Blocking receptors also blocks tissue inflammatory responses.

Montelukast (Singulair) is a leukotriene receptor antagonist. This drug is indicated for the prophylaxis and chronic treatment of asthma. Montelukast has been shown to reduce incidence of daytime asthma and nocturnal awakenings due to asthma attacks. It can also decrease the need for beta-adrenergic agonists. Montelukast should not be used to treat acute attacks. Unlike the other leukotriene modifiers, which can be prescribed only for adults or older children, montelukast has been approved for use in children over the age of 12 months. Montelukast also has the benefit of a once-daily dosage, as opposed to the other leukotriene inhibitors, which must be dosed two to four times per day. A headache is the most common side effect associated with montelukast. This drug is also approved to treat seasonal allergic rhinitis. Asthma and hay fever are treated with the same dose.

Zafirlukast (Accolate), like montelukast, antagonizes leukotriene receptors, thus reducing edema, mucus, and vascular permeability. It is intended for prophylaxis and long-term treatment in patients 5 years of age or older. Side effects are headache, rhinitis (inflammation of the nasal membranes), and cough. Good results are reported with few side effects.

Zileuton (Zyflo) is a leukotriene inhibitor that reduces the production of leukotrienes rather than blocking leukotriene receptors. Zileuton carries strong warnings about liver toxicity. It can also double theophylline levels if the patient is taking that drug. It is approved only for patients 12 years of age or older.

Corticosteroids A **corticosteroid** resembles certain chemicals naturally produced by the adrenal gland. Corticosteroids inhibit inflammatory cells by stimulating adenylate cyclase. They act as an anti-inflammatory agent to suppress the immune response. Inhaled corticosteroids may be successful when other drugs are not.

Nevertheless, many persons with asthma still are not using inhaled corticosteroids because they fear potential side effects. The primary side effects of these drugs, if inhaled, are oral candidiasis (a fungal infection), irritation and burning of the nasal mucosa, hoarseness, and dry mouth. This irritation can sometimes lead to episodes of coughing. To reduce the likelihood of these effects, the patient should always be advised to rinse the mouth thoroughly with water after using a corticosteroid inhaler. Improper technique when using a metered dose inhaler can result in inadequate response, but this problem can be avoided with proper instruction.

If corticosteroids are taken orally for a long period in a dosage exceeding 10 mg/day, they can cause growth of facial hair in females, breast development in males, "buffalo hump," "moon face," edema, weight gain, and easy bruising. A short-term course of high-dose corticosteroid will not cause these side effects.

Another concern is that corticosteroids may stunt a child's growth. Evidence indicates, however, that inhaled steroids do not affect long-term growth in children. Initially, there may be a slowdown of half an inch in growth in the first year, but the children eventually reach normal adult height. Controlling the asthma is more important to achieving normal growth and development.

Patients should always use the lowest effective dose of a corticosteroid. A $beta_2$ agonist such as salmeterol (Serevent) should be added to inhaled corticosteroid if needed to decrease the steroid dose necessary for control. The $beta_2$ agonist helps open the airway, thus allowing more of the inhaled steroid to reach its site of action in the lungs.

Fluticasone (Flovent) is the same drug found in the nasal spray Flonase. Flovent comes in three strengths. The lowest is for mild asthma, and the highest is used to wean patients off oral corticosteroids. It should be used twice daily and may take up to 1 to 2 weeks to reach maximum benefit.

Budesonide (Entocort EC, Pulmicort Respules, Pulmicort Turbuhaler, Rhinocort) is a corticosteroid with unique administration techniques. As with other drugs in this class, patients should be instructed to rinse their mouth after each dose. Inadequate response to budesonide is often the result of an improper inhalation technique. The pharmacist can help correct this problem by providing appropriate instructions to the patient. Pulmicort Turbuhaler uses a novel, dry-powder, propellant-free inhalant that is breath activated. This formulation requires less hand-lung coordination than other forms. As a result, it is easier to use. Moreover, the Turbuhaler needs to be primed only prior to the initial use rather than before each dose as is necessary with other corticosteroid inhalers. Pulmicort is associated with a lower frequency of coughing episodes than other inhaled corticosteroids. Pulmicort Respules was the first formulation of budesonide for use in home nebulizers. This formulation has made possible the treatment of children as young as 12 months of age.

Beclomethasone (Beconase AQ, QVAR, Vanceril) is a steroid inhaler that uses the propellant hydrofluoroalkane (HFA) instead of chlorofluorocarbons. HFA particles are smaller and improved delivery is provided to the smaller airways of the lungs, so a lower dose may be effective. Patients should rinse their mouth after using beclomethasone, as they should with any steroid inhaler.

Mometasone (Asmanex) is a dry powder for inhalation. It should be dosed once daily in the evening. The dispenser is called a Twisthaler and has a dose counter. When the dose counter gets to 00 or the package has been open 45 days, the package needs to be disposed of. Pharmacy technicians should write the date opened on the dispenser and make sure the patient knows when to dispose of the drug. Mometasone can be used for prophylactic therapy, but maximum benefit may take 2 weeks or longer. It is not to be used in acute episodes. Headache is the major side effect. Mometasone has high potency and little systemic bioavailability.

Other steroids are **prednisone (Deltasone)**, **hydrocortisone (Solu-Cortef)**, **methylprednisolone (Medrol Dose Pack, Solu-Medrol)**, **dexamethasone (Decadron)**, **prednisolone (Orapred, Pediapred)**, **triamcinolone (Azmacort, Nasacort AQ)**, and **flunisolide (AeroBid)**.

Mast Cell Stabilizers A **mast cell stabilizer** protects mast cell membranes against rupture caused by antigenic substances. As a result, less histamine, leukotrienes, and prostaglandins are released in airway tissue.

Cromolyn sodium (Crolom, Gastrocrom, Intal, Nasalcrom, Opticrom) works topically in the airways. It is a prophylactic drug with no benefit for acute reactions. Cromolyn sodium stabilizes mast cell membranes and directly inhibits other inflammatory cells. The airways must be open before administration, so a bronchodilator is often given first. This is a very effective drug, but patient compliance is a big problem. The drug is dosed four times a day, and most patients have difficulty fitting the four doses into their daily routine. Moreover, cromolyn sodium has an unpleasant taste after inhalation, and side effects include hoarseness, dry mouth, and stuffy nose. The drug has many dosage forms, so care must be taken to select the correct one.

Nedocromil (Tilade) is used for maintenance therapy in patients with mild-to-moderate asthma. It inhibits early and late bronchoconstrictive response to inhaled antigens, exercise, cold air, fog, and sulfur dioxide. The few side effects, including arthritis, rash, and tremors, are rare.

Monoclonal Antibody A **monoclonal antibody** is an antibody produced in a laboratory from an isolated specific lymphocyte that produces a pure antibody against a known specific antigen.

Omalizumab (Xolair) is a monoclonal antibody for treatment of asthma not controlled with inhaled steroids. It is used for adults and children older than 12 years of age. It is not to be used acutely, as in status asthmaticus or asthma exacerbations. It is administered subcutaneously. Omalizumab blocks the immunoglobulin IgE, which is a major cause of allergic asthma. This drug should be reserved for cases that have proven difficult to treat with other medications.

Combination Drugs Combination drugs typically combine a short-acting and a long-acting drug. Combinations for asthma are designed for maintenance therapy and work better than monotherapy to decrease exacerbations and control symptoms. The efficacy is similar to using the two drugs separately.

Budesonide-formoterol (Symbicort) is indicated for maintenance therapy for asthma. Budesonide-formoterol is approved for acute symptoms in Canada, but not in the United States. The budesonide-formoterol inhaler must be primed, and patients are directed to take two puffs twice daily, with mouth rinsing afterward. The combination works better than either drug alone.

Fluticasone-salmeterol (Advair Diskus) is an anti-inflammatory and beta$_2$-adrenergic agonist used for maintenance treatment of asthma and COPD for patients older than 12 years of age. It is a powder for oral inhalation. Fluticasone, a corticosteroid, is a potent vasoconstrictor and anti-inflammatory. Salmeterol relaxes bronchial smooth muscle with little effect on heart rate. Together, the two drugs act synergistically to improve pulmonary function more than either agent used alone. Fluticasone-salmeterol should not be used with a spacer.

Chronic Obstructive Pulmonary Disease

Chronic obstructive pulmonary disease (COPD) encompasses emphysema and chronic bronchitis.

Emphysema

Emphysema is characterized by destruction of the tiny alveoli, or air sacs, of the lungs (shown in Figure 9.1). As a result, air accumulates in tissues and organs. Typically, air spaces distal to (farther away from) the terminal bronchioles are enlarged. Inflammation destroys these air sacs, which then lose their ability to expand and contract and their ability to pass oxygen into the blood and remove carbon dioxide. In the early stages, shortness of breath occurs only after heavy exercise. As the disease progresses, walking even a short distance can make the patient gasp for air. Patients with emphysema have **tachypnea** (very rapid respiration), which gives them a flushed appearance. Major risk factors are cigarette smoking (which destroys the walls of the lungs), occupational exposure, air pollution, and genetic factors.

Bronchitis

Bronchitis is a condition in which the lining of the bronchial airways becomes inflamed, causing the patient to experience obstruction of air flow on expiration. This disease is characterized by a cough that produces sputum (phlegm) that may be purulent (containing pus), green, or blood streaked. Acute bronchitis is caused by an infection, usually viral; it runs a brief course and is corrected by the body, often with the aid of antibiotics to prevent or treat secondary bacterial infections; it generally does not return. Chronic bronchitis is a serious disease, defined as excessive production of tracheobronchial mucus sufficient to cause cough with expectoration of at least 30 mL of sputum per 24 hours for 3 months of the year for more than two consecutive years. Patients usually are overweight, have a barrel chest, and tend to retain carbon dioxide. Most persons have a morning cough resulting from irritation to the lungs.

Several factors can contribute to the development of chronic bronchitis. The most prominent of these include cigarette smoke; exposure to occupational dusts, fumes, and environmental pollution; and bacterial infection. Studies of lungs from smoking and nonsmoking subjects clearly demonstrate that those who smoke cigarettes have more bronchial inflammation and substantially increased numbers of alveolar macrophages.

Drug Treatments for COPD

To understand the treatment for emphysema and chronic bronchitis, you must also understand the lungs' natural defense system. When this system is functioning properly, the host defenses of the respiratory tract provide good protection against pathogen invasion and remove potentially infectious agents from the lungs. The lungs are normally sterile below the first branch. It is when organisms breach this region that infection and inflammation are initiated.

The body's defenses include a number of different types of cells.

- The ciliary carpet consists of minute hairlike processes, called cilia, that beat rhythmically to propel fluid or mucus, and any inhaled particles that have become trapped in the fluid, over the inner surface of the airway, upward and out.
- Goblet cells secrete mucus.
- Clara cells, unciliated cells at the branching of the alveolar duct into the bronchioles, secrete enzymes that break down airborne toxins.
- Epithelial cells produce a protein-rich exudate in the small bronchi and bronchioles.
- Type I pneumocytes in the alveolar membranes act as the phagocytes of the lung. They clear trash and organisms from the lung.
- Type II pneumocytes synthesize and secrete surfactant.

Figure 9.4 demonstrates the relationship of cells composing the alveolus and blood supply.

Emphysema and chronic bronchitis sometimes occur together, and their pharmacologic treatment is similar. Table 9.2 lists the drugs commonly used to treat emphysema and chronic bronchitis. The pharmacologic management of emphysema and bronchitis is still largely empirical, with methylxanthines, corticosteroids, beta agonists, and ipratropium forming the foundation of therapy, as in asthma. Oxygen administration and physiotherapy play an important role in treating both lung diseases. In both emphysema and chronic bronchitis, antibiotic therapy is sometimes needed if either sputum changes from yellow to green or fever is present. Expectorants (discussed in greater detail later in the chapter) are sometimes used to stimulate respiratory secretions and counter dryness, which stimulates irritation and coughing. Drinking large amounts of water helps to break up mucus and enables the patient to cough up secretions; water is the expectorant of choice. Patients with COPD should always be encouraged to get influenza and pneumococcal vaccinations annually, because this disease state predisposes them to flu and pneumonia.

Bronchodilators Some of the same bronchodilators used in the long-term treatment of asthma are also used in COPD.

Formoterol (Perforomist) and **arformoterol (Brovana)** are different isomers of the same compound. Formoterol is a solution form of the drug and is used for COPD as well as for asthma. Arformoterol is also used for long-term maintenance treatment in COPD. Both need to be refrigerated until dispensed, after which time they can be stored outside the refrigerator but must be protected from heat and moisture. These medications must not be used after the "Use By" date, which is filled in by the pharmacy staff. The "Use By" date is either 4 months after purchase or the expiration date, whichever comes first. Both formoterol and arformoterol are beta agonists, and both are used for maintenance therapy, not acute events. Both agents are used in a nebulizer and are ideal for patients who may not be able to use an inhaler.

Ipratropium-albuterol (Combivent) is a combination inhaler that should be used for patients who require a second

FIGURE 9.4
Cellular Makeup of an Alveolus and Capillary Supply

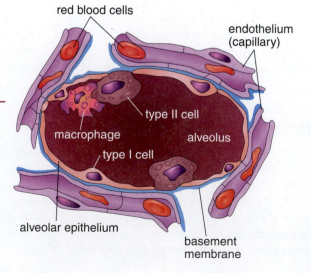

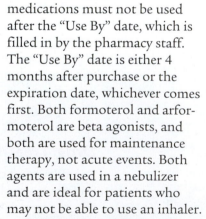

red blood cells

endothelium (capillary)

type II cell

macrophage

alveolus

type I cell

alveolar epithelium

basement membrane

TABLE 9.2 Most Commonly Used Agents for COPD

Generic Name	Pronunciation	Dosage Form	Brand Name	Dispensing Status
Mucolytics				
acetylcysteine	a-see-til-SIS-teen	inhalation solution, IV, oral liquid	Acetadote, Mucomyst	Rx
dornase alfa	DOR-nayse AL-fa	inhalation	Pulmozyme	Rx
Anticholinergic				
tiotropium	tye-oh-TROE-pee-um	inhalation	Spiriva	Rx
Beta Agonists				
arformoterol	ar-for-MOE-ter-awl	inhalation	Brovana	Rx
formoterol	for-MOE-ter-awl	inhalation	Perforomist	Rx
isoproterenol*	eye-soe-proe-TER-e-nawl	inhalation, IV	Isuprel	Rx
metaproterenol*	met-a-proe-TER-e-nawl	inhalation, oral liquid, tablet	Alupent	Rx
Combinations				
ipratropium-albuterol	i-pra-TROE-pee-um al-BYOO-ter-awl	inhalation	Combivent	Rx
fluticasone-salmeterol	floo-TIK-a-sone sal-ME-te-rawl	inhalation	Advair Diskus	Rx

*These products are produced in forms other than inhalants, such as liquids (for use in nebulizers), syrups, and injections. Pharmacists and pharmacy technicians should always carefully read the prescription and choose the correct dosage form.

inhaler. The pharmacy technician should determine whether the patient has a peanut allergy if this drug is prescribed, because, as previously stated, the propellent is based on soy lecithin, which can trigger a cross-reaction in persons with peanut allergies.

Tiotropium (Spiriva) is similar to ipratropium (Atrovent) but is dosed only once daily, although it works for approximately 36 hours. It is indicated only for long-term maintenance therapy for bronchospasms associated with emphysema and bronchitis. Dry mouth is a very common side effect. Tiotropium is provided by the manufacturer as a capsule for inhalation. One capsule should be placed in the HandiHaler and the button pressed to disperse the powder into the inhaler. After the inhaler is used, the drug should be emptied into a disposable container. The dry powder should not be touched. This drug is very sensitive to moisture and heat, so the capsule should not be exposed before the patient is ready to use it. Therefore, the patient needs to know that the package should be peeled back only to the STOP mark.

Warning

Watch for injectable acetylcysteine (Acetadote) versus oral (Mucomyst), as they come in vials that look alike and are the same strength. Confusion could result in a very serious error.

Mucolytics Another treatment for chronic bronchitis is the use of a **mucolytic** (an agent that destroys or dissolves mucus), such as **acetylcysteine (Acetadote, Mucomyst)**, which breaks apart glycoproteins, thereby reducing viscosity and promoting easier movement and removal of secretions.

Another mucolytic, **dornase alfa (Pulmozyme)**, is discussed in the next section concerning cystic fibrosis.

Other Lung Diseases

In addition to the diseases already discussed, there are many other forms of lung infections. Several measures can be taken to control and prevent lung disease. Not smoking is the very best protection against the risk of lung disease. Avoiding secondhand smoke and air pollution is also important. Influenza and pneumococcal pneumonia can be prevented with vaccination. Most infections occur when people come into contact with fluids, sneezes, and coughs that contain bacteria, viruses, or fungi. It has long been thought that respiratory infections are transmitted through inhalation, but recent studies have shown that hand contact is the most frequent culprit. Thus, frequent hand washing and avoiding of close contact with infected hosts are the best defense.

Pneumonia

Pneumonia is a common lung infection that affects persons of all ages. The microorganisms that cause pneumonia gain access to the lower respiratory tract by the following three routes:

- inhalation as aerosolized particles
- entry through the bloodstream
- aspiration in oropharyngeal contents

Aspiration, which involves inhalation of fluids from the mouth and throat, is a common occurrence in both healthy and ill persons during sleep. It is the major mechanism by which pulmonary pathogens gain access to the normally sterile lower airways and alveoli. Pneumonia is treated with antibiotics, depending on the causative organism.

Cystic Fibrosis

Cystic fibrosis (CF) is a hereditary disease that involves the gastrointestinal and pulmonary systems. It is a fatal disease, but some patients survive into early adulthood. The morbidity and mortality of the disease are associated with disorders in the pulmonary system. The GI involvement is due to increased viscosity of secreted mucus, causing bile duct blockage, and a relative deficiency of pancreatic digestive enzymes.

Patients with cystic fibrosis experience hypoxia (lack of adequate oxygen) with resultant cyanosis and digital clubbing (enlarged fingertips with loss of normal angle at the nailbed) are common. A patient's respiratory status follows a cyclic pattern, from a state of relative well-being to one of acute pulmonary deterioration. Management of the pulmonary aspect of this disease can be broken down into two areas: respiratory therapy and antibiotic therapy.

The cornerstone of respiratory therapy is **percussion**, a tapping movement to induce cough and expectoration of sputum from the lungs. This is often preceded by nebulizer therapy, during which nebulized sterile water or normal saline is breathed to liquefy pulmonary secretions.

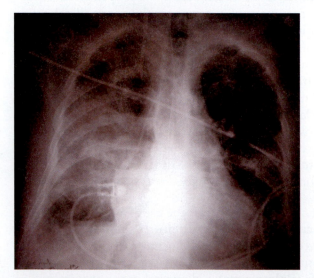

An X-ray of a patient with pneumonia that shows fluid in the right lung.

Acetylcysteine or other bronchodilators may be added to the nebulizer solution to prevent bronchospasm and further liquefy the secretions. Oral Mucomyst has a very unpleasant taste and odor, though, and many patients prefer not to use it. Normal asthmatic bronchodilators are appropriate for CF. Theophylline may be of benefit; however, theophylline clearance in CF patients may differ from that in asthmatics, so clearance and dosage should be carefully monitored. Acetylcysteine and dornase alfa, already listed in Table 9.2 in connection with COPD, are the most commonly used agents for CF.

Dornase alfa (Pulmozyme) selectively breaks down DNA that is released by degenerating leukocytes. The leukocytes collect in response to infection. By destroying DNA in the mucus, dornase alfa helps reduce secretion viscosity (resistance to flow, thickness).

Most CF patients are at high risk for complications from influenza, so influenza vaccine should be given yearly. Most clinicians treat pulmonary exacerbations with antibiotics, although this may be controversial because microorganisms may develop a resistance to the antibiotic.

Respiratory Distress Syndrome

Respiratory distress syndrome (RDS) occurs in newborns during the first few hours of life. It is characterized by inadequate production of pulmonary **surfactant**—a fluid that, like soap, lowers the surface tension between the air and alveolar surfaces. Lack of surfactant leads to collapse of the alveoli along with acute asphyxia with hypoxia and acidosis. Prematurity and maternal diabetes are two known causative factors of RDS. If RDS occurs, a replacement surfactant is administered. Table 9.3 lists the most commonly used agents for RDS.

Beractant (Survanta) is the drug of choice for RDS. It is a natural agent extracted from cattle lung and supplied as a suspension for intratracheal administration. Beractant replaces deficient or ineffective endogenous lung surfactant in neonates and prevents the alveoli from collapsing during expiration by lowering the surface tension between the air and alveolar surfaces. Beractant is used for prophylactic therapy in high-risk infants and rescue therapy within 8 hours of birth.

Colfosceril palimate (Exosurf Neonatal) is a lung surfactant that, by reducing surface tension in the lung, stabilizes the alveoli from collapsing in infants. Once reconstituted, the drug must be used immediately.

Calfactant (Infasurf) replaces deficient endogenous lung surfactant and is indicated for neonates who are less than 72 hours of age. When on this drug, infants require less oxygen than with other RDS drugs. The drug should be stored in the

TABLE 9.3	Most Commonly Used Surfactants for Respiratory Distress Syndrome			
Generic Name	Pronunciation	Dosage Form	Brand Name	Dispensing Status
beractant	ber-AKT-ant	injection	Survanta	Rx
calfactant	kal-FAK-tant	injection	Infasurf	Rx
colfosceril palimate	kohl-FOS-ser-il PAL-i-mate	injection	Exosurf Neonatal	Rx
poractant alfa	por-AKT-ant AL-fa	injection	Curosurf	Rx

refrigerator. The suspension settles and should be swirled gently but not shaken to redisperse the medication. It is not necessary to warm calfactant before administration. Vials that have been stored unopen at room temperature for less than 24 hours may be safely returned to the refrigerator.

Poractant alfa (Curosurf) may be preferred for very tiny babies because it requires much less fluid than the other cystic fibrosis drugs and can be administered in one dose. With some of the other drugs, a partial dose must be administered, followed by a 2- or 3-hour wait, and then another partial dose.

Tuberculosis

Tuberculosis (TB) is caused by the bacterium *Mycobacterium tuberculosis*. The disease most commonly affects the lungs, but it may also infect other body tissues and organs. TB is transmitted by respiratory droplets inhaled into the lungs of persons at risk. The droplets are produced when infected persons with active TB cough, sneeze, speak, kiss, or spit. Suspended in the air, these droplets descend under the influence of gravity at the relatively slow rate of 1 to 2 inches (2.5–5 cm) per hour. Once inhaled, *M. tuberculosis* may spread throughout the body in the bloodstream and in lymphatic fluids. A follicle forms and is surrounded by epithelial cells. The mass may spread or liquefy, forming a cavity filled with fluid and teeming with organisms. The fluid may move in the direction of least resistance, spreading organisms and disease within the organ, and thereby destroying more tissue (formation of a fibrosis). The *M. tuberculosis* bacterium thrives in areas of high oxygen, so resulting lesions concentrate primarily in the lung, but they may also occur in bone and kidney tissue.

Tuberculosis is seen primarily in alcoholics, the prison population, the immuno-compromised, and the elderly. It should be included in the differential diagnosis of patients with fever of unknown origin, subacute meningitis, or chronic infection at any site.

Two groups of tuberculosis patients are recognized based on disease symptoms and antibody production:

1. Exposed but showing no disease. If time has elapsed since exposure, these patients produce TB antibodies and may test positive to the TB skin test. This does not mean they have active disease.
2. Exposed and having active organisms. These patients may or may not produce antibodies depending on the competence of their immune system. Significant signs and symptoms of active disease include weight loss, spitting blood, night sweats and night fever, chest pain, and malaise.

The agent in the TB test is purified protein derivative (PPD) from killed bacteria. This product is injected intradermally. Persons who have been exposed to or have the disease show a circular area of hardened tissue (induration) at the injection site within 48 to 72 hours. A false-negative reaction may occur in persons recently exposed and in older persons who have delayed-type hypersensitivity. If the reading is positive, the patient is directed to have a chest X-ray taken so as to detect the presence of a lung shadow, which, if present, may indicate active disease.

Tuberculosis generally develops slowly and may take as long as 20 years to develop from the time of exposure. The highest incidence of infection occurs 1 to 2 years after exposure. Even if the disease is arrested early (4 to 10 weeks after exposure), patients still have a risk of reactivity for the remainder of their life. The organism can lie dormant for years until the immune system is depressed, when it will reemerge as an active infection. The medical history of the patient should be watched for disease symptoms such as weight loss, fever, night sweats, malaise, and loss of appetite.

The goals of TB therapy are to

- initiate treatment promptly
- convert the sputum culture from positive to negative as soon as possible
- achieve cure without relapse
- prevent emergence of drug-resistant strains

Table 9.4 describes the most commonly used agents for treating TB. The primary agents used are isoniazid, rifampin, ethambutol, streptomycin, and pyrazinamide. Isoniazid and rifampin are highly effective if used in combination. Streptomycin is recommended as a third drug, especially because it can be injected twice weekly to guarantee compliance.

The treatment regimen for TB varies depending on the patient's symptoms. For patients with no symptoms, a positive PPD skin test, and a positive X-ray, the disease is treated with a single agent, usually isoniazid (INH), 300 mg once daily for 12 months. For patients with the clinical disease, at least two agents to which the organism is susceptible will be administered.

Rifampin plus pyrazinamide is recommended only for treatment of active TB, not latent TB. Pyrazinamide seems to be the most hepatotoxic of all the first-line drugs for TB. For latent TB, isoniazid or rifampin can be prescribed. Isoniazid is often written INH by prescribers on prescriptions.

Active tuberculosis should be treated with a combination of drugs. In contrast, a prophylaxis drug therapy should include only one drug. This limit is an effort to

TABLE 9.4 Most Commonly Used Agents for Tuberculosis

Generic Name	Pronunciation	Dosage Form	Brand Name	Dispensing Status
capreomycin	kap-ree-oh-MYE-sin	injection	Capastat	Rx
ciprofloxacin	sip-roe-FLOX-a-sin	injection, IV, oral liquid, tablet	Cipro	Rx
cycloserine	sye-kloe-SER-een	capsule	Seromycin	Rx
ethambutol	e-THAM-byoo-tawl	tablet	Myambutol	Rx
ethionamide	e-thye-ON-am-ide	tablet	Trecator-SC	Rx
isoniazid (INH)	eye-soe-NYE-a-zid	injection, oral liquid, tablet	Laniazid, Nydrazid	Rx
isoniazid-pyrazinamide-rifampin	eye-soe-NYE-a-zid peer-a-ZIN-a-mide rif-AM-pin	tablet	Rifater	Rx
isoniazid-rifampin	eye-soe-NYE-a-zid rif-AM-pin	capsule	Rifamate	Rx
ofloxacin	oe-FLOX-a-sin	IV, tablet	Floxin	Rx
pyrazinamide	peer-a-ZIN-a-mide	tablet	(none)	Rx
rifampin	rif-AM-pin	capsule, IV	Rifadin, Rimactane	Rx
rifapentine	RIF-a-pen-teen	tablet	Priftin	Rx
streptomycin	strep-toe-MYE-sin	injection, IV	(none)	Rx

prevent the development of drug-resistant bacteria. Nevertheless, a new strain of *M. tuberculosis* that is very resistant to many currently used drugs and difficult to treat has now emerged. Defined as multidrug-resistant tuberculosis (MDR-TB), this new strain of *M. tuberculosis* constitutes a serious health problem. The organisms show resistance to the commonly used therapeutic agents. Risk factors for developing MDR-TB include being exposed to MDR-TB, failing to complete therapy, being prescribed inappropriate agents, having immune deficiencies, and having a recurrence of TB. Successful therapy for MDR-TB may require 18 to 24 months of treatment. First-line therapy includes capreomycin and cycloserine.

Most patients receive the drug isoniazid. If resistance to isoniazid develops, rifampin is the drug of choice. When the disease exhibits resistance to both these agents, the following combinations are recommended: pyrazinamide plus ethambutol (Myambutol); pyrazinamide plus ciprofloxacin (Cipro) or ofloxacin (Floxin).

Rifampin (Rifadin, Rimactane) is an antitubercular agent that works through the inhibition of bacterial RNA synthesis. Side effects include the discoloration of urine, tears, sweat, and other body fluids, which turn reddish orange. This discoloration can permanently stain soft contact lenses. The IV and oral dosages are the same. Rifampin interferes with oral contraceptives; thus, female patients taking this drug must be advised to seek alternative forms of birth control. Rifampin must be taken on an empty stomach.

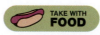

Rifapentine (Priftin) has a longer duration of action than rifampin and, therefore, has the advantage of a less frequent administration schedule, leading to improved patient compliance. Rifapentine is always used as an adjunctive therapy. This drug has the same side effect profile as rifampin. It must be taken with food.

Patient compliance is a major problem in treating this disease. The severe side effect profile, the length of time required for treatment of active TB, and the number of medications required all contribute to noncompliance. Patients being treated for active TB should avoid alcohol.

Histoplasmosis

Another pulmonary disease, **histoplasmosis,** is caused by a fungus that most commonly occurs in accumulated droppings from chickens, pigeons, starlings, other birds, and bats. When the fungus-bearing dust is inhaled, spores are transported into the bronchial tubes. The lymph tissue reacts to this invasion and sensitivity develops; as a result, tissue becomes inflamed. This disease is most prevalent in the valleys of the Missouri and Ohio Rivers.

Histoplasmosis is often referred to as the summer flu because it produces flu-like symptoms. Although the disease mimics tuberculosis, most patients recover on their own without treatment. Histoplasmosis is usually self-limiting and is serious only if there is a very large number of fungi. In the disseminated form, however, it can be fatal without treatment. Amphotericin B and itraconazole appear to be the only effective drugs for the more serious disseminated form. Surgery may sometimes be indicated.

Cough, Cold, and Allergy

The most prevalent form of respiratory tract infection is the common cold, which is a mild self-limited viral infection. Symptoms are readily recognized by the patient and include mild malaise, rhinorrhea (runny nose), sneezing, scratchy throat, and fever. Bacterial sinusitis and otitis media are frequent complications necessitating antimicrobial therapy. Antibiotics and sometimes antivirals are used in treating these problems. However, viruses are the most common cause of infections to the respiratory system.

Symptoms of some allergies are the same as those of colds—runny nose and itchy eyes—so these allergies can be misidentified as a cold. In contrast to the viral cause of the common cold, an allergy results from a state of hypersensitivity induced by exposure to a particular antigen. Both colds and many allergies are treated with the same medications.

The vast majority of colds are self-limiting, but people seek self-treatment to relieve the symptoms and often to prevent complications. Ordinarily, the common cough and cold are treated with four groups of drugs, either alone or in combination: antitussives, expectorants, decongestants, and antihistamines. A large number of the drugs in these four groups are available as OTC products. Consequently, this is an area where technicians can put their drug knowledge to use. Although the technician must still refer to the pharmacist in areas requiring judgmental decisions, the

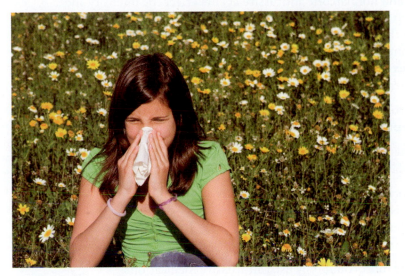
Millions of American are affected by allergies, including hay fever.

OTCs have directions printed on the package. The technician will be the person who most frequently directs the patient to OTC remedies. Although recommendations should not be made, the technician can definitely make the patient aware of the proper uses and side effects of these drugs. Tavist (clemastine) is the only drug approved by the FDA to treat a cold.

For the most part, colds can be successfully avoided if a few simple precautions are taken. Colds are transmitted from an infected person to other people (1) directly when an infected person sneezes or coughs and (2) indirectly by contact with surfaces such as telelphones, doorknobs, or toys. A sneeze or cough should be covered by turning the head and coughing into the shoulder, *not the hand*. Many people contract a cold by rubbing their eyes or nose after touching contaminated surfaces or people with colds. Washing one's hands is the best preventive measure—this cannot be stressed enough. Use of a telephone right after an infected person has used the phone is a frequent way a cold is transmitted. In the pharmacy it is very important to wipe the phones with alcohol on a regular basis.

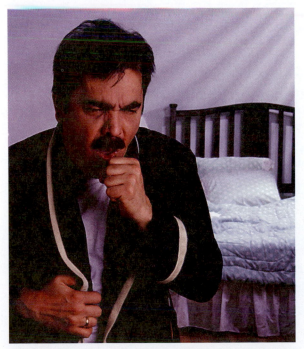
Stimulating receptors in the airways and lungs produces a cough.

Antitussives

Coughing is a mechanism for clearing the airways of excess secretions and foreign materials. Intense, frequent coughing with lack of sputum production can be annoying to the patient. In these instances, an **antitussive** can be therapeutic. An antitussive is an agent that suppresses coughing and is indicated when cough frequency needs to be reduced, especially when the cough is dry and nonproductive. The mechanism by which the narcotic and nonnarcotic antitussive agents affect the intensity and frequency of a cough depends on the principal site of action: (1) CNS depression of the cough center in the medulla (cough reflex) or (2) suppression of the nerve receptors within the respiratory tract.

The **cough reflex** involves two types of receptors found in the lungs and airways. These receptors, when stimulated, can initiate the events leading to a cough.

- A **stretch receptor** responds to elongation of muscle.
- An **irritant receptor** responds to coarse particles and chemicals.

Theoretically, the cough reflex can be stopped at several points. The antitussive products are formulated to act on one or more of the events in this series by

- correcting or blocking the irritation of receptors
- blocking transmission to the brain
- increasing the cough center threshold
- blocking the action of the expiratory muscles

Table 9.5 lists the most commonly used antitussive medications.

TABLE 9.5   Most Commonly Used Antitussive Medications

Generic Name	Pronunciation	Dosage Form	Brand Name	Dispensing Status	Control Schedule
benzonatate	ben-ZOE-na-tate	capsule	Tessalon	Rx	
codeine	KOE-deen	oral liquid	(various combinations)	OTC	C-V
dextromethorphan	dex-troe-meth-OR-fan	oral liquid, tablet	Delsym	OTC	
diphenhydramine	dye-fen-HYE-dra-meen	capsule, oral liquid, tablet	Benadryl	OTC	
hydrocodone-chlorpheniramine	hye-droe-KOE-done klor-fen-EER-a-meen	liquid	Tussionex	Rx	CIII
promethazine-codeine	proe-METH-a-zeen KOE-deen	oral liquid	Phenergan with codeine	Rx	C-V
Dextromethorphan Combinations					
dextromethorphan-pseudoephedrine-brompheniramine	dex-troe-meth-OR-fan soo-doe-e-FED-rin bro-em-fen-EER-a-meen	oral liquid	Bromfed-DM, Myphetane DX	Rx	
guaifenesin-dextromethorphan	gwye-FEN-e-sin dex-troe-meth-OR-fen	capsule, oral liquid, tablet	Mucinex DM	OTC	
promethazine-dextromethorphan	proe-METH-a-zeen dex-troe-meth-OR-fan	oral liquid	(none)	Rx	

Codeine is considered the "gold standard" against which the efficiency of other antitussive therapies is measured. Codeine's average adult dose is 15 mg every 4 to 6 hours. By itself, codeine is a Schedule II controlled substance, but, depending on the drug with which it is paired, it can have other control schedules. Codeine is a CNS depressant, and this effect is additive if taken with other CNS depressants, such as alcohol. Codeine is also thought to have a drying effect on the respiratory mucosa; this would be detrimental to patients with asthma or emphysema. The most common side effects are nausea, drowsiness, lightheadedness, and constipation, especially if the recommended dose is exceeded. Codeine should be taken with food to decrease stomach upset.

When used at the recommended dosage, codeine has low potential for dependency. As a result of their misuse, stringent controls have been placed on codeine-containing products. They may be purchased without a prescription in some states, but the purchaser must sign for them, be an adult according to state law, and show identification. The products may be dispensed only by the pharmacist, because the pharmacist is required to place his or her initial by the patient's signature.

Hydrocodone-chlorpheniramine (Tussionex) is a very popular medication and often a "drug of abuse." Hydrocodone is a derivative of codeine with many of the same qualities and side effects. It is prescribed for cough and upper respiratory symptoms of allergies and colds. This drug has a very high street value and even though it is Schedule III, most pharmacies will store it under lock and key. It is a very addictive. A prescription for this drug should be checked carefully to make sure it is a legal prescription.

Diphenhydramine (Benadryl) is an antitussive and an antihistamine. The usual adult dose is 25 mg every 4 hours. The main side effect is drowsiness, which is additive if the drug is taken with other CNS depressants.

Benzonatate (Tessalon) is a prescription drug used for a nonproductive cough. It locally anesthetizes the stretch receptors in the airway, lungs, and pleura (membrane that lines the thoracic cavity) but does not affect the respiratory center. The medication should carry a warning label telling the patient not to chew the capsule, because chewing the drug would cause a very unpleasant effect with pronounced salivation. Fluid intake is especially encouraged to help liquefy sputum. The main side effects are sedation, headache, and dizziness.

Dextromethorphan (Delsym) is considered equivalent to codeine, without its analgesic properties, and does not depress respiration. Furthermore, dextromethorphan acts on the same receptors as codeine, which is why it is a good cough suppressant. Dextromethorphan is a nonopioid derivative of morphine and acts on the cough center to suppress the cough reflex. If a patient is allergic to morphine, the pharmacy database on the technician's computer will flag the patient as also being allergic to dextromethorphan. The average adult dose is 10 mg to 20 mg every 4 hours. Dextromethorphan, which is commonly combined with other drugs, interacts with monoamine oxidase inhibitors (MAOIs). If large quantities of dextromethorphan are consumed it can produce hallucinations; this is known as "robo-tripping," which is popular with teenagers. For this reason, dextromethorphan has become a recreational drug. Because of misuse, the purchaser must show proof of age and be over 18 years old.

Expectorants

The purpose of an **expectorant** is to enable the patient to rid the lungs and airway of mucus when coughing. Expectorants decrease the thickness and viscosity (stickiness) of mucus so that a cough will eject mucus and other fluids from the bronchi. Such a cough is called a productive cough. Expectorants are used for both dry, unproductive coughs and productive coughs.

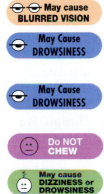

Warning

Diphenhydramine (Benadryl) and dicyclomine (Bentyl) have both similar generic names and similar brand names. Dicyclomine is a stomach antispasmodic and has many of the same side effects as diphenhydramine. Diphenhydramine is dosed at 12.5 mg, 25 mg, and 50 mg. Dicyclomine is dosed at 10 mg and 20 mg.

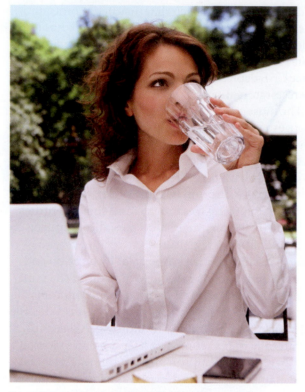
Sometimes maintaining good fluid intake is all that is needed to allow the respiratory tract to clear itself through coughing.

If a patient is well hydrated, coughing up mucus is not a problem. Fluid intake and adequate humidity in the inspired air are important to liquefy mucus in the respiratory tract and, therefore, are essential in cold therapy. This can be accomplished by drinking 6 to 8 glasses of water a day, which can be as effective as an expectorant or even more so. Table 9.6 lists commonly used expectorants.

The most commonly used OTC expectorant is **guaifenesin**, which can be taken in caplet, capsule, liquid, syrup, tablet, or sustained-release form. This drug is also frequently combined with other drugs. It is derived from tree bark extract and is a common component of many cough and cold remedies. It loosens phlegm (mucus) and thins bronchial secretions to make coughs more productive and rid the respiratory tract of mucus. Guaifenesin is especially indicated in patients with a persistent or chronic cough (from smoking, asthma, or emphysema) with excessive secretions. For example, **Mucinex** is a tablet form of guaifenesin. Guaifensesin is also manufactured in chewable form and alternate brand names as well. The side effects include vomiting, nausea, GI upset, and drowsiness.

Potassium iodide (Iosat, Lugol solution) is a useful expectorant when mucus complicates respiratory problems, as in patients with cystic fibrosis. Each dose should be diluted with at least a glass of liquid (fruit juice, water, or milk). Stomach pain is the primary side effect.

Decongestants

Vasodilation of blood vessels in the nasal mucosa allows fluids to leak into these tissues, resulting in swelling and stuffiness. A **decongestant** stimulates the alpha-adrenergic receptors of the vascular smooth muscle, constricting the dilated arteriolar

TABLE 9.6   Most Commonly Used Expectorants

Generic Name	Pronunciation	Dosage Form	Brand Name	Dispensing Status	Control Schedule
guaifenesin	gwye-FEN-e-sin	capsule, oral liquid, tablet	Mucinex	OTC	
potassium iodide	poe-TAS-ee-um EYE-oh-dide	oral liquid, tablet	Iosat, Lugol Solution	OTC	
Combinations					
guaifenesin-codeine	gwye-FEN-e-sin KOE-deen	oral liquid	Robitussin A-C	OTC, Rx	C-V
guaifenesin-pseudoephedrine	gwye-FEN-e-sin soo-doe-e-FED-rin	tablet	Mucinex D	OTC	behind the counter

network within the nasal mucosa. This constriction shrinks the engorged mucous membranes, which promotes drainage, improves nasal ventilation, and relieves the feeling of stuffiness. Shrinking the mucous membranes not only makes breathing easier but also permits the sinus cavities to drain. Topical agents are more immediately effective but of shorter duration than systemic agents. Decongestants should not be given to patients who cannot tolerate sympathetic nervous system stimulation. Sympathetic nervous system stimulation causes increased heart rate and blood pressure and heightened CNS stimulation. Decongestants are often combined with antihistamines in an effort to offset the antihistamine side effect of drowsiness. Most decongestants are OTC drugs.

Following the label directions regarding the frequency and duration of use is very important. Topical nasal application of these drugs over prolonged periods is often followed by a rebound phenomenon called **rhinitis medicamentosa**. It is thought to be caused by severe nasal edema and reduced receptor sensitivity. Patients with this condition use more spray more often with less response. Patients should be counseled on the use of topical decongestants to prevent rhinitis medicamentosa. Duration of therapy of a nasal decongestant should be limited to 3 to 5 days.

These drugs should be used with caution in the elderly and in patients with hypertension, diabetes, or cardiovascular disease. They can be dangerous if overdosed. They directly stimulate the alpha-adrenergic receptors of respiratory mucosa, causing vasoconstriction to relieve congestion. When they do so, it also affects blood pressure and the heart.

Table 9.7 describes the most commonly used decongestants. Decongestants can be administered topically or orally. Topical administration takes the form of drops, sprays, and vapors that are applied nasally. Oral administration takes the form of capsules, syrups, and tablets. Administering a decongestant orally distributes the drug through the systemic circulation to the vascular bed of the nasal mucosa.

Therapeutic Uses of Decongestants Decongestants are used for temporary symptomatic relief of nasal congestion due to the common cold, upper respiratory allergies, and sinusitis. They promote nasal sinus drainage and are useful in providing vascular constriction of blood vessels in the nasal mucosa. Vessel constriction allows excess tissue fluids to be carried away in circulation, thus reducing swelling in the mucosa, opening air passageways, and allowing the patient to breathe more freely.

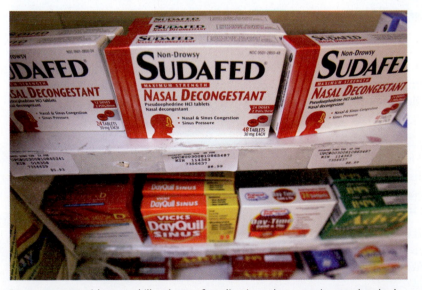

In response to wide spread illegal use of medications that contain pseudoephedrine, all products that contain this compound are now sold behind the counter.

TABLE 9.7   Most Commonly Used Decongestants

Generic Name	Pronunciation	Dosage Form	Brand Name	Dispensing Status
pseudoephedrine	soo-doe-e-FED-rin	capsule, oral liquid, tablet	Sudafed	OTC
phenylephrine	fen-il-EFF-rin	cream, nasal spray, ointment, ophthalmic, suppository, suspension, tablet	Sudafed PE, Neo-Synephrine, others	OTC
phenylephrine	fen-il-EFF-rin	IV	none	Rx
Pseudoephedrine Combinations				
cetirizine-pseudoephedrine	se-TEER-a-zeen soo-doe-e-FED-rin	tablet	Zyrtec-D	OTC
fexofenadine-pseudoephedrine	fex-o-FEN-a-deen soo-doe-e-FED-rin	tablet	Allegra-D	Rx
guaifenesin-pseudoephrine	gwye-FEN-e-sin soo-doe-e-FED-rin	tablet	Mucinex D	OTC
ibuprofen-pseudoephedrine,	eye-byoo-PROE-fen soo-doe-e-FED-rin	tablet	Advil Cold and Sinus	OTC
ibuprofen-pseudoephedrine chlorpheniramine	eye-byoo-PROE-fen soo-doe-e-FED-rin klor-fen-EER-a-meen	tablet	Advil Allergy and Sinus	OTC
loratidine-pseudoephedrine	lor-AT-a-deen soo-doe-e-FED-rin	tablet	Claritin D	OTC
naproxen-pseudoephedrine	na-PROX-en soo-doe-e-FED-rin	tablet	Aleve Cold and Sinus	OTC
triprolidine-pseudoephedrine	trye-PROE-li-deen soo-doe-e-FED-rin	tablet	Actifed Cold and Allergy	OTC

*Any drugs containing pseudoephedrine are sold behind the counter.

Side Effects and Dispensing Issues of Decongestants Decongestants should *not* be taken if the patient is using other sympathomimetic drugs. They should also be avoided if the following conditions exist.

- diabetes
- heart disease
- uncontrolled hypertension
- hyperthyroidism
- prostatic hypertrophy
- Tourette syndrome

Both oral and topical agents have side effects, which are listed in Table 9.8. Some of these are relatively minor, though unpleasant, but other side effects can be serious. These effects differ for oral agents and topical agents.

Pseudoephedrine (Sudafed) is by far the most-used and most effective decongestant and is combined with many other drugs. In the past, patients with hypertension were advised to avoid this drug. Current evidence shows that if the hypertension is controlled, by whatever means, then pseudoephedrine is not contraindicated for short term use. The results of clinical trials cited in the scientific literature indicate that pseudoephedrine works best combined with an antihistamine.

Pseudoephedrine has strong abuse potential because it is a derivative of ephedrine, which is a controlled substance in some states, and can be made into methamphetamine. Because of illegal methamphetamine production, the amount of pseudoephedrine a consumer may purchase at one time is limited. Products containing pseudoephedrine are kept behind the counter, and the consumer must specifically ask for them and present identification.

Phenylephrine (Sudafed PE) has replaced pseudoephedrine in most decongestant combinations because it cannot be made into methamphetamine and therefore does not require the security measures required by law for pseudoephedrine. Phenylephrine is, however, significantly less effective than pseudoephedrine as a decongestant. Both drugs seem to work better in combination with an antihistamine. Phenylephrine is used extensively IV to treat hypotension because of the arterial vasoconstriction it causes. It is also used in eye drops and nasal sprays. The sprays should not be used more than 3 days in a row in order to prevent rebound. The eye drops are also used extensively in the treatment of allergies. This drug is used over the counter primarily to treat symptoms of cold and allergies and itchy, watery eyes.

Combinations of ingredients in OTC preparations change frequently without notice to consumers or health care professionals. When purchasing any OTC medications, it is very important to read the labels.

Antihistamines

Histamine is found in all body tissue. It induces capillary dilation and increases capillary permeability, both of which help to decrease blood pressure. It contracts most smooth muscle, increases gastric acid secretion, increases heart rate, and mediates hypersensitivity. Basically, two types of drugs block the histamine receptors. The drugs

TABLE 9.8   Side Effects of Decongestants

Oral Agents	Topical Agents
anxiety	burning sensation
CNS stimulation (can be used to avoid sleep)	contact dermatitis
dizziness	dry mouth
hallucinations	rhinitis medicamentosa
headache	sneezing
increased blood pressure	stinging sensation
increased heart rate	
insomnia	
tremor	

commonly referred to as **antihistamines** block the H_1 receptors in the upper respiratory system. The other group of antihistamines is referred to as H_2 blockers, and they affect the cells in the gastrointestinal tract. This chapter discusses the H_1 blockers.

Antihistamines are well absorbed in tissues and widely distributed across the blood-brain barrier and placenta. Sedation occurs when they penetrate the blood-brain barrier. Pregnant mothers are warned not to take antihistamines, because these products can cross the placenta and adversely affect the fetus. Table 9.9 lists the most commonly used antihistamines.

Therapeutic Uses of Antihistamines The drugs normally thought of as antihistamines (H_1 blockers) provide symptomatic relief by acting on the H_1 receptors to prevent histamine binding. They have many uses including

- treatment of allergies and rashes
- treatment of insomnia
- symptomatic relief of urticarial lesions (rash), edema, and hay fever
- control of cough
- alleviation of vertigo
- alleviation of nausea and vomiting
- relief of serum sickness (hypersensitivity reaction that may occur several days to 2 to 3 weeks after receiving antisera or following drug therapy)
- control of venom reactions (venom contains histamine and other substances causing histamine release)
- mitigation of the extrapyramidal side effects of antipsychotic medication

TABLE 9.9 Most Commonly Used Antihistamines

Generic Name	Pronunciation	Dosage Form	Brand Name	Dispensing Status
azatadine	a-ZAT-a-deen	tablet	Optimine	Rx
azelastine	a-ZEL-a-steen	nasal spray, ophthalmic	Astelin, Optivar	Rx
cetirizine	se-TEER-a-zeen	oral liquid, tablet	Zyrtec	OTC
chlorpheniramine	klor-fen-EER-a-meen	tablet	Chlortrimeton	OTC
clemastine	KLEM-as-teen	oral liquid, tablet	Tavist Allergy	OTC
cyproheptadine	si-proe-HEP-ta-deen	oral liquid, tablet	Periactin	Rx
desloratadine	des-lor-AT-a-deen	oral liquid, tablet	Clarinex	Rx
diphenhydramine	dye-fen-HYE-dra-meen	injection, IV	Benadryl	Rx
		tablet, capsule		OTC
fexofenadine	fex-o-FEN-a-deen	capsule, tablet	Allegra	Rx
hydroxyzine	hye-DROX-i-zeen	capsule, injection, oral liquid, tablet	Atarax, Vistaril	Rx
levocetirizine	lee-vo-se-TEER-a-zeen	tablet	Xyzal	Rx
loratadine	lor-AT-a-deen	oral liquid, tablet	Claritin	OTC
meclizine	MEK-li-zeen	capsule, chewable, tablet	Antivert	OTC
promethazine	proe-METH-a-zeen	suppository, tablet	Phenergan	Rx

- prophylaxis for certain drug reactions
- prophylaxis for certain drug allergies

Antihistamines can also be used in the treatment of hypersensitivity reactions. Hypersensitivity is a state of altered reactivity in which the body reacts with an exaggerated immune response to a foreign agent. This response can range from quite serious, as in serum sickness, to a slight rash or low-grade fever. **Promethazine (Phenergan)** and **meclizine (Antivert)** are the antihistamines used most frequently for nausea and motion sickness. (In low doses, promethazine is an antihistamine, even though it is a derivative of phenothiazine. In high doses promethazine can function as an antipsychotic; however, it is rarely used this way.) Some antihistamines are promoted for specific indications even though the therapeutic uses of these drugs overlap considerably. The side effect profile is also the same even though there may be varying degrees for each drug. Antihistamines are more effective at preventing some allergic reactions from occurring than in reversing these actions once they have taken place.

The second-generation antihistamines produce less drowsiness. They are cetirizine, clemastine, desloratidine, fexofenadine, levocetirizine, and loratadine. Cetirizine and levocetirizine both tend to lean toward more sedation than the other second-generation antihistamines. Levocetirizine (Xyzal) is being promoted as a faster-onset and longer acting drug than the others. It is first-line for itching and rashes. It is also approved for allergies.

Side Effects and Dispensing Issues of Antihistamines The most common side effects of the currently available antihistamines include anticholinergic responses, hyperactivity (in children), and sedation. The anticholinergic responses include atropine-like dry mouth, drying of the mucosa of the upper respiratory tract, blurred vision, constipation, and urinary retention. Sedation is the most common side effect of antihistamines. Some antihistamines are actually prescribed to induce sleep. In fact, almost every OTC sleeping pill contains the antihistamine **diphenhydramine**. This effect is synergistic with alcohol use. Dizziness is also a common side effect. The newer drugs on the market have fewer side effects.

Antihistamines are very versatile drugs, used for many different maladies. Some are better than others at treating specific problems. The following drugs are used primarily in the following ways:

- Azelastine: (Astelin, Optivar) seasonal allergies
- Brompheniramine: runny noses
- Cetirizine (Zyntek): alergies
- Chlorpheniramine: upper respiratory symptoms
- Clemastine: (Tavist) common cold
- Desloratadine: (Clarinex) allergies
- Diphenhydramine: (Benadryl) allergic reactions and sleep promotion
- Fexofenadine: (Allegra) allergies
- Levocetirizine: (Xyzal) rashes and itching
- Loratadine: (Claritin) allergies
- Meclizine: (Antivert) motion sickness

Azelastine (Astelin, Optivar) was the first antihistamine nasal spray. It is indicated in seasonal allergic rhinitis and seems to work as well as the oral antihistamines for itchy, runny nose and sneezing. It tastes bitter. Even though the drug has a low incidence of sedative side effects, the bottle should carry a sticker warning of potential drowsiness. It is stable for 3 months after the bottle is opened.

Clemastine (Tavist Allergy) is the only drug approved by the FDA for cold symptoms and is the least-sedating OTC antihistamine.

Fexofenadine (Allegra) is not as sedating as many of the other antihistamines. Studies have not reported any arrhythmias or other serious reactions having occurred with this drug.

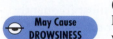

Loratadine (Claritin) has been an OTC drug since 2002, but **desloratadine (Clarinex)** does require a prescription. Desloratadine is a long-acting metabolite of loratadine. It has additional anti-inflammatory properties and should not be given with erythromycin or ketoconazole.

Nasal Corticosteroids A new group of drugs has emerged to treat allergies: nasal corticosteroids. They must be used daily for maximum benefit. They can cause nasal irritation and bleeding. The spray should be directed away from the septum to avoid this. Local infections of *Candida albicans* may occur in the nose of patients using nasal steroids long-term. Nasal steroids are now the most effective monotherapy for allergic rhinitis. The most commonly prescribed nasal corticosteroids are listed in Table 9.10.

Ciclesonide (Omnaris) is a prodrug that is converted to the active form (desisobutyryl ciclesonide) by an enzyme in the nasal mucosa. This process is known as target activation. Theoretically, target activation should reduce side effects; however, systemic exposure is negligible in the nasal inhalations.

Fluticasone is used in two different forms. **Veramyst** has a stronger binding affinity than **Flonase** and the device is easier to use.

Mometasone (Nasonex) depresses the release of endogenous chemical mediators of inflammation (kinin, histamine, and prostaglandins). It reverses the dilation and permeability of vessels in the area and decreases access of cells to the site of injury. It may be used in children who are over 12 years of age to prevent symptoms of allergic rhinitis.

TABLE 9.10   Most Commonly Prescribed Nasal Corticosteroids

Generic Name	Pronunciation	Dosage Form	Brand Name	Dispensing Status
beclomethasone	be-kloe-METH-a-sone	nasal spray	Beconase AQ	Rx
budesonide	byoo-DES-oh-nide	nasal spray	Rhinecort Aqua	Rx
ciclesonide	sye-KLES-oh-nide	nasal spray	Omnaris	Rx
flunisolide	floo-NISS-oh-lide	nasal spray	Nasarel	Rx
fluticasone (furoate)	floo-TIK-a-sone	nasal spray	Veramyst	Rx
fluticasone (propionate)	floo-TIK-a-sone	nasal spray	Flonase	Rx
mometasone	moe-MET-a-sone	nasal spray	Nasonex	Rx
triamcinolone	trye-am-SIN-oh-lone	nasal spray	Nasacort AQ	Rx

Smoking Cessation

Cigarette smoking poses a wide variety of risks to health. On average, cigarette smokers live approximately 15 years less than nonsmokers. Cigarette smoke contains more than 4000 identified chemical compounds, including at least 43 carcinogens. In addition to lung cancer, leukemia and cancers of the mouth, pharynx, larynx, esophagus, pancreas, cervix, kidney, and bladder are associated with smoking. Evidence also links smoking with other cancers, such as ovarian, uterine, and prostate. Tobacco is the single largest cause of preventable death.

Smoking also increases the risk of heart disease, COPD, and stroke. The acute risks include shortness of breath, aggravation of asthma, impotence, infertility, and increased serum carbon monoxide concentration.

Environmental (secondhand) tobacco smoke also poses a substantial health threat because it contains all the carcinogens and toxins present in inhaled cigarette smoke. Children living in a household with smokers have a higher risk of respiratory infection, asthma, and middle-ear infection than those who live with nonsmokers. Birth defects may be related to the mother's smoking during pregnancy.

The physical benefits of smoking cessation include a longer life and better health (i.e., decreased risk of lung, laryngeal, esophageal, oral, pancreatic, bladder, and cervical cancers; coronary heart disease; and other diseases aggravated by smoking). A few personal benefits from smoking cessation are listed in Table 9.11.

Nicotine, the addictive component of tobacco, is readily absorbed in the lungs from inhaled smoke. Nicotine from smokeless tobacco products, such as chewing tobacco and snuff, is absorbed across the oral or nasal mucosa, respectively. In the body, nicotine is extensively metabolized in the liver and to a lesser extent in the kidneys and lungs. One major urinary metabolite, **cotinine**, has a longer half-life (15 to 20 hours) and a tenfold higher concentration than nicotine. Presence of this metabolite indictes that a person is a smoker.

Nicotine and polycyclic aromatic hydrocarbons in cigarette smoke induce the production of hepatic (liver) enzymes responsible for metabolizing caffeine, theophylline, imipramine, and other drugs. Smoking increases plasma cortisol (a major natural glutocorticoid) and catecholamine (sympathomimetic amines, including dopamine, epinephrine, and norepinephrine) concentrations, which affect treatment with adrenergic agonists and adrenergic-blocking agents.

TABLE 9.11   Personal Benefits to Smoking Cessation

Improved performance in sports and sex
Better-smelling home, car, clothing, and breath
Economic savings
Freedom from addiction
Healthier babies
Improved health
Improved self-esteem
Improved sense of taste and smell
No concern about exposing others to smoke
Setting a good example for children and young adults

Nicotine itself is a ganglionic cholinergic-receptor agonist with dose-related, pharmacologic effects. These effects include central and peripheral nervous system stimulation and depression, respiratory stimulation, skeletal muscle relaxation, catecholamine release by the adrenal medulla, peripheral vasoconstriction, and increases in blood pressure, heart rate, cardiac output, and oxygen consumption. Chronic nicotine ingestion leads to physical and psychological dependence. Consequently, smoking cessation results in withdrawal symptoms, usually within 24 hours. These symptoms are listed in Table 9.12.

Planning to Stop Smoking

One of the reasons that stopping smoking is difficult is that nicotine has many behavior-reinforcing properties. These properties include relaxation, increased alertness, decreased fatigue, improved cognitive performance, and a "reward" effect (pleasure or euphoria). Increased alertness and cognitive performance result from stimulation of the cerebral cortex, which can occur at low doses. The reward effect, mediated by the limbic system, occurs at high doses.

To combat these properties, smoking cessation treatment involves three main elements: training in general problem-solving skills, social support from the clinician, and nicotine replacement therapy. Nicotine replacement therapy is recommended as first-line pharmacotherapy for smokers without contraindications to therapy (myocardial infarction in the previous 4 weeks, serious arrhythmias, severe or worsening angina pectoris). Patients must understand, however, that nicotine replacement therapy is not a substitute for behavior modification and that success is greatest when the two modes of therapy are used concomitantly. Individual or group counseling is highly recommended.

The steps in establishing a plan for quitting are as follows.

1. Set a date.
2. Inform family, friends, and coworkers of the decision and request understanding and support.
3. Remove cigarettes from the environment and avoid spending a lot of time in places where smoking is prevalent.
4. Review previous attempts to quit, if applicable, and analyze the factors that caused relapse.
5. Anticipate challenges, particularly during the critical first few weeks.

The key to smoking cessation is total abstinence. Patients can help by rewarding abstinence and avoiding situations that serve as smoking triggers. Because drinking

TABLE 9.12	Symptoms of Nicotine Withdrawal
Anxiety	Gastrointestinal disturbances
Craving for tobacco	Headache
Decreased blood pressure and heart rate	Hostility
Depression	Increased appetite and weight gain
Difficulty in concentrating	Increased skin temperature
Drowsiness	Insomnia
Frustration, irritability, impatience, restlessness	

alcohol is strongly associated with relapse to tobacco use, smokers should reduce their alcohol consumption or abstain from drinking altogether during the quitting process.

One major reason smokers are reluctant to quit is fear of weight gain. Although weight gain does occur, most smokers gain less than 10 pounds. The weight gain is caused by both increased caloric intake and metabolic adjustments; it can occur even if caloric intake remains constant or is restricted.

Smoking Cessation Drug Therapy

The most commonly used agents for smoking cessation are listed in Table 9.13. Patients must be strongly advised to stop smoking when initiating nicotine replacement therapy. Those who continue to smoke may show signs of nicotine excess. The symptoms of nicotine excess are listed in Table 9.14; note that they often overlap with withdrawal symptoms. Dizziness and perspiration are more often associated with excessive nicotine levels; anxiety, depression, and irritability are common symptoms of withdrawal.

All the listed drugs except the **nicotine** nasal spray and inhalant **(Nicotrol), varenicline (Chantix),** and the antidepressant **buproprion (Wellbutrin SR, Zyban)** have been approved for OTC drug use.

Nicotine nasal spray mimics the effects of cigarette smoking more closely than the transdermal systems or chewing gum because nicotine is absorbed more rapidly after nasal administration. Adverse effects from the nasal spray include nasal irritation, runny nose, throat irritation, watering eyes, sneezing, and cough. Regular use of the spray during the first week of treatment may help patients adapt to its irritating effects. If patients complain of irritation at first, they should not be told to stop using the drug.

The nicotine lozenge is based on the "time" of the first cigarette instead of the number per day. The lozenge should not be chewed. The full dose of nicotine is

TABLE 9.13 Most Commonly Used Agents for Smoking Cessation

Generic Name	Pronunciation	Dosage Form	Brand Name	Dispensing Status
bupropion	byoo-PROE-pee-on	tablet	Wellbutrin SR, Zyban	Rx
nicotine	NIK-oh-teen	gum, lozenge, transdermal patch	Commit, Habitrol, Nicoderm CQ, Nicorette, ProStep	OTC
		inhaler, nasal spray	Nicotrol	Rx
varenicline	var-EN-i-kleen	tablet	Chantix	Rx

TABLE 9.14 Symptoms of Nicotine Excess

Abdominal pain	Hypersalivation
Confusion	Nausea
Diarrhea	Perspiration
Dizziness	Visual disturbances
Headache	Vomiting
Hearing loss	Weakness

released as the smoker sucks on it, and it completely dissolves. The lozenge appears to work as well as other first-line agents. Daily cost is about the same as a pack of cigarettes. As with other agents, behavioral counseling should be a part of the regimen for best results.

The gum is recommended for users of smokeless tobacco. Common adverse effects from nicotine chewing gum (usually mild and transient) include mouth soreness, hiccups, dyspepsia, and jaw ache.

Compared with a placebo, transdermal nicotine doubles abstinence rates at 6 and 12 months after initiation of therapy. The patch should be applied daily to a nonhairy, clean, dry site on the upper body or outer arm. Skin reactions from the patches may be prevented by rotating the application site.

Varenicline (Chantix) blocks nicotine binding to pleasure receptors and reduces the severity of craving and withdrawal symptoms. Smoking while on Chantix does not provide the same sense of satisfaction. Foods also do not provide as much satisfaction while a patient is taking varenicline, so weight gain is usually not a problem while using this drug for smoking cessation.. This is an important factor, because weight gain is a common side effect of smoking cessation that causes many patients to resume smoking. Varenicline needs to be started a week before the quit date. It should be taken with food and a full glass of water so as to decrease nausea, which is one of the primary side effects. Varenicline should be taken for 24 weeks, and the patient should attend a smoking cessation program. This drug has been the most successful pharmacotherapy treatment developed at this time. The most prominent side effect is unusual dreams.

Chapter Terms

antihistamines common term for drugs that block the H_1 receptors

antitussives drugs that block or suppress the act of coughing

aspiration inhalation of fluids from the mouth and throat

asthma a reversible lung disease with intermittent attacks in which inspiration is obstructed; provoked by airborne allergens

bronchitis a condition in which the inner lining of the bronchial airways becomes inflamed, causing the expiration of air from the lungs to be obstructed

bronchodilator an agent that relaxes smooth-muscle cells of the bronchioles, thereby increasing airway diameter and improving the movement of gases into and out of the lungs

bronchospasm spasmodic contraction of the smooth muscles of the bronchiole

corticosteroid a drug that chemically resembles substances produced by the adrenal gland and acts as an anti-inflammatory agent to suppress the immune response by stimulating adenylate cyclase

cotinine a major metabolite of nicotine

cough reflex a coordinated series of events, initiated by stimulation of receptors in the lungs and airways, that results in a cough

cystic fibrosis (CF) a hereditary disorder of infants, children, and young adults that involves widespread dysfunction of the gastrointestinal and pulmonary systems

decongestant an agent that causes the mucous membranes to shrink, thereby allowing the sinus cavities to drain

emphysema an irreversible lung disease characterized by destruction of the alveoli in the lungs, which allows air to accumulate in tissues and organs

expectorant an agent that decreases the thickness and stickiness of mucus, enabling the patient to rid the lungs and airway of mucus when coughing

histoplasmosis a respiratory tract infection caused by a fungus, most often found in accumulated droppings from birds and bats; often called the summer flu

irritant receptor a nerve cell in the lungs and airways that responds to coarse particles and chemicals to trigger a cough

leukotriene inhibitor an agent that blocks the body's inflammatory responses to the leukotrienes or blocks their synthesis

mast cell stabilizer an agent that stabilizes mast cell membranes against rupture caused by antigenic substances and thereby reduces the amount of histamine and other inflammatory substances released in airway tissues

metered dose inhaler (MDI) a device that delivers a specific amount of medication (as for asthma) in a fine enough spray to reach the innermost parts of the lungs using a puff of compressed gas

monoclonal antibody an antibody produced in a laboratory from an isolated specific lymphocyte that produces a pure antibody against a known, specific antigen

mucolytic an agent that destroys or dissolves mucus

nebulizer a device used in the administration of inhaled medications, using air flowing past a liquid to create a mist

nicotine the addictive component of tobacco

peak expiratory flow rate (PEFR) the maximum flow rate generated during a forced expiration, measured in liters per minute

peak flow meter a device used to measure the PEFR as an indication of respiratory status; usually used twice a day by asthma patients

percussion a therapy used for cystic fibrosis (CF) patients involving a tapping movement to induce cough and expectoration of sputum from the lungs; usually preceded by nebulizer therapy during which nebulized sterile water or normal saline is breathed to liquefy pulmonary secretions

pneumonia a common lung infection, caused by microorganisms that gain access to the lower respiratory tract

respiratory distress syndrome (RDS) a syndrome occurring in newborns that is characterized by acute asphyxia with hypoxia and acidosis

rhinitis medicamentosa a condition of decreased response that results when nasal decongestants are used over prolonged periods

spacer a device used with a metered dose inhaler (MDI) to decrease the amount of spray deposited on the back of the throat and swallowed

status asthmaticus a medical emergency that begins as an asthma attack but does not respond to normal management; can result in loss of consciousness and death

stretch receptor a nerve cell in the lungs and airways that responds to elongation of muscle to trigger a cough

surfactant a fluid that reduces surface tension between the air in the alveoli and the inner surfaces of the alveoli, allowing gas to be exchanged between the lung and the air

tachypnea very rapid respiration causing a flushed appearance; a characteristic of emphysema

tuberculosis (TB) a disease of the lungs and other body tissues and organs caused by *Mycobacterium tuberculosis*

xanthine derivative a drug that causes relaxation of airway smooth muscle, thus causing airway dilation and better air movement

Chapter Summary

Asthma

- Asthma is a disease in which inflammation causes the airways to tighten; asthma is a reversible condition.
- The asthmatic lung is more sensitive and responds to lower doses of challenge from allergens than do normal lungs.
- Asthma is a pulmonary condition with the following characteristics: reversible small airway obstruction, progressive airway inflammation, and increased airway responsiveness to stimuli.
- The most useful measure for assessing severity and following the course of asthma is the peak expiratory flow rate (PEFR).
- Drug therapy is the mainstay of asthma management.

- In 2008 the FDA mandated that all inhalers will no longer use the ozone-depleting propellant chlorofluorocarbon (CFC).
- A rescue course of corticosteroids may be needed at any time.
- Exercise-induced asthma is best treated with the inhalation of terbutaline or albuterol before exercising. This will provide protection for 2 hours after inhalation.
- Asthmatics should not use antihistamines in acute attacks and should always avoid beta blockers. Other drugs to be avoided include aspirin, NSAIDs, penicillins, cephalosporins, and sulfas.
- With an MDI, the patient inhales slowly, whereas with a dry-powder inhaler the patient breathes in quickly to activate the inhaler.

- Nebulizers are effective delivery systems, for children too young to use inhalers.
- Home nebulizers can easily become contaminated, leading to bronchitis, if not cleaned properly on a daily basis.
- A spacer is recommended with an MDI to decrease the amount of spray that is deposited on the back of the throat and swallowed. It improves the penetration of drug into the lungs.
- Epinephrine is the drug of choice for an acute attack of asthma. Many patients with asthma carry an EpiPen for this purpose.
- Short-acting inhaled bronchodilators are albuterol, isoproterenol, metaproterenol, and pirbuterol.
- Levalbuterol, one of two isomers of albuterol, is more effective than the other isomer and has fewer side effects.
- Salmeterol and terbutaline are long-acting inhaled bronchodilators.
- Salmeterol (Serevent) should be used exactly as directed and never for acute situations.
- Formoterol (Foradil) is a long-acting bronchodilator with an onset of action of just a few minutes. It should be refrigerated before it is dispensed, but it does not have to be refrigerated after dispensing. The pharmacy team must put a date on it to indicate that after that date it cannot be used and should be thrown away.
- Theophylline should be used only in lung diseases unresponsive to other drugs because of its high interaction profile.
- Leukotrienes are 100 to 1000 times more potent than histamine; therefore, when these receptors are antagonized, inflammatory responses do not take place.
- Zafirlukast (Accolate) is a leukotriene receptor antagonist that has shown very good results.
- Zileuton (Zyflo) is a leukotriene inhibitor that carries strong warnings about liver toxicity and can double theophylline levels.
- Montelukast (Singulair) is indicated for prophylaxis and chronic treatment of asthma. It is approved for use in adults and children 12 months and older.
- Corticosteroids are reserved for the more difficult cases of asthma and are usually prescribed on an alternate-day basis or as tapering doses when short-term therapy is indicated. when the liquid or pill form is prescribed. The primary side effect of inhaling these drugs is oral candidiasis. The patient should always be advised to rinse the mouth after using these inhalers.
- Many asthmatics still are not using corticosteroids.
- Always use the lowest effective dose of a corticosteroid.
- Add salmeterol to inhaled corticosteroids if needed to decrease the dose of corticosteroid needed for control.
- Fluticasone (Flovent) is a corticosteroid inhaler that comes in three strengths.
- Budesonide (Pulmicort Turbuhaler) is a dry-powder inhalant with no propellant because it is breath activated. Pulmicort Respules is the first formulation of budesonide for home nebulizers.

Chronic Obstructive Pulmonary Disease

- Chronic obstructive pulmonary disease (COPD) encompasses emphysema and chronic bronchitis. COPD is irreversible.
- Emphysema is characterized by destruction of the tiny alveoli, walls, or air sacs of the lungs.
- Chronic bronchitis can be caused by cigarette smoke; exposure to occupational dusts, fumes, and environmental pollution; and bacterial infection.
- Pharmacologic management of bronchitis and emphysema is still largely empirical, with methylxanthines, corticosteroids, beta agonists, and ipratropium forming the foundation of therapy.
- One of the best expectorants is water.
- Tiotropium (Spiriva) is similar to ipratropium (Atrovent) but is dosed only once daily; it is used for treatment of COPD.
- Other drugs indicated only for COPD are Combivent, DuoNeb, Brovana, and Perforomist.

Other Lung Diseases

- Respiratory distress syndrome occurs in newborns and is treated with surfactants.
- The treatment regimen for TB varies depending on the patient's symptoms.
- Histoplasmosis is often referred to as the summer flu. It is usually benign, but some rare cases can be life threatening. The only drug that is effective is amphotericin B.

Cough, Cold, and Allergy

- Antitussives, expectorants, decongestants, and antihistamines each have a different mechanism of action and purpose. Most are OTC products.

Antitussives

- Antitussives are indicated to reduce the frequency of a cough, especially when dry and nonproductive.
- The cough reflex can be stopped at several points in the reflex pathway.
- Codeine, commonly referred to as the "gold standard of antitussives," is the antitussive against which all others are compared.
- Dextromethorphan may be as effective as codeine.
- One must be over 18 years old and show proof of age to purchase dextromethorphan.

Expectorants

- Expectorants decrease the thickness and stickiness of mucus by decreasing viscosity.
- Guaifenesin is the most-used expectorant, but water may work as well.

Decongestants

- Decongestants stimulate the alpha-adrenergic receptors of the vascular smooth muscle, constricting the dilated arteriolar network and shrinking the engorged mucous membranes. This promotes drainage of the sinus cavities and makes breathing easier. This sympathetic nervous system stimula-tion also increases heart rate and blood pressure and stimulates the CNS. Patients sometimes take decongestants to overcome drowsiness; these drugs should not be taken by those who cannot tolerate sympathetic stimulation.
- Topical application of decongestants (nasal sprays and drops) can cause a rebound phenomenon, rhinitis medicamentosa.
- Pseudoephedrine is the most effective decongestant but now may be purchased only in limited quantities and by someone who is over 18 years old and by showing identification.

Antihistamines

- Antihistamines are used primarily to combat allergic reactions, nausea, vertigo, and insomnia. They prevent binding of histamine to the receptor sites.
- The most common side effects of antihistamines are sedation and anticholinergic responses (dry mouth, constipation, urinary retention).
- Many antihistamines are sold OTC.
- Diphenhydramine is the major ingredient in OTC sleep medications.
- Fexofenadine (Allegra) is less sedating than most other antihistamines currently available. Clemastine (Tavist Allergy) is the least-sedating OTC antihistamine. It has been approved by the FDA for treatment of symptoms of the common cold.
- The most effective treatment for allergic rhinitis is application of nasal steroids.

Smoking Cessation

- Benefits of smoking cessation include a longer life and better health. The key to smoking cessation is total abstinence.
- Most nicotine cessation drugs are OTC.
- Chantix has been the most successful.

Drug List

The following drugs were discussed in this chapter. Each generic drug name is followed in parentheses by one or more brand names.

Antiasthma Agents

Bronchodilators
albuterol (Proventil, Proventil HFA, Ventolin, ProAir HFA)*
epinephrine (EpiPen, Primatene Mist)
formoterol (Foradil)
ipratropium (Atrovent)*
isoproterenol (Isuprel)
levalbuterol (Xopenex)
metaproterenol (Alupent)
pirbuterol (Maxair)
salmeterol (Serevent)
terbutaline (Brethine)
tiotropium (Spiriva)*

Xanthine Derivatives
aminophylline (Truphylline)
theophylline (Theo 24, TheoAir)

Leukotriene Inhibitors
montelukast (Singulair)*
zafirlukast (Accolate)
zileuton (Zyflo)

Corticosteroids
beclomethasone (Beconase AQ, QVAR, Vanceril)
budesonide (Entocort EC, Pulmicort Respules, Pulmicort Turbuhaler, Rhinocort)*
dexamethasone (Decadron)
flunisolide (AeroBid)
fluticasone (Flonase, Flovent)
hydrocortisone (Solu-Cortef)
methylprednisolone (Medrol Dose Pack, Solu-Medrol)
mometasone furoate (Asmanex)
prednisolone (Orapred, Pediapred)
prednisone (Deltasone)
triamcinolone (Azmacort*, Nasacort AQ)

Monoclonal Antibody
omalizumab (Xolair)

Mast Cell Stabilizers
cromolyn sodium (Crolom, Gastrocrom, Intal, Nasalcrom, Opticrom)
nedocromil (Tilade)

Combination
budesonide-formoterol (Symbicort)
fluticasone-salmeterol (Advair Diskus)*

COPD Agents

Beta Agonists
arformoterol (Brovana)
formoterol (Perforomist)
isoproterenol (Isuprel)
metaproterenol (Alupent)

Mucolytics
acetylcysteine (Acetadote, Mucomyst)
dornase alfa (Pulmozyme)

Anticholinergic
tiotropium (Spiriva)

Combinations
ipratropium/albuterol (Combivent)*
fluticasone/salmeterol (Advair)*

Surfactants
beractant (Survanta)
calfactant (Infasurf)
colfosceril palimate (Exosurf Neonatal)
poractant alfa (Curosurf)

Tuberculosis Agents
capreomycin (Capastat)
ciprofloxacin (Cipro)
cycloserine (Seromycin)
ethambutol (Myambutol)
ethionamide (Trecator-SC)
isoniazid, INH (Laniazid, Nydrazid)
isoniazid-pyrazinamide-rifampin (Rifater)
isoniazid-rifampin (Rifamate)
ofloxacin (Floxin)
pyrazinamide
rifampin (Rifadin, Rimactane)

rifapentine (Priftin)
streptomycin

Antitussives
benzonatate (Tessalon)
codeine (various combinations)
dextromethorphan (Delsym)
diphenhydramine (Benadryl)
hydrocodone-chlorpheniramine
(Tussionex)*
promethazine-codeine*

Dextromethorphan Combinations
dextromethorphan-pseudoephedrine-
brompheniramine (Bromfed-DM,
Myphetane DX)
guaifenesin-dextromethorphan
(Mucinex DM)
promethazine-dextromethorphan

Expectorants
guaifenesin (Mucinex)*
potassium iodide (Iosat, Lugol solution)

Combinations
guaifenesin-codeine (Robitussin A-C)*
guaifenesin-pseudoephedrine (Mucinex D)*

Decongestants
pseudoephedrine (Sudafed)
phenylephrine (Sudafed PE,
Neo-Synephrine)
cetirizine-pseudoephedrine (Zyrtec-D)*
fexofenadine-pseudoephedrine (Allegra-D)*
guaifenesin-pseudoephedrine (Mucinex D)
ibuprofen-pseudoephedrine (Advil Cold and
Sinus, Sine-Aid IB)
ibuprofen-pseudoephedrine-chlorphe-
niramine (Advil Allergy & Sinus)

loratadine-pseudoephedrine (Claritin D)
naproxen-pseudoephedrine (Aleve Cold and
Sinus)
triprolidine-pseudoephedrine (Actifed Cold
and Allergy)

Antihistamines
azatadine (Optimine)
azelastine (Astelin, Optivar)
cetirizine (Zyrtec)*
clemastine (Tavist Allergy)
cyproheptadine (Periactin)
desloratadine (Clarinex)*
diphenhydramine (Benadryl)
fexofenadine (Allegra)*
hydroxyzine (Atarax, Vistaril)
levocetirizine (Xyzal)
loratadine (Claritin)
meclizine (Antivert)
promethazine (Phenergan)

Nasal Corticosteroids
beclomethasone (Beconase AQ)
budesonide (Rhinecort Aqua)
ciclesonide (Omanaris)
flunisolide (Nasarel)
fluticasone furoate (Veramyst)
fluticasone propionate (Flonase)
mometasone (Nasonex)*
triamcinolone (Nasacort AQ)

Smoking Cessation Agents
bupropion (Wellbutrin SR, Zyban)
nicotine (Commit, Habitrol, Nicoderm CQ,
Nicorette, Nicotrol, ProStep)
varenicline (Chantix)

Chapter Review

Pharmaceuticals and Body Functions

Select the best answer from the choices given.

1. Which of the following diseases is reversible?
   a. asthma
   b. chronic bronchitis
   c. emphysema
   d. all of the above

2. The date is 1-10-2010. Foradil is dispensed. The expiration date on the box is 3-21-2010. Which "do not use after" date should the technician put on the box?
   a. 5-10-2010
   b. 3-21-2010
   c. 1-10-2010
   d. none of the above

3. Patients with asthma should avoid
   a. beta blockers.
   b. albuterol.
   c. Tilade.
   d. Accolate.

4. Which drug is a natural agent extracted from cattle lung and used in newborns for RDS?
   a. Accolate
   b. Survanta
   c. Mucomyst
   d. Pulmozyme

5. A major metabolite of nicotine is
   a. magnesium.
   b. calcium.
   c. potassium.
   d. cotinine.

6. Which smoking cessation product does not contain nicotine?
   a. Nicorette
   b. Habitrol
   c. Zyban
   d. Nicoderm

7. The drug most used in OTC sleep medications is
   a. pseudoephedrine.
   b. diphenhydramine.
   c. guaifenesin.
   d. dextromethorphan.

8. A controlled substance used to relieve cough is
   a. codeine.
   b. dextromethorphan.
   c. a and b.
   d. Benadryl.

9. The most used antitussive is
   a. dextromethorphan.
   b. diphenhydramine.
   c. benzonatate.
   d. codeine.

10. Diphenhydramine is often prescribed for its
    a. diuretic effects.
    b. decongestant effects.
    c. sedating qualities.
    d. ability to help students remain alert and test better.

The following statements are true or false. If an item is false, rewrite the statement so it is true.

_____ 1. The most useful way to assess severity and follow the course of asthma on a regular basis is the peak expiratory flow rate (PEFR).

_____ 2. Albuterol is the drug of choice for acute attacks of asthma.

_____ 3. Serevent is indicated for an acute asthma attack.

_____ 4. Status asthmaticus is never life threatening.

_____ 5. Asthma, chronic bronchitis, and emphysema are all reversible.

_____ 6. Cystic fibrosis is a disease that involves only the pulmonary system.

_____ 7. Rhinitis medicamentosa may result from overuse of topical decongestants.

_____ 8. A cough involves two types of receptors—stretch and irritant.

_____ 9. Drinking eight glasses of water a day may be more effective than an expectorant.

_____ 10. Antihistamines are prescribed for many reasons, including vertigo, insomnia, allergic reactions, and birth control.

Diseases and Drug Therapies

1. Develop educational materials for patients to teach them to use MDIs and dry-powder inhalers.

2. List the six goals of asthma care.

3. List four classes of drugs used for maintenance therapy for asthma.

4. Explain how antihistamines, decongestants, antitussives, and expectorants differ.

5. Which drug is approved by the FDA for treating symptoms of the common cold?

6. Make "stop smoking" posters for your school.

Dispensing Medications

1. Create a smoking cessation plan.

2. Mrs. Jones cannot seem to control her asthma. She brings in this new prescription. Where do problems exist in this regimen?

> ℞ **MT. HOPE MEDICAL PARK**
> **ST. PAUL, MN (651) 555-3591**
>
> DEA# _____
>
> Pt. name _Mary Lou Jones_ Date _6-01-07_
>
> Address _____
>
> Serevent use as directed prn
>   # three (3)
> Azmacort use as directed prn
>   # three (3)
> Ventolin use as directed
>   3–4 Times daily
>
> _____ Dispense as written
> ✓ Fills _five_ times (no refill unless indicated)
> _____ _Kathy Grad_ _____ M.D.

3. The physician orders "Vistaril one hundred (100) mg IM q4h prn." How much will you draw up per dose?

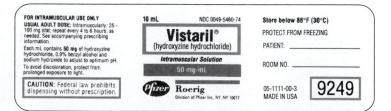

4. Identify a drug discussed in this chapter that is commonly prescribed for its side effects. Explain.

5. When is the best time to take an antihistamine for an allergy? Why?

Internet Research

Use the Internet to complete the following assignments.

1. Find statistics related to tuberculosis in the United States. How many new cases (incidents) are reported each year? Is this number increasing or decreasing? What is the prevalence (number of existing cases) of tuberculosis in the United States? Which segment of the population has the highest risk of contracting tuberculosis and why? List your Internet sources.

2. Select three prescription medications discussed in the chapter. Locate the manufacturer's Web site for each. Describe your process for finding the manufacturer: Did you need to go to another Web site first, or did a search on the drug name lead you directly to the site? What type of information was available on the manufacturer's site? Did it list side effects? Did it list indications and contraindications? Create a table with the manufacturer's Web site address and a brief description of the site's information related to that particular drug.

What Would You Do?

1. You are dispensing Foradil. The pharmacist tells you not to bother with putting the "do not use after" date on the box. Just go ahead and dispense it.

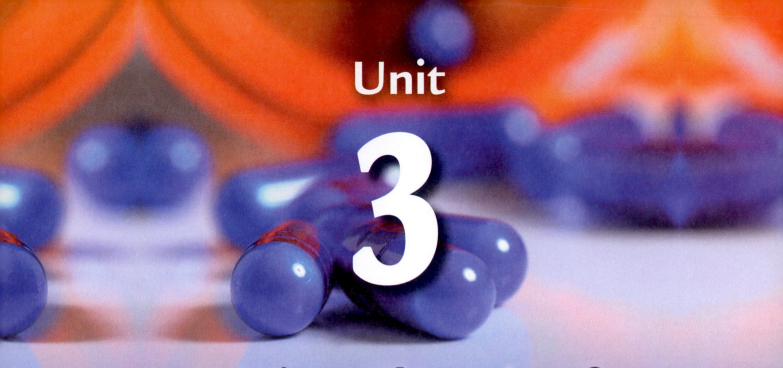

Unit

3

Major Classes of Pharmaceutical Products II

Drugs for Gastrointestinal and Related Diseases

10

Learning Objectives

- Describe gastrointestinal physiology and how it affects GI diseases.
- Be aware of drug treatments for GI diseases.
- Understand gastroesophageal reflux disease and its ramifications.
- Discuss antidiarrheal agents and explain how they work.
- Describe the role of fiber in the digestive process.
- Discuss laxatives and their mechanisms of action.
- Identify the chemoreceptor trigger zone (CTZ) and discuss its role in nausea.

- Know which antiemetics act on the CTZ and their mechanisms of action.
- Know the definition of obesity and how to calculate ideal body weight and body mass index.
- Recognize medications used to treat malaria and the side effects of these drugs.
- Understand the measures to prevent and treat hepatitis.

STUDY PARTNER

Preview chapter terms and definitions.

This chapter will discuss the diseases and disorders of the gastrointestinal (GI) tract. Problems examined range from gastroesophageal reflux disease (GERD) to obesity which has become a major health problem. Among the GI disorders discussed are ulcers and the triggers that can cause them; malabsorption syndrome, gastritis, and Crohn disease; GERD and the lifestyle factors that may contribute to it; gallstones and their dissolution; diarrhea, including traveler's diarrhea; and constipation and the role that a low-fiber diet can play in causing it. Next, the chapter examines vomiting and explains how the chemoreceptor trigger zone in the brain can be involved in initiating it. The discussion of obesity considers the role of heredity in its development as well as behavioral modifications that may be helpful in treating it. The chapter concludes with an examination of the drugs used to treat parasites, malaria, and hepatitis.

The Gastrointestinal System

The **gastrointestinal (GI) tract** is a continuous tube that begins in the mouth, extends through the pharynx, esophagus, stomach, small intestine, and large intestine, and ends at the anus (see Figure 10.1). It varies considerably in diameter. The major function of the GI tract is to convert complex food substances into simpler compounds that can be absorbed into the bloodstream and used by the cells of the body. It also excretes solid waste from the body.

GI transit time is the time it takes for material to pass from one end of the GI tract to the other. It is subdivided into gastric emptying time and small intestine and colon transit time. Reducing transit time by speeding the movement of material through the intestines decreases the absorption of nutrients and water. Slowing intestinal transit time increases absorption because nutrients and water spend more time at the absorptive surfaces.

The stomach is composed of layers of smooth muscle lined with glands that secrete gastric juice, containing enzymes and hydrochloric acid, which help break down food and mucus. Most absorption takes place in the small intestine. In the large intestine, the material that has not been absorbed is exposed to bacteria, which continue some limited digestion. Mucous membranes protect the entire digestive system against abrasion and strong digestive enzymes.

FIGURE 10.1
The Gastrointestinal System

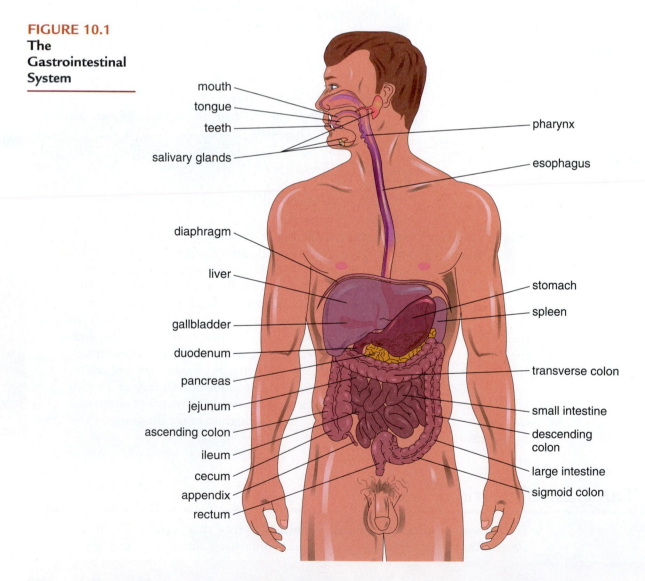

mouth
tongue
teeth
salivary glands
pharynx
esophagus
diaphragm
liver
gallbladder
duodenum
pancreas
jejunum
ascending colon
ileum
cecum
appendix
rectum
stomach
spleen
transverse colon
small intestine
descending colon
large intestine
sigmoid colon

Gastrointestinal Diseases

A wide variety of diseases can affect the GI tract. Although gastroesophageal reflux disease (GERD, or heartburn) and the various conditions known collectively as peptic disease may be the most common, several other diseases, including gastritis and inflammatory bowel disease, are also important.

Gastroesophageal Reflux Disease (GERD)

Gastroesophageal reflux disease (GERD), also called heartburn, is a common problem. Symptoms include radiating burning or pain in the chest and an acid taste. GERD patients also have recurrent abdominal pain, which may move about in the epigastric area. They may have nonspecific epigastric discomfort (gnawing or burning) that is worse before meals and may awaken the patient from sleep.

The primary mechanism responsible for meal-related symptoms of esophagitis (irritation of the esophagus) is the **reflux** (backflow) of acidic stomach contents through an incompetent lower esophageal sphincter. This sphincter is normally in a state of relative contraction. During swallowing, it relaxes enough to allow the forward passage of food and drink into the stomach; then it contracts again, preventing the reflux of the stomach contents. Heartburn occurs when the sphincter becomes incompetent (unable to keep itself sufficiently contracted). Figure 10.2 shows a normal sphincter retaining the stomach contents and an incompetent sphincter allowing reflux of the stomach contents up into the esophagus. Even with a competent sphincter, the likelihood of reflux increases during pregnancy as the uterus exerts upward pressure on abdominal organs, including the stomach; the gastric contents are pushed toward the lower esophageal sphincter and up into the esophagus. GERD may also result from physical conditions such as a hiatal hernia.

Factors that may contribute to the malfunctioning of the lower esophageal sphincter include overeating, eating on the run, eating late at night, drinking alcohol, smoking cigarettes, and consuming various foods. Foods known to trigger reflux symptoms include those with a high fat content and those containing caffeine (in particular, chocolate, coffee, tea, and colas), citric and other acids, and spices. Gas-producing foods may also contribute to heartburn. Alcohol, caffeine, and smoking are complicating and precipitating factors in GERD. Alcohol is the most common cause of gastritis, mucosal irritation, and esophageal varices (swollen veins). Caffeine stimulates acid secretion. Smoking reduces bicarbonate production in pancreatic juice, which neutralizes some acid.

Symptomatic relief of mild to moderate GERD can be obtained by using a combination of lifestyle modifications and medications. The main premise underlying treatment is that many patients have a lifelong problem. Ideally, persons prone to reflux will adopt preventive behavior, but compliance is difficult to achieve. Patient education remains the cornerstone of therapy. Preventive dietary changes include weight loss, if the patient is overweight, and restricted intake of foods that tend to

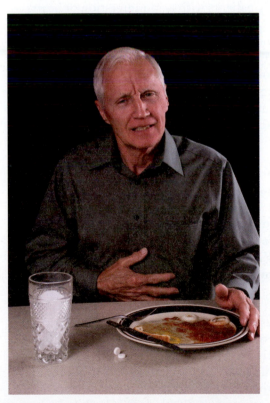

Millions of Americans suffer from various types of gastrointestinal ailments.

FIGURE 10.2
Function of
the Esophageal
Sphincter

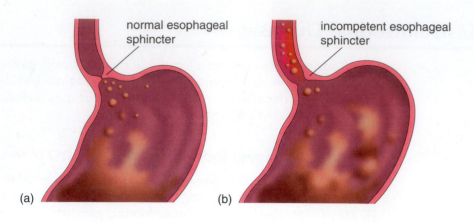

normal esophageal sphincter

incompetent esophageal sphincter

(a)   (b)

(a) The normal esophageal sphincter closes between swallowings. (b) The incompetent esophageal sphincter does not close completely, allowing the gastric contents to be ejected upward into the esophagus.

produce symptoms. Medications that promote reflux (e.g., theophylline and nifedipine) should be avoided. Patients should be advised to stop smoking. To reduce discomfort, patients should be advised not to lie down for at least 3 hours after a meal.

Patients with GERD typically describe it as mild heartburn associated with anxiety. However, anxiety has little or nothing to do with the formation of ulcers—a cause-and-effect relationship that was medical dogma for many years before disproven in the 1980s.

Pharmacologic Treatment of GERD

Table 10.1 lists the agents commonly used to treat GERD and several other GI disorders.

Treatments for GERD are categorized as phase I and phase II treatments. Phase I includes lifestyle modifications and/or use of an antacid. Antacids neutralize the acidic stomach contents so that if reflux does occur, the contents will be less irritating to the esophageal lining. Fortunately, many patients with acid indigestion or heartburn respond to phase I interventions.

Phase II treatments employ medications to try to improve gastric motility and decrease acid production in the stomach. Examples of phase II drugs include acid reducers, proton pump inhibitors, and prokinetic agents. The first two categories of these drugs are used to stimulate cholinergic receptors and to reduce stomach acid production (the H_2 blockers or proton pump inhibitors) in order to block secretion of hydrogen ions into gastric contents. Sometimes, combinations of phase I and phase II medications are used.

Antacids Antacid therapy has several shortcomings, including the need for frequency of dosing and patient compliance. For patients with an active bleed (that is, the GI tract is bleeding somewhere), antacids must be given every hour between meals for 6 to 8 weeks. If there is no active bleed, they must be dosed 1 hour before meals and at bedtime. Patient compliance is a major problem. **Magnesium hydroxide (Phillips Milk of Magnesia)** has good neutralizing capacity, but diarrhea can be a side effect. In contrast, **aluminum hydroxide (AlternaGel)** can have the side effect of constipation; it also contains aluminum, which can be a problem for some disease states.

H_2 Histamine Receptor Antagonists Gastric acid secretion and pepsin secretion occur in response to histamine, gastrin, foods, distention, caffeine, or cholinergic stimulation. When these processes result from histamine, they can be blocked by an **H_2 histamine receptor antagonist**. The mechanism of action is competitive inhibition of histamine at H_2 receptors on the stomach's gastric-secreting cells, which inhibits gastric acid secretion. All of these antagonists are available in OTC strengths, but

TABLE 10.1   Most Commonly Used Agents for GERD

Generic Name	Pronunciation	Dosage Form	Brand Name	Dispensing Status
Antacids				
aluminum hydroxide	a-LOO-mi-num hye-DROX-ide	capsule, oral liquid, tablet	ALternaGel	OTC
aluminum hydroxide–magnesium carbonate	a-LOO-mi-num hye-DROX-ide mag-NEE-zhum KAR-bon-ate	oral liquid, tablet	Gaviscon Extra Strength	OTC
aluminum hydroxide–magnesium hydroxide–simethicone	a-LOO-mi-num hye-DROX-ide mag-NEE-zhum hye-DROX-ide si-METH-i-kone	oral liquid, tablet	Mylanta	
magnesium hydroxide	mag-NEE-zhum hye-DROX-ide	oral liquid, tablet	Phillips Milk of Magnesia	OTC
H₂ Histamine Receptor Antagonists				
cimetidine	sye-MET-i-deen	IV, tablet	Tagamet	Rx
			Tagamet HB	OTC
famotidine	fa-MOE-ti-deen	capsule, IV, oral liquid, tablet	Pepcid	Rx
			Pepcid AC	OTC
nizatidine	ni-ZAT-i-deen	capsule, oral liquid, tablet	Axid	Rx
			Axid AR	OTC
ranitidine	ra-NIT-i-deen	capsule, IV, oral liquid, tablet	Zantac	Rx
			Zantac 75	OTC
Proton Pump Inhibitors				
esomeprazole	es-oh-MEP-ra-zole	capsule	Nexium	Rx
lansoprazole	lan-SOE-pra-zole	capsule, IV, oral liquid, tablet	Prevacid	Rx
omeprazole	oh-MEP-ra-zole	capsule, tablet	Prilosec	Rx
			Prilosec OTC	OTC
pantoprazole	pan-TOE-pra-zole	IV, tablet	Protonix	Rx
rabeprazole	ra-BEP-ra-zole	tablet	Aciphex	Rx
Combinations				
calcium carbonate–famotidine–magnesium hydroxide	KAL-see-um KAR-bon-ate fa-MOE-ti-deen mag-NEE-zhum hye-DROX-ide	tablet	Pepcid Complete	OTC
lansoprazole-naproxen	lan-SOE-pra-zole na-PROX-en	capsule, tablet	Prevacid NapraPAC	Rx
Coating Agent				
sucralfate	soo-KRAL-fate	oral liquid, tablet	Carafate	Rx
Prostaglandin E Analog				
misoprostol	mye-soe-PROS-tawl	tablet	Cytotec	Rx
Cholinergic Agent				
bethanechol	be-THAN-e-kawl	tablet	Urecholine	Rx

some dosages are by prescription only. The bedtime dose is the most important one for H₂ antagonists.

Cimetidine (Tagamet, Tagamet HB) is indicated for treating ulcers and benign gastric ulcers, gastric hypersecretory states, GERD, postoperative ulcers, and upper GI bleeds and for preventing stress ulcers. It reduces hydrogen ion concentration in gastric secretions by 70% (i.e., it increases pH by 0.5). Four to 6 weeks of therapy are required for ulcers to heal. Reduced doses are necessary in renal disease. Because it can inhibit the cytochrome P-450 system, cimetidine has many interactions.

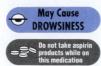

Nizatidine (Axid, Axid AR) is used for treating duodenal ulcers and GERD. It may take several days before the patient gets any relief. If an antacid is added to the regimen, the doses of the two agents should be taken at least 30 minutes apart. A 100 mg dose of nizatidine is equivalent to 300 mg of cimetidine. The patient should avoid aspirin, alcohol, caffeine, cough and cold preparations, and black pepper and other spices while taking this drug. Drowsiness is a side effect.

Ranitidine (Zantac, Zantac 75) is used for active duodenal ulcers and benign gastric ulcers, long-term prophylaxis of duodenal ulcers, gastric hypersecretory states, GERD, postoperative ulcers, and upper GI bleeding and for preventing stress ulcers. It has fewer interactions than some of the other H₂ blockers. Concomitant administration of an antacid should be separated by 30 to 60 minutes. Constipation seems to be the primary side effect.

Warning

Ranitidine may be misread as amantadine or rimantadine (antivirals). Zantac and Xanax (alprazolam, antianxiety medication) can also be confused.

Famotidine (Pepcid, Pepcid AC) is indicated for treating duodenal ulcers, gastric ulcers, stress ulcers, GERD, and hypersecretory conditions. It relieves heartburn, acid indigestion, and sour stomach. The dose should be modified if the patient's kidney function is impaired, and it should be used cautiously in patients taking a calcium channel blocker.

Proton Pump Inhibitors Acidity in gastric secretions is maintained by an enzyme known as the parietal cell H⁺, K⁺-ATPase pump (hydrogen ion–potassium ion pump). The term indicates that this enzyme pumps acidic hydrogen ions (H⁺), or protons, into the stomach; pumps nonacidic potassium (K⁺) ions out; and uses up energy (ATP) to do so. A **proton pump inhibitor,** a drug that blocks this enzyme, reduces stomach acidity. Proton pump inhibitors (PPIs) must be taken on a daily basis, not as needed, in order for them to work properly.

Omeprazole (Prilosec, Prilosec OTC) is indicated for short-term treatment of severe erosive esophagitis, GERD, and hypersecretory conditions. It should be taken before meals. It is also indicated for peptic disease caused by the bacterium *Helicobacter pylori*, in which case it is used in combination with tetracycline, clarithromycin, and an H₂ antagonist. Diarrhea is a primary side effect, and patients can dehydrate quickly.

Lansoprazole (Prevacid) has the same mechanism of action and indications as omeprazole. It is used for short-term treatment of ulcers (4 weeks) and esophagitis (8 weeks). It is also used in long-term treatment of hypersecretory conditions and Zollinger-Ellison syndrome (hypersecretion from a tumor). H₂ blockers and other proton pump inhibitors can also be used in this syndrome.

Esomeprazole (Nexium) is an isomer of omeprazole, and is thus very similar to it. Esomeprazole is metabolized more slowly, which leads to higher and more prolonged drug concentrations and longer acid suppression. It relieves heartburn faster than omeprazole and is slightly more effective for healing erosive esophagitis. Esomeprazole is used for GERD and in combination with amoxicillin and clarithromycin to treat *H. pylori*. It should be taken on an empty stomach. The capsules can be opened and mixed with a small amount of apple sauce if patients have difficulty swallowing pills.

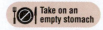

Pantoprazole (Protonix) may be less expensive than most other proton pump inhibitors. It is the drug of choice at many hospitals because it has an IV form, which facilitates switching the patient from IV to oral dosage forms.

Rabeprazole (Aciphex) is a proton pump inhibitor supplied as a delayed-release tablet. It works best if taken in the morning before breakfast.

Combinations **Calcium carbonate–famotidine–magnesium hydroxide (Pepcid Complete)** is indicated for heartburn due to acid indigestion. **Lansoprazole-naproxen (Prevacid NapraPAC)** is provided by the manufacturer in a blister pack. This combination of drugs is intended for patients with a history of ulcers who need a nonsteroidal anti-inflammatory drug (NSAID). It is not known whether this combination is safer than any other combination.

Coating Agent **Sucralfate (Carafate)** is a complex of aluminum hydroxide and sulfated sucrose with an affinity for proteins. It is used to treat duodenal ulcers. It adheres to proteins at the ulcer site, forming a protective coat or shield over the ulcer that resists degradation by gastric acid, pepsin, and bile salts. It also inhibits pepsin, exhibits a cytoprotective effect (protecting cells from noxious chemicals), and forms a viscous, adhesive barrier on the surface of the intact intestinal mucosa and stomach. Sucralfate is dosed every 6 hours (the duration of the coating action's effectiveness). Patients are often awakened from sleep by the ulcer, so around-the-clock dosing is recommended for the first few days. Once the ulcer is relieved, dosing can be twice daily for better compliance. Sucralfate should be taken on an empty stomach and should not be taken within 2 hours of other medications.

Take on an empty stomach

Prostaglandin E Analog **Misoprostol (Cytotec)** is a synthetic prostaglandin E analog for NSAID-induced gastric ulcers. It replaces the protective prostaglandins consumed by such therapies. The primary side effects of this drug are diarrhea and abdominal pain. In other countries it is used for ulcers other than those caused by NSAIDs. It is very important that pregnant women not take this drug or even handle it with their bare hands, because misoprostol is also used to induce labor.

Do not take this drug if pregnant or planning to become pregnant

Cholinergic Agent **Bethanechol (Urecholine)** stimulates cholinergic receptors in the GI tract as well as the urinary tract, resulting in increased peristalsis. It is used primarily for its effect on the urinary tract, but it is sometimes used to treat GERD.

Peptic Disease

The term **peptic disease** is used to refer to a broad spectrum of disorders of the upper GI tract caused by the action of acid and pepsin, a stomach enzyme that assists in degrading food proteins.

An **ulcer** is a local defect or excavation of the surface of an organ or tissue. A **peptic ulcer** is an ulcer formed along any part of the GI tract exposed to acid and the enzyme pepsin. There are three common types of peptic ulcers: gastric, duodenal, and stress ulcers. Many factors, including bacterial infection and severe physiological stress, can contribute to the development of ulcers. Medications can also cause ulcers.

Gastric Ulcers A **gastric ulcer** is a local excavation in the gastric mucosa. These lesions have malignant potential, occur more often in men than women, and become more frequent with aging. They are prevalent in smokers and in populations in the Western Hemisphere. Gastric ulcers do not necessarily occur in persons who are high acid secretors. A family history of gastric ulcers represents a risk factor. As discussed later, a contributing factor for many patients is the bacterium *H. pylori*.

Duodenal Ulcers A **duodenal ulcer** is a peptic lesion situated in the duodenum. Duodenal ulcers occur more in hypersecretors and are more difficult to treat than gastric ulcers because of the difficulty of getting medication into the duodenum.

Stress Ulcers A **stress ulcer** is a peptic ulcer, usually gastric, that occurs in the clinical setting in patients who are under severe physiological stress from serious illness, such as sepsis, burns, major surgery, chronic disease, or chronic infection. Usually, the patient is in the intensive care unit (ICU). Stress ulcers are caused by the breakdown of natural mucosal resistance. The patient usually has no clinical symptoms but can experience acute hemorrhage. Inserting a nasogastric tube yields blood in the aspirate of the stomach contents. Perforations of the stomach wall occur in 8 to 18% of patients, with severe pain radiating toward the back. Therapy includes antacids every 3 to 4 hours, H_2 histamine receptor antagonists or blockers intravenously by continuous infusion or every 3 to 6 hours, or proton pump inhibitors intravenously or through a feeding tube. The potential for developing stress ulcers is why almost everyone in the ICU receives an H_2 blocker.

Drug-Induced Ulcers Several drugs can cause ulcers. They are listed in Table 10.2. Aspirin is the most common cause of drug-induced ulcers.

Pharmacologic Treatment of *H. pylori*

Research has shown that **Helicobacter pylori** is responsible for the majority of peptic ulcers. It also plays a role in chronic active gastritis and gastric cancer. Therefore, treatment regimens aim at eradication of the bacterium. The mainstays of therapy for ulcers include antacids, H_2 receptor antagonists, and proton pump inhibitors. Once a positive diagnosis has been made, *H. pylori* is treated with the drugs listed in Table 10.3. *H. pylori* is able to survive in stomach acid because it secretes enzymes that neutralize the acid. This allows the bacterium to make its way to the protective mucous lining. Once there, the spiral shape helps it burrow through the lining. Triple therapy is recommended; if that is unsuccessful, then quadruple therapy is used as a

TABLE 10.2	Drugs That May Cause Ulcers
Drug	**Adverse Effect**
alcohol	irritating to the GI tract
aspirin	irritating to the GI tract
anti-inflammatory drugs, ibuprofen, fenoprofen, naproxen, tolmetin solution	reduce production of mucus
corticosteroids (often used in inflammatory bowel disease)	reduce the mucosal barrier
potassium chloride (KCl)	irritating to the GI tract
methotrexate	irritating to the GI tract, ulceration, hemorrhage
iron	causes esophageal ulceration (must be taken with food, milk, or lots of water)

rescue treatment. Triple therapy involves a proton pump inhibitor (PPI) and two antibiotics. The drugs are taken for a 2 week period. When drug or other therapies are unsuccessful, surgery is the last resort to treat peptic ulcers.

Many combinations of the drugs listed in Table 10.3 are being used to eradicate *H. pylori*. Treatment usually consists of one or two antibiotics combined with an antacid or proton pump inhibitor. The antibiotic is the mainstay of therapy since the target is bacteria.

Bismuth subsalicylate–metronidazole–tetracycline (Helidac) is a drug combination used to treat *H. pylori*. Bismuth subsalicylate exhibits both antisecretory and antimicrobial action. It may even provide some anti-inflammatory action. It also has some antacid properties. This bismuth compound exhibits antimicrobial action, and the subsalicylate provides the antisecretory effect. The other two drugs in the combination are antibiotics. The combination comes in a 14 day supply kit.

Bismuth subcitrate potassium, metronidazole, and tetracycline (Pylera) combined with a PPI is approved to treat *H. pylori*. The advantage of this drug in contrast to Helidac is that the bismuth subcitrate is a not a salt of salicylic acid and therefore can be used in people with an aspirin allergy.

Warning

Metronidazole and macrodantin (nitrofurantoin, prescribed for urinary tract infections) can be confused.

Other GI Diseases and Pharmacologic Treatment

Gastritis is an irritation and superficial erosion of the stomach lining. In contrast to gastric ulcer, the damage is spread over large areas in the gastric mucosa rather than focused on specific lesions. Alcohol is a common causative factor.

TABLE 10.3   Most Commonly Used Agents for *H. pylori*

Generic Name	Pronunciation	Dosage Form	Brand Name	Dispensing Status
Antibiotics				
amoxicillin	a-mox-i-SIL-in	capsule, oral liquid, tablet	Amoxil, Trimox	Rx
clarithromycin	kla-rith-roe-MYE-sin	oral liquid, tablet	Biaxin	Rx
metronidazole	me-troe-NYE-da-zole	capsule, IV, tablet	Flagyl, Flagyl I.V.	Rx
tetracycline	te-tra-SYE-kleen	capsule, oral liquid, tablet	Sumycin	Rx
Histamine² Receptor Antagonists (see Table 10.1)				
Proton Pump Inhibitors (see Table 10.1)				
Combinations				
bismuth subsalicylate–metronidazole–tetracycline	BIS-muth sub-sa-LIS-a-late me-troe-NYE-da-zole te-tra-SYE-kleen	capsule, tablet	Helidac	Rx
bismuth subcitrate potassium-metronidazole-tetracycline	BIS-muth-sub-SIT-rate poe-TASS-ee-um me-troe-NYE-da-zole te-tra-SYE-kleen	capsule	Pylera	Rx
lansoprazole-amoxicillin-clarithromycin	lan-SOE-pra-zole a-mox-i-SIL-in kla-rith-roe-MYE-sin	capsule, tablet	Prevpac	Rx

Inflammatory bowel disease has two forms. The first of these, **ulcerative colitis,** is an irritation and inflammation of the large bowel, causing it to appear scraped; the disease is characterized by bloody mucus leading to watery diarrhea that contains blood, mucus, and pus. Ulcerative colitis is confined to the rectum and colon. The second inflammatory bowel disease, **Crohn disease,** is similar in some ways to ulcerative colitis but can affect any portion of the tubular GI tract. Therefore, Crohn disease cannot be cured by surgical resection.

Cystic fibrosis (CF), mentioned in Chapter 9, is a GI disease as well as a pulmonary disease. Involvement of the GI tract is due to increased viscosity of mucous secretions and to a relative deficiency of pancreatic enzymes. The backbone of GI therapy in cystic fibrosis is pancreatic enzyme replacement and vitamin supplementation.

Table 10.4 lists the agents commonly used to treat these gastrointestinal diseases. Agents used to treat specific gastrointestinal diseases will be discussed in the following sections.

Mast Cell Stabilizer As noted previously, gastric acid secretion and pepsin secretion occur in response to histamine, among other factors. Histamine is released from the

TABLE 10.4   Most Commonly Used Agents for Gastrointestinal Diseases

Generic Name	Pronunciation	Dosage Form	Brand Name	Dispensing Status
Mast Cell Stabilizer				
cromolyn sodium	KROE-moe-lin SOE-dee-um	inhalation, nebulizing solution, ophthalmic solution, oral liquid	Crolom, Gastrocrom, Intal, Opticrom	Rx
Pancreatic Enzyme				
pancrelipase	pan-kre-LIP-ase	capsule, tablet	Creon-10, Pancrease, Viokase	Rx
Immunosuppression				
azathioprine	ay-za-THYE-oh-preen	tablet	Imuran	Rx
Monoclonal Antibody				
infliximab	in-FLIX-i-mab	IV	Remicade	Rx
Anti-inflammatory Medications				
balsalazide	bal-SAL-a-zide	capsule	Colazal	Rx
budesonide	byoo-DES-oh-nide	capsule	Entocort EC	Rx
mesalamine	me-SAL-a-meen	capsule, enema, tablet	Asacol, Lialda, Pentasa, Rowasa	Rx
olsalazine	ole-SAL-a-zeen	capsule	Dipentum	Rx
sulfasalazine	sul-fa-SAL-a-zeen	tablet	Azulfidine	Rx
Gallstone Dissolution Agent				
ursodiol	ER-soe-dye-ole	capsule	Actigall	Rx
Antiemetic				
metoclopramide	met-oh-KLOE-pra-mide	injection, IV, tablet	Reglan	Rx

membranes of mast cells. The mast cell stabilizer **cromolyn sodium (Crolom, Gastrocrom, Intal, Opticrom),** discussed in Chapter 9 in relation to the treatment of asthma, inhibits release of histamine in the GI tract and is indicated for abdominal pain. It is used to treat inflammatory bowel disease and symptoms of food allergies.

Pancreatic Enzyme   Enzymes secreted into the duodenum of the small intestine by the pancreas play an important role in the digestive process (see Figure 10.3, which shows the relationship between the pancreas and the small intestine). Without these enzymes, **malabsorption syndrome** (impaired absorption of nutrients) can result. **Pancrelipase (Creon-10, Pancrease, Viokase)** is indicated for replacement therapy in symptomatic treatment of malabsorption syndrome caused by pancreatic insufficiency. It is also often used in cystic fibrosis patients. It should be taken before or with meals. Nausea, cramps, constipation, and diarrhea can all be side effects. At higher doses, this drug can trigger gout attacks because of the resulting high blood levels of purine, which is converted to uric acid, which in turn causes hyperuricemia.

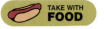

Immunosuppression   **Azathioprine (Imuran)** is an immunosuppressive agent that interferes with nucleic acid synthesis in both normal and precancer cells. The overall action is the suppression of the immune system. This drug is approved for treatment of severe arthritis and to prevent the rejection of organ transplants. It is also used as an anti-inflammatory agent in Crohn disease, ulcerative colitis, and chronic active hepatitis. It can cause serious but reversible forms of bone marrow depression. An allergic response is chills, fever, and arthralgias up to 1 month after therapy. Rash, alopecia (hair loss), hepatotoxicity, and increased risk of infection are side effects.

Monoclonal Antibody   **Infliximab (Remicade)** binds to tumor necrosis factor (TNF) alpha and neutralizes its activity by preventing it from binding to the cell membrane and in the blood. It decreases infiltration of inflammatory cells and TNF alpha production in inflamed areas of the intestines. Infliximab is indicated in the treatment of active Crohn disease and ulcerative colitis and is generally reserved for moderate-to-severe cases. It is also indicated for rheumatoid arthritis because of its action on TNF alpha. Like azathioprine, infliximab is an immunosuppressant.

Infliximab is given either as a single infusion or, for more complicated outbreaks, as a three-dose infusion series. The vials should be refrigerated but not frozen. Infliximab is reconstituted with sterile water that is *directed to the glass wall of the vial*. The powder should be *gently swirled* by rotating the vial. *It should not be shaken*. It should then be admixed with normal saline. After it is mixed, it has a 24 hour expiration date. Because it is incompatible with polyvinyl chloride (PVC), it must be prepared *only* in glass bottles or polypropylene or polyolefin infusion bags and administered through polyethylene-lined administration sets.

Anti-inflammatory Medications   **Mesalamine (Asacol, Pentasa, Rowasa, Lialda)** is used in Crohn disease and ulcerative colitis. **Rowasa** is given as a rectal enema. It can cause abdominal pain, headache, flatulence, nausea, and flu-like symptoms. It works topically by blocking prostaglandin production and inhibiting inflammation. **Lialda** is the first available once-daily oral mesalamine for ulcerative colitis. Two to four tablets are taken once daily with food.

Sulfasalazine (Azulfidine) is believed to be a prodrug, inactive until colon bacteria convert it into two metabolites: mesalamine, responsible for the anti-inflammatory effect as described in the preceding paragraph, and sulfapyridine, responsible for the antibacterial action and most of the adverse effects. These effects are dose related.

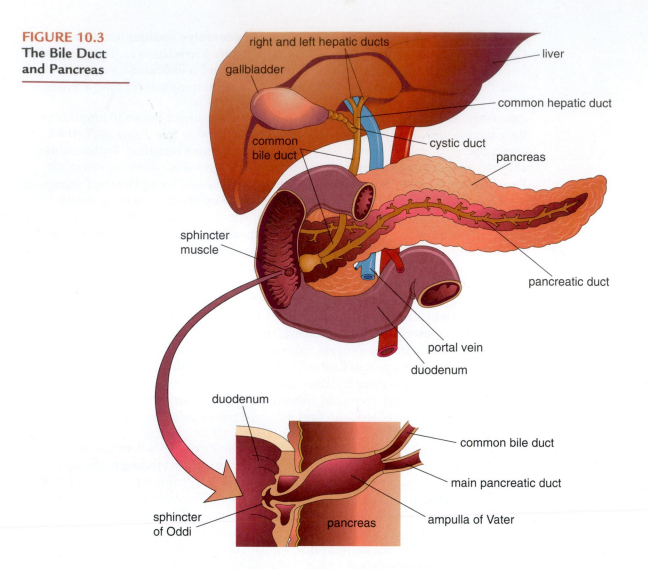

FIGURE 10.3
The Bile Duct and Pancreas

Labels on upper figure: right and left hepatic ducts; liver; gallbladder; common hepatic duct; common bile duct; cystic duct; pancreas; sphincter muscle; pancreatic duct; portal vein; duodenum

Labels on lower figure: duodenum; common bile duct; main pancreatic duct; sphincter of Oddi; pancreas; ampulla of Vater

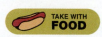

Sulfasalazine is contraindicated in patients allergic to sulfa or salicylates. It should not be given within 1 hour of iron, as it will bind the iron. Patients should maintain proper fluid intake and take the drug after meals. The drug can change urine, perspiration, tears, and semen to an orange-yellow color that may permanently stain soft contact lenses yellow. Other side effects of sulfasalazine are nausea, vomiting, fever, headache, rash, and arthralgias. It can also cause bronchospasm, hepatotoxicity, pancreatitis, neuropathies, and severe anemias. The patient should avoid the sun. Sulfasalazine therapy usually is limited to 2 years.

Olsalazine (Dipentum) maintains remission of ulcerative colitis and Crohn disease in patients who are resistant to sulfasalazine. This drug should be taken with food in evenly divided doses.

Balsalazide (Colazal) is broken down by bacteria in the colon to release mesalamine. It works as well as mesalamine and is better tolerated than sulfasalazine because there is no sulfa entity. It is used to treat ulcerative colitis.

Budesonide (Entocort EC) is a steroid indicated for acute attacks of Crohn disease. It has beneficial effects on the inflammatory abnormalities of the acute disease. Budesonide is not indicated for maintenance therapy, however, and will not prevent relapse. It is a capsule of coated granules that are released in the small intestine, its site of action. Budesonide is subject to a high first-pass effect, which reduces systemic glucocorticoid exposure and side effects. Budesonide causes less severe symptoms of hypercorticism than other glucocorticoids, but can still cause adrenal suppression.

Gallstone Dissolution **Ursodiol (Actigall)** is a naturally occurring bile acid used as an oral agent to dissolve cholesterol gallstones that form in the gallbladder or bile duct (see Figure 10.3). It decreases the cholesterol content of bile and bile stones by reducing the secretion of cholesterol from the liver and the fractional reabsorption of cholesterol by the intestines. Frequent blood work is necessary to follow the drug's effects. Persistent nausea, vomiting, and abdominal pain should be reported. Gallstone dissolution can take several months; for some patients, however, gallstones are never dissolved. Even for cases of successful dissolution, recurrence of stones within 5 years has been observed in 50% of patients.

Antiemetic **Metoclopramide (Reglan)** is described in a later section as an agent to prevent vomiting, but it is also a prokinetic agent that increases contraction in the GI tract. It increases the pressure closing the lower esophageal sphincter, thus decreasing the likelihood that stomach contents will move into the esophagus. Metoclopramide also helps peristalsis (the squeezing movements of the GI tract) and increases the rate at which the stomach empties. Metoclopramide is more likely to be efficacious if dosed more than once daily. It has fewer side effects than other promotility agents, but it can cause sedation.

Diarrhea

Diarrhea has many causes. Acute diarrhea can be the result of a bacterial and viral infection, a **parasite** (an organism that feeds off another organism, such as a human, referred to as its host), or medications. Chronic diarrhea is the production of loose stools for more than 4 weeks. It is usually caused by a disease state such as Crohn disease or ulcerative colitis.

Diarrhea can be dangerous because it can quickly lead to dehydration. It decreases GI transit time and will impair absorption of drugs, vitamins, nutrients, and toxins. The most commonly used antidiarrheal agents are listed in Table 10.5. Specifically, the antimotility drugs should be used in managing chronic disease states, such as inflammatory bowel disease, postvagotomy diarrhea, and ileostomy. They should not be used to manage short-term, self-limiting diarrhea. They can also be hazardous in infectious diarrhea by prolonging fever and delaying clearance of organisms.

Adsorbent

Bismuth subsalicylate (Pepto-Bismol, Kaopectate) is safe to use as an antidiarrheal because it acts as an adsorbent, soaking up water from the fecal matter, rather than by reducing intestinal motility. If diarrhea is not controlled within 24 hours, the patient should contact a physician.

Antimotility Drugs

Antimotility drugs for diarrhea work by slowing peristalsis, the smooth muscle contractions that propel fecal matter along the colon. Water absorption from the feces is improved as the colon contents spend more time in transit. Most of these drugs contain opiates and therefore are controlled substances. Recall that long-term use of

TABLE 10.5   Most Commonly Used Antidiarrheal Agents

Generic Name	Pronunciation	Dosage Form	Brand Name	Dispensing Status	Control Schedule
Adsorbent					
bismuth subsalicylate	BIS-muth sub-sa-LIS-i-late	oral liquid, tablet	Pepto-Bismol Kaopectate	OTC OTC	
Antimotility Drugs					
difenoxin-atropine	dye-fen-OX-in AT-roe-peen	tablet	Motofen	Rx	C-IV
diphenoxylate-atropine	dye-fen-OX-i-late AT-roe-peen	oral liquid, tablet	Lomotil	Rx	C-V
loperamide	loe-PAIR-a-mide	capsule, oral solution, tablet	Imodium, Imodium A-D	OTC	
paregoric	pair-e-GOR-ik	oral liquid	(none)	Rx	C-III
Drugs for Infectious Diarrhea					
nitazoxanide	nye-tah-ZOX-ah-nide	oral liquid, tablet	Alinia	Rx	
rifaximin	rye-FAX-i-min	tablet	Xifaxan	Rx	

narcotics for pain leads to constipation; the use of narcotics to control diarrhea is an example of using a drug for its side effects to treat another condition.

Diphenoxylate-atropine (Lomotil) is a combination of 0.25 mg of diphenoxylate and 0.25 mg of atropine. Diphenoxylate is derived from the narcotic meperidine, which is why the medication is a Schedule V controlled substance. Atropine is added to discourage abuse; it also reduces peristalsis, but in excessive doses it produces anticholinergic side effects (dry mouth, blurred vision, flushing, and urinary retention). Further side effects include constipation, paralytic ileus, respiratory depression, and sedation. Care should be taken in infectious diarrhea with fever; acute diarrhea; toxic megacolon, which can result in perforation; and advanced liver disease.

Both of these drugs slow peristaltic action, which produces bulking of fecal matter.

Difenoxin-atropine (Motofen) contains a metabolite of diphenoxylate and is classified as Schedule IV. The side effect profile and usage are the same as for diphenoxylate-atropine (Lomotil).

Loperamide (Imodium, Imodium A-D) is a synthetic opioid similar to diphenoxylate. It acts on the intestinal nerves with antiperistaltic activity, but it does not act on the central nervous system. Loperamide has been used for prolonged periods (18 months or longer) without loss of efficacy or signs of toxicity. Side effects are drowsiness, constipation, and dry mouth. It is available OTC and is replacing diphenoxylate-atropine because it seems to be as efficacious without the potentially addictive side effect profile.

Paregoric (also called camphorated tincture of opium) increases smooth-muscle tone in the GI tract, decreases motility and peristalsis, and diminishes digestive secretions. The patient should avoid alcohol when taking any opium derivative. Paregoric may cause drowsiness, may impair judgment or coordination, and may cause physical and psychological dependence with prolonged use. It is a Schedule III controlled substance.

Drugs for Infectious Diarrhea

Nitazoxanide (Alinia) is indicated for the treatment of infectious diarrhea caused by the waterborne **protozoan** (single-celled animal) parasites *Giardia lamblia* and *Cryptosporidium parvum*. It may be used in patients aged 1 year or older. Nitazoxanide interferes with an enzyme-dependent electron transfer that is essential for anaerobic energy metabolism. Nitazoxanide is provided by the manufacturer as a powder that is to be mixed with water. Both the powder and oral suspension should be refrigerated. The reconstituted suspension should be discarded after 7 days. Diabetics should be aware that this drug contains 1.48 g of sucrose per 5 mL. It is strawberry flavored. Other drugs used against GI parasites are described in a later section of this chapter.

REFRIGERATE

Rifaximin (Xifaxan) represents a significant addition to the antimicrobial therapy for the treatment of **traveler's diarrhea**. This condition poses a significant risk to U.S. citizens who travel to some foreign countries; it is acquired through ingestion of food or water contaminated with the fecal bacterium *Escherichia coli*. To avoid contamination, travelers should limit their consumption to well-cooked foods, peeled fruits and vegetables, and bottled water. Previously, systemic antibiotics were commonly prescribed, but due to increased antibiotic resistance, this practice is no longer recommended. The only people who should use systemic antibiotics to combat traveler's diarrhea are "critical travelers" such as Olympic athletes and politicians. If prophylaxis is warranted, some physicians recommend taking quinolone and loperamide with the first loose stool. Rifaximin inhibits bacterial RNA synthesis. The significant advantage of this drug is that it is not absorbed into the body, so there is little risk of developing long-term resistance to it. It is indicated for patients 12 years and older. It should not be used in diarrhea complicated by fever or blood.

Constipation and Related GI Diseases

Constipation and several gastrointestinal diseases are intricately related to the dietary fiber. In this section we discuss what fiber is, how to supplement dietary fiber, constipation and its treatment, and other ailments of the GI tract and their treatment.

Fiber

Fiber is defined as the undigested residue of fruits, vegetables, and other foods of plant origin after digestion by the human GI enzymes. The most important classification of fiber is by water solubility. Fruits, vegetables, and grains contain both soluble and insoluble fibers. Total fiber is the sum of soluble and insoluble fiber. Dietary fiber consists of relatively large-molecule carbohydrates. The term "fiber" is a bit misleading, as many of these molecules are not actually *fibrous* in form. Figure 10.4 illustrates the colon, or large intestine, an organ that depends on dietary fiber to function normally.

In addition to solubility, fiber is characterized by fermentability (ability to be converted into other compounds by bacteria in the colon), water-holding capacity, and stool-bulking capacity. The bacteria in the colon are able to ferment some types of fiber. Soluble fibers are fermented to a greater extent than insoluble ones. The end products of fermentation are short-chain fatty acids, gases, water, and energy. The water-holding and stool-bulking capacities of fiber are related in that absorbing and holding water is how fiber bulks (increases the volume of) fecal material. Insoluble fibers hold less water than soluble ones. Bacterial growth in the colon provides additional bulking. Most dietary fiber reaches the colon unaltered; there it increases colon content, reduces colon

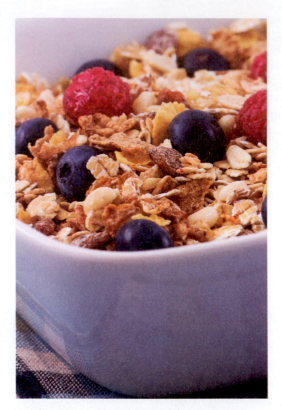

Foods such as many grains and fruits contain abundant fiber that helps to decrease the incidence of constipation.

pressure, and increases propulsive motility (forward motion). These effects account for fiber's role in preventing or relieving constipation. Chronic constipation has often been associated with low-fiber diets. It is a common problem among the elderly in the United States and other Western countries, but does not appear to be a problem in less developed countries.

Extended transit time in the colon permits more water to be absorbed from the GI tract into the body, thus producing smaller, harder stools. Shortening the transit time produces looser, more watery stools because less water is absorbed.

Insoluble fibers reduce GI transit time. Some soluble fibers, such as psyllium (the common name of a group of plants whose seeds yield fiber), work to regulate the speed of transit of waste. Soluble fibers form gels when mixed with water. In the GI tract, they act more like solids than like liquids and thus delay emptying. This is why psyllium can be used as an antidiarrheal as well as a laxative. Inactivity or confinement to bed can actually cause constipation when combined with these products. Fiber also provides lubrication.

Dietary fiber offers benefits aside from those associated with constipation. Soluble fibers exert metabolic effects that can lower the risk of diabetes and coronary artery disease. In addition to delaying emptying, natural soluble fibers slow the absorption of glucose from the

FIGURE 10.4
The Large Intestine

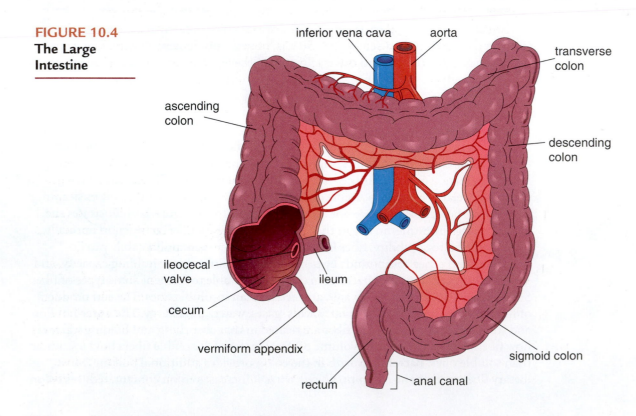

small intestine. Fiber may also increase tissue sensitivity to insulin by increasing the number of insulin receptors on target cells. For these reasons, high-fiber diets or fiber supplements can have a positive effect on diabetes.

In addition, psyllium, fruit and vegetable fiber, and other soluble fibers bind to bile acids in the small intestine. The liver makes bile acids from cholesterol and other circulating lipids and stores the acids in the gallbladder, from which they are released into the duodenum, where they help to break masses of dietary fats into small droplets that can be absorbed. Most of the bile acids are reabsorbed in the ileum (the lowest section of the small intestine) and recycled in a process known as enterohepatic circulation. By binding bile acids and transporting them onward into the stool, fiber interrupts the enterohepatic circulation. The removed bile acids must be replaced to ensure fat metabolism. Making more bile acids removes cholesterol from the pool of lipoproteins circulating in the bloodstream. The end result is to maintain or increase blood levels of high-density lipoproteins (HDLs) and to reduce blood levels of low-density lipoproteins (LDLs)—an effect that lowers the risk of coronary artery disease.

Fiber also plays a role in lowering the risk of colorectal cancer. Colon cancer is more likely to develop when the diet has a high fat content and a low fiber content (the latter raises the risk even more). As dietary fiber increases, risk of colon cancer is reduced. Everyone over 55 years should have a rectal examination to screen for cancer or potentially cancerous tissue.

Fiber Supplementation

The most widely accepted therapeutic use of high-fiber foods is in managing constipation, but fiber supplementation is also widely used to suppress appetite and achieve weight loss. Fiber helps to produce feelings of satiety (fullness). The most effective diets are low-calorie, high-residue (high-fiber) ones. The beneficial fiber intake threshold is approximately 40 g/day. Most Americans consume only 15 to 20 g/day. Doubling the daily fiber intake could produce a significant health benefit.

The adverse effects of fiber are distention, excessive gas, and flatulence, but these symptoms usually subside after the first few weeks of increased fiber consumption. These symptoms may also be associated with esophageal, gastric, or small-bowel or rectal obstruction, especially in patients with intestinal stricture or stenosis. They may also interfere with absorbing some drugs and nutrients.

Pharmacologic Treatment of Constipation

Although, as described above, constipation is often associated with a low-fiber diet, it has many other causes, including certain medications. Another cause of constipation is dehydration, which can be due to fever, hot dry temperature, vomiting, and diarrhea. It is very important to drink six to eight glasses of fluids daily. This alone can often prevent constipation. In addition, regular exercise will often help prevent constipation. Bed rest and mucosal damage can also lead to constipation.

Sometimes medications are needed to treat constipation and for bowel cleansing prior to colorectal examination. Medications used to treat constipation and its effects include hydrating agents (including osmotic laxatives, saline laxatives, and bowel evacuants), irritant/stimulants, surfactants, bulk-forming agents, and antiflatulents. Table 10.6 lists the most commonly used laxatives as well as other agents to treat constipation.

Osmotic Laxatives An **osmotic laxative** is an organic substance that draws water into the colon and thereby stimulates evacuation. For example, glycerin draws fluid

TABLE 10.6 Most Commonly Used Agents to Treat Constipation

Generic Name	Pronunciation	Dosage Form	Brand Name	Dispensing Status
Osmotic Laxatives				
glycerin	GLIS-er-in	suppository	Fleet Glycerin Suppositories	OTC
lactulose	LAK-tu-los	oral liquid	Enulose	Rx
polyethylene glycol 3350	pol-ee-ETH-il-een GLYE-kawl 3350	powder for oral solution	MiraLax	OTC
Saline Laxatives				
magnesium hydroxide	mag-NEE-zhum hye-DROX-ide	oral liquid, tablet	Phillips Milk of Magnesia	OTC
magnesium sulfate (Epsom salts)	mag-NEE-zhum SUL-fate	granules	(none)	OTC
Irritant/Stimulant				
bisacodyl	bis-a-KOE-dil	suppository, tablet	Dulcolax	OTC
Surfactants				
docusate	DOK-yoo-sate	capsule, oral liquid, tablet	Colace	OTC
			Ex-Lax Stool Softener, Surfak	OTC
docusate-senna	DOK-yoo-sate SEN-na	tablet	Senokot-S	OTC
Bulk-Forming Agent				
psyllium	SIL-ee-um	oral liquid, wafer	Fiberall, Metamucil, Perdiem Fiber Therapy	OTC
Antiflatulent				
aluminum hydroxide–magnesium hydroxide–simethicone	a-LOO-mi-num hye-DROX-ide mag-NEE-zhum hye-DROX-ide si-METH-i-kone	oral liquid, tablet	Mylanta	OTC
calcium carbonate–simethicone	kal-see-um-KAR-bun-ate-si-METH-i-kone	oral liquid, tablet	Maalox	OTC
simethicone	si-METH-i-kone	oral liquid,tablet	Gas Aid, Mylanta Maximum Strength, Mylicon Drops	OTC
Bowel Evacuants				
polyethylene glycol 3350 and electrolytes	pol-ee-ETH-il-een GLYE-kawl 3350 and ee-LEK-tro-lytes	powder	GoLYTELY, HalfLytely	Rx
sodium phosphate	SOE-dee-um FOS-fate	oral liquid, tablet	Fleet Phospho-Soda, Visicol	Rx
Miscellaneous				
lubiprostone	loo-bi-PROS-tone	capsule	Amitiza	Rx

into the colon and stimulates evacuation of the lower bowel, so few nutrients are lost. Glycerin suppositories are a fairly quick, effective method to relieve constipation.

Lactulose (Enulose) is metabolized by bacteria in the colon; this metabolic process reduces fecal pH (that is, increases acidity), reduces absorption of ammonia and toxic nitrogenous substances, and has a cathartic (emptying of the bowel) effect. Lactulose delivers osmotically active molecules to the colon. It is used to prevent and treat hepatic-induced encephalopathy. Normally the liver removes nitrogen waste by-products that the blood has picked up from the intestines, including ammonia from protein breakdown. When the liver is not functioning properly, as in alcoholism, these nitrogen by-products build up in the blood, destroying brain cells, which results in encephalopathy. Lactulose is thought to offset this process by reducing ammonia production and absorption from the GI tract. The side effects include nausea and vomiting, cramps, diarrhea, and anorexia.

Polyethylene glycol 3350 (MiraLax) is an OTC product and stool softener. This product uses the same active ingredient as GoLYTELY, discussed below under bowel evacuants, but in MiraLax a much smaller quantity of the drug, 17 g, is taken daily to maintain a soft stool and to avoid constipation. MiraLax is frequently used in children.

Saline Laxatives A **saline laxative** is an inorganic salt that, like an osmotic laxative, attracts water into the intestinal lumen (the hollow portion of the bowel through which fecal material passes) and increases intraluminal pressure.

Magnesium hydroxide (Milk of Magnesia) is a laxative as well as an antacid. Magnesium is supplied as the citrate, hydroxide, and sulfate (epsom salts) forms. It promotes evacuation of the bowel by causing osmotic retention of fluid, which distends the colon and increases peristaltic activity. It also reacts with hydrochloric acid in the stomach, which enables it to produce the antacid effects. Caution should be used in renal patients.

Irritant and Stimulant Laxatives A **stimulant laxative** increases gut activity by irritating the mucosa. **Bisacodyl (Dulcolax)** works in this way. Technicians should be watchful for patients on long-term narcotic pain medication. A common side effect is constipation, and such patients should be on a stimulant laxative. If they are not, the technician should bring this to someone's attention.

Surfactant Laxatives A **surfactant laxative** is a substance that acts as a detergent, helping fatty and watery components of the intestinal contents to mix, thus making the stool soft and mushy. **Docusate (Colace, Ex-Lax)** and **docusate-senna (Senokot-S)** are examples of this type of drug.

Bulk-Forming Agents Bran and other bulking agents—dietary fiber, as previously discussed—are the most natural and safest materials to use. Eating bran is an excellent way to increase fiber in the diet and promote normal gut peristalsis. Bran as a dietary supplement can be acquired by including whole grains and grain products in the diet. These naturally occurring bulk materials appeal to many patients who want to return to natural foods. Bulk-producing products should be taken with a full glass of water about a half hour before eating.

Psyllium (Fiberall, Metamucil, Perdiem Fiber Therapy) increases nonabsorbable bulk to promote soft stools and easy defecation in patients who should avoid straining (e.g., postoperative, post-myocardial infarction, elderly, pregnant). Patients should drink six to eight glasses of water a day. Psyllium is classified as an antidiarrheal as well as a laxative. It adsorbs water in the intestine, producing a viscous liquid that promotes peristalsis and reduces transit time. Patients must be active for it to work; as mentioned earlier, psyllium can cause constipation in a bedridden patient. It is also an excellent cholesterol-lowering agent.

Miscellaneous Agent **Lubiprostone (Amitiza)** is the only drug approved for chronic idiopathic constipation. It is a prostaglandin derivative that activates the chloride channel locally in the small intestine, which increases intestinal fluid secretion. Nausea is the primary side effect. Patients may want to take this drug with food in order to minimize this side effect.

Antiflatulent **Simethicone (Gas Aid, Mylicon Drops, and Mylanta Maximum Strength)** is an inert silicon polymer for gastric defoaming. By reducing surface tension, the drug causes gas bubbles to brake or to coalesce into a foam that can be eliminated more easily by belching or passing flatus. Simethicone relieves flatulence and functional gastric bloating and postoperative gas pains. Dosage recommendations should not be exceeded, especially in children. Mylicon Drops is the only OTC product for babies with colic.

Bowel Evacuants In contrast to laxatives, which are used to restore normal bowel function, a **bowel evacuant** such as **polyethylene glycol 3350 with electrolytes (GoLYTELY)** is indicated for bowel cleansing prior to GI examination (colonoscopy or X-ray with barium enema) or in rare cases following toxic ingestion. GoLYTELY increases the osmolarity of bowel contents, thus drawing large amounts of water into the lumen so as to flush the bowel contents out. The recommended dose is 4 L. The patient should fast 3 to 4 hours prior to administration and for 2 hours following administration; 240 mL (8 oz) should be consumed every 10 minutes until the 4 L are gone. The doctor or manufacturer usually supplies a printed informational sheet for the patient with explicit instructions. A powder is dispensed in a 4 L container. HalfLYTELY is sometimes used instead of GoLYTELY. It consists of 2 L (half the amount of GoLYTELY) of solution that is to be combined with bisacodyl (a stimulant laxative) delayed release tablets.

   Sodium phosphate (Fleet Phospho-Soda) is indicated for evacuation of the colon and for treating and testing of hypophosphatemia. Like saline laxatives, sodium phosphate draws water into the colon. **Visicol** is a sodium phosphate tablet indicated for bowel preparation prior to colonoscopy. The tablets are tasteless and can be taken with any clear liquid such as water, lemonade, or ginger ale. This drug has been proved to be associated with significantly less nausea, vomiting, and bloating than other preparations. It is much better tolerated by patients than other bowel evacuants.

Other GI Diseases That May Accompany Constipation

Low amounts of fiber in the diet not only produce a state of constipation but can increase the likelihood that a patient will encounter a number of other gastrointestinal diseases. Several of these diseases are discussed here.

Diverticular Disease **Diverticular disease** occurs when an outpocketing (diverticulum) from the bowel wall forms (diverticulosis) and/or becomes inflamed (diverticulitis; see Figure 10.5). It is believed to result from a deficiency of fiber over time. Vegetarians, whose average daily intake of fiber (40 g) is approximately twice that of nonvegetarians, have approximately one-third the incidence of diverticular disease. Diverticular disease seems to be related to the predominance of more highly refined carbohydrates and other processed foods in the modern diet. Colonic segmentation

FIGURE 10.5
Portion of the Colon with Diverticula

In diverticular disease, herniations form along the mucous membranes, and the muscular layers of the colon wall may become inflamed, causing pain.

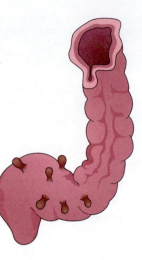

(in which the colon acts as if it is divided into small parts that move independently of each other rather than contributing to an integrated overall motion) is accompanied by an increase in pressure inside the colon, prolonged GI transit time, and low fecal weight. All of these factors contribute to herniation (protrusion through a weakened muscular wall) of the colon lining, with accompanying inflammation and pain. Fiber may reduce the pressure generated in the colon.

Hiatal Hernia **Hiatal hernia** is related to chronic constipation. Straining to pass small, firm stools can significantly raise intra-abdominal pressures. Over a period of several years, daily straining to pass stools can force the gastroesophageal junction upward into the thoracic cavity (Figure 10.2) through the esophageal hiatus (the opening in the diaphragm through which normally only the esophagus passes).

Irritable Bowel Syndrome (IBS) **Irritable bowel syndrome (IBS)** is the most common of the GI disorders. Many patients with GI complaints are diagnosed with IBS. IBS is a functional disorder in which the lower GI tract does not have the appropriate tone or spasticity to regulate bowel activity. Some evidence also suggests that patients presenting with IBS have an abnormal sensitivity to a neurotransmitter within the GI tract. This disorder affects twice as many women as men. Patients with IBS have an increased rate of hospital stays, abdominal surgery, and absenteeism from work. Criteria for diagnosis include the following:

- abdominal distention
- gas
- increased colonic mucus
- irregular bowel habits (diarrhea or constipation more than 25% of the time)
- pain

Hemorrhoids **Hemorrhoids** result from pressure exerted on anal veins while straining to pass a stool, which causes engorgement of the vascular cushions situated within the sphincter muscles. Passing a small, hard stool through the anal canal can abrade the overlying mucosa, causing hemorrhoidal bleeding. Prolapse (displacement) of the vascular cushions may occur from rupture of their attachments to the surrounding sphincter.

Hemorrhoids are treated with suppositories, ointments, and sometimes surgery. Most medications for hemorrhoids include **hydrocortisone**, a synthetic preparation used to treat inflammation (see Table 10.7). Modifying the diet by increasing fiber can help prevent hemorrhoids.

TABLE 10.7	Most Commonly Used Hemorrhoidal Agent				
Generic Name	Pronunciation	Dosage Form	Brand Name	Dispensing Status
hydrocortisone	hye-droe-KOR-ti-sone	topical	Anusol HC	Rx

Nausea and Vomiting

The vomiting center in the brain is located in the medulla (see Figure 10.6). It receives input from the **chemoreceptor trigger zone (CTZ)** via the vagus nerve or the tenth cranial nerve. The CTZ, which is located below the floor of the fourth ventricle of the brain, receives its input from the cerebral cortex and hypothalamus and also from blood-borne stimuli (such as bacterial toxins and drugs that have access to the brain via the blood vascular systems). The main neurotransmitters that cause nausea and vomiting are acetylcholine, dopamine, and serotonin.

Vomiting (also referred to as **emesis**) can be initiated in two ways: by stimulating the CTZ, which in turn stimulates the GI tract via the vomiting center (e.g., narcotics stimulate brain receptors), or by stimulating the vagal receptors in the stomach with no CTZ involvement.

Vomiting can cause dehydration, electrolyte imbalance leading to alkalosis (loss of acid from the body), and possible aspiration pneumonia. It may also cause bradycardia or other arrhythmias resulting from an electrolyte imbalance.

FIGURE 10.6
Chemoreceptor Trigger Zone and Vomiting Center

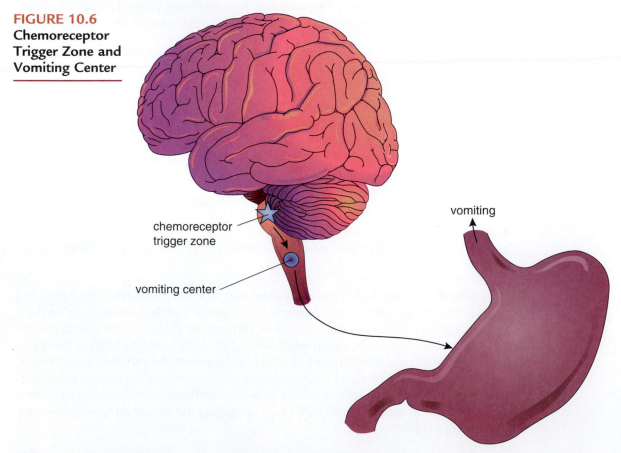

chemoreceptor trigger zone

vomiting center

vomiting

Emesis often occurs as a result of narcotic intake. Morphine and its derivatives stimulate the CTZ. Vomiting is dose related. Narcotics also increase the vomiting center's sensitivity to stimuli from the vestibular nucleus of the ear, which is near the vomiting center.

Stimulating the labyrinth system of the inner ear produces impulses that are transmitted via cholinergic and adrenergic tracts to the vestibular nucleus. This is common in car sickness. **Vertigo**, the sensation of the room spinning when one gets up or changes positions, is treated with anticholinergic agents.

An **antiemetic** is a drug that works primarily in the vomiting center to inhibit impulses that cause vomiting from going to the stomach. Table 10.8 presents the most commonly used antiemetics.

Antihistamines and Related Compounds

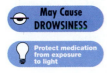

Antihistamines can serve as antiemetics because they inhibit cholinergic spread of impulses from the vestibular nucleus to the vomiting center. **Meclizine (Antivert, Dramamine II)** is used primarily for vertigo. **Trimethobenzamide (Tigan)** is structurally related to the antihistamines. It has antinausea activity and is used in patients with prochlorperazine allergies.

TABLE 10.8   Most Commonly Used Antiemetic Medications

Generic Name	Pronunciation	Dosage Form	Brand Name	Dispensing Status
Antihistamines and Related Compounds				
diphenhydramine	dye-fen-HYE-dra-meen	capsule, cream, injection, IV, lotion, oral liquid, tablet	Benadryl	OTC, Rx
hydroxyzine	hye-DROX-i-zeen	capsule, injection, oral liquid	Atarax, Vistaril	Rx
meclizine	MEK-li-zeen	capsule, tablet	Antivert	Rx
trimethobenzamide	trye-meth-oh-BEN-za-mide	capsule, injection	Tigan	Rx
Serotonin Receptor Antagonists				
dolasetron	dol-AS-e-tron	IV, tablet	Anzemet	Rx
granisetron	gra-NI-se-tron	IV, oral solution, tablet	Kytril	Rx
ondansetron	on-DAN-se-tron	IV, oral solution, tablet	Zofran	Rx
Phenothiazines				
prochlorperazine	proe-klor-PAIR-a-zeen	injection, IV, oral liquid, suppository, tablet	Compazine	Rx
promethazine	proe-METH-a-zeen	suppository, tablet	Phenergan	Rx
Other Antiemetic Medications				
aprepitant	ap-REP-i-tant	capsule, IV	Emend	Rx
metoclopramide	met-oh-KLOE-pra-mide	injection, IV, tablet	Reglan	Rx

Serotonin Receptor Antagonists

Dolasetron (Anzemet) was designed to be used for chemotherapy-induced nausea. Serotonin is released from the gut cells, which stimulates those receptors and cause vomiting when chemotherarpy is administered. Dolasetron is also used for surgery-related nausea. The intravenous form can be given IVP (IV push, over 15 minutes) or diluted (over 30 minutes). Also, the IV form can be diluted in apple or apple-grape juice and taken orally. If given for chemotherapy, it should be administered 1 hour before; if given for postsurgery nausea it should be given 15 minutes before stopping anesthesia or as soon as needed.

Granisetron (Kytril) binds to serotonin (5-HT) receptors with little or no affinity for dopamine D_2, benzodiazepine, or opiate receptors. It blocks the 5-HT receptors both peripherally on vagal nerve terminals and centrally in the CTZ. Side effects of granisetron include headache, asthenia (weakness), drowsiness, and diarrhea. It is usually given by the IV route. Granisetron must be protected from light.

Ondansetron (Zofran) blocks serotonin (5-HT) receptors in either the CTZ or small-bowel vagal nerve terminals. It is used for chemotherapeutic-induced emesis. Headache is a major side effect. Ondansetron can also cause either constipation or diarrhea.

Phenothiazines

Phenothiazine compounds, related to the typical antipsychotics described in Chapter 7, inhibit the CTZ. They act as a sedative, antiemetic, and anticholinergic (causing dry mouth, blurred vision, and urinary retention). To avoid hypotension, these drugs should not be given by IV push. **Prochlorperazine (Compazine)** is the prototype phenothiazine. It is administered orally, by rectal suppository, IM injection, or IV. It must be used with caution in children and is easily overdosed, precipitating seizures. **Promethazine (Phenergan),** a phenothiazine, is probably the most widely used anti-emetic. It is usually given as an IV push but if the dose is greater than 100 mg, it should be diluted *in the pharmacy* to a maximum concentration of 25 mg/mL and infused over 15 to 30 minutes. Promethazine has a black box warning regarding the use of the drug in children less than 2 years. Side effects are much more unpleasant than the 5HT receptors. Suppositories are stored in the refrigerator.

Other Antiemetic Medications

Aprepitant (Emend) works at the substance P receptor to prevent vomiting and augments the 5-HT receptor antagonists. It is used to treat postoperative and chemotherapy-related nausea. Aprepitant should be administered within 3 hours prior to either of these procedures.

Metoclopramide (Reglan) is used in **gastric stasis** (lack of stomach motility), GI reflux, and chemotherapy-induced emesis. It inhibits or reduces nausea and vomiting by blocking dopamine receptors in the CTZ. As described earlier, it relieves esophageal reflux by improving the tone of the lower esophageal sphincter and reduces gastric stasis by stimulating motility of the upper GI tract, thus reducing gastric emptying time. The side effects are extrapyramidal symptoms (EPS, which are Parkinson-like, especially in children), drowsiness, and depression. Diphenhydramine is used to reduce EPS. Metoclopramide should not be used longer than 12 weeks.

Obesity

Obesity is defined as a state in which an individual's total body weight includes greater quantities of fat than is considered normal. Obesity in males is 25% of total body weight over ideal body weight; in females the figure is 35%. Normal weight is defined as the ideal body weight (IBW), which is calculated as follows:

Male IBW kg = 50 + (2.3 × height in inches over 5 feet)
Female IBW kg = 45.5 + (2.3 × height in inches over 5 feet)

Note that IBW is calculated in kilograms even though the patient's height is measured in feet and inches. To convert kg to pounds, multiply by 2.2. **Morbid obesity** is a weight that is two or more times the IBW; it is so called because it results in many serious and life-threatening disorders. Obesity has become a major health problem of today's society.

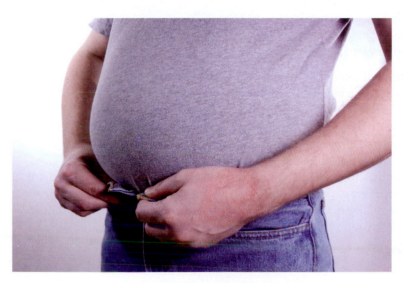

Millions of Americans are obese. Obesity increases the odds of diabetes, heart disease, and psychological problems.

Obesity can lead to both physiological and psychological problems. Obese persons tend to have a higher incidence of cardiovascular disease and non-insulin-dependent diabetes. In addition, obese individuals may experience anxiety, stress, and poor self-image. External factors such as social repugnance and intolerance, discrimination, and emotional reactions to social pressure also correlate with obesity.

Genetic factors play an important role in obesity. A child with one obese parent has a 50% chance of being obese, but that chance increases to 80% if both parents are obese. Adipocyte cells, or fat cells, are determined in childhood. The number and size of these cells is set by age 2. Consequently, childhood obesity is a concern because it may persist into adulthood and lead to high cholesterol, cardiovascular disease, and diabetes. An obese adult who was not overweight in childhood is more likely to be able to sustain a weight loss.

Furthermore, those who strongly believe they can change their eating habits are more likely to be successful in losing weight than those who do not. If patients believe weight loss depends on external circumstances, they are less likely to lose weight. Individuals with weight disorders (obesity, anorexia, bulimia) generally have low self-esteem. External psychological factors include family traits, lifestyle, and customs. Food is usually substituted for manual and oral craving. There may also be cravings for certain foods such as sweets or carbohydrates.

Obesity can be managed by diet, behavioral modification, prescription and nonprescription medications, surgical procedures, and other nondrug therapy. To be effective and permanent, weight loss requires permanent changes in eating habits, behavioral modification, and regular exercise. Types of diet include

- calorie restriction
- manipulation of amounts of protein, carbohydrate, and fats but no calorie restriction
- decrease in grams of fat consumed

When a weight-loss diet is initiated, the first loss is retained water, up to 6 pounds in the first week. Later decrease in basal metabolic rate and activity levels neutralizes the diet's effectiveness. There is also a roller-coaster syndrome:

1. weight loss
2. plateau
3. cessation of dieting
4. resumption of regular eating habits
5. increase in weight

This syndrome can be disheartening, but behavior modification can help to overcome it. The most important type of behavior modification for weight loss is increasing exercise. However, other types of behavior modifications such as the following can be helpful:

- keeping records of what is eaten daily
- restricting cues that signal eating
- slowing the rate of eating
- rewarding appropriate eating behaviors

The decision to treat obesity with drug therapy must be carefully considered. Patients must be aware that a balanced diet is always needed along with drug therapy. The **body mass index (BMI)**, which is determined by dividing the patient's weight in kilograms by the square of the patient's height in meters (kg/m^2), is used as a guide in deciding whether to initiate pharmacologic treatment for this disorder. Appetite suppressants are the drugs used to treat obesity.

Surgical treatment methods are available but have significant side effects and are expensive. These include jaw-wiring (about 50% success), jejunoileal bypass, gastroplasty, and intragastric balloon.

The most commonly used pharmacologic agents to treat obesity are listed in Table 10.9.

Stimulants

Stimulants are the most commonly used agents for weight reduction. They work in several ways. **Diethylpropion (Tenuate)** and **phentermine (Adipex-P, Ionamin)**

TABLE 10.9 Most Commonly Used Agents to Treat Obesity

Generic Name	Pronunciation	Dosage Form	Brand Name	Dispensing Status	Control Schedule
Stimulants					
dextroamphetamine	dex-troe-am-FET-a-meen	capsule, tablet	Dexedrine	Rx	C-II
diethylpropion	dye-eth-il-PROE-pee-on	tablet	Tenuate	Rx	C-IV
methamphetamine	meth-am-FET-a-meen	tablet	Desoxyn	Rx	C-II
phentermine	FEN-ter-meen	capsule, tablet	Adipex-P, Ionamin	Rx	C-IV
sibutramine	si-BYOO-tra-meen	capsule	Meridia	Rx	C-IV
Lipase Inhibitor					
orlistat	OR-li-stat	capsule	Xenical, Alli	Rx, OTC	

stimulate adrenergic pathways. **Dextroamphetamine (Dexedrine)** and **methamphetamine (Desoxyn)** act on norepinephrine and dopaminergic pathways. **Sibutramine (Meridia)** inhibits the reuptake of norepinephrine, serotonin, and dopamine. Preparations usually work for 3 to 4 hours. Long-acting or sustained-release forms work up to 12 hours. Short-acting agents should be taken 30 to 60 minutes before each meal. Long-acting ones should be taken 12 hours before retiring to prevent insomnia. These drugs are all controlled substances and subject to the laws governing their dispensing. The purpose of these drugs is to "jump start" the weight loss process; they should be used only for the short term.

The adverse effects of these drugs are

- central nervous system stimulation, dizziness, euphoria, dysphoria, fatigue, and insomnia
- GI symptoms of dry mouth, nausea, abdominal discomfort, and constipation
- cardiovascular hypertension, palpitations, and arrhythmias

Withdrawal from these drugs can cause tremor, confusion, and headache. Most should not be given within 14 days of a monoamine oxidase inhibitor (MAOI) and are contraindicated in pulmonary hypertension.

Lipase Inhibitor

Orlistat (Xenical, Alli) has a unique mechanism of action. This drug binds with and inhibits the action of gastric and pancreatic lipases in the lumen of the stomach and in the small intestine. This prevents the fat in the diet from being hydrolyzed and absorbed, but it also means that the fat-soluble vitamins (i.e., A, D, E, and beta-carotene) required to maintain good health are not absorbed. Consequently, most patients will need to add a multivitamin supplement to their diet. A BMI of at least 30 is required to initiate treatment with this drug; in the presence of other risk factors (e.g., hypertension, diabetes, dyslipidemia), a BMI of at least 27 is required.

Orlistat and sibutramine have different mechanisms of action, so these agents are often used in combination. Patients on orlistat should be on a balanced diet and should spread their fat intake in relatively equal portions over three meals in order to decrease adverse GI events such as oily spotting from the anus, flatus with discharge, fecal urgency, fatty or oily stools, increased defecation, and fecal incontinence. In fact, orlistat aims at behavior modification. If a patient does consume fat while taking orlistat, these side effects are so unpleasant that the patient will learn to avoid those foods that cause the diarrhea and other GI distress. Success lies in eating a low-fat diet and changing lifestyle patterns. Patients should be on a balanced diet that provides no more than 30% of calories from fat. This drug has been shown to decrease LDL cholesterol slightly and to increase HDL cholesterol.

Fiber Agents

Bulk-producing products, which contain fibers from natural grain components as the active ingredients, provide a sense of fullness. The results are a lessened desire to eat and a decrease in calorie intake. These ingredients are not absorbed systemically and are, therefore, considered safe. However, they must be consumed with large quantities of water. They may actually increase peristalsis by moving food faster, but can also have the opposite effect. The accumulation of bulk may result in esophageal, gastric, or small-intestine or rectal obstruction. Bulking agents should not be used by patients who have preexisting intestinal problems or by those on restricted carbohydrate diets.

Most importantly, weight loss can only be brought about by lifestyle changes. Most over the counter products make false claims and are unsafe to one degree or another. For most OTC weight-loss products, risks outweigh benefits. In contrast, diet medications that are prescribed by a healthcare provider are tools that can help bring about these changes when used appropriately.

Parasites and Protozoa

Animal parasites live in the body of another animal (their **host**), which they utilize for nutrition, either by consuming the tissues of the host itself or by diverting the food intake of the host. Many parasites spend part of their life cycle in one host, such as a human, and another part of the cycle in another animal. Each parasite has its own particular animal hosts, and these hosts are not interchangeable.

The life cycle of most parasites is complex, passing through several developmental stages that may have very different appearances before the individual parasite becomes an adult. During the larval stage or stages, the parasite passes through its intermediate host. The definitive host is the one in which the parasite reaches maturity and and becomes capable of reproducing. An intermediate host is also referred to as a **vector,** whose role is primarily to transfer the parasite to another host. Many parasites spend part of their life cycle in the gut; they exit the body through the anus, enter the body through the mouth, or both. Poor hygiene and sanitation promote the spread of these parasites.

Parasites can be single-celled animals (protozoa) or multicellular organisms, often with common names that end in "worm," although they belong to several different taxonomic groups and most are not related to the common earthworm.

Parasitic infections are a worldwide health problem, particularly in less developed countries, where they affect a large percentage of the human population. In these countries, parasitic diseases are among the most pressing and serious, yet most neglected, public health problems. Factors supporting infection include overcrowding, poor sanitation, a warm climate, inadequate health education, poor control of vectors (such as fleas, ticks, mosquitoes, and flies), and reservoirs of infection.

Antiparasitic Drugs

Table 10.10 presents the drugs most commonly used against multicellular parasites.

Albendazole (Albenza) is approved by the FDA for tapeworm (*Taenia*) infestations, and it is also used to treat microsporidiasis (infections caused by single-celled

TABLE 10.10	Most Commonly Used Antiparasitic Drugs			
Generic Name	**Pronunciation**	**Dosage Form**	**Brand Name**	**Dispensing Status**
albendazole	al-BEN-da-zole	tablet	Albenza	Rx
mebendazole	me-BEN-da-zole	tablet	Vermox	Rx
praziquantel	pray-zee-KWON-tel	tablet	Biltricide	Rx
pyrantel	pye-RAN-tel	oral liquid	Pin-X	OTC
thiabendazole	thye-a-BEN-da-zole	suspension, tablet	Mintezol	Rx

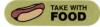
TAKE WITH FOOD

organisms called Microsporidia). Albendazole causes selective degeneration of microtubules in the cells and walls of the parasite, preventing the parasite from absorbing glucose. Liver enzyme levels must be watched carefully, and if they are significantly elevated, drug administration must be terminated.

Praziquantel (Biltricide) is indicated for intestinal tapeworms (*Taenia*). It increases the permeability of worm cells to calcium, causing contractions and paralysis of worm musculature and leading to detachment of suckers from the blood vessel walls and to dislodgment. The tablets should be taken with food. The drug may impair judgment and coordination, so caution should be taken when performing tasks that require mental alertness.

Mebendazole (Vermox) binds to tubular proteins in the pinworm parasite (*Enterobius*) and inhibits glucose uptake. It also is used to treat ascarides (flukes), hookworms, whipworms, and threadworms.

Pyrantel (Pin-X) is also used in the treatment of pinworms. It paralyzes the worm by acting as a neuromuscular blocker.

Thiabendazole (Mintezol) inhibits ATP synthesis within the *Trichinella* parasite. This action blocks cellular metabolism (energy production) and thus leads to the death of the organism. Thiabendazole was formerly also used to treat infestations of threadworms (*Strongyloides*).

Protozoan Infections

Protozoa are single-cell organisms that inhabit water and soil. Generally these organisms feed on bacteria and small particles of nutrients and are harmless to humans. However, some protozoa are responsible for human diseases. For example, the protozoan that causes malaria has an insect vector, the anopheles mosquito. In contrast, intestinal protozoa are spread by the feces-to-mouth route. Furthermore, two protozoa are the cause of many GI infections. *Trichomonas* is parasite that occurs in intestinal and genitourinary tracts of humans and *Giardia* commonly occurs in the human intestine. These two organisms are treated with many of the same drugs.

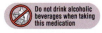
Do not drink alcoholic beverages when taking this medication

Nitazoxanide (Alinia) was previously mentioned as a treatment for the protozoa *Giardia* and *Cryptosporidium*, which cause infectious diarrhea. Table 10.11 lists other drugs used to treat protozoan infections.

Metronidazole (Flagyl, Flagyl I.V.), first mentioned in Chapter 4 as an antibiotic that is useful against fungi as well as bacteria, is effective against some protozoa as well. Metronidazole is used to treat amebiasis caused by *Entamoeba histolytica* and infections caused by *Trichomonas*. Patients must avoid alcohol while taking this medication because it causes a disulfiram reaction.

Sulfamethoxazole-trimethoprim (Bactrim, Bactrim DS, Cotrim, Cotrim DS, Septra, Septra DS) is used to treat isosporiasis and cyclosporiasis, diarrheal infections caused by *Isospora belli* and *Cyclospora cayetanensis*, respectively.

TABLE 10.11 Most Commonly Used Drugs to Treat Protozoan Infections

Generic Name	Pronunciation	Dosage Form	Brand Name	Dispensing Status
metronidazole	met-roe-NYE-da-zole	capsule, IV, tablet	Flagyl, Flagyl I.V.	Rx
sulfamethoxazole-trimethoprim	sul-fa-meth-OX-a-zole trye-METH-oh-prim	IV, oral liquid, tablet	Bactrim, Bactrim DS, Cotrim, Cotrim DS, Septra, Septra DS	Rx

Malaria

An infection of **malaria** is acquired from the bite of an infected *Anopheles* mosquito, a blood transfusion from an infected donor, or shared syringe use by drug addicts. It is uncommon in the United States, but prevalent in many countries. Travelers to less developed countries should take precautions.

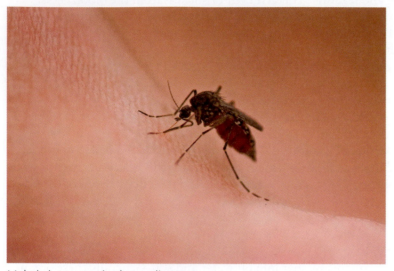

Malaria is a mosquito-borne disease.

In a human host, the parasite first multiplies asexually within a red blood cell (RBC). The cell ruptures, releasing organisms to infect additional RBCs. As the infection is prolonged, the spleen and liver exhibit signs of the infection. The incubation period is 10 to 35 days. Symptoms include high fever, recurrent chills, sweating, and jaundice. Medication is used to treat the disease or as prophylaxis to prevent infection. The drugs commonly used are listed in Table 10.12. Some medications stop the organism from entering the liver by destroying the organism as it enters the bloodstream. Other medications stop the organism's multiplication.

Atovaquone-proguanil (Malarone) is a combination drug that is effective for both prevention and treatment of malaria. It is better tolerated than most other antimalarial drugs. Atovaquone-proguanil should be taken at the same time each day with food. For prevention, it should be taken 1 to 2 days before entering the malaria area and continued for 7 days after leaving.

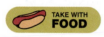

Chloroquine (Aralen) and **hydroxychloroquine (Plaquenil)** belong to the quinoline family. They are related drugs with different therapeutic uses. These drugs have also been expanded for nonmalarial uses, such as arthritis and lupus. Chloroquine has an affinity for pigment (melanin-containing structures), and with prolonged exposure will accumulate in the retina. These drugs are well tolerated and are used for both prophylaxis and treatment of malaria.

TABLE 10.12   **Most Commonly Used Drugs to Treat and Prevent Malaria**

Generic Name	Pronunciation	Dosage Form	Brand Name	Dispensing Status
atovaquone-proguanil	a-TOE-va-kwone pro-GWAN-il	tablet	Malarone	Rx
chloroquine	KLOR-oh-kwin	tablet	Aralen	Rx
doxycycline	dox-i-SYE-kleen	capsule, IV, oral liquid	Vibramycin	Rx
hydroxychloroquine	hye-drox-ee-KLOR-oh-kwin	tablet	Plaquenil	Rx
mefloquine	ME-floe-kwin	tablet	Lariam	Rx
primaquine	PRIM-a-kween	tablet	(none)	Rx
quinine	KWYE-nine	tablet	Qualaquin	Rx

Doxycycline (Vibramycin) is as efficacious as mefloquine. It can be used to treat forms of the disease that are resistant to mefloquine.

Mefloquine (Lariam) is used to treat and prevent malaria. It kills the organisms that cause malaria. A problem is that vomiting frequently occurs after dosing, particularly in pediatric patients. If the patient vomits again in less than 30 minutes after taking the medication, then another full dose should be taken. If vomiting occurs between 30 and 60 minutes after ingesting the drug, a half dose should be taken. In addition to this distasteful side effect, mefloquine is associated with some psychiatric side effects ranging from nightmares to psychosis. If taken for a long period of time, it can affect the eyes. Mefloquine should not be given to patients with a history of psychiatric illness.

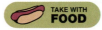

Primaquine is used to prevent relapse. The tablet is so bitter that this drug has to be taken with food.

Quinine (Qualaquin), which was used by natives of South America to treat malaria and has been known to European civilization since the seventeenth century, is now used in combination with other drugs. It inhibits the organism that causes malaria from entering the bloodstream. Combined with another medication, quinine is the drug of choice for chloroquine-resistant malaria. (Tonic water also contains quinine, but only a small amount.) Quinine can cause severe blood disorders, hearing loss, cardiac arrhythmias, visual disturbances and death.

For prevention of malaria, the Centers for Disease Control (CDC) now recommends mefloquine, doxycycline, or atovaquone-proguanil. The latter is probably the most effective and has the fewest side effects.

Hepatitis

Hepatitis is a liver disease that has several forms, A through G. The three most common, A, B, and C, will be discussed. Each can damage liver cells and cause the liver to become swollen and tender. Some can cause permanent damage. Hepatitis has many causes; some forms are viral, but others are caused by medications, long-term alcohol use, or exposure to certain industrial chemicals.

Types of Hepatitis

Hepatitis A is a viral infection that can be spread from one person to another. It can be transmitted through blood and body fluids. It is the most common and least dangerous form of hepatitis; it usually runs its course with no permanent damage. Hepatitis A often produces epidemics due to its feces-to-mouth route of transmission. The highest rates occur in children. Treatment is supportive (no drugs, just food and rest). Hepatitis A can be prevented by a vaccine. If people know they have been exposed, they should be protected with immune globulin (IG) within two weeks of exposure. IG can be given intramuscularly or intravaneously. If it is ordered as an IV, it will be written **IVIG**. It provides passive immunity by increasing the antibody titer and antigen-antibody reaction potential.

There are two types of **hepatitis B:** acute and chronic. Acute hepatitis B usually clears up on its own without treatment. The patient develops antibodies that provide lifelong protection. Chronic hepatitis B, which is the most dangerous form of hepatitis, continues to be present for 6 months or more. It can be the cause of serious liver disease such as cirrhosis or liver cancer. The patient may require a liver transplant. Chronic hepatitis B is treated with antiviral medications, depending on antigens in the blood. The vaccines for Hepatitis B are given in a three dose series over 6 months. The vaccines are **Recombivax HB** and **Enegerix B**. Most health care workers should receive these vaccines, including pharmacy technicians. These vaccines are stored in the refrigerator.

Hepatitis C is an infection that cannot be spread from one person to another by casual contact. The acute form should be treated to prevent the disease from becoming chronic. It can progress to liver fibrosis and end-stage liver disease. It is most commonly transmitted through blood transfusions or illicit drug use.

Pharmacologic Treatment and Prevention of Hepatitis

Prevention of hepatitis is achieved through vaccination. Anyone who works in a hospital must be vaccinated against hepatitis B. The CDC now recommends that travelers who are going to endemic areas or who are otherwise high-risk patients should be vaccinated against hepatitis B in two to three doses over the 6 months prior to travel and against hepatitis A 2 to 4 weeks before travel. Babies and school children must also have hepatitis B vaccine with their other immunizations. Anyone who is immuno-compromised should also be vaccinated against hepatitis.

Table 10.13 lists the drugs used to treat and prevent hepatitis.

The mainstays of therapy for hepatitis B, once infection occurs, are **lamivudine (Epivir-HBV)** and interferon, depending on the hepatitis B virus (HBV) DNA concentrations in the blood. Interferon is associated with many adverse effects, including flu-like symptoms. It is given subcutaneously and is more expensive than lamivudine. Both of these drugs have been discussed in earlier chapters. **Interferon alfa-2a (Roferon A)** and **interferon alfa-2b (Intron A)** are used for treating hepatitis.

Adefovir (Hepsera) is an antiviral medication for hepatitis B. It was originally developed to treat HIV, but the high doses required were nephrotoxic. It has now been approved for hepatitis B. Adefovir blocks the replication of the virus in the body. It may cause nausea and GI upset. This drug must be stored at room temperature away from moisture and heat. It is very important that each dose be taken with a full glass of water.

Entecavir (Baraclude) is indicated to treat chronic hepatitis B. It blocks an enzyme responsible for replication of the virus in the body. The major advantage of

---

TABLE 10.13   **Most Commonly Used Drugs Used to Treat and Prevent Hepatitis**

Generic Name	Pronunciation	Dosage Form	Brand Name	Dispensing Status
adefovir	a-DEF-oh-veer	tablet	Hepsera	Rx
entecavir	en-TEK-a-vir	oral liquid, tablet	Baraclude	Rx
immune globulin	i-MYOON GLOB-yoo-lin	injection, IV	Gamunex	Rx
interferon alfa-2a	in-ter-FEER-on AL-fa 2A	injection	Roferon A	Rx
interferon alfa-2b	in-ter-FEER-on AL-fa 2B	injection	Intron A	Rx
lamivudine	la-MIV-yoo-deen	oral liquid, tablet	Epivir, Epivir-HBV	Rx
peginterferon alfa-2a	peg-in-ter-FEER-on AL-fa 2A	injection	Pegasys	Rx
ribavirin	rye-ba-VYE-rin	tablet	Copegus, Rebetol	Rx
telbivudine	tel-BIV-you-deen	tablet	Tyzeka	Rx

entecavir is that it can be used in HIV-positive patients. It is taken once a day and should be taken on an **empty stomach**; that is, 2 hours before or after eating.

Peginterferon alfa-2a (Pegasys) is interferon linked to a high-molecular-weight branched polyethylene glycol (PEG) molecule. This linkage increases the half-life, allowing once weekly dosing. It is indicated for patients with hepatitis C and chronic hepatitis B. Peginterferon alfa-2a works better when combined with ribavirin. It requires a medication guide when dispensed from an outpatient (retail) pharmacy. The advantage of peginterferon alfa-2a over regular interferon is its long half-life. The most serious adverse events include neuropsychiatric disorders (suicidal ideation). The prefilled syringes should be stored in the refrigerator. They can safely be left out for 24 hours but no longer. The drug should be injected subcutaneously into the abdomen or thigh, using a different spot each time to avoid tissue damage or irritation. Peginterferon alfa-2a (the longer-acting form of interferon) and ribavirin are the drugs used to treat hepatitis C. The combination of these drugs has been shown to be the most effective treatment and has become the standard of care. Peginterferon alpha-2a is given as an injection, and ribavirin is taken by mouth. Neither is safe in pregnancy.

Ribavirin (Copegus, Rebetol) can be used for respiratory synctial virus (RSV) infections as well as hepatitis C. It is used as an inhalation for RSV and orally for hepatitis C. For hepatitis C, it should always be taken with peginterferon alpha-2a, never alone. It inhibits the replication of RNA and DNA in the virus.

Telbivudine (Tyzeka) is used to treat chronic hepatitis B virus infection. It blocks replication of the virus in the body. Muscle aches and pains can occur even months after treatment with this drug.

Chapter Terms

antiemetic a drug that inhibits impulses that cause vomiting from going to the stomach

body mass index (BMI) a guide to use in determining whether to initiate pharmacologic treatment for obesity; calculated by dividing the patient's weight (in kilograms) by the patient's height (in meters) squared (kg/m^2)

bowel evacuant an agent used to empty the colon prior to GI examination or after toxic ingestion

chemoreceptor trigger zone (CTZ) an area below the floor of the fourth ventricle of the brain that can trigger nausea and vomiting when certain signals are received

Crohn disease an inflammatory bowel disease affecting the entire GI tract from mouth to anus

diverticular disease formation and inflammation of an outpocketing from the colon wall

duodenal ulcer a peptic lesion situated in the duodenum

emesis vomiting

empty stomach 2 hours before or after eating

fiber the undigested residue of fruits, vegetables, and other foods of plant origin that remains after digestion by the human GI enzymes; characterized by fermentability and may be either water soluble or insoluble

gastric stasis lack of stomach motility

gastric ulcer a local excavation in the gastric mucosa

gastritis irritation and superficial erosion of the stomach lining

gastroesophageal reflux disease (GERD) a GI disease characterized by radiating burning or pain in the chest and an acid taste, caused by backflow of acidic stomach contents across an incompetent lower esophageal sphincter; also referred to as heartburn

gastrointestinal (GI) tract a continuous tube that begins in the mouth and extends through the pharynx, esophagus, stomach, small intestine, and large intestine to end at the anus

GI transit time the time it takes for material to pass from one end of the GI tract to the other; the slower the GI transit time, the greater the amounts of nutrients and water absorbed

H_2 histamine receptor antagonist an agent that blocks acid and pepsin secretion in response to histamine, gastrin, foods, distention, caffeine, or cholinergic stimulation; used to treat GERD and *H. pylori*

Helicobacter pylori (H. pylori) a bacterium that contributes to the development of many gastric ulcers

hemorrhoids engorgements of the vascular cushions situated within the sphincter muscles; result from pressure exerted on anal veins while straining to pass a stool

hepatitis a disease of the liver that causes inflammation, can be acute or chronic, and has several forms A through G

hepatitis A a viral form of hepatitis that is usually mild and transient and can be spread from one person to another

hepatitis B the most dangerous form of hepatitis, accompanied by jaundice and easily spread from one person to another

hepatitis C an infection of the liver that cannot be spread from one person to another by contact; most commonly transmitted by blood transfusions or illicit drug use

hiatal hernia a protrusion through the esophageal hiatus of the diaphragm

host the animal on which a parasite feeds

irritable bowel syndrome (IBS) a functional disorder in which the lower GI tract does not have appropriate tone or spasticity to regulate bowel activity

IVIG the notation for immune globulin that is given intravenously

malabsorption syndrome impaired intestinal absorption of nutrients

malaria an infectious febrile disease caused by the protozoan *Plasmodium* and transmitted by the *Anopheles* mosquito

morbid obesity a state in which an individual's weight is two or more times the ideal body weight (IBW)

obesity a state in which an individual's total body weight includes greater quantities of fat than is considered normal (25% of total body weight for men and 35% for women)

osmotic laxative an organic substance that draws water into the colon and thereby stimulates evacuation

parasite an organism that lives on or in another organism (known as the host), surviving by drawing nourishment from the food or the tissues of the host; the parasite lives within the intermediate host during the larval stage and within the definitive host at maturity

peptic disease disorders of the upper GI tract caused by the action of acid and pepsin; includes mucosal injury, erythema, erosions, and frank ulceration

peptic ulcer an ulcer formed at any part of the GI tract exposed to acid and the enzyme pepsin

phenothiazine a drug, related to the typical antipsychotics, that controls vomiting by inhibiting the CTZ

proton pump inhibitor a drug that blocks gastric acid secretion by inhibiting the enzyme that pumps hydrogen ions into the stomach

protozoan single-celled animal

reflux backflow; specifically in GERD, the backflow of acidic stomach contents across an incompetent lower esophageal sphincter

saline laxative an inorganic salt that attracts water into the hollow portion (lumen) of the colon, increasing intraluminal pressure to cause evacuation

stimulant laxative a laxative that increases gut activity by irritating the mucosa

stress ulcer a peptic ulcer, usually gastric, that occurs in a clinical setting; caused by a breakdown of natural mucosal resistance

surfactant laxative a stool softener that has a detergent activity that facilitates mixing of fat and water, making the stool soft and mushy

traveler's diarrhea diarrhea caused by ingesting contaminated food or water; so called because it is often contracted by travelers in countries where the water supply is contaminated

ulcer a local defect or excavation of the surface of an organ or tissue

ulcerative colitis irritation and inflammation of the large bowel, causing it to look scraped; characterized by bloody mucus leading to watery diarrhea containing blood, mucus, and pus

vector an animal that transfers a parasite to a host

vertigo the sensation of the room spinning when one gets up or changes positions; can be treated with anticholinergic agents

Chapter Summary

The Gastrointestinal System

- The gastrointestinal (GI) tract is a tube that begins in the mouth; extends through the pharynx, esophagus, stomach, small intestine, and large intestine; and ends at the anus.
- The digestive and absorptive processes take place in the GI tract.
- Mucous membranes protect the entire digestive system against abrasion and strong digestive chemicals.

Gastrointestinal Diseases

- GERD is commonly known as heartburn. Alcohol, nicotine, and caffeine exacerbate GERD.
- Phase I medications for GERD are antacids that exert their action by neutralizing the acidic stomach contents so that if reflux does occur, the contents will be less irritating to the esophageal lining. Phase II medications serve two functions. First, they improve gastric motility. Second, they decrease acid production in the stomach (H_2 blockers, proton pump inhibitors).
- The bedtime dose of the H_2 blockers is the most important one.
- The three types of ulcers are gastric, duodenal, and stress.
- There are drug regimens for the treatment of *Helicobacter pylori* (*H. pylori*), understood to be a factor to be eradicated in treating ulcers. Helidac therapy is a kit with a 14 day supply of tetracycline, metronidazole, and bismuth subsalicylate to treat ulcers.
- Gastritis is an irritation and superficial erosion of the stomach lining. Ulcerative colitis is an irritation of the large bowel.
- Infliximab (Remicade) is an agent used for moderate-to-severe cases of Crohn disease. It will affect the normal immune response.
- Mesalamine (Asacol, Pentasa, Rowasa) is used in Crohn disease and ulcerative colitis.

- Sulfasalazine (Azulfidine) should not be taken for longer than 2 years. It decreases inflammatory response in the colon. It can change the color of the urine and stain soft contact lenses.
- Olsalazine (Dipentum) is used for patients resistant to sulfasalazine.
- Balsalazide (Colazal) is better tolerated than sulfasalazine because there is no sulfa entity.
- Ursodiol (Actigall) is used to dissolve gallstones, but it can take several months.

Diarrhea

- Diphenoxylate-atropine (Lomotil) is a combination drug and a controlled substance used for diarrhea.
- Loperamide (Imodium) has been found to be as effective as diphenoxylate-atropine and is available OTC.

Constipation and Related GI Diseases

- Dietary fiber increases colon content, decreases colon pressure, and increases propulsive motility.
- Chronic constipation is often associated with low-fiber diets.
- Aluminum hydroxide–magnesium hydroxide–simethicone is a gastric defoaming antiflatulent agent. It reduces surface tension, causing bubbles to be broken or to coalesce into a foam that can be eliminated more easily by belching or passing flatus.
- Constipation can be relieved with osmotic laxatives, saline laxatives, irritant/stimulant laxatives, surfactant laxatives, bulk-forming agents
- Constipation and lack of dietary fiber increase the likelihood of other diseases including diverticular disease, hiatal hernia, and hemorrhoids.

Nausea and Vomiting

- The chemoreceptor trigger zone (CTZ) is involved in vomiting.
- Some antiemetics bind to serotonin (5-HT) receptors to prevent nausea.

Obesity

- Male ideal body weight (IBW) in kg = 50 + (2.3 × height in inches over 5 feet)
- Female IBW in kg = 45.5 + (2.3 × height in inches over 5 feet)
- Morbid obesity is the condition of weighing two or more times the ideal body weight; it is so called because it results in many serious and life-threatening disorders.
- Obesity has become a major health problem.
- BMI (body mass index) is determined by dividing the patient's weight in kilograms by the patient's height in meters squared (kg/m²). The BMI is used as a guide to determine whether pharmacologic treatment should be used for obesity.
- Stimulants are the most commonly used agents for weight reduction.
- A BMI of at least 30 or, in the presence of other risk factors, 27 is required to initiate pharmacologic intervention with orlistat (Xenical).

Parasites and Protozoa

- Praziquantel (Biltricide) rids the body of tapeworms.
- Albendazole (Albenza) is used to treat tapeworms and microsporidiosis. Liver enzymes must be watched carefully when taking this drug.

- Mebendazole (Vermox) is used in the treatment of pinworms, whipworms, hookworms, and ascarides.
- Pyrantel (Pin-X) is used to treat pinworms.
- Thiabendazole (Mintezol) is used for treatment of *Trichinella* and *Strongyloides*.
- Intestinal protozoa are spread by the feces-to-mouth route.
- Amebiasis is treated with metronidazole (Flagyl, Flagyl I.V.).
- Sulfamethoxazole-trimethoprim (Bactrim, Bactrim DS, Cotrim, Septra, Septra DS) treats isosporiasis and cyclosporiasis.
- Malaria is acquired by the bite of an infected *Anopheles* mosquito. There are various treatments, but the most effective is probably atovaquone-proguanil (Malarone). It is used for prevention and treatment.

Hepatitis

- Hepatitis has several forms; A, B, and C are the most common.
- Hepatitis A and B can be transmitted from one person to another through contact, blood and body fluids, or the fecal-oral route.
- Hepatitis C can be transmitted only through blood and body fluids.
- Adefovir (Hepsera) is an effective treatment for hepatitis B.
- Peginterferon alfa-2a (Pegasys) and ribavirin (Copegus) are the drugs most effective for hepatitis C. They must be used together.

Drug List

The following drugs were discussed in this chapter. Each generic drug name is followed in parentheses by one or more brand names.

GERD

Antacids
aluminum hydroxide (ALternaGel)
aluminum hydroxide–magnesium carbonate (Gaviscon Extra Strength)
aluminum hydroxide–magnesium hydroxide–simethicone (Mylanta)
magnesium hydroxide (Phillips Milk of Magnesia)

H_2 Histamine Receptor Antagonists
cimetidine (Tagamet, Tagamet HB)
famotidine (Pepcid, Pepcid AC)*
nizatidine (Axid, Axid AR)
ranitidine (Zantac, Zantac 75)*

Proton Pump Inhibitors
esomeprazole (Nexium)*
lansoprazole (Prevacid)*
omeprazole (Prilosec, Prilosec OTC)*
pantoprazole (Protonix)*
rabeprazole (Aciphex)*

Combinations
calcium carbonate–famotidine–magnesium hydroxide (Pepcid Complete)
lansoprazole-naproxen (Prevacid NapraPAC)

Coating Agent
sucralfate (Carafate)

Prostaglandin E Analog
misoprostol (Cytotec)

Cholinergic Agent
bethanechol (Urecholine)

H. pylori

Antibiotics
amoxicillin (Amoxil, Trimox)*
clarithromycin (Biaxin)
metronidazole (Flagyl, Flagyl I.V.)
tetracycline (Sumycin)

Combinations
bismuth subsalicylate–metronidazole–tetracycline (Helidac)
bismuth subcitrate potassium–metronidazole-tetracycline (Pylera)
lansoprazole–amoxicillin–clarithromycin (Prevpac)

Gastrointestinal Diseases

Mast Cell Stabilizer
cromolyn sodium (Crolom, Gastrocrom, Intal, Opticrom)

Pancreatic Enzyme
pancrelipase (Creon-10, Pancrease, Viokase)

Immunosuppression
azathioprine (Imuran)

Monoclonal Antibody
infliximab (Remicade)

Anti-Inflammatory
balsalazide (Colazal)
budesonide (Entocort EC)
mesalamine (Asacol, Lialda, Pentasa, Rowasa)
olsalazine (Dipentum)
sulfasalazine (Azulfidine)

Gallstone Dissolution Agent
ursodiol (Actigall)

Antiemetic
metoclopramide (Reglan)

Antidiarrheals
bismuth subsalicylate (Pepto-Bismol, Kaopectate)
difenoxin-atropine (Motofen)
diphenoxylate-atropine (Lomotil)
loperamide (Imodium, Imodium A-D)
nitazoxanide (Alinia)
paregoric
rifaximin (Xifaxan)

Constipation

Osmotic Laxatives
glycerin (Fleet Glycerin Suppositories)
lactulose (Enulose)
polyethylene glycol 3350 (MiraLax)*

Saline Laxatives
magnesium hydroxide (Phillips Milk of Magnesia)
magnesium sulfate

Irritant/Stimulant Laxatives
bisacodyl (Dulcolax)

Surfactant Laxatives
docusate (Colace, Ex-Lax Stool Softener, Surfak)
docusate-senna (Senokot-S)

Bulk-Forming Agent
psyllium (Fiberall, Metamucil, Perdiem Fiber Therapy)

Antiflatulent
aluminum hydroxide–magnesium hydroxide–simethicone (Mylanta)
calcium carbonate–simethicone (Maalox)
simethicone (Gas Aid, Mylanta, Maximum Strength, Mylicon Drops)

Bowel Evacuants
polyethylene glycol 3350 and electrolytes (GoLYTELY, HalfLytely)
sodium phosphate (Fleet Phospho-Soda, Visicol)

Miscellaneous
lubiprostone (Amitiza)

Hemorrhoidal Agent
hydrocortisone (Anusol HC)

Antiemetics

Antihistamines and Related Compounds
diphenhydramine (Benadryl)
hydroxyzine (Atarax, Vistaril)
meclizine* (Antivert, Dramamine II)
trimethobenzamide (Tigan)

Serotonin Receptor Antagonists
dolasetron (Anzemet)
granisetron (Kytril)
ondansetron (Zofran)

Phenothiazines
prochlorperazine (Compazine)
promethazine (Phenergan)*

Other Antiemetic Medications
aprepitant (Emend)
metoclopramide (Reglan)

Weight Loss Drugs

Stimulants
dextroamphetamine (Dexedrine)
diethylpropion (Tenuate)
methamphetamine (Desoxyn)
phentermine (Adipex-P, Ionamin)
sibutramine (Meridia)

Lipase Inhibitor
orlistat (Xenical, Alli)

Antiparasitic Drugs
albendazole (Albenza)
mebendazole (Vermox)
praziquantel (Biltricide)
pyrantel (Pin-X)
thiabendazole (Mintezol)

Drugs for Protozoan Infections
metronidazole (Flagyl, Flagyl I.V.)
sulfamethoxazole-trimethoprim (Bactrim, Bactrim DS, Cotrim, Cotrim DS, Septra, Septra DS)

Antimalarials
atovaquone-proguanil (Malarone)
chloroquine (Aralen)
doxycycline (Vibramycin)
hydroxychloroquine (Plaquenil)
mefloquine (Lariam)
primaquine
quinine (Qualaquin)

Hepatitis Drugs
adefovir (Hepsera)
entecavir (Baraclude)
immune globulin (Gamunex)
interferon alfa-2a (Roferon A)
interferon alfa-2b (Intron A)
lamivudine (Epivir, Epivir-HBV)
peginterferon alfa-2a (Pegasys)
ribavirin (Copegus)
telbivudine (Tyzeka)

Chapter Review

Pharmaceuticals and Body Functions

Select the best answer from the choices given.

1. A common cause of gastritis is
   a. food.
   b. alcohol.
   c. medicine.
   d. all of the above

2. The most common cause of drug-induced ulcers is
   a. alcohol.
   b. aspirin.
   c. prednisone.
   d. methotrexate.

3. Which drug is a bowel motility stimulant?
   a. Cytotec
   b. Carafate
   c. Dulcolax
   d. Prevacid

4. Which drug is a coating agent?
   a. Cytotec
   b. Carafate
   c. Axid
   d. Prevacid

5. Which antidiarrheal is a controlled substance?
   a. Lomotil
   b. Imodium
   c. Alinia
   d. loperamide

6. Which drug is used in cystic fibrosis?
   a. Actigall
   b. Dulcolax
   c. Imuran
   d. Creon-10

7. Which drug is used in Crohn disease?
   a. cyclizine
   b. aspirin
   c. Actigall
   d. sulfasalazine

8. Which drug is used to treat gallstones?
   a. Imuran
   b. Actigall
   c. Rowasa
   d. Azulfidine

9. Which drug should not be touched by a pregnant technician?
   a. Imuran
   b. Actigall
   c. Rowasa
   d. Cytotec

10. Malaria is transmitted through
    a. person-to-person contact.
    b. worms.
    c. intestinal protozoa.
    d. *Anopheles* mosquito.

The following statements are true or false. If the answer is false, rewrite the statement so it is true.

_____ 1. Imuran is an enema.

_____ 2. Actigall is an immunosuppressive agent.

_____ 3. Fiber has no adverse effects.

_____ 4. If a child has two obese parents, the percentage chance of that individual being overweight is 20%.

_____ 5. Diethylpropion is a diet medication that stimulates adrenergic pathways.

_____ 6. Loperamide is a narcotic antidiarrheal.

_____ 7. Hepatitis A cannot be transmitted from person to person.

_____ 8. Morbid obesity is body weight 30% over the ideal.

_____ 9. Even with drug therapy, diet modification plays an essential role in weight reduction.

_____ 10. Chronic constipation is often associated with low-fiber diets.

Diseases and Drug Therapies

1. Describe the roller-coaster syndrome.

2. Explain why fiber agents may help weight loss.

3. The three forms of hepatitis are A, B and C. Under each heading list the drugs to treat that form.

4. List the symptoms of GERD.

5. Discuss the agents used to treat obesity listed in the chapter and their mechanism of action.

Dispensing Medications

1. List the OTC products to treat GERD.

2. Explain to a patient why an OTC drug has different ingredients than the last time the patient bought it.

3. Which are the most common forms of hepatitis? Which forms should one be vaccinated against? What is meant by at risk?

4. Figure ideal body weight for a male 6 feet 3 inches tall.

5. Figure ideal body weight for a female 5 feet 6 inches tall.

6. Figure the BMI for the above female patient with a weight of 200 pounds. (1 kg = 2.2 lbs; 1 inch = 2.5 cm; 100 cm = 1 m)

Internet Research

Use the Internet to complete the following assignments.

1. Locate information related to ongoing clinical trials aimed at the development of new treatments for Crohn disease. Create a table listing at least three experimental therapies. Indicate the phase (one through three) of testing presently under way and where (institution and country) the trials are taking place. List your Internet sources.

2. Identify two Internet sites that discuss the role of *Helicobacter pylori* in gastrointestinal disease. What specific disorders does this bacterium affect? List your Internet source(s).

What Would You Do?

1. An epidemic of Hepatitis A has broken out in your school. You will be doing your hospital rotation next month.

Renal System Drugs

11

The kidneys, ureters, bladder, and urethra are all part of the **urinary tract**. Disease in any of these areas of the tract can upset the delicate balance of the body and result in many problems, some of them serious. Kidney disease, in particular, has disastrous implications because the kidneys regulate the balance of body chemistry. Although the kidneys are most often thought of as an excretory organ, most of their metabolic work is directed toward the reclamation of filtered solutes. In addition, the kidneys play an important role in the metabolism of various peptide hormones and are active biosynthetically in the production of renin, ammonia, erythropoietin, and 1-alpha, 25-dihydroxy-vitamin D_3.

Function of the Renal System

The primary function of the kidneys is to maintain the balance of water, electrolytes, and acids and bases in the extracellular fluid (plasma and tissue fluid) environment of the body. They accomplish this function through the formation of urine, which is a modified filtrate of plasma. Urine formation is essential for normal body function because it enables the blood to reabsorb necessary nutrients, water, and electrolytes. Large molecules, such as plasma proteins, cannot cross the glomerular membranes to filter from the blood, whereas small molecules, such as water, ions, and glucose, do pass through the membranes, later to be reabsorbed into the blood. Figure 11.1 illustrates the urinary system and renal anatomy. In the process of urine formation, the kidneys regulate (1) the volume of blood plasma (thus contributing significantly to the regulation of blood pressure); (2) the concentration of waste products in the blood; (3) the concentration of electrolytes—sodium (Na^+), potassium (K^+), bicarbonate (HCO_3^-), calcium (Ca^{2+}), and phosphate (PO_4^{3-})—in the plasma; and (4) the pH, or acid-base balance, of plasma.

The Kidneys

The working unit of the kidneys is the **nephron.** The normal human kidney contains two million of these functionally integrated glomerulotubular units (see Figure 11.2). The nephrons work in a highly consistent manner to produce urine and thereby maintain constancy in the body's internal environment. The renal tubules of the nephrons produce urine through three processes: filtration, reabsorption, and secretion.

- **Filtration**, or the removal of substances from the blood, takes place in the glomeruli.
- During **reabsorption**, filtered substances are selectively pulled back into the blood. Sodium is the principal (99%) cation (positively charged ion) of extracellular fluid transported (exchanged for hydrogen and potassium ions), and chloride is the principal anion (negatively charged ion) transported. In the loop of Henle, sodium is absorbed along with chloride. In the distal tubule, potassium is secreted into the urine in exchange for sodium. This exchange is promoted by aldosterone.
- **Secretion** of hydrogen ions, potassium ions, weak acids, and weak bases also takes place in the tubules. Hydrogen ion secretion regulates acid-base balance and acidification of urine (blood pH is normally between 7.32 and 7.42, which is slightly basic).

Acute renal failure is a rapid reduction in kidney function, resulting in accumulation of nitrogen and other waste. It may be caused by renal ischemia, trauma, pregnancy, volume depletion, hemorrhage, surgery, or shock. **Uremia** is the clinical

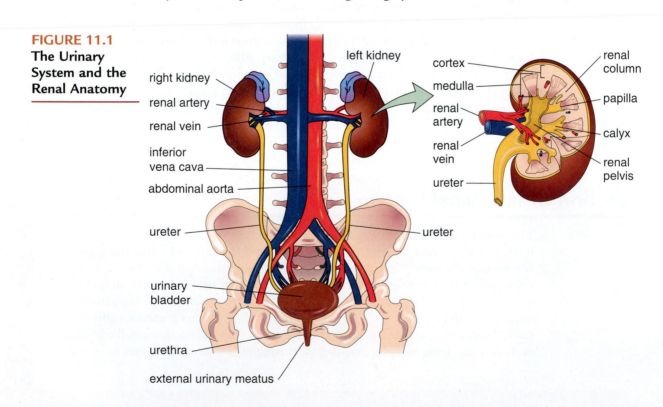

FIGURE 11.1
The Urinary System and the Renal Anatomy

right kidney
renal artery
renal vein
inferior vena cava
abdominal aorta
ureter
urinary bladder
urethra
external urinary meatus

left kidney
ureter

cortex
medulla
renal artery
renal vein
ureter

renal column
papilla
calyx
renal pelvis

FIGURE 11.2
Anatomy of the
Nephron

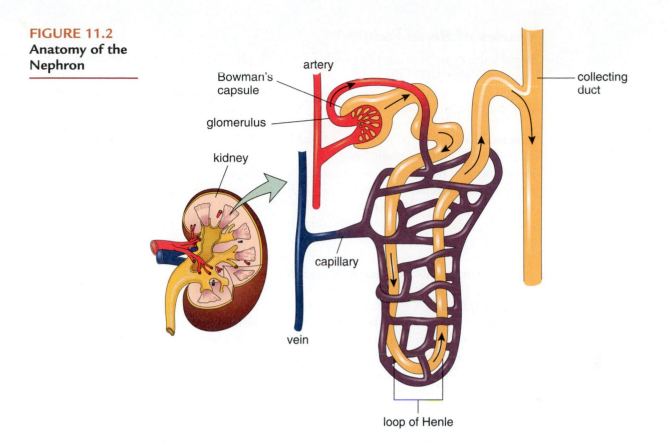

syndrome resulting from renal dysfunction. In this syndrome, excessive products of protein metabolism (e.g., urea) are retained in the blood, and the toxic condition produced is marked by nausea, vomiting, vertigo, convulsions, and coma.

Stages of Renal Disease

The clinical course of progressive renal disease is classified into four stages.

1. **Loss of Renal Reserve:** Patients are generally asymptomatic.
2. **Renal Insufficiency:** Patients are still asymptomatic for the most part but may have **nocturia** (excess urination at night, sometimes during sleep) secondary to a loss of urinary concentrating ability, hypertension secondary to volume expansion from impaired sodium excretion, or both. Blood urea nitrogen (BUN) level is mildly elevated, serum creatinine level is increased, and mild anemia is present.
3. **Chronic Renal Insufficiency:** Patients are easily fatigued, are intolerant of cold, and have abnormal taste sensation and anorexia. The anemia worsens, and laboratory abnormalities develop, including hyperphosphatemia, hypocalcemia, hyperkalemia, and metabolic acidosis. Uremia develops at this stage. Creatinine clearance drops below 40 mL/min, and the patient has malaise, generalized pruritus (itching), nausea, vomiting, and leg cramps. At this stage before the full syndrome develops, dialysis is indicated to remove the by-products of protein metabolism thought to be responsible for this symptom complex.
4. **End-Stage Renal Disease (ESRD):** The patient requires chronic dialysis.

Causes of Renal Failure

Renal failure can be caused by problems with fluids before they reach the kidneys, from problems within the kidneys, or due to problems with anatomical parts downstream from the kidneys. The causes are referred to, respectively, as prerenal, intrarenal, and postrenal events.

Prerenal Events Renal problems caused by fluids before they reach the kidneys are referred to as prerenal events. Body fluid volume problems other than those caused by the kidney can be due to diuretics, vomiting, nasogastric suction, diarrhea, hemorrhage, burns, adrenal insufficiency, or diabetic ketoacidosis. A decreased effective volume may be caused by congestive heart failure (CHF), myocardial infarction (MI), cirrhosis (liver disease), sepsis (infection that is very difficult to treat), vasodilators, or pulmonary edema (fluid in the lungs). The result is reduced renal blood flow. The kidney usually receives 20% of the cardiac output. Reduction in renal blood flow can cause ischemia, cell dysfunction, or even death.

Intrarenal Events Changes inside the kidney, such as rapidly progressive glomerulonephritis, renal vein thrombosis, vascular obstruction, vasculitis, and hypertension, can all contribute to declining renal function. These renal problems are called intrarenal events. Causes of ischemia are surgery, hypotension, shock, radiocontrast dyes, emboli, and thrombi. Nephrotoxins can be antibiotics, nonsteroidal anti-inflammatory drugs (NSAIDs), radiocontrast dyes, mismatched transfusions, myoglobin, and mineral precipitates. Glomerular inflammation can cause the glomerular membrane to rupture, allowing filtrates and blood to flow back into the capsular (Bowman) space and stimulating fibrin formation (see Figure 11.2 for the glomerulus). Macrophages are attracted, and permanent damage results.

Damage to the glomerulus generally results from the following causes.

- **Damage to the vascular tree** (the branching structure of capillaries in the kidney that distributes blood from the incoming renal artery to the individual nephrons): This can result in occlusive disease, completely cutting off blood flow to some nephrons.
- **Change in glomerular permeability:** Damage allows protein and cellular debris to enter the urine and is believed to obstruct blood flow.
- **Autoimmune reactions:** The glomerular membrane may act as an antigen, causing a circulating antibody to become trapped in the glomerular membrane and initiate an immune reaction.
- **Radiocontrast dyes:** These dyes are used for diagnostic tests to highlight areas on x-ray images and help the physician make a more accurate diagnosis. However, they are also the third most common cause of renal failure in hospitalized patients. This can be easily avoided in many cases. Technicians need to be on the alert for patients undergoing tests using radiocontrast dyes. When orders are received for such a test, make sure (1) the patient is well hydrated; (2) nephrotoxic drugs such as NSAIDs, aminoglycosides, and cyclosporines are held, at least temporarily, until the test is administered; (3) metformin is stopped and not restarted for 48 hours after the test; (4) acetylcysteine is begun a day before the test (it provides some protection against the dye without interfering with the test). If the orders do not make these provisions for the patient, make the pharmacist or prescriber aware.

Postrenal Events Disease can also occur in the structures below the kidney. These probems are collectively referred to as postrenal events. The urethra and ureter can be damaged by crystals, clots, stones, tumor, fibrosis, infection, endometriosis, and papillary necrosis. Bladder disease can be serious, as in prostatic hyperplasia and cancer. Blockage to urine flow may be partial or complete and could involve the renal pelvis, ureters, bladder, or urethra. Initially, the obstruction causes vasoconstriction of affected arteries as a result of feedback signals from increased hydrostatic pressure in the tubules. If not corrected, it can lead to defects in the tubules.

Renal Drug Therapy

A diagnosis of renal disease is made by two indicators: signs and evaluations. Signs include orthostatic blood pressure, skin turgor (swelling), temperature, color, edema, weight loss, changes in urine volume (which may not relate directly to disease severity), and bad urine odor. Evaluations of renal disease include filtration rate, urine volume, electrolyte levels and osmolality, urine protein level, measuring of other urine contents, serum creatinine level, and blood urea level (BUN).

Renal therapy is aimed at reestablishing an appropriate intravascular fluid volume and pressure, restricting fluids in volume-overload cases, and treating the underlying problem (fluids, sodium, potassium, calcium, phosphorus, magnesium, and pH).

Anemia due to renal failure is caused by decreased erythropoietin. This hormone, which is secreted by the kidneys, stimulates the production of red blood cells. Most renal patients show evidence of erythropoietin deficiency. Inhibitors of erythropoiesis exist in the blood and other body fluids. Patients undergoing hemodialysis or peritoneal dialysis may have a rise in **hematocrit** (proportion of red blood cells), indicating that inhibiting substances are being removed by dialysis. Patients undergoing dialysis must also be watched closely for aluminum intoxication, which interferes with the incorporation of iron into erythrocytes. Sucralfate and aluminum-containing antacids can be causes. Antacids can also cause iron deficiency by reducing the absorption of iron. Blood loss and reduced dietary intake also lead to iron deficiency. Vitamins are lost, especially the water-soluble ones; pyridoxine (B_6) and folic acid (B_9) are both removed by dialysis.

Table 11.1 presents the most commonly used agents in renal disease. Drugs that may be used include diuretics, antihypertensives, corticosteroids, and even some cytotoxic agents. Some are discussed in other chapters. Appropriate pharmacologic intervention can markedly enhance the quality of life for patients with this disease. Although drugs can often be the cause of renal disease, they can also be helpful in treatment. Once a patient is on dialysis, most drugs have to be dosed differently. The technician must be aware of this. If a patient has renal disease, the dosing should always be checked.

Cinacalcet (Sensipar) lowers parathyroid hormone, calcium, and phosphate levels and is indicated for the treatment of secondary hyperparathyroidism in adult patients on dialysis. It is also indicated for hypercalcemia. Cinacalcet can be given alone or in combination with vitamin D. It reduces serum calcium, so calcium levels should be monitored. Beneficial effects of cinacalcet have been demonstrated in dialysis patients regardless of the severity of the disease.

Warning

Aranesp and Aricept (donepezil, used in treating Alzheimer disease) look very much alike.

Darbepoetin alfa (Aranesp) is a longer-acting erythropoietin analog for anemia. It is approved for anemia associated with chronic renal failure. Its half-life is three times that of erythropoietin.

Epoetin alfa, erythropoietin (Epogen, Procrit) is used to treat anemia associated with end-stage renal disease. This drug induces release of **reticulocytes** (immature red blood cells) from bone marrow into the bloodstream, where the reticulocytes mature to erythrocytes. The result is a rise in hematocrit and hemoglobin levels. Frequent

TABLE 11.1   Most Commonly Used Agents in Renal Disease

Generic Name	Pronunciation	Dosage Form	Brand Name	Dispensing Status
cinacalcet	sin-a-KAL-set	tablet	Sensipar	Rx
darbepoetin alfa	dar-be-POE-e-tin AL-fa	injection	Aranesp	Rx
epoetin alfa (erythropoietin)	eh-POE-e-tin AL-fa	injection, IV	Epogen, Procrit	Rx
ergocalciferol (vitamin D)	er-goe-kal-SIF-e-rawl	capsule, oral liquid, tablet	(none)	Rx
folic acid (vitamin B$_9$)	FOE-lik AS-id	injection, IV, tablet	(many)	OTC, Rx
iron dextran	EYE-ern DEX-tran	injection, IV	INFeD	Rx
iron sucrose	EYE-ern SOO-krose	injection, IV	Venofer	Rx
levocarnitine	lee-voe-KAR-ni-teen	injection, oral liquid, tablet	Carnitor	Rx
methoxy polyethylene glycol–epoetin beta	meth-OX-i pol-ee-ETH-i-leen-GLYE-kawl-eh-POE-e-tin-BAY-ta	injection	Mircera	Rx
multiple vitamin complex	MUL-ti-ple VYE-ta-min KOM-plex	IV, oral liquid, tablet	(many)	OTC, Rx
pyridoxine (vitamin B$_6$)	peer-i-DOX-een	injection, IV, tablet	(many)	OTC, Rx
sevelamer	se-VEL-a-mer	tablet	Renagel, Renvela	Rx

blood tests are needed to determine the correct dose. The patient should notify the physician if frequent headaches occur. The drug is produced by animal cell cultures into which the human erythropoietin gene has been placed. Adverse effects are hypertension, seizures, increased clotting potential, and allergic reactions.

Ergocalciferol, a **vitamin D** supplement, is determined by serum calcium concentrations. Ergocalciferol is not routinely given to patients until they begin dialysis. **Folic acid (vitamin B$_9$)** should be administered to renal patients daily, because it is required for forming new erythrocytes. Nephrocaps is a vitamin especially formulated for dialysis patients. It has folic acid, other B vitamins and vitamin C.

Iron dextran (INFeD) releases iron from the plasma and eventually replenishes the iron stores in bone marrow, where it is incorporated into hemoglobin. This complex can be given by deep IM injection into the upper-outer quadrant of the buttocks (never in the arm or other area) using the Z-track technique, or by IV. It must be used with caution, and a test dose should be given before the full dose is administered.

Iron sucrose (Venofer) is used to replenish iron body stores in patients on chronic hemodialysis who have iron deficiency. Anemia is a chronic problem for dialysis patients. Iron sucrose is eliminated mainly by urinary excretion. A significant amount of the iron distributes in the liver, spleen, and bone marrow. Iron sucrose is administered one to three times a week, either intravenously or by slow infusion. Most IV iron needs a test dose, but iron sucrose does not. It appears to be a safer alternative than the other iron supplements, especially for those patients who have had a reaction to iron dextran. Patients still need to be monitored for hypotension, which is the most common side effect. Slowing the infusion may help.

Levocarnitine (Carnitor) is an amino acid derivative involved in metabolism. It is a cofactor needed for the transformation of long-chain fatty acids. A deficiency of levocarnitine leads to fatigue. It is thought that dialysis reduces circulating levels of levocarnitine. The most common side effects are gastrointestinal and include nausea, vomiting, cramps, and diarrhea. It is used primarily for deficiency states and hemodialysis patients.

Methoxy polyethylene glycol–epoetin beta (Mircera) is an erythropoiesis (red blood cell formation) stimulating agent for anemia associated with chronic renal failure. The receptor-binding and extended half-life allow continuous stimulation with one monthly dose. It may take as long as 6 weeks before symptoms improve. Methoxy polyethylene glycol–epoetin beta is usually given as a subcutaneous injection in the upper arm, thigh, or lower abdomen or intravenously. The vial must not be shaken and must be stored in the original container until immediately before use.

Multiple vitamins are necessary because of the imbalance of electrolytes (and other substances) that coincides with renal disease, which depletes vitamin stores.

Pyridoxine, vitamin B$_6$, should also be administered daily. It is removed by dialysis and must be replaced.

Sevelamer (Renagel, Renvela) binds phosphate in the intestinal lumen, limiting its absorption. The drug has the ability to decrease serum phosphate concentrations without altering calcium, aluminum, or bicarbonate concentrations. Sevelamer can interfere with the absorption of other drugs. Therefore, patients should take other medications at least 1 hour before or 3 hours after the administration of this drug. Serum calcium, bicarbonate, and chloride concentrations should be monitored. Renagel is in the form of a hydrochloride salt. Renvela has the advantage of a carbonate salt, which serves as a buffer and may be better tolerated.

Renal Transplants

When the kidneys fail completely, the patient may receive a renal transplant, a treatment that has been very successful. When a renal transplant is performed, the patient must be given drugs that prevent the body from rejecting the foreign organ (see Table 11.2). The doses may be adjusted, usually lowered, but these drugs must be taken for the rest of the patient's life. Mycophenolic acid is approved specifically to prevent the rejection of transplanted kidneys.

Mycophenolic acid (Myfortic) is an immunosuppressant used to prevent the body from rejecting a kidney transplant. It is usually combined with **cyclosporine**

TABLE 11.2	Most Commonly Used Renal Transplant Drugs			
Generic Name	Pronunciation	Dosage Form	Brand Name	Dispensing Status
cyclosporine	SYE-kloe-spor-een	capsule, IV, oral liquid	Sandimmune	Rx
mycophenolate	my-koe-FEN-oh-late	capsule, IV, oral liquid, tablet	CellCept	Rx
mycophenolic acid	my-koe-fen-AW-lik AS-id	tablet	Myfortic	Rx

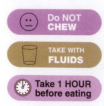

(**Sandimmune**) and a steroid. Mycophenolic acid may increase risk of infection and the development of cancer. The patient should never receive live vaccines when on this drug. It should be taken with a full glass of water, on an empty stomach 1 hour before or 2 hours after a meal. The patient should avoid the sun. The tablet should not be crushed, cut, or chewed because it has a special coating to protect the stomach.

Mycophenolate (CellCept) is another immunosuppressant. It is used prophylactically in patients with kidney, heart, or liver transplants. It is usually administered with cyclosporine (Sandimmune). The advantage of mycophenolate is that it comes in an IV dosage form. It is compatible only with D_5W. The oral dosage form should be taken 1 to 2 hours before or after meals.

Drugs for Urinary Tract Diseases and Disorders

In addition to renal disease, the urinary tract can be affected by several other diseases and disorders. These include urinary problems such as spastic bladder and frequent urination, urinary tract infections caused by bacteria, and benign prostatic hyperplasia, an abnormal enlargement of the prostate gland that occurs in men as they age. The symptoms in each case may include bothersome urination, but they are treated with different classes of drugs. Postmenopausal women and elderly men are frequently prone to incontinence (inability to control urination). A variety of diapers for adults are available.

A common malady of the elderly is what is called overactive bladder (voiding eight or more times in a 24 hour period or awakening two or more times during the night). The detrusor muscle, or bladder muscle, contracts prior to the bladder being full, which produces an urgent sense to urinate. This problem can affect the quality of life. Patients often avoid social events in order to prevent embarrassment. Overactive bladder can limit travel; long trips where bathrooms are not available for several hours become a serious problem. There are numerous medications available; behavioral techniques for this condition should also be considered.

Urinary Problems

Table 11.3 lists the most commonly used agents for urinary problems such as spastic bladder and frequent urination.

Bethanechol (Urecholine) stimulates cholinergic receptors in the smooth muscle of the urinary bladder and gastrointestinal (GI) tract, resulting in increased peristalsis, increased GI and pancreatic secretions, bladder muscle contraction, and increased ureteral peristaltic waves. This drug should be taken 1 hour before meals or 2 hours after meals. It may cause abdominal discomfort, salivation, sweating, or flushing. The patient should notify the physician if these symptoms become pronounced.

Darifenacin (Enablex) blocks the cholinergic receptor in the bladder and limits contractions, which reduces the symptoms of ugency and frequency. The drug must be protected from light. As with all other agents in this class, the primary side effect is dry mouth.

Duloxetine (Cymbalta), a medication described in Chapter 7 as a treatment for depression, also helps contract the sphincter to prevent urine from leaking from the bladder. When duloxetine is used for treatment of depression, a hesitancy to urinate is reported as a side effect. Duloxetine is marketed under the name Yentreve in countries where it is approved for **stress incontinence** (urine leakage during physical movements).

TABLE 11.3   Most Commonly Used Agents for Urinary Problems

Generic Name	Pronunciation	Dosage Form	Brand Name	Dispensing Status
bethanechol	be-THAN-e-kawl	tablet	Urecholine	Rx
darifenecin	dar-i-FEN-a-sin	tablet	Enablex	Rx
duloxetine	doo-LOX-e-teen	capsule	Cymbalta	Rx
flavoxate	fla-VOX-ate	tablet	Urispas	Rx
oxybutynin	ox-i-BYOO-ti-nin	oral liquid, patch, tablet	Ditropan, Oxytrol	Rx
pentosan polysulfate sodium	PEN-toe-san pol-i-SUL-fate SOE-dee-um	capsule	Elmiron	Rx
propantheline	proe-PAN-the-leen	tablet	Pro-Banthine	Rx
solifenacin	sol-i-FEN-a-sin	tablet	Vesicare	Rx
tolterodine	tole-TAIR-oh-deen	capsule, tablet	Detrol	Rx
trospium	TROSE-pee-um	tablet	Sanctura	Rx

Flavoxate (Urispas) exerts a direct spasmolytic effect on smooth muscle, primarily in the urinary tract. Acting on the detrusor muscle by cholinergic blockage, this agent increases bladder capacity in patients with bladder spasticity. It also has local anesthetic and analgesic effects. It can cause drowsiness, blurred vision, and GI upset.

Oxybutynin (Ditropan, Oxytrol) is a urinary antispasmodic agent used to decrease frequent urination. The antispasmodic works to inhibit the action of acetylcholine (ACh). It decreases spasms in smooth muscle without affecting skeletal muscles. This drug also increases bladder capacity and decreases urgency and frequency. Dry mouth is a side effect. **Oxytrol** is a transdermal patch composed of three layers: (1) backing film that protects the middle adhesive/drug layer; (2) the adhesive/drug layer; and (3) the release liner that is pulled off prior to application. The patch is applied twice a week to dry, intact skin on the abdomen, hip, or buttock. The site should be rotated with each application, and a patch should not be reapplied to the same site within 7 days. It should be stored away from humidity and moisture at room temperature. The transdermal form minimizes the side effects of dry mouth and constipation, possibly because the transdermal patch is constantly releasing the drug. Thus, first-pass metabolism is avoided. The patch also avoids high peak concentration.

Pentosan polysulfate sodium (Elmiron) is the first oral therapy for interstitial cystitis (inflammation of the urinary bladder), which causes a painful condition whereby patients need to urinate very frequently. It is used for relief of bladder pain, presumably by exerting a protective effect on the bladder wall to reduce irritation and inflammation. Patients need to take it for up to 6 weeks before they get relief; this can be discouraging and often leads to poor compliance. It also has a weak anticoagulant effect.

Propantheline (Pro-Banthine) is used to treat bladder spasms. It competitively blocks the action of ACh at postganglionic parasympathetic receptor sites. It should be taken 30 minutes before meals and at bedtime. It may cause blurred vision and decreased salivation. Skin rash, flushing, eye pain, difficulty in urination, or sensitivity to light should be reported to the physician.

Solifenacin (Vesicare) is an anticholinergic agent used for the treatment of overactive bladder. It is more selective for the muscarinic receptors and should have fewer side effects such as dry mouth. Maximum dose should not exceed 5 mg per day.

Tolterodine (Detrol) is a competitive muscarinic receptor antagonist similar to oxybutynin. It differs in its selectivity for urinary bladder receptors over salivary receptors. As a result, dry mouth effects of tolterodine are significantly less than those of oxybutynin. This drug also decreases detrusor muscle pressure.

Trospium (Sanctura) is an antispasmodic agent. It does not cross the blood brain barrier, so it will not cause drowsiness as do most of the drugs in this class. It should be taken on an empty stomach. It is dosed twice a day, whereas most of the other agents have once-daily dosing. It relaxes the smooth muscle tissue in the bladder, decreasing bladder contractions.

Urinary Tract Infections

A **urinary tract infection (UTI)** occurs when bacteria, most often *Escherichia coli*, enter the opening of the urethra and multiply. The infection usually begins in the lower tract (urethra and bladder) and, if not treated, progresses to the upper tract (ureters and kidneys). Even when the urinary tract is healthy, *E. coli* or other bacteria may enter. In UTIs, many more organisms than normal are found. The presence of bacteria in the urine with localized symptoms is considered symptomatic of UTI. Blood may appear in the urine, and urination may be difficult or painful. Fever is common. Community-acquired UTIs account for over five million physician visits per year.

The highest incidence of UTIs occurs in sexually active women. Incidence is related to the ability of intestinal bacteria to colonize the vagina, ascend the short urethra, and gain access to the bladder. UTIs become a problem for males after age 50 because of prostatic obstruction, instrumentation, or surgery.

UTIs are classified according to their anatomic location in the urinary tract. The classifications are

- cystitis
- urethritis (lower tract infection)
- prostatitis
- pyelonephritis (upper tract infection)

UTIs can be described as

- **uncomplicated:** no evidence of underlying structural or neurologic problems of the urinary tract
- **complicated:** a predisposing lesion of the urinary tract, such as a stone, stricture, neurogenic bladder, prostate hyperplasia, or obstruction

UTIs are most commonly treated with one of the antibiotics listed in Table 11.4. Treatment may involve a single dose of medicine or a 3 to 14 day course. Usually, a short course (1 to 3 days) is all that is needed to clear the infection. If several infections occur in sequence, an antibiotic may be prescribed for 6 to 12 months to prevent recurrence. A female patient with recurrent UTIs may be instructed to urinate and take one dose of an antibiotic immediately after sexual intercourse.

Amoxicillin (Amoxil) is taken without regard for food; the primary side effect is skin rash. It is dosed three times a day.

Amoxicillin-clavulanate (Augmentin) should be taken with food to avoid stomach upset. Diarrhea is the primary side effect.

TABLE 11.4 Most Commonly Used Medications to Treat UTIs

Generic Name	Pronunciation	Dosage Form	Brand Name	Dispensing Status
Antibiotics				
amoxicillin	a-mox-i-SIL-in	capsule, oral liquid, tablet	Amoxil	Rx
amoxicillin-clavulanate	a-mox-i-SIL-in klav-yoo-LAN-ate	oral liquid, tablet	Augmentin	Rx
ampicillin	am-pi-SIL-in	capsule, injection, IV, oral liquid	Principen	Rx
ciprofloxacin	sip-roe-FLOX-a-sin	IV, oral liquid, tablet	Cipro	Rx
methenamine	meth-EN-a-meen	tablet	Cystex, Hiprex, Urex	Rx
nitrofurantoin	nye-troe-fyoor-AN-toyn	capsule	Macrobid, Macrodantin	Rx
sulfamethoxazole-trimethoprim	sul-fa-meth-OX-a-zole trye-METH-oh-prim	IV, oral liquid, tablet	Bactrim, Bactrim DS, Cotrim, Cotrim DS, Septra, Septra DS	Rx
Urinary Analgesic				
phenazopyridine	fen-az-oh-PEER-i-deen	tablet	Azo-Standard, Uristat	OTC

Ampicillin (Principen) should be taken on an empty stomach; the primary side effects are diarrhea and skin rash. It is dosed four times a day.

Ciprofloxacin (Cipro) is indicated for the treatment of uncomplicated UTIs. Quinolones such as ciprofloxacin should not be taken with antacids, theophylline, warfarin, magnesium, or calcium. It should be administered at least 2 hours before or 6 hours after antacids containing magnesium or aluminum or other products containing metal cations. The tablet should not be split, crushed, or chewed. Since this drug increases sensitivity to the sun, it is very important to use sunscreen to protect the skin, even if one has minimum exposure to the sun.

Methenamine (Cystex, Hiprex, Urex) has a local anesthetic effect on urinary tract mucosa in addition to its antimicrobial effect. It is classified as a miscellaneous antibiotic. Methenamine should be taken with food to minimize GI upset and with sufficient fluids to ensure adequate urine flow. Cranberry juice, which is a weak germicide when used as a mild genitourinary antiseptic, is a good fluid to drink when taking methenamine. Alkaline foods, antacids, and other alkalinizing medication (e.g., bicarbonate) should be avoided. Skin rash, painful urination, or excessive abdominal pain should be reported to the physician. Administration with sulfonamides is contraindicated. If a dye is used in the formulation of Hiprex, it can turn urine blue and can cause allergic reactions.

Do not take with ANTACIDS

Sulfamethoxazole-trimethoprim (Bactrim, Bactrim DS, Cotrim, Cotrim DS, Septra, Septra DS) should be taken with plenty of water. A sunscreen should be used because this drug increases sensitivity to the sun.

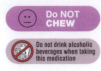

Nitrofurantoin (Macrobid, Macrodantin) should be taken with food or milk; it may turn urine brown or dark yellow, and alcohol should be avoided. This drug has side effects resembling those of disulfiram (Antabuse), discussed in Chapter 7.

Phenazopyridine (Azo-Standard, Uristat) is an OTC agent that has a local anesthetic effect on urinary tract mucosa. It colors the urine orange and stains anything it contacts. It should not be used for more than 2 days and should be taken with an antibiotic, because phenazopyridine by itself does not have antimicrobial activity. It is used for symptomatic relief of urinary burning, itching, frequency, and urgency in association with urinary tract infection or following urologic procedures.

Benign Prostatic Hyperplasia

Benign prostatic hyperplasia (BPH) is one of the most common medical conditions occurring in older men. This abnormal enlargement of the prostate gland appears to occur with aging in combination with certain pathophysiologic influences. An enlarged prostate becomes a problem when it obstructs urine outflow from the bladder. The prostate is involved primarily in reproduction but may sometimes protect against UTIs through the secretion of prostatic antibacterial factor (PAF). Figure 11.3 shows the organs of the male reproductive system.

Increasing evidence shows that nonsurgical interventions, especially drug therapy, may be effective as a primary treatment for selected patients with BPH. Alpha blockers and 5-alpha-reductase inhibitors represent promising and innovative approaches to pharmacologic management. The future challenge is to evaluate critically all therapeutic alternatives to identify the optimal treatment for each patient.

Alpha blockers were originally developed for treating hypertension, which, like BPH, is a common disorder in aging men. They cause relaxation of smooth muscles, especially in prostatic tissue, reducing urinary symptoms in BPH. Many older men have both conditions. In such cases, it is reasonable to consider using an alpha blocker to treat both the hypertension and the BPH.

Certain types of drugs affect bladder function and should not be used for patients with BPH. Table 11.5 lists both the classes of drugs that should not be used and the preferred alternatives. Table 11.6 lists the most commonly used agents for BPH.

FIGURE 11.3
The Male Reproductive System

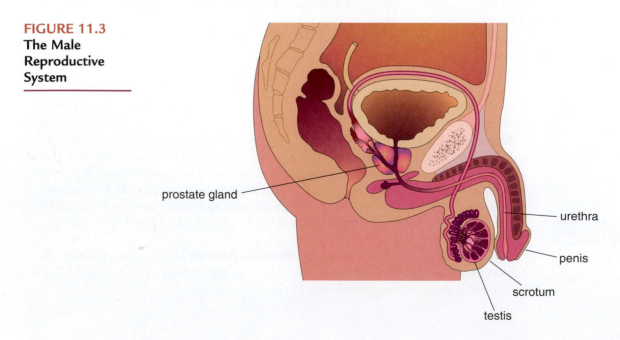

prostate gland

urethra

penis

scrotum

testis

Male hormones are commonly indicated in prostatic carcinomas. Therefore, female hormones or drugs that mimic them are used to slow the progress of this disease. These drugs are listed with the drugs used for BPH in Table 11.6. The discussions of the drugs will differentiate them. In some cases these drugs will be used together.

Alfuzosin (Uroxatral) is an alpha blocker. Because alfuzosin has fewer side effects alfuzosin is much better tolerated than other alpha blockers. It does not need to be titrated, and decreased ejaculation is not reported as a problem. Because it is an alpha blocker, the primary side effects are hypotension and dizziness. Alfuzosin helps relax the muscles in the prostate gland and the opening of the bladder, which improves the passage of urine. It should be taken with the same meal each day, and never on an empty stomach. Because it is a long-acting tablet, alfuzosin is dosed once per day. Therefore, the coating of the tablet must remain intact, and patients should not split, chew, or crush the tablets.

May cause **DIZZINESS**

TAKE WITH **FOOD**

Do NOT **CHEW**

TABLE 11.5   Contraindicated and Alternative Drugs for BPH Patients

Classes That Should Not Be Used	Preferred Alternatives
anticholinergics	sucralfate, antacids, proton pump inhibitors (PPIs)
oral bronchodilators	inhalation bronchodilators
tricyclic antidepressants (TCAs)	selective serotonin reuptake inhibitors (SSRIs)
calcium channel blockers	alpha blockers
disopyramide	quinidine
antihistamines	(discontinue)

TABLE 11.6   Most Commonly Used Agents for Prostatic Disease

Generic Name	Pronunciation	Dosage Form	Brand Name	Dispensing Status
alfuzosin	al-FYOO-zoe-sin	tablet	Uroxatral	Rx
doxazosin	dox-AY-zoe-sin	tablet	Cardura	Rx
dutasteride	du-TAS-tur-ide	capsule	Avodart	Rx
finasteride	fin-AS-tur-ide	tablet	Propecia, Proscar	Rx
flutamide	FLOO-ta-mide	capsule	Eulexin	Rx
goserelin	GOE-se-rel-in	implant	Zoladex	Rx
leuprolide	LOO-proe-lide	implant, injection	Eligard, Lupron Depot, Viadur	Rx
megestrol	me-JES-trawl	oral liquid, tablet	Megace	Rx
nilutamide	nye-LOO-ta-mide	tablet	Nilandron	Rx
prazosin	PRAZ-oh-sin	capsule	Minipress	Rx
tamsulosin	tam-SOO-loe-sin	capsule	Flomax	Rx
terazosin	ter-AY-zoe-sin	capsule, tablet	Hytrin	Rx

Doxazosin (Cardura) is an alpha blocker which prevents the constriction of blood vessels. It lowers blood pressure in this way; it was also found to relax the muscles around the prostate gland, which makes urination easier. First doses can cause excessive lowering of blood pressure, so it is often recommended that these doses be taken at bedtime to prevent dizziness and fainting. It may cause swelling of the ankle and fatigue.

Dutasteride (Avodart) has been shown to shrink the prostate, keep it smaller, improve symptoms, and decrease the risk of long-term symptoms. It has also shown excellent results in the treatment and reversal of male pattern baldness. Women should not handle this drug if pregnant. It blocks both type one and type two 5-alpha-reductase. It may take up to 6 months before there is an improvement in urinary symptoms.

Finasteride (Propecia, Proscar) blocks the enzyme that converts testosterone to dihydrotestosterone (DHT). The inhibition affects only DHT and not testosterone, so the side effects of general androgen blockade are minimized. The drug results in an increase in intracellular testosterone levels, thereby minimizing sexual dysfunction, the primary drawback of hormonal therapy. Advantageous effects are

Warning

Proscar, Prozac (antidepressant), and ProSom (estazolam, a sleep inducer, now discontinued) could easily be confused.

- reduction in prostate size, similar to that with other forms of androgen withdrawal
- improved urine flow and symptom relief, similar to those with other forms of androgen withdrawal
- minimal drug-related adverse effects
- decrease in male pattern baldness

Finasteride is provided in film-coated tablets. Crushed finasteride tablets or finasteride powder should not be handled by a woman who is or may become pregnant because of risk to a male fetus.

Flutamide (Eulexin) is an antiandrogen that inhibits androgen uptake or binding of androgen in target tissues. It is used in combination with leuprolide, and both drugs need to be started simultaneously. Over half of study patients reported breast pain or breast enlargement (gynecomastia). Half also experienced GI side effects. Flutamide is currently approved for treating symptomatic prostate cancer when used in conjunction with a luteinizing hormone blocker such as leuprolide or goserelin.

Goserelin (Zoladex) is a gonadotropin-releasing hormone used to treat carcinoma of the prostate, breast cancer, and endometriosis. It is a synthetic hormone that causes serum testosterone to fall to levels comparable with the results of surgical castration. The manufacturer provides goserelin in a 1 month and a 3 month implant in a disposable syringe. The implant is injected subcutaneously in the abdomen every 28 days or 3 months, depending on the dose.

Leuprolide (Eligard, Lupron Depot, Viadur) is a luteinizing hormone blocker that inhibits production of androgen. Monthly injections are necessary for leuprolide. Improvement in symptoms is slow, and after cessation of therapy the prostate returns to pretreatment size within 6 months. Viadur is an implant that is surgically inserted subcutaneously every 12 months. It is used to treat carcinoma of the prostate. Chronic administration can result in serum testosterone levels comparable to surgical castration.

Megestrol (Megace) is a progestational antiandrogen. It centrally inhibits luteinizing hormone. This inhibition in turn reduces testosterone production, resulting in reduced serum levels and consequently in the adverse effects of decreased libido and impotence.

Nilutamide (Nilandron) is indicated for use in advanced prostate cancer. It is an antiandrogen similar to flutamide. It helps reduce metastatic bone pain and improves survival. It is dosed once daily, in contrast to three times daily for flutamide.

Nilutamide causes visual disturbances—mainly a delay in adjusting from light to dark. Patients may need to avoid night driving. It can also cause a disulfiram-like reaction.

Prazosin (Minipress) is a selective alpha-1 adrenergic antagonist approved for treating hypertension. Several studies have shown benefit in patients with BPH, and the number of patients using this drug is increasing. Orthostatic hypotension is common, but this effect can sometimes be minimized by initiating the therapy at bedtime.

Tamsulosin (Flomax) is an alpha-1 blocker, but it is more selective than other alpha blockers. It has little effect on blood pressure but works well for BPH.

Terazosin (Hytrin) is a long-acting selective alpha-1 blocker approved for use as an antihypertensive agent. It produces significant improvement in obstructive symptoms and urinary flow rates. Its primary advantage over prazosin is a longer half-life that allows for once-daily dosing and presumably better rates of compliance. The side effects of tiredness, dizziness, and orthostatic hypotension can be minimized by giving the drug at bedtime. Headache has also been reported. Prophylactic administration of acetaminophen, 650 to 675 mg, a half hour before the terazosin dose may lessen the severity of headache, which usually subsides after several weeks of treatment.

Diuretics

A **diuretic** is a substance that increases the urine output. The primary purpose of using diuretics is to rid the body of excess fluid and electrolytes. A diuretic is often the first drug chosen to treat high blood pressure and may also be used to treat the various causes of edema. In addition, the effectiveness of certain drugs may be enhanced by combination with a diuretic. Table 11.7 presents the most commonly used diuretics.

A **thiazide diuretic** is based on benzothiadiazine (a molecule with two fused rings of which one contains two nitrogen atoms and a sulfur atom in place of carbon). Thiazides work by blocking a molecular pump that pulls sodium and chloride back into the blood from the distal tubule. Therefore, thiazides promote sodium and water excretion in the urine, lower the sodium level in the blood, and reduce vasoconstriction. These drugs are about equivalent in potency but may differ in onset, peak, and duration of action. The increased sodium concentrations in the urine lead to increased exchange of potassium for sodium, so potassium is lost too. Therefore, side effects of thiazide diuretics include hypokalemia, and patients should be told to ingest potassium (bananas, orange juice, citrus fruits) daily. Hypomagnesia, hyperuricemia, hyperglycemia, and hypercalcemia are other side effects. A few patients become more sensitive to sunlight when taking a thiazide.

A **loop diuretic** inhibits reabsorption of sodium and chloride in the ascending loop of Henle and distal renal tubules, thus causing increased urinary excretion of water, sodium, chloride, magnesium, calcium, and potassium, as with the thiazides. The high degree of efficacy of loop diuretics is due to this unique site of action.

A **potassium-sparing diuretic** inhibits the exchange of sodium from the urine for potassium from the blood. This type of diuretic should be administered with caution to patients on angiotensin-converting enzyme (ACE) inhibitors because these drugs also have a potassium-sparing effect. The side effects are hyperkalemia and gynecomastia in men. Hyperkalemia can lead to serious arrhythmias. Spironolactone is an antagonist of aldosterone, which in itself will promote potassium sparing.

A **carbonic anhydrase inhibitor** acts in the proximal tubule to cause an increase in the urine volume and a change to an alkaline pH, with a subsequent decrease in the excretion of titratable acid and ammonia.

TABLE 11.7 Most Commonly Used Diuretics

Generic Name	Pronunciation	Dosage Form	Brand Name	Dispensing Status
Thiazide Diuretics				
hydrochlorothiazide (HCTZ)	hye-droe-klor-oh-THYE-a-zide	tablet	Esidrix	Rx
methyclothiazide	meth-ee-kloe-THYE-a-zide	tablet	Enduron	Rx
Drug Related to the Thiazides				
chlorthalidone	klor-THAL-i-done	tablet	Hygroton	Rx
Combinations				
atenolol-chlorthalidone	a-TEN-oh-lawl chlor-THAL-i-done	tablet	Tenoretic	Rx
bisoprolol-hydrochlorothiazide	bis-OH-proe-lawl hye-droe-klor-oh-THYE-a-zide	tablet	Ziac	Rx
lisinopril-hydrochlorothiazide	lyse-IN-oh-pril hye-droe-klor-oh-THYE-a-zide	tablet	Zestoretic	Rx
losartan-hydrochlorothiazide	loe-SAR-tan hye-droe-klor-oh-THYE-a-zide	tablet	Hyzaar	Rx
triamterene-hydrochlorothiazide	trye-AM-ter-een hye-droe-klor-oh-THYE-a-zide	capsule, tablet	Dyazide, Maxzide	Rx
Loop Diuretics				
bumetanide	byoo-MET-a-nide	injection, tablet	Bumex	Rx
ethacrynic acid	eth-a-KRIN-ik AS-id	injection, tablet	Edecrin	Rx
furosemide	fur-OH-se-mide	injection, IV, oral liquid, tablet	Lasix	Rx
torsemide	TORE-se-mide	IV, tablet	Demadex	Rx
Potassium-Sparing Diuretics				
amiloride	a-MIL-oh-ride	tablet	Midamor	Rx
eplerenone	ep-LAIR-a-none	tablet	Inspra	Rx
spironolactone	speer-on-oh-LAK-tone	tablet	Aldactone	Rx
triamterene	trye-AM-ter-een	capsule	Dyrenium	Rx
Carbonic Anhydrase Inhibitors				
acetazolamide	a-seet-a-ZOLE-a-mide	capsule, injection, IV, tablet	Diamox	Rx
methazolamide	meth-a-ZOLE-a-mide	tablet	Neptazane	Rx
Osmotic Diuretics				
mannitol	MAN-i-tawl	IV	Osmitrol	Rx
Miscellaneous Diuretics				
indapamide	in-DAP-a-mide	tablet	Lozol	Rx
metolazone	me-TOLE-a-zone	tablet	Zaroxolyn	Rx

An **osmotic diuretic** increases the osmotic pressure of glomerular filtrate, which inhibits tubular reabsorption of water and electrolytes and increases urinary output. **Mannitol (Osmitrol)** is the only osmotic diuretic on the market. It is primarily used for cerebral edema or to decrease intraocular pressure. It is usually stored in a warmer to prevent precipitation. However, if it does precipitate, it can be warmed by running hot water over the bottle. It should be infused with a filter set.

More pharmaceutical companies are combining hypertensive and diuretic agents to improve compliance by decreasing the pill load. A diuretic is probably the best first step in blood pressure control. It has fewer unpleasant side effects and may even make the patient feel better by preventing bloating.

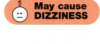

Atenolol-chlorthalidione (Tenoretic) is a cardioselective beta blocker combined with a diuretic, which is used to treat hypertension.

Bisoprolol-hydrochlorothiazide (Ziac) is a beta blocker combined with a diuretic. It can cause dizziness, headache, diarrhea, and fatigue.

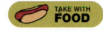

Chlorthalidone (Hygroton) inhibits sodium and chloride reabsorption in the cortical-diluting segment of the ascending loop of Henle. The primary side effect is hypokalemia. Chlorthalidone should be taken with food or milk early in the day; with multiple doses, the last should be taken no later than 6 P.M. so as to avoid nocturia.

Eplerenone (Inspra) is a selective aldosterone blocker. It is 100 times more specific in its affinity for aldosterone than spironolactone (Aldactone), a first-generation aldosterone blocker. Eplerenone prevents sodium and water retention in the kidneys, thereby reducing blood volume and blood pressure. It is used for the treatment of hypertension alone or in combination with other drugs and is also indicated for congestive heart failure after an acute myocardial infarction. Potassium levels should be monitored when this drug is being taken. Patients should avoid foods containing salt and bananas. Hyperkalemia is the primary side effect.

Furosemide (Lasix), a loop diuretic, should be given in two doses per day of 20 mg to 40 mg at a 6 to 8 hour interval. The name was designed to indicate the 6 hour interval (La*six*). This dosage schedule gets a better area under the curve than other dosing. Also, if the first dose is a morning dose and the next is given 6 hours later, the patient will not be up going to the bathroom all night.

Indapamide (Lozol) enhances sodium, chloride, and water excretion by interfering with the transport of sodium ions across the renal tubular epithelium. The effect is localized at the proximal segment of the distal tubule of the nephron.

Lisinopril-hydrochlorothiazide (Zestoretic) is a combination ACE inhibitor and thiazide diuretic used for the treatment of hypertension, CHF, and acute MI.

Losartan-hydrochlorothiazide (Hyzaar) is an angiotensin II receptor blocker combined with a thiazide diuretic used for treatment of hypertension and stroke risk reduction.

Warning

Hyzaar is easily confused with Cozaar, which is simply losartan, the angiotensin II receptor blocker component.

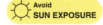

Metolazone (Zaroxolyn) inhibits sodium reabsorption in the distal tubules, causing increased excretion of sodium, water, and potassium and hydrogen ions. It should be taken with food early in the day to avoid nocturia; the last dose should be taken no later than 6 P.M. It may increase sensitivity to sunlight.

Triamterene-hydrochlorothiazide (Dyazide, Maxzide) is a widely used combination diuretic. It is among the safest drugs on the market. Even though this is a thiazide combination, it is claimed not to waste potassium because of the triamterene. The reality is that almost all diuretics do waste potassium, and people on diuretics will need potassium supplements. It is very important that physicians order appropriate labs on a regular basis. The tablet form (Maxzide) is absorbed better than the Dyazide capsules. Triamterene can change the urine color to blue-green.

Chapter Terms

acute renal failure rapid reduction in kidney function resulting in accumulation of nitrogen and other wastes

benign prostatic hyperplasia (BPH) abnormal enlargement of the prostate gland, usually associated with aging

carbonic anhydrase inhibitor a diuretic that acts in the proximal tubule to increase urine volume and change the pH to alkaline

diuretic a substance that rids the body of excess fluid and electrolytes by increasing the urine output

filtration the removal of substances from the blood as part of the formation of urine by the renal tubules

hematocrit the proportion of volume of red blood cells to the total volume of blood

loop diuretic a drug that inhibits reabsorption of sodium and chloride in the loop of Henle, thereby causing increased urinary output

nephron glomerulotubular units that are the working units of the kidney

nocturia urinary frequency at night

osmotic diuretic a drug that increases the osmotic pressure of glomerular filtrate, thereby inhibiting tubular reabsorption of water and electrolytes and increasing urinary output

potassium-sparing diuretic a drug that promotes excretion of water and sodium but inhibits the exchange of sodium for potassium

reabsorption the process by which substances are pulled back into the blood after waste products have been removed during the formation of urine

reticulocytes immature red blood cells

secretion the release of cell products, including hydrogen and potassium ions and acids and bases, into urine being formed

stress incontinence urine leakage during physical movements

thiazide diuretic a drug based on benzothiadiazine that blocks a pump that removes sodium and chloride together from the distal tubule

uremia the clinical syndrome resulting from renal dysfunction in which excessive products of protein metabolism are retained in the blood

urinary tract the group of organs that include the kidneys, ureters, bladder, and urethra, and that is involved in the production and transportation of urine

urinary tract infection (UTI) an infection caused by bacteria, usually *E. coli,* that enter via the urethra and progress up the urinary tract; characterized by the presence of bacteria in the urine with localized symptoms

Chapter Summary

Function of the Renal System

- Acute renal failure is a rapid reduction in kidney function resulting in accumulation of nitrogen and other waste. Uremia is the clinical syndrome resulting from renal dysfunction.

- Renal disease is divided into four stages: (1) loss of renal reserve, (2) renal insufficiency, (3) chronic renal failure, and (4) end-stage renal disease.
- Contrast dyes are the third most common cause of renal failure in hospitalized patients.

- Renal failure is commonly caused by prerenal, intrarenal, or postrenal events.
- Most renal patients show evidence of erythropoietin deficiency.
- Sucralfate and aluminum-containing antacids can cause aluminum toxicity in a patient on dialysis.
- Folic acid (vitamin B_9) is required for erythropoiesis.
- If a renal transplant is necessary, the patient must take drugs to prevent the rejection of the new organ. Mycophenolic acid (Myfortic) is indicated specifically to prevent rejection of the kidney.

Drugs for Urinary Tract Diseases and Disorders

- Methenamine (Cystex, Hiprex, Urex) has a local anesthetic effect on urinary tract mucosa.
- Pentosan polysulfate sodium (Elmiron) is the first oral therapy for interstitial cystitis. It is used for relief of bladder pain, presumably by exerting a protective effect on the bladder wall to reduce irritation and inflammation.
- Oxybutynin (Ditropan, Oxytrol) and tolterodine (Detrol) are urinary antispasmodics used to decrease urinary frequency. Tolterodine has greater selectivity for urinary bladder receptors than salivary receptors.
- UTIs are treated with antibiotics, some of which require only a short course to clear the infection.
- Used for prostatic disease, tamsulosin (Flomax) is an alpha-1 blocker but is more selective than terazosin (Hytrin).
- Nilutamide (Nilandron) is used for advanced prostate cancer.
- Flutamide (Eulexin) can cause gynecomastia.

Diuretics

- The primary action of diuretics is to rid the body of excess fluid and electrolytes.
- Diuretics have different mechanisms of action. They are classified by where and how they work in the kidney: thiazide diuretics, loop diuretics, potassium-sparing diuretics, carbonic anhydrase inhibitors, osmotic diuretics, and miscellaneous.
- Triamterene-hydrochlorothiazide (Dyazide, Maxzide) theoretically does not waste potassium. The tablet, Maxzide, is better absorbed than the capsule, Dyazide.

Drug List

The following drugs were discussed in this chapter. Each generic drug name is followed in parentheses by one or more brand names.

Renal Disease
cinacalcet (Sensipar)
darbepoetin alfa (Aranesp)
epoetin alfa, erythropoietin (Epogen, Procrit)
ergocalciferol, vitamin D
folic acid, vitamin B_9
iron dextran (INFeD)
iron sucrose (Venofer)
levocarnitine (Carnitor)
methoxy polyethylene glycol–epoetin beta (Mircera)
multiple vitamin complex

pyridoxine, vitamin B_6
sevelamer (Renagel, Renvela)

Renal Transplant Drugs
cyclosporine (Sandimmune)
mycophenolate (CellCept)
mycophenolic acid (Myfortic)

Urinary Problems
bethanechol (Urecholine)
darifenecin (Enablex)
duloxetine (Cymbalta)
flavoxate (Urispas)

oxybutynin (Ditropan*, Oxytrol)
pentosan polysulfate sodium (Elmiron)
propantheline (Pro-Banthine)
solifenacin (Vesicare)
tolterodine (Detrol)*
trospium (Sanctura)

Medications for UTIs

Antibiotics
amoxicillin (Amoxil, Trimox)
amoxicillin-clavulanate (Augmentin)
ampicillin (Principen)
ciprofloxacin (Cipro)
methenamine (Cystex, Hiprex, Urex)
nitrofurantoin (Macrobid, Macrodantin)
sulfamethoxazole-trimethoprim (Bactrim,
    Bactrim DS, Cotrim, Cotrim DS, Septra,
    Septra DS)

Urinary Analgesic
phenazopyridine (Azo-Standard, Uristat)

Prostatic Disease
alfuzosin (Uroxatral)
doxazosin (Cardura)
dutasteride (Avodart)
finasteride (Propecia, Proscar*)
flutamide (Eulexin)
goserelin (Zoladex)
leuprolide (Eligard, Lupron Depot, Viadur)
megestrol (Megace)
nilutamide (Nilandron)
prazosin (Minipress)
tamsulosin (Flomax)*
terazosin (Hytrin)

Diuretics

Thiazides
hydrochlorothiazide, HCTZ (Esidrix)*
methyclothiazide (Enduron)

Drugs Related to Thiazides
chlorthalidone (Hygroton)

Combinations
atenolol- hydrochlorothiazide (Tenorectic)*
bisoprolol-hydrochlorothiazide (Ziac)*
lisinopril-hydrochlorothiazide (Zestoretic)*
losartan-hydrochlorothiazide (Hyzaar)*
triamterene-hydrochlorothiazide (Dyazide,
    Maxzide)*

Loop Diuretics
bumetanide (Bumex)
ethacrynic acid (Edecrin)
furosemide (Lasix)*
torsemide (Demadex)

Potassium-Sparing Diuretics
amiloride (Midamor)
eplerenone (Inspra)
spironolactone* (Aldactone)
triamterene (Dyrenium)

Carbonic Anhydrase Inhibitors
acetazolamide (Diamox)
methazolamide (Neptazane)

Osmotic Diuretics
mannitol (Osmitrol)

Miscellaneous Diuretics
indapamide (Lozol)
metolazone (Zaroxolyn)

Chapter Review

Pharmaceuticals and Body Functions

Select the best answer from the choices given.

1. Anemia due to renal failure is caused by decreased
   a. somatostatin.
   b. erythropoietin.
   c. pyridoxine.
   d. folic acid.

2. Which drug listed is an implant?
   a. Zoladex
   b. Lupron Depot
   c. Megace
   d. Proscar

3. Elmiron is used as
   a. an aluminum-coating antacid.
   b. a urinary agent to relieve bladder pain.
   c. an alpha-1 blocker to decrease blood pressure.
   d. a diuretic to rid the body of excess fluid.

4. The primary action of diuretics is on the
   a. feet and hands.
   b. kidneys.
   c. heart.
   d. all of the above

5. Which class of diuretics blocks the reabsorption of sodium and chloride together in the distal tubule?
   a. carbonic anhydrase inhibitors
   b. loop diuretics
   c. thiazide diuretics
   d. potassium-sparing diuretics

6. Which class of diuretics inhibits reabsorption of sodium and chloride in the ascending loop of Henle and distal renal tubule?
   a. carbonic anhydrase inhibitors
   b. loop diuretics
   c. thiazide diuretics
   d. potassium-sparing diuretics

7. Which diuretic acts as an antagonist of aldosterone?
   a. acetazolamide
   b. furosemide
   c. hydrochlorothiazide
   d. spironolactone

8. Which diuretic has a brand name that indicates the time between doses?
   a. furosemide
   b. indapamide
   c. metolazone
   d. trichloromethiazide

9. Diuretics are combined with other drugs that lower blood pressure because
   a. the combination saves money
   b. the combination improves compliance
   c. drug companies do fewer trials
   d. prescribers only have to remember one name

10. Which class of drugs should not be used in BPH?
    a. diuretics
    b. alpha blockers
    c. TCAs
    d. antibiotics

The following statements are true or false. If the answer is false, rewrite the statement so it is true.

_____ 1. Maxzide turns the urine orange.

_____ 2. Minipress has a longer half-life than Hytrin.

_____ 3. It is a good idea to give a patient on dialysis an aluminum-containing antacid to prevent stress ulcers.

_____ 4. Renal disease has three stages.

_____ 5. Erythropoietin treats cystic fibrosis.

_____ 6. Patients in end-stage renal disease generally do not need iron replacement.

_____ 7. Methenamine works primarily as a bactericidal.

_____ 8. Urispas exerts a direct spasmolytic effect on smooth muscle, primarily in the urinary tract.

_____ 9. Urecholine is the first oral therapy for interstitial cystitis.

_____ 10. Some antibiotics require only a short course to treat a UTI.

Diseases and Drug Therapies

1. Define filtration, secretion, excretion, and reabsorption.

2. Why would a patient in end-stage renal disease need iron and folic acid?

3. List the four stages of renal disease.

4. Explain the difference between Urispas and Pro-Banthine.

5. Fill in the following chart with names of appropriate medications.

Thiazide Diuretics
Loop Diuretics
Potassium-Sparing Diuretics
Osmotic Diuretics
Carbonic Anhydrase Inhibitors
Miscellaneous Diuretics

Dispensing Medications

1. The following orders are sent from the ER.

    John Doe furosemide 40 mg STAT
    Pricilla Perkins Lasix 20 mg stat
    Peter Pumpkin 30 mg furosemide STAT

    The technician needs to draw up the doses and label them. How many mLs will each patient receive? Can all of the doses be drawn up from this bottle?

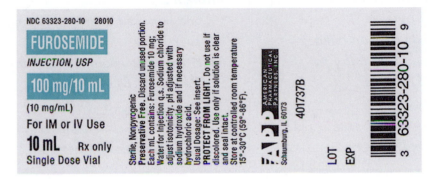

2. Dr. J. Bland has prescribed Macrodantin 100 mg four times daily to Ms. Belinda Bold. You need to dispense a 10 day supply with four refills. How many will you dispense, and which stickers will you put on the bottle? Prepare the label. You have only the 50 mg Macrodantin available.

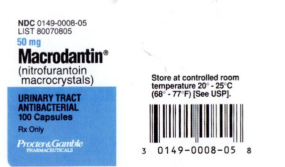

3. You receive the following prescriptions for a dialysis patient. What has the physician left off? How many of each of the following medications will you dispense for 8 weeks?
    Folic acid comes in tablets of 1 mg.
    B_6 comes in 180 mg doses.
    # of folic acid ___
    # of B_6 ___

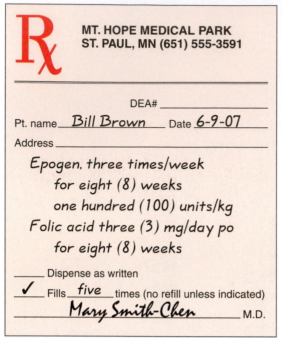

Rx MT. HOPE MEDICAL PARK
ST. PAUL, MN (651) 555-3591

DEA# _____

Pt. name _Bill Brown_ Date _6-9-07_

Address _____

Epogen, three times/week
   for eight (8) weeks
   one hundred (100) units/kg
Folic acid three (3) mg/day po
   for eight (8) weeks

____ Dispense as written
✓ Fills _five_ times (no refill unless indicated)
Mary Smith-Chen M.D.

Rx MT. HOPE MEDICAL PARK
ST. PAUL, MN (651) 555-3591

DEA# _____

Pt. name _Bill Brown_ Date _6-9-07_

Address _____

Vitamin B_6
   one hundred eighty (180) mg po
   every day
multi-purpose vitamin every day
   for eight (8) weeks

____ Dispense as written
✓ Fills _five_ times (no refill unless indicated)
Mary Smith-Chen M.D.

Internet Research

Use the Internet to complete the following assignments.

1. Benign prostatic hyperplasia (BPH) is a medical condition that is common in older men. Importantly, this condition must be differentiated from prostate cancer. Use the Internet to find information on prostate cancer screening programs. What is the screening test called, and how does it work? Who should be screened? Does BPH affect screening? List your Internet sources.

2. Diuretics are often used to treat high blood pressure. Find one or more Internet sites that describe how diuretics help to treat this condition. Write a paragraph summarizing that information. List your Internet sources.

What Would You Do?

1. Every time you fill Ms. Smith's Dyazide, the computer alerts you that she is also taking potassium and this is very serious interaction.

Drugs for Cardiovascular Diseases

12

Learning Objectives

- Understand the cardiovascular system.
- Know the drugs and treatment for each type of heart disease.
- Recognize anticoagulant and antiplatelet drugs and know their functions.

- Discuss stroke and the drugs used to treat it.
- Identify drugs used to treat hyperlipidemia and understand its role in heart disease and stroke treatment.

Preview chapter terms and definitions.

Cardiovascular diseases (those affecting the heart and blood vessels) account for significant morbidity and mortality. Cardiovascular problems include arrhythmias, congestive heart failure, myocardial infarction, angina, hypertension, coagulation, and excessive cholesterol in the blood. Many causative factors can be modified by lifestyle changes, and some are amenable to prophylaxis. Drugs have been developed to help manage these diseases. Drug therapy discussed in this chapter includes antiarrhythmic, antianginal, antihypertensive, anticoagulant, antiplatelet, and antihyperlipidemic agents. Many of these drugs can be used to treat more than one cardiovascular problem.

The Heart and Causative Factors of Cardiovascular Disease

The heart has three functional parts: the cardiac muscle (myocardium), conducting system, and blood supply. Figure 12.1 shows the functional anatomy of the heart, and Figure 12.2 shows the internal heart structure and vessels leading to and exiting from the heart. Cardiovascular (CV) disease can involve any or all of these functional parts.

FIGURE 12.1
Functional Anatomy of the Heart

(a) cardiac muscle (b) conducting system (c) blood supply.

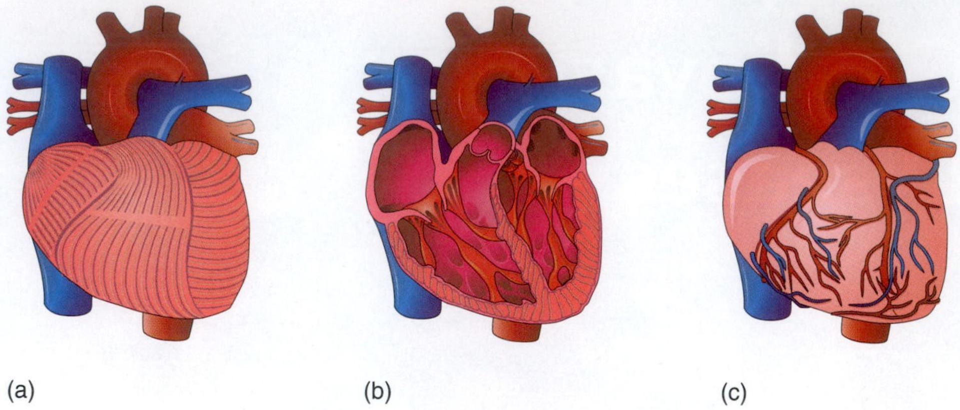
(a)
(b)
(c)

FIGURE 12.2
Internal Structures of the Heart

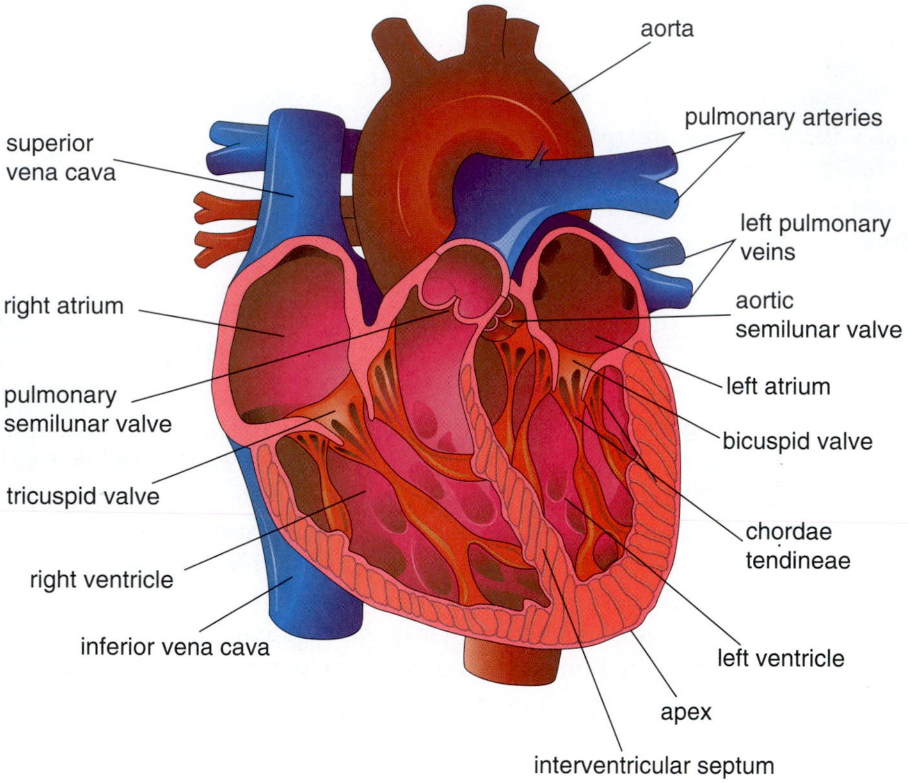
aorta
pulmonary arteries
superior vena cava
left pulmonary veins
aortic semilunar valve
right atrium
left atrium
pulmonary semilunar valve
bicuspid valve
tricuspid valve
chordae tendineae
right ventricle
inferior vena cava
left ventricle
apex
interventricular septum

A normal heartbeat is the result of a coordinated series of electrical events. It begins in the membranes of cells in the **sinoatrial (SA) node,** often called the pacemaker. Between beats these membranes are polarized; that is, the inside of the cell is at a negative voltage relative to the outside. The beat originates when ion channels in the cell membrane open to allow positively charged sodium and calcium ions to flow into the cell, making the voltage positive instead of negative (**depolarization**). Other channels then open to allow positively charged potassium ions to flow out of the cell, making the voltage negative again (**repolarization**). The resulting electrical burst, known as an **action potential,** propagates through the conduction system to the muscle cells of the myocardium. When the action potential arrives at a myocardial cell, it too depolarizes with a rapid inflow of sodium and a slower inflow of calcium (which is what triggers the muscle to contract) and repolarizes with an outflow of potassium.

If the depolarizing and repolarizing flows were the only ion flows, the cell would run out of potassium and accumulate huge amounts of sodium and calcium. Other proteins in the cell membrane continually restore the balance by using energy to pump sodium and calcium out and potassium in simultaneously.

The conduction system is arranged so that the action potential first arrives at the atria, which contract and pump blood received from veins into the ventricles, and then travels through the **atrioventricular (AV) node** to reach the ventricles, which pump blood out into the arteries. The first arteries to branch off the main artery from the left ventricle are the coronary arteries, which carry oxygen and nutrients to the various parts of the heart itself.

Various factors contribute to the development of heart disease. Some are genetically inherited, whereas others are within the individual's control. Many cardiovascular problems develop because of poor health habits; however, one can be genetically predisposed to develop these problems. Even if a person has a genetic tendency toward heart disease, proper diet, exercise, and rest can facilitate healthy heart functioning and prolong good health and extend life for a long time.

Predetermined factors include heredity, gender, and increasing age.

- **Heredity:** Children of parents with CV disease have a higher risk of developing heart disease. Ethnicity also plays a role. For example, African Americans are two to three times more likely than other ethnic groups to have high blood pressure.
- **Gender:** Men face a greater risk of heart attack than women until age 55. At age 55, a woman's risk increases tenfold and may surpass a man's if she smokes or has other conditions that cause CV disease.
- **Increasing age:** Almost 55% of all heart attack victims are age 65 or older. Of those who die, more than 80% are over age 65.

The following factors can be influenced by lifestyle modification.

- **Cigarette smoking:** Smokers have more than twice the risk of heart attack as nonsmokers. A smoker who has a heart attack is also more likely to die from it.
- **High blood pressure:** High blood pressure stresses the heart over time and increases the risk of stroke and heart attack. However, a nutritious diet, regular exercise, weight loss, reduction of salt intake, and drugs can lower blood pressure.
- **High blood cholesterol levels:** Heart disease is related to rising levels of blood cholesterol. Too much cholesterol in the blood contributes to a buildup of plaque on the inner walls of the arteries that feed the heart and reduces blood flow to the heart. A diet low in cholesterol and fats helps to lower blood cholesterol levels. Drugs can also lower blood cholesterol.

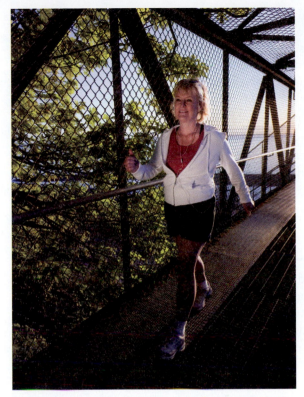

Regular exercise, a healthy diet, and adequate rest facilitate heart health and extended life expectancy.

- **Obesity:** Obesity puts added strain on the heart. It can also increase blood pressure and blood cholesterol levels and lead to diabetes. When a person is obese, the blood volume increases, putting additional strain on the heart.
- **Diabetes:** Diabetics are prone to develop heart disease because diabetes leads to vascular problems. The disease sharply increases the risk of heart attack. Proper diet and weight as well as exercise and drugs can help keep diabetes in check.

As this list indicates, lifestyle modification plays a critical role in reducing the risk of heart disease. The value of smoking cessation, dietary modifications, weight control, physical exercise, and adherence to a drug regimen should not be underestimated. The treatment of cardiovascular diseases requires permanent changes in lifestyle as well as drug therapy.

Angina

Angina pectoris (sometimes referred to simply as *angina*) is chest pain due to an imbalance between oxygen supply and oxygen demand. Oxygen demand is directly related to heart rate, strength of contraction, and resistance to blood flow. In angina, the diminished blood supply to the heart does not cause irreversible changes related to obstruction or narrowing of coronary arteries as occur in atherosclerosis, arterial spasm, pulmonary hypertension, or cardiac hypertrophy (enlargement of the heart).

There are three types of angina.

- **Stable angina** is characterized by effort-induced pain from physical activity or emotional stress. This pain is relieved by rest and is usually predictable and reproducible.
- **Unstable angina** is characterized by pain that occurs with increasing frequency, diminishes the patient's ability to work, and has a decreasing response to treatment. It may signal an oncoming myocardial infarction.
- **Variant angina** is characterized by pain due to coronary artery spasm. This pain may occur at certain times of the day, but it is not induced by stress.

Symptoms and Risk Factors of Angina

The characteristic symptom of angina is severe chest discomfort, which may be described as heaviness, pressure, tightness, choking, a squeezing sensation, or a combination of these. Other symptoms may include sweating, dizziness, and dyspnea (shortness of breath). Diagnosis is made from the physical examination, resting and exercise ECGs, coronary angiogram, and radioisotope study. The ECG may be normal, but usually the T wave, discussed later in the chapter, is flat or inverted. Anginal pain is usually brief and precipitated by exercise or emotional stress.

The risk factors for angina are

- advanced age
- coronary artery disease
- hypertension
- increased serum glucose levels (diabetes)
- increased serum lipoprotein levels
- obesity
- smoking
- type A personality

Factors that may initiate an attack of angina include

- cold weather
- emotions
- heavy meals, which cause blood flow to the gut to increase, resulting in decreased flow to the brain and heart
- hypoglycemia
- pain
- smoking (nicotine causes arterial constriction and contributes to arteriosclerosis)

Angina is characterized by chest discomfort that occurs predictably and is relieved with rest or nitroglycerin. Treatment goals are to reduce symptoms and prevent heart attacks.

Antianginal Drugs

There are three major classes of drugs that are used in the treatment of angina: beta blockers, calcium channel blockers, and nitrates. A fourth type of drug, ranolazine (Ranexa), is a metabolic modifier and is distinct from the drugs of the other three groups. These drugs are listed in Table 12.1.

Beta Blockers As described in Chapter 6, in response to increased anxiety, physical activity, or emotional stress, the sympathetic nervous system stimulates the release of catecholamines (the class of neurotransmitters that includes epinephrine and norepinephrine). The action of these neurotransmitters on the beta-1 receptors, in particular, increases heart rate and contractile force. A **beta blocker** is a drug that inhibits this response; beta blockers are similar in molecular structure to catecholamines and compete for the same receptor sites. Beta blockers are used in angina pectoris because of their effectiveness in slowing the heart rate, decreasing myocardial contractility, and lowering blood pressure, particularly during exercise. All of these actions reduce oxygen demand; thus, beta blockers reduce the frequency and severity of angina attacks.

There are two types of beta receptors—beta-1 and beta-2—and a drug that blocks both is considered to be nonselective. In choosing a drug for the heart, a drug with more beta-1 than beta-2 blockage is preferred, as beta-1 receptors are found more abundantly in the heart. Drugs that block beta-2 receptors can adversely affect respiration in asthmatic patients. Beta blockers that are selected more readily by beta-1 receptors than by beta-2 receptors are referred to as cardioselective. Certain agents in this class exhibit membrane-stabilizing and intrinsic sympathomimetic activity.

Beta blockers are also used to treat arrhythmias and hypertension and are most commonly used following a myocardial infarction. They have been shown to improve morbidity and mortality rates. While most are contraindicated in congestive heart failure (CHF), carvedilol (Coreg) has been approved even for that disease state.

Most adverse reactions to beta blockers are mild and transient and rarely require withdrawal of therapy. The most common is tiredness. Beta blockers should not be withdrawn abruptly. Dosage should be reduced gradually over 1 to 2 weeks.

The primary side effect of beta blockers is **bradycardia** (slowed heart rate); they also mask symptoms of hypoglycemia and hyperthyroidism. Diabetics should avoid beta blockers because of their hypoglycemia-masking effects. Beta blockers should also be used with caution in patients with bronchospastic disease because they may inhibit the bronchodilating effects of endogenous catecholamine.

Acebutolol (Sectral) and **pindolol (Visken)** are beta blockers that have intrinsic sympathomimetic activity and so produce less reduction in heart rate than other beta blockers. Side effects are bradycardia, increased airway resistance, fluid retention, masked signs of hypoglycemia, and depression.

TABLE 12.1 Most Commonly Used Drugs in the Treatment of Angina

Generic Name	Pronunciation	Dosage Form	Brand Name	Dispensing Status
Beta Blockers				
acebutolol	a-se-BYOO-toe-lawl	capsule	Sectral	Rx
atenolol	a-TEN-oh-lawl	IV, tablet	Tenormin	Rx
betaxolol	be-TAX-oh-lawl	ophthalmic, tablet	Kerlone	Rx
bisoprolol	bis-OE-proe-lawl	tablet	Zebeta	Rx
carvedilol	KAR-ve-dil-awl	tablet	Coreg	Rx
esmolol	ES-moe-lawl	IV	Brevibloc	Rx
labetalol	la-BET-a-lawl	IV, tablet	Normodyne, Trandate	Rx
metoprolol	me-TOE-proe-lawl	IV, tablet	Lopressor, Toprol-XL	Rx
nadolol	naye-DOE-lawl	tablet	Corgard	Rx
nebivolol	neh-BIV-oe-lawl	tablet	Bystolic	Rx
pindolol	PIN-doe-lawl	tablet	Visken	Rx
propranolol	proe-PRAN-oh-lawl	capsule, IV, oral liquid, tablet	Inderal	Rx
sotalol	SOE-ta-lawl	tablet	Betapace	Rx
timolol	TYE-moe-lawl	tablet	Blocadren	Rx
Nitrates				
isosorbide dinitrate	eye-soe-SOR-bide dye-NYE-trate	capsule, tablet	Dilatrate-SR, Isordil	Rx
isosorbide mononitrate	eye-soe-SOR-bide mon-oh-NYE-trate	tablet	Imdur, Ismo	Rx
nitroglycerin	nye-troe-GLISS-er-in	IV, ointment, pump spray, tablet, trans-dermal patch	Minitran, Nitrolingual, Nitrostat, NitroDur	Rx
Calcium Channel Blockers				
amlodipine	am-LOE-di-peen	tablet	Norvasc	Rx
diltiazem	dil-TYE-a-zem	capsule, IV, tablet	Cardizem, Dilacor XR	Rx
felodipine	fe-LOE-di-peen	tablet	Plendil	Rx
isradipine	iz-RAD-i-peen	capsule	DynaCirc	Rx
nicardipine	nye-KAR-de-peen	capsule, injection	Cardene	Rx
nifedipine	nye-FED-i-peen	capsule	Procardia	Rx
nisoldipine	nye-SOLE-di-peen	tablet	Sular	Rx
verapamil	ver-AP-a-mil	capsule, IV, tablet	Calan, Covera HS, Isoptin, Verelan	Rx
Metabolic Modifier				
ranolozine	ra-NOE-la-zeen	tablet	Ranexa	Rx

Carvedilol (Coreg), the first beta blocker approved for congestive heart failure, is a nonselective beta blocker with vasodilating effects. Physicians usually avoid beta blockers when treating congestive heart failure because these drugs slow the heart and worsen the condition. However, studies indicate that beta blockers can improve left ventricular function by blocking excessive adrenergic stimulation in patients with mild to moderate CHF. The patient is started on a low dose, which is slowly increased. If the drug is taken with food, dizziness will be reduced. It can be used alone or in conjunction with other agents, especially thiazide diuretics, in the management of hypertension. Beta blockers are contraindicated in patients with severe CHF.

Labetalol (Normodyne, Trandate) is an alpha blocker and nonspecific beta blocker. Pharmacy technicians should watch for a patient with prescriptions for both of these brands of labetalol. Prescribers often do not realize that the two brands are the same drug, so a patient could risk getting a double dose. Side effects are the same as for acebutolol and pindolol.

Nebivolol (Bystolic) causes vasodilation by increasing the production of nitric acid. In this way it is different from other beta blockers. Nebivolol is approved only for hypertension. It reduces vascular resistance and large-artery stiffness. The dosage should be reduced gradually when the patient stops taking the drug. Nebivolol cannot be discontinued abruptly.

Sotalol (Betapace) is indicated for the treatment of documented ventricular arrhythmia (e.g., sustained ventricular tachycardia, discussed later in this chapter) that, in the judgment of the physician, is life threatening. The side effects are bradycardia, mental depression, and decreased sexual ability.

Nitrates The drugs most used for angina are nitrates. They relax vascular smooth muscle (venous more than arterial), which reduces venous return to the heart (**preload**) and cardiac filling and decreases tension in the heart walls. Nitrates dilate coronary vessels, allowing blood flow to redistribute to ischemic tissues. Because peripheral vasodilation decreases preload, nitroglycerin is also beneficial in the treatment of pulmonary edema in congestive heart failure. Arterial vasodilation decreases arterial impedance (**afterload**), thereby lessening left ventricular work and aiding the failing heart.

Technicians need to be on the alert for patients who get prescriptions for any form of nitrate and any of the drugs for erectile dysfunction (ED): sildenafil (Viagra, also branded as Revatio for use in treating hypertension), vardenafil (Levitra), or tadalafil (Cialis). These patients typically use different prescribers to get the drugs for ED and do not tell those prescribers they are on nitrates as well. This omission can result in a deadly interaction.

Nitroglycerin is the drug of choice for acute attacks of angina and is taken sublingually. If the pain does not subside within 5 minutes after taking nitroglycerin, the patient should call 911. The spray is applied under the tongue, one to two sprays every 3 to 5 minutes, with a maximum of three doses in a 15 minute period. Both the spray and the tablets produce a stinging sensation under the tongue. Only the sublingual and translingual routes should be used for acute attacks. Nitroglycerin may also be used as a prophylaxis; in this case, the drug is taken a few minutes before the activity or stress that might cause an attack.

Nitroglycerin patches (NitroDur) should not remain on the skin for more than 24 hours. There should be a patch-free time, usually when the patient is sleeping, or tolerance will develop. The label should instruct the patient in this procedure.

Nitroglycerin can cause severe headaches when first taken by a patient; aspirin or acetaminophen may provide relief. To avoid headaches, the dose of nitroglycerin can be reduced or, if taken as a patch or ointment, it can be placed lower on the body and gradually moved to the chest as the patient acclimates to the medication. Nitroglycerin can also cause orthostatic hypotension when first used, so patients should be advised to move slowly, especially when changing from a sitting or lying position. The drug can also cause flushing. When nitroglycerin must be discontinued, the drug should be tapered and not stopped abruptly.

Nitroglycerin whether capsules or sublingual tablets is sold in the original amber glass container. *Do not repackage this drug,* because it adheres to soft plastic, which causes nitroglycerin to lose its effectiveness. The patient should replenish the sublingual tablets every 3 months whether any have been used or not and discard any remaining drug.

Isosorbide dinitrate (Dilatrate-SR, Isordil) is used for the same purposes as nitroglycerin—the prevention of angina and CHF. It is easily confused with Dilacor XR, which is diltiazem, a calcium channel blocker. The technician should be careful, as they are very different drugs.

Calcium Channel Blockers A **calcium channel blocker** impedes the movement of calcium ions into cardiac muscle cells through slow channels during depolarization. Blockage of the slow channels thus reduces calcium influx. Because the calcium is what triggers the actual contraction of the muscle, the calcium channel blocker thereby reduces cell contractility and thus reduces the requirements of the cell for energy and oxygen. Moreover, calcium channel blockers also relax coronary vascular smooth muscle, allowing coronary arteries and arterioles to dilate, which in turn increases oxygen delivery. Thus the oxygen demand of heart muscle tissue are reduced while the oxygen supply is increased.

Calcium channel blockers are the agents of choice for most supraventricular tachyarrhythmias (rapid, irregular atrial beats) and successfully convert most to normal (sinus) rhythm. Some calcium channel blockers slow conduction through the atrio-ventricular (AV) node, slow sinoatrial (SA) node action, and relax coronary artery smooth muscle. They are used to control fast ventricular rates in patients with atrial flutter and atrial fibrillation. Side effects include bradycardia, hypotension, heart block, cardiac failure, nausea, constipation, headache, dizziness, and fatigue, all of which lead to poor compliance. The patient does not understand the drug is helping them because he or she feels worse after taking these drugs.

Some of these drugs should be taken with food, and caffeine should be limited. The most common side effect is constipation. The patient should notify the physician in the event of swelling hands and feet or shortness of breath. Some patients experience drowsiness when they begin taking a calcium channel blocker.

Calcium channel blockers are also first-line therapy for hypertension. They reduce blood pressure by dilating the arterioles, which leads to reduced peripheral resistance to blood flow and reduced energy consumption and oxygen requirements. Diltiazem and verapamil also slow calcium movement into myocardial cells, thus reducing contraction ability, coupled with lower energy and oxygen usage. Other channel blockers act only on vascular smooth muscle and lack antiarrhythmic activity. Calcium channel blockers or diuretics are also used to treat isolated systolic hypertension.

Verapamil (Covera HS) is a timed-release product designed for bedtime dosing. It is approved for either angina or hypertension. The tablets do not release medication until approximately 4 to 5 hours after they have been swallowed. The drug is pumped out of two laser holes in the tablet. Patients may see a ghost tablet in the stool.

Metabolic Modifier **Ranolazine (Ranexa)** is indicated for chronic angina. Conventional angina drugs reduce cardiac oxygen demand, but ranolazine is a metabolic modifier; that is, it assists the heart to generate energy more efficiently by allowing

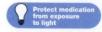
Protect medication from exposure to light

Warning

Dilatrate-SR and Dilacor XR (a calcium channel blocker) are often confused.

Warning

Nicardipine, nifedipine (two calcium channel blockers used in cardiovascular disease), and nimodipine (a calcium channel blocker used in stroke) could easily be confused.

Warning

Cardene (nicardipine) and Cardizem (diltiazem) are often confused.

Warning

Cardene can look (or sound) like codeine.

the heart to function despite a decrease in oxygen. Ranolazine is used as add-on therapy for patients for whom the other drugs do not work. It should be used with amlodipine, beta blockers, or nitrates. Ranolazine is produced as a light orange, oblong shaped, extended release tablet, which cannot be cut or broken in half and must be swallowed whole. It may be taken without regard to meals. Because ranolazine has many interactions, it is not used as first-line therapy. Ranolazine should not be given with simvastatin, because it can double plasma concentration of the latter drug.

Arrhythmia

An **arrhythmia** is any variation from the normal rhythm of the heart. Heart rate and/ or rhythm abnormalities occur when the heartbeat is too slow or too fast or when the contractions of the ventricles and atria are not synchronized.

Heart Rates and Rhythms

Normal cardiac rhythm is generated by the sinoatrial (SA) node at a rate of approximately 70 to 80 beats per minute. This rate exceeds the rate that can be produced by other potential pacemaking automatic (spontaneously depolarizing) cells, such as the atrioventricular (AV) node, the AV bundle (also called the bundle of His), and the Purkinje fibers (see Figure 12.3). An electrocardiogram (ECG) records and documents the signals sent through the conducting system of the heart, as shown in Figure 12.4. The QT interval, shown in the electrocardiographic recording in the figure, is a period in which the heart is refractory (nonresponsive) to all but the most powerful signals, if at all.

FIGURE 12.3
Conduction System of the Heart

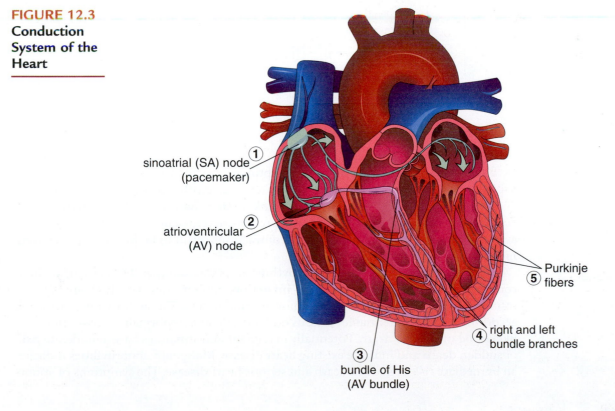

sinoatrial (SA) node (1) (pacemaker)

atrioventricular (2) (AV) node

Purkinje (5) fibers

right and left (4) bundle branches

bundle of His (3) (AV bundle)

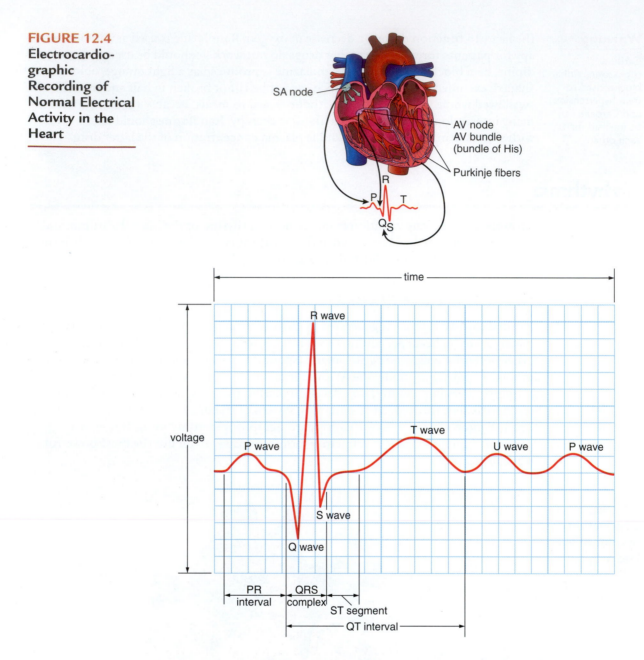

FIGURE 12.4
Electrocardio-graphic Recording of Normal Electrical Activity in the Heart

When the SA node works at less than optimal capacity, when conduction is interrupted, or when other areas become hyperexcitable, another discharging area may become the dominant pacemaker. A pacemaker other than the SA node is termed an **ectopic pacemaker.** Figure 12.5 shows a premature ventricular contraction, one example of an ectopic focus. Premature contractions result in **tachycardia** (excessively high heart rate), flutter, or fibrillation.

Table 12.2 shows abnormal heart rhythms and rates and their ECG tracings. These conditions may be caused by ischemia, infarction, or alteration of body chemicals resulting in nonautomatic cells becoming automatic cells. The abnormalities are rated according to their potential for serious outcome. Benign abnormalities have a low likelihood of sudden death. Potentially malignant abnormalities have a moderate risk of sudden death and indicate existing heart disease. Malignant abnormalities indicate an immediate risk of sudden death and serious heart disease. The symptoms of abnor-

FIGURE 12.5
Premature Ventricular Contraction

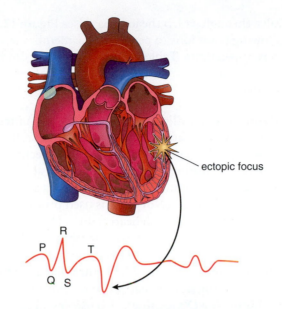

ectopic focus

TABLE 12.2   Abnormal Heart Rhythms

Arrhythmia	Beats per Minute	Electrocardiogram
tachycardia	150–250	
bradycardia	<60	
atrial flutter	200–350	
atrial fibrillation	>350	
premature atrial contraction	variable	
premature ventricular contraction	variable	
ventricular fibrillation	variable	

mal heart rhythms or rates include palpitations, syncope (loss of consciousness), light-headedness, visual disturbances, pallor (paleness), cyanosis (bluish skin discoloration), weakness, sweating, chest pain, and hypotension.

Pharmaceutical Treatment of Abnormal Heart Rates and Rhythms

Pharmaceutical treatment for arrhythmias is directed at preventing these life-threatening conditions by restoring sinus (normal) rhythm. The various classes of antiarrhythmic drugs have characteristic electrophysiologic effects on the myocardium and the conducting system. Some drugs influence the heart rate directly or indirectly by affecting the movement of ions into or out of the cell. The excitability of the cells of the SA node is influenced by the permeability of the cell membrane to sodium and calcium ions. The sodium and calcium ions cross the cell membrane through openings called ion channels, which are actually protein molecules that are sensitive to specific electrical and chemical conditions. In effect, one can think of an ion channel as a gate or valve through which the ions pass (see Figure 12.6). Drugs may act to close the valve, allowing fewer ions to penetrate the membrane, or to open the valve, allowing more ions to penetrate. Table 12.3 lists the most commonly used antiarrhythmic agents.

Beta blockers and calcium channel blockers were discussed in the discussion of angina.

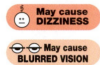
Membrane-Stabilizing Agents (Class I) A **membrane-stabilizing agent** slows the movement of sodium ions into myocardial cells, thus requiring a stronger signal to trigger an action potential, which is the electrical transmission developed in a muscle or nerve cell during activity. The reduced ability to generate an action potential will dampen out potential abnormal rhythms and heartbeats.

Disopyramide (Norpace) is used primarily on ventricular arrhythmias but is avoided in patients with heart failure. Disopyramide is an anticholinergic, so dry mouth, urinary retention, constipation, and blurred vision are side effects.

Flecainide (Tambocor) prolongs refractory periods, action potential duration, and QT interval. It is used for ventricular arrhythmias. The side effects are dizziness, blurred vision, tremor, nausea, and vomiting.

Lidocaine (Xylocaine), also used as a local anesthetic, reduces the ability of myocardial cells to respond to stimulation. It is the drug of choice for emergency IV therapy. Lidocaine is effective on the ventricles but has little effect on the atria. It must be given intravenously for premature ventricular contractions (PVCs) associated with myocardial infarction (MI).

Mexiletine (Mexitil) has action similar to lidocaine. It is used for ventricular tachycardia but is more effective when used with another drug. Adverse effects include gastrointestinal and neurologic symptoms and elevated liver enzyme levels.

Moricizine (Ethmozine) is used only in life-threatening ventricular arrhythmias. It slows conduction through the nodes and bundle; however, it may cause new arrhythmias, hypotension, tremor, anxiety, urinary retention, hyperventilation, apnea, and asthma.

Phenytoin (Dilantin) decreases the refractory period (time the myocardium is unresponsive to input signals), action potential duration, and the repolarization of the ventricles, called the QT interval (shown in Figure 12.4). It is used on resistant arrhythmias and arrhythmias caused by digoxin toxicity. Adverse effects include cardiovascular collapse and central nervous system (CNS) and respiratory depression. Phenytoin is also an anticonvulsant agent.

FIGURE 12.6
The "Gatekeeper" Role of Cardiovascular Drugs

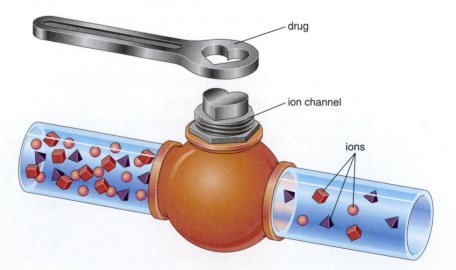

drug

ion channel

ions

Procainamide (Procanbid, Pronestyl) is very similar to quinidine, which is discussed below.

Propafenone (Rythmol) is used only for life-threatening arrhythmias, because it may cause new arrhythmias or worsen existing ones. Propafenone may also worsen congestive heart failure (CHF) and alter pacemakers. Patients should be on a cardiac monitor at the beginning of therapy or with any increase in dosage.

Quinidine acts to slow the SA node rate and AV conduction in atrial and ventricular arrhythmias. Adverse effects include **thrombocytopenia** (a decrease in the bone marrow production of blood platelets) and cinchonism (headache, blurred vision, tinnitus, confusion, and nausea). Disopyramide and procainamide, discussed above, are similar to quinidine. Procainamide and quinidine are so similar that sometimes they can be used interchangeably. However, procainamide is less effective for atrial arrhythmias than quinidine.

👓👓 **May cause BLURRED VISION**

TABLE 12.3   Most Commonly Used Antiarrhythmic Agents

Generic Name	Pronunciation	Dosage Form	Brand Name	Dispensing Status
Membrane-Stabilizing Agents (Class I)				
disopyramide	dye-soe-PEER-a-mide	capsule	Norpace	Rx
flecainide	FLEK-a-nide	tablet	Tambocor	Rx
lidocaine	LYE-doe-kane	IV	Xylocaine	Rx
mexiletine	mex-IL-a-teen	capsule	Mexitil	Rx
moricizine	mor-ISS-iz-een	tablet	Ethmozine	Rx
phenytoin	FEN-i-toyn	capsule, IV, oral liquid, tablet	Dilantin	Rx
procainamide	proe-KANE-a-mide	capsule, injection, IV, tablet	Procanbid, Pronestyl	Rx
propafenone	proe-pa-FEE-none	tablet	Rythmol	Rx
quinidine	KWIN-i-deen	injection, IV, tablet	(none)	Rx
tocainide	toe-KAY-nide	tablet	Tonocard	Rx
Beta Blockers (Class II), see Table 12.1				
Potassium Channel Blockers (Class III)				
amiodarone	am-ee-OH-da-rone	IV, tablet	Cordarone	Rx
dofetilide	doe-FET-il-ide	capsule	Tikosyn	Rx
Calcium Channel Blockers (Class IV), see Table 12.1				
Other Antiarrhythmic Agents				
atropine	AT-roe-peen	injection, IV, tablet	(none)	Rx
digoxin	di-JOX-in	capsule, IV, tablet	Lanoxicaps, Lanoxin	Rx
isoproterenol	eye-soe-proe-TER-e-nawl	IV	Isuprel	Rx
Antidote for Digoxin Toxicity				
digoxin immune Fab	di-JOX-in i-MYUN fab	injection (powder to be dissolved in liquid)	Digibind	Rx

Tocainide (Tonocard) suppresses and prevents symptomatic life-threatening ventricular arrhythmias. It blocks both the initiation and the conduction of nerve impulses by decreasing the neuronal membrane's permeability to sodium ions, which inhibits depolarization with a resultant blockade of conduction. The primary side effects of tocainide are tremor, nausea, dizziness, and confusion.

Potassium Channel Blockers (Class III) Potassium channel blockers delay repolarization of atrial and ventricular fibers by blocking the flow of potassium across cell membranes.

Amiodarone (Cordarone) is used for atrial and ventricular arrhythmias that do not respond to other medications. It is very effective, but it is not considered a first-line drug, because of the high incidence of significant and potentially fatal toxicities. It is best reserved for patients with ventricular arrhythmias and should not be used routinely in CHF. Establishing control may take several days to several weeks with the IV and up to 1 to 4 weeks with the oral dose. Many patients experience hypotension. The IV drip must be mixed in a glass bottle in D₅W, unless the facility uses the polyolefin bags. During a crisis, the "push" will be put in a bag of D₅W; then the drip will be mixed in glass. Interactions can occur for several weeks or longer after cessation of amiodarone. Some patients will develop a slate blue rash from this drug. Because some of the side effects can be fatal, it is imperative that the prescriber carefully monitor the patient and order appropriate lab work.

Dofetilide (Tikosyn) is used to maintain normal sinus rhythm in patients with atrial fibrillation/atrial flutter of greater than 1 week duration and who have been converted to normal sinus rhythm. The drug itself can induce arrhythmias. Dofetilide must be initiated or reinitiated in a hospital setting. The patient must be placed in a facility that can provide monitoring and resuscitation for a period of 3 days. Dofetilide is available only to hospitals and to prescribers who have received training in the dosing and initiation of this drug. T.I.P.S. (Tikosyn in Pharmacy Systems) is the pharmacy system designed to allow retail pharmacies to dispense the drug, once the patient has been initiated in the hospital. Pharmacies must educate their staff, document that the prescriber is enrolled in the program, and document that the patient has been properly initiated before dispensing the drug.

Other Agents Other agents used to treat abnormal heart rates have different mechanisms of action.

Atropine is an anticholinergic agent that decreases the effect of vagal mediated parasympathetic tone (see Chapter 6), allowing sympathetic action to take over. It is used in bradycardia, or heart rates below 60 beats per minute. Low doses may worsen the bradycardia, whereas high doses may cause cardioacceleration (a rate that is too high), which increases oxygen demand, resulting in ischemia and leading to arrhythmias. Atropine is also used as a preoperative medication to inhibit salivation and secretions during surgery.

Digoxin (Lanoxicaps, Lanoxin) is the most important drug in managing atrial flutter and fibrillation. It does not convert atrial fibrillation to sinus rhythm, but it slows ventricular rate and treats cardiac failure. Digoxin is a much-used drug for treating CHF as well as atrial fibrillation and flutter. It has the following mechanisms of action.

- It increases the force of contraction.
- It increases the effective refractory period of the AV node (slows AV node stimulation).
- It affects the SA node, increasing automaticity due to ion imbalance (direct stimulation).

Digoxin is used to restore the force of myocardial contraction without increasing oxygen demands and to slow ventricle response to stimulation by reducing AV node stimulation.

Digoxin should be used with caution because of the possibility of systemic accumulation of the drug. Patients who take digoxin commonly experience "digitalis" toxicity, commonly referred to as "dig" (pronounced "didge") toxicity. This is especially true of elderly patients. The patient becomes nauseated, has vertigo, experiences general weakness, and may see yellow-green halos around objects. The three primary signs of digitalis toxicity are nausea, vomiting, and arrhythmias. If these occur, the drug should be withdrawn immediately. **Digoxin immune Fab (Digibind)** is an antidote for digitalis toxicity. It is an antibody fragment that binds to digoxin, inactivating the drug, and is then excreted by the kidneys.

Isoproterenol (Isuprel) dilates coronary vessels. It is used parenterally in ventricular arrhythmias due to AV nodal block, or bradyarrhythmias (slow, irregular heartbeats). It may be used temporarily in third-degree AV block until pacemaker insertion. It increases heart rate and contractility.

Congestive Heart Failure

Figure 12.7 shows the normal flow of blood through the heart. In **congestive heart failure** (**CHF**), a form of heart failure (HF), the pumping ability of the heart can no longer meet the metabolic needs of the body's tissues. The heart pumps less blood than it receives. Consequently, blood accumulates in the chambers and stretches the walls. Less blood circulates to the body organs. The kidneys, which are sensitive to reduced oxygen, retain water and electrolytes, which resuts in an increase in blood

FIGURE 12.7
Blood Flow Through the Heart

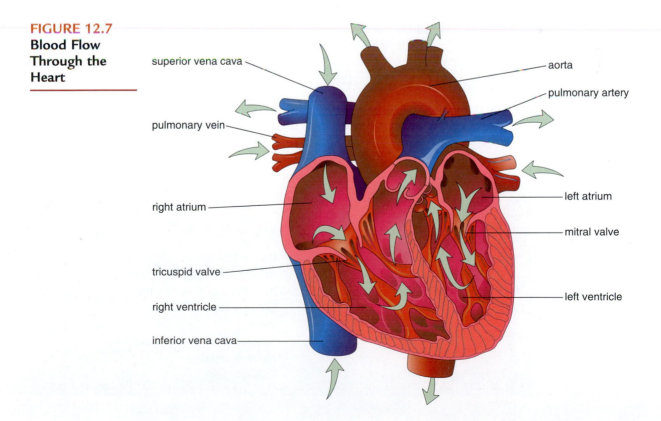

superior vena cava

aorta

pulmonary artery

pulmonary vein

right atrium

left atrium

mitral valve

tricuspid valve

right ventricle

left ventricle

inferior vena cava

volume. The result is edema, or the accumulation of fluid in the body tissues, especially the pulmonary vessels or the abdominal organs. Congestive heart failure affects 10% of the population over 75 years of age. It can result in death from either progressive failure of the heart or sudden cardiac death.

In the normal heart, contraction is directly proportional to the length or stretch of the cardiac muscle cells. Conditions leading to HF cause the heart to work unusually hard (see Table 12.4). As a result of this overstimulation and/or excessive ventricular filling, two changes will occur in the heart. In **cardiomegaly**, the heart becomes enlarged because of overwork. The muscle stretches and loses elasticity. In **myocardial hypertrophy**, the heart muscle thickens in response to the overstimulation. In this text CHF and HF will be used interchangeably since the drugs and goals of therapy are so similar.

The goals of therapy are to prolong survival, relieve symptoms, improve quality of life, and prevent progression of disease. Most patients will be managed with a combination of drugs. Current guidelines recommend angiotensin-converting enzyme (ACE) inhibitors and beta blockers as first-line agents. Diuretics are recommended for patients who retain fluid, and digoxin is recommended for patients who continue to experience symptoms after receiving optimal treatment with other drugs. Most patients are also placed on an anticoagulation or antiplatelet drug such as aspirin or warfarin.

When HF results in left-sided failure of the heart, fluid accumulates in the lungs, causing pulmonary edema, reduced gas exchange, shortness of breath, cough, memory loss and confusion, anorexia, and profuse sweating. Failure on the right side of the heart results in **ascites** (fluids collecting in abdominal organs and the lower extremities), which causes weight gain, anorexia, and nausea.

Treatment involves the use of combinations of diuretics, digoxin, and ACE inhibitors. Clinical studies have shown that ACE inhibitors reduce the risk of mortality and morbidity in patients with chronic heart failure. It is thought that ACE inhibitors are beneficial in CHF because they inhibit the formation of angiotensin II, which is a potent vasoconstrictor, thus helping blood vessels to dilate and lower the resistance against which the heart must work. The most commonly used agents for HF that have not been previously discussed in this text are listed in Table 12.5.

Antiarrhythmic Medications

Digoxin (Lanoxicaps, Lanoxin) is a much-used drug for treating HF as well as atrial fibrillation and flutter; it was previously described in the section on arrhythmias.

TABLE 12.4   Causes of Heart Failure

Primary Causes	Secondary Causes
cardiomyopathy	high salt intake
coronary artery disease	noncompliance with treatment
hypertension	side effects of drug therapy
	kidney failure
	stress
	infection and inflammation
	cigarette smoking
	obesity

Vasodilators

Drugs that cause blood vessels to dilate are used in HF because dilating the vessels reduces the resistance against which the heart must work. Some vasodilators are described here; others are discussed in the section on hypertension.

Milrinone (Primacor) is a phosphodiesterase inhibitor that causes vasodilation and increases the force of myocardial contraction. It is used for short-term IV therapy of HF and for calcium channel blocker intoxication.

Isosorbide-hydralazine (BiDil) is a combination drug used to supplement standard therapy in the African American population. It is the first drug approved for a specific race. Both drugs are vasodilators. They enhance the relaxation of vessels by nitric oxide, which is thought to be produced in lower levels in the African American population. BiDil is dosed three times a day. It can cause headaches and dizziness. It is a film-coated tablet containing 20 mg of isosorbide dinitrate and 37.5 mg of hydralazine. This drug is usually reserved for HF patients with clinically significant renal dysfunction who cannot tolerate ACE inhibitors. It is also approved for a form of angina.

ACE Inhibitors

An ACE inhibitor is a drug that competitively inhibits the conversion of angiotensin I to angiotensin II. (Angiotensin II is a potent vasoconstrictor that will be further

---

TABLE 12.5 Most Commonly Used Agents for Treating Heart Failure (Not Previously Discussed)

Generic Name	Pronunciation	Dosage Form	Brand Name	Dispensing Status
Vasodilators				
milrinone	MIL-ri-none	IV	Primacor	Rx
nitroprusside	nye-troe-PRUS-ide	IV	Nitropress	Rx
isosorbide-hydralazine	eye-soe-SOR-bide hye-DRAL-a-zeen	tablet	BiDil	Rx
ACE Inhibitors				
benazepril	ben-AZ-eh-pril	tablet	Lotensin	Rx
captopril	KAP-toe-pril	tablet	Capoten	Rx
enalapril	e-NAL-a-pril	IV, tablet	Vasotec	Rx
fosinopril	foe-SIN-oh-pril	tablet	Monopril	Rx
lisinopril	lyse-IN-oh-pril	tablet	Prinivil, Zestril	Rx
moexipril	moe-EX-i-pril	tablet	Univasc	Rx
perindopril	per-IN-doe-pril	tablet	Aceon	Rx
quinapril	KWIN-a-pril	tablet	Accupril	Rx
ramipril	RA-mi-pril	capsule	Altace	Rx
trandolapril	tran-DOE-la-pril	tablet	Mavik	Rx
Human B-Type Natriuretic Peptide (hBNP)				
nesiritide	ni-SIR-i-tide	IV	Natrecor	Rx

discussed in the later section on hypertension.) The result is lower levels of angiotensin II and therefore less constriction of blood vessels, reducing resistance to blood flow. Lowering blood pressure puts less stress on the heart, allowing it to work more effectively. HF is especially responsive to ACE inhibitors. ACE inhibitors have been clearly shown to decrease the risk of cardiovascular events for patients with hypertension or HF and for patients post-MI. This class of drug is also considered to preserve potassium. If an ACE inhibitor is combined with other drugs with this same characteristic or with potassium supplementation, the patient can become hyperkalemic. One would not expect these patients to need potassium supplementation, but often they do, especially if they are on a diuretic, even a potassium-sparing one. The important issue here is that potassium blood levels must be checked. If the prescription for the ACE inhibitor and that for the potassium supplement are written by the same prescriber, then it is most likely labs are being checked and the patient is being watched. However, if more than one prescriber is involved, all prescribers need to be made aware of the possible interactions.

A persistent cough seems to be the most troublesome side effect of ACE inhibitors. It is a dry, unproductive cough that is extremely annoying. The cough may be the result of buildup of bradykinin, the breakdown of which is inhibited by the ACE inhibitor. As a result of the cough, compliance with ACE inhibitors is poor. The most dangerous side effect is angioedema. It most commonly presents as swelling of the face and tongue, which may begin a few hours after initiation of therapy or may not occur for several years into the treatment. The drug may cause dizziness, especially during the first few days. The patient should be told to stand up slowly to prevent orthostatic hypotension and to avoid salt substitutes, which contain potassium. ACE inhibitors should be given with caution to patients taking lithium.

Human B-Type Natriuretic Peptide (hBNP)

Nesiritide (Natrecor) is one of a class of drugs that bind to guanylate cyclase–linked receptors on vascular smooth muscle, causing relaxation and thereby lowering blood pressure. It is a product of DNA recombinant technology. Nesiritide improves circulation, shortness of breath, and fatigue in patients with acute HF. It should be used only in hospitalized patients with acute HF. Nesiritide is used as an alternative to IV nitroglycerin, milrinone, or nitroprusside. It is better tolerated than IV nitroglycerin and does not increase heart rate or cause arrhythmias.

Hypertension

Blood pressure (BP) is defined as the product of cardiac output and total peripheral resistance. Cardiac output, which is the product of heart rate and stroke volume, is determined by three parameters: **preload** (the amount of blood being delivered to the heart), **afterload** (the force against which cardiac muscle shortens), and **contractility** (the capacity of the cardiac muscle for becoming shorter in response to a stimulus). Additional factors that affect blood pressure are blood viscosity, blood volume, and various nerve controls.

Blood pressure is expressed as the **systolic blood pressure** reading, which measures the pressure when the heart ejects blood, and the **diastolic blood pressure** reading, which measures the pressure when the heart relaxes and fills. Cardiac output is the major determinant of systolic pressure, while total peripheral resistance largely determines the level of diastolic pressure. Both readings are in millimeters of mercury (abbreviated "mm Hg"), that is, the height of a mercury column whose weight offsets the pressure. The reading is stated as systolic "over" diastolic pressure. 120 mm Hg systolic, 80 mm Hg diastolic is written "120/80" and read "120 over 80." This reading is often considered normal, even though there is really no "normal" reading. **Hypertension** is defined arbitrarily as a disease in which the systolic blood pressure is greater than 140 mm Hg and the diastolic pressure is greater than 90 mm Hg. Table 12.6 describes the staging of blood pressure in adults. Fatal events double for every 20 mm Hg systolic and every 10 mm Hg diastolic over these numbers.

The underlying basis of most cases of hypertension is unknown, although family history, cigarette smoking, and a high-fat diet are definite factors. Other factors include kidney disease, decreased pressure or delayed pulse in the lower extremities, obesity, adrenal tumor, and drugs such as oral contraceptives, corticosteroids, nonsteroidal anti-inflammatory drugs (NSAIDs), nasal decongestants, and appetite suppressants.

Untreated Hypertension

Untreated hypertension can have devastating results. A variety of diseases can develop or be worsened, including the following;

- Cardiovascular disease develops, characterized by enlargement of the heart (cardio-megaly), cardiac hypertrophy, and thickening of the cardiac wall, with loss of elasticity. Cardiac output is reduced, along with the ability of the heart to push blood through the body to perfuse tissue, leading to HF.
- HF results in inadequate perfusion, cold extremities (toes and fingers), pitting or whole-body edema (especially in the feet and legs), and accumulation of fluid in the lungs.
- Renal insufficiency can also result. The higher the blood pressure, the more the kidneys reduce renal blood flow and renal function.
- Accelerated cardiac and peripheral vascular disease can also result from high blood pressure.

In general, the higher the pressure, the greater the risk. Hypertension alters capillaries, venules, and arterioles. Blood cholesterol collects in arterial walls, reducing the size of the lumen and, therefore, the blood flow, leading to increased potential for infection, vascular problems (as in diabetes), and deterioration of nerves from diminished blood supply.

TABLE 12.6	Staging of Blood Pressure in Adults	
Category	**Systolic (mm Hg)**	**Diastolic (mm Hg)**
Normal	<120	<80
Prehypertension	120–139	80–89
Hypertension		
Stage 1	140–159	90–99
Stage 2	>160	>100

Hypertension Therapy

Hypertension control begins with detection and continued surveillance. Initial readings should be confirmed with subsequent readings for several weeks, unless the pressure is dangerously high at the first reading.

The goal of therapy is to prevent the morbidity and mortality associated with high blood pressure and to reduce blood pressure by the least intrusive means possible. A four-step regimen, presented in Table 12.7, is needed to reduce blood pressure.

Antihypertensive Therapeutics

Table 12.8 gives an overview of the main drug classes used in the treatment of hypertension, and Table 12.9 lists the most commonly prescribed agents for this disease state.

Beta blockers, calcium channel blockers, and ACE inhibitors are important drugs used to treat hypertension. They have all been discussed previously in this chapter.

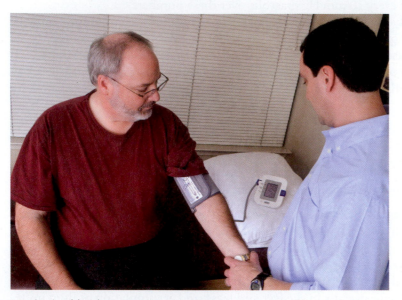

Monitoring blood pressure is an important component of hypertension therapy.

TABLE 12.7	Regimen for Reducing Blood Pressure		
Step 1	**Modify lifestyle factors**		
	high sodium intake	to	moderate sodium intake
	excess consumption of calories	to	weight reduction
	physical inactivity	to	regular aerobic physical activity
	excess alcohol consumption	to	moderate alcohol consumption
	nicotine usage	to	cessation of nicotine usage
	high stress	to	control of stress
Step 2	Monotherapy: use a single drug, usually a diuretic, beta blocker, ACE inhibitor, angiotensin II receptor antagonist, or calcium channel blocker.		
Step 3	Add a diuretic, if it was not the drug used to begin therapy in step 2 of the regimen.		
Step 4	Add a third agent that will be synergistic with the other two in reducing blood pressure.		

TABLE 12.8   Pharmacologic Antihypertensive Therapies

Drug Class	Mechanism of Action
diuretics	First-line therapy. These drugs, discussed in Chapter 11, reduce total peripheral resistance. It is often difficult to get good control of moderate to severe hypertension without a diuretic.
selective aldosterone receptor antagonists	These drugs act as diuretics by binding to mineralocorticoid receptors, blocking aldosterone action, thereby decreasing sodium retention and decreasing blood pressure.
calcium channel blockers	First-line therapy. These drugs, discussed earlier under angina, dilate the aterioles, thereby reducing peripheral resistance, energy consumption, and oxygen requirements.
ACE (angiotensin-converting enzyme) inhibitors	These drugs, discussed earlier under HF, are first line therapy. They act by blocking angiotensin-converting enzymes to prevent the conversion of angiotensin I to angiotensin II, which is a potent vasoconstrictor. The decrease in blood pressure is accompanied by a reduction in peripheral resistance and an increase in the elasticity of the large arteries, suggesting a direct effect on arterial smooth muscle. Diabetics should be on ACE inhibitors to treat hypertension if present.
ARBs (angiotensin II receptor blockers)	These drugs bind to the angiotensin II receptors, thereby blocking the vasoconstriction effects of these receptors. Unlike ACE inhibitors, ARBs do not affect bradykinin-altered responses (therefore, no cough).
beta blockers	These drugs block beta receptor response to adrenergic stimulation, thereby decreasing heart rate, myocardial contractility, blood pressure, and myocardial oxygen demand. Agents selective to beta-1 receptors act specifically on the heart and are said to be cardio-specific. Agents that act at both beta-1 and beta-2 receptors are said to be nonselective.
CNS agents	These drugs stimulate the alpha-2 adrenergic receptors in the brain and thereby reduce the sympathetic outflow from the vasomotor center in the brain. Thus, heart rate is decreased, cardiac output decreases slightly, and total peripheral resistance is lowered as a result of reduced stimulation of vascular muscle.
peripheral acting agents (alpha blockers)	These drugs block alpha receptor–induced constriction of blood vessels, leading indirectly to vasodilation and hypotension.
vasodilators	These drugs relax arterial smooth muscle and lower peripheral resistance via direct mechanism.
combination drugs	Second-line therapy. Additive effects lower blood pressure. Two low doses of different drugs usually cause fewer side effects than pushing the dose of either drug.

Diuretics Diuretics are first-line drugs for treating hypertension. They reduce the cardiac output by increasing the elimination of urine and reducing the volume of fluid in the body, thereby reducing preload. Their ability to reduce the sodium load, however, is probably their most important effect on lowering blood pressure. Diuretics are discussed in Chapter 11.

Angiotensin Receptor Blockers Angiotensin receptor blockers (ARBs) seem to work as well as ACE inhibitors in lowering blood pressure. Whereas ACE inhibitors reduce the production of angiotensin II, ARBs block the action of angiotensin II at its receptors. When chemically bound, angiotensin II is not able to exert its effects. The

TABLE 12.9 Most Commonly Used Antihypertensive Therapeutic Agents

Generic Name	Pronunciation	Dosage Form	Brand Name	Dispensing Status
Calcium Channel Blockers, see Table 12.1				
ACE Inhibitors, see Table 12.5				
Angiotensin Receptor Blockers (ARBs)				
candesartan	kan-de-SAR-tan	tablet	Atacand	Rx
eprosartan	ep-roe-SAR-tan	tablet	Teveten	Rx
irbesartan	ir-be-SAR-tan	tablet	Avapro	Rx
losartan	loe-SAR-tan	tablet	Cozaar	Rx
olmesartan	ohl-me-SAR-tan	tablet	Benicar	Rx
telmisartan	tel-me-SAR-tan	tablet	Micardis	Rx
valsartan	val-SAR-tan	capsule, tablet	Diovan	Rx
Beta Blockers, see Table 12.1				
CNS Agents				
clonidine	KLON-i-deen	IV, tablet, transdermal patch	Catapres, Catapres-TTS, Duraclon	Rx
guanfacine	GWAHN-fa-seen	tablet	Tenex	Rx
methyldopa	meth-il-DOE-pa	IV, tablet	Aldomet	Rx
Peripheral Acting Agents (Alpha Blockers)				
alfuzosin	al-FYOO-zoe-sin	tablet	Uroxatral	Rx
doxazosin	dox-AY-zoe-sin	tablet	Cardura	Rx
phentolamine	fen-TOLE-a-meen	IV	Regitine	Rx
prazosin	PRAY-zoe-sin	capsule	Minipress	Rx
terazosin	ter-AYE-zoe-sin	capsule, tablet	Hytrin	Rx
Vasodilators (see also Table 12.5)				
epoprostenol	e-poe-PROST-en-awl	IV	Flolan	Rx
fenoldopam	fe-NOL-doe-pam	IV	Corlopam	Rx
hydralazine	hye-DRAL-a-zeen	IV, tablet	Apresoline	Rx
minoxidil	mi-NOX-i-dil	tablet, topical	Loniten	Rx
			Rogaine	OTC
treprostinil	treh-PROST-in-il	injection, subcutaneous infusion	Remodulin	Rx
sildenafil	sil-DEN-a-fil	tablet	Revatio, Viagra	Rx
Direct Renin Inhibitors (DRIs)				
aliskiren	a-lis-KYE-ren	tablet	Tekturna	Rx
Combination Drugs				
amlodipine-benazepril	am-LOE-di-peen ben-AYE-ze-pril	capsule	Lotrel	Rx
amlodipine-valsartan	am-LOE-di-peen val-SAR-tan	tablet	Exforge	Rx

Generic Name	Pronunciation	Dosage Form	Brand Name	Dispensing Status
atenolol-hydrochlorothiazide	a-TEN-oh-lawl hye-droe-klor-oh-THYE-a-zide	tablet	Tenorectic	Rx
benazepril-hydrochlorothiazide	ben-AZ-eh-pril hye-droe-klor-oh-THYE-a-zide	tablet	Lotensin HCT	Rx
bisoprolol-hydrochlorothiazide	bis-OE-proe-lawl hye-droe-klor-oh-THYE-a-zide	tablet	Ziac	Rx
enalapril-diltiazem	e-NAL-a-pril dil-TYE-a-zem	tablet	Teczem	Rx
enalapril-hydrochlorothiazide	e-NAL-a-pril hye-droe-klor-oh-THYE-a-zide	tablet	Vaseretic	Rx
irbesartan-hydrochlorothiazide	ir-be-SAR-tan hye-droe-klor-oh-THYE-a-zide	tablet	Avalide	Rx
lisinopril-hydrochlorothiazide	lyse-IN-oh-pril hye-droe-klor-oh-THYE-a-zide	tablet	Zestoretic	Rx
losartan-hydrochlorothiazide	loe-SAR-tan hye-droe-klor-oh-THYE-a-zide	tablet	Hyzaar	Rx
trandolapril-verapamil	tran-DOE-la-pril ver-AP-a-mil	tablet	Tarka	Rx
valsartan-hydrochlorothiazide	val-SAR-tan hye-droe-klor-oh-THYE-a-zide	tablet	Diovan HCT	Rx

antagonists do not affect bradykinin, they result in less coughing and angioedema, and are thus better tolerated. ACEs and ARBs both affect the renin-angiotensin system but work at different points in the cascade.

Angiotensin II–receptor blockers (ARBs) can be given alone or in combination therapy with other drugs. ARBs should be used for patients who cannot tolerate ACEs. Theoretically, ARBs should be a safer alternative for patients with ACE induced angioedema. ARBs have been shown to improve renal outcomes in patients with type 2 diabetes.

There are some conditions in which the combination of an ARB and an ACE may provide greater therapeutic benefit than either alone. This synergy is because of the different ways in which the two classes of drug block the angiotensin-renin system. There will be times when prescribers will have a patient on both drug classes. Watch for this combination but do not be alarmed. If the patient has prescriptions for these drugs from two different prescribers, then the prescribers should be made aware that the patient is on both classes of drug. ARBS, like ACEIs, are potassium savers, so electrolytes must be monitored in these patients.

Candesartan (Atacand) has received the FDA approval to state that it lowers blood pressure more than losartan (Cozaar). There is a 2 mm Hg drop. Some clinicians may feel this small lowering of blood pressure is nonetheless important, because it may reduce incidence of strokes and heart attacks. Candesartan is also approved for heart failure when used with an ACE.

Eprosartan (Teveten) is indicated for the treatment of hypertension alone or in combination with other drugs. It is provided by the manufacturer in 400 mg oval,

Warning

Many of these drug names end in -sartan (e.g., losartan and valsartan), so technicians must pay close attention to the first letters of these drug names.

scored, pink tablets. Eprosartan tablets may be cut or broken in half. The 600 mg tablet is white and capsule–shaped and is dosed without regard to meals.

Irbesartan (Avapro) is approved for hypertension and diabetic nephropathy in patients with type II diabetes. It slows the progression of kidney disease.

Losartan (Cozaar) is approved for hypertension, diabetic nephropathy, and stroke prevention. Research data shows that twice-daily dosing may be more effective than once-daily dosing. The pharmacy technician may want to verify advantage in twice-daily dosing with the prescriber.

Olmesartan (Benicar) is a selective ARB agent. It is a prodrug that is converted to its active form during absorption in the GI tract. Olmesartan is indicated for the treatment of hypertension and may be used alone or with additional antihypertensive agents.

Telmisartan (Micardis) may be used alone or in combination with other antihypertensive agents. It is specific and selective and maintains blood pressure reduction over a 24 hour period. Telmisartan has the longest half-life of all the ARBs. It is so sensitive to moisture that it is provided by the manufactuer in a foil blister pack. Because of this sensitivity to moisture, a telmisartan tablet cannot be cut in half. Pharmacy technicians should be aware that telmisartan will loose potency when the pack is opened.

Valsartan (Diovan) is approved for hypertension and heart failure. It may be dosed without regard for food.

Central Nervous System Agents Central nervous system (CNS) agents stimulate the alpha-2 adrenergic receptors in the brain. This leads to a reduction in the sympathetic outflow from the vasomotor center in the brain and an associated increase in parasympathetic activity (vagal tone). As a consequence of these effects, heart rate is decreased, cardiac output decreases slightly, total peripheral resistance is lowered, plasma renin activity is reduced, and baroreceptor reflexes are blunted.

Warning

Catapres and Cataflam (diclofenac, a drug for arthritis pain) are similar.

Clonidine (Catapres, Catapres-TTS, Duraclon) is the only antihypertensive supplied as a transdermal delivery system. The patch is worn for 7 days. This delivery form seems to have fewer side effects than the other forms. Clonidine is also used to treat hypertension in patients experiencing withdrawal symptoms, especially alcoholics.

Guanfacine (Tenex) has less sedative effect than clonidine. Its side effects are drowsiness, fatigue, dry mouth, depression, and fluid retention.

Peripheral Acting Agents (Alpha Blockers) Peripheral acting agents block alpha constriction of blood vessels. This action leads indirectly to vasodilation and hypotension.

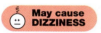

Prazosin (Minipress) blocks impulses at the neurovascular junction and vascular smooth muscle. The side effect is orthostatic hypotension, which is severe for the first few doses. Because of this side effect, patients should take the drug at bedtime. Other side effects are dizziness, weakness, and headache.

Terazosin (Hytrin) blocks impulses at vascular smooth muscle. The side effects are orthostatic hypotension with the first dose.

Doxazosin (Cardura), like prazosin and terazosin, selectively blocks alpha-1 receptors, which results in vasodilation of veins and arterioles. On a weight-to-weight basis, however, doxazosin is 50% more potent than prazosin.

Vasodilators Vasodilators have a direct relaxant effect on arterial smooth muscle, which reduces peripheral resistance. Several of these drugs have been discussed in the section on congestive heart failure.

Hydralazine (Apresoline) has to be given three to four times a day, so compliance is a problem. Side effects are reflex sympathetic stimulation associated with vasodilation, which leads to tachycardia, palpitations, flushing, and headache. Patients often complain of a racing heart. Less common is an autoimmune disorder with high dosage. Somehow the drug stimulates the production of antibodies that cause the symptoms of lupus (butterfly rash, joint pain, and stiffness). This antibody may also attack the kidneys. If any of these symptoms occur, the drug must be stopped immediately.

Minoxidil (Loniten, Rogaine) relaxes arteriolar smooth muscle with little effect on veins. It also stimulates hair growth, though this effect is secondary to vasodilation. Other side effects are temporary edema, nausea, vomiting, and rash. The topical forms of Rogaine are now available over-the-counter for both male pattern baldness and female baldness. The topical forms do not affect blood pressure as much as the oral dosage forms.

Epoprostenol (Flolan) is a prostacyclin (PGI-2) used only in pulmonary hypertension. It is a strong vasodilator of all vascular beds, including the pulmonary vessels. In addition, it is a potent endogenous inhibitor of platelet aggregation, so it can prevent thrombogenesis and platelet clumping in the lungs. Epoprostenol is used for hemodialysis patients.

Fenoldopam (Corlopam) is a dopamine D_1 receptor agonist that exhibits a vasodilating action. It is indicated for the in-hospital, short-term (up to 48 hours) management of severe hypertension when rapid, but quickly reversible, emergency reduction of blood pressure is clinically indicated. It increases renal blood flow and diuresis. The most common adverse events are hypotension, headache, flushing, and nausea. Fenoldopam should not be used concurrently with a beta blocker. An infusion can be abruptly stopped or tapered. Oral antihypertensive agents can be administered during an infusion. Fenoldopam has an elimination half-life of approximately 5 minutes. It can be mixed with either D_5W or normal saline and is stable under normal light and temperature for 24 hours. Fenoldopam contains metabisulfite, which may cause an allergic reaction.

Sildenafil (Revatio, Viagra) reduces blood pressure by vasodilator effects. It reduces mean pulmonary arterial pressure and pulmonary vascular resistance while increasing cardiac index. Caution should be exercised not to use with nitrates. There is also concern for the potential for medication errors with sildenafil now that it has two different names. Technicians should be careful when receiving a prescription for either of these brands to make sure the patient is not on both forms of this drug (or on both Revatio and Levitra or Cialis). Revatio is a white round tablet containing 20 mg of sildenafil, whereas Viagra is a blue, diamond-shaped tablet in 25, 50, or 100 mg strengths.

Treprostinil (Remodulin) reduces hypertension through direct vasodilation of pulmonary and systemic arterial beds and inhibition of platelet aggregation. It is a solution that must be infused SC or IV using a special pump. Headache and infusion site pain are the primary side effects.

Direct Renin Inhibitor **Aliskiren (Tekturna)** inhibits renin, which controls the first rate-limiting step of the renin-angiotensin-aldosterone system. It is indicated for the treatment of hypertension. The medication should not be taken with meals because a high-fat meal can reduce the absorption of this drug. Diarrhea appears to be the primary side effect.

Combination Drugs Combination drugs have additive effects to relax blood vessels and lower pressure. Two low doses of different drugs usually cause fewer side effects than pushing the dose of either drug. This is still second-line therapy. More and more manufacturers are combining drugs to improve compliance.

Most frequently, drugs from different classes are combined to get the additive effects of the two. Many hypertensive medications require more than one drug. Combining two drugs of lower strength should provide an additive effect as far as reduction of blood pressure and decrease side effects of both drugs.

Amlodipine-valsartan (Exforge) is a calcium channel blocker and an ARB. The ARB should decrease edema caused by the calcium channel blocker as well as lower blood pressure. Amlodipine-valsartan is manufactured in four strengths and is approved only to treat hypertension. It is not indicated for initial treatment, but can be used as monotherapy when the two classes need to be combined. Amlodipine-valsartan tablets may be halved. Because there are other combination products that contain these drugs, the pharmacy technician must make sure that the patient is not receiving the same drug from two different sources.

Myocardial Infarction

Myocardial infarction (MI), most commonly known as a heart attack, is the leading cause of death in industrialized nations. When the heart muscle is deprived of oxygen because of reduced blood supply, muscle cells die (necrosis). The damaged area is known as an *infarct*. Lesser infarcts undergo healing, in which muscle is replaced by scars made of connective tissue. The contractility of the heart is reduced around the scarring.

Causes of a Heart Attack

A myocardial infarction may occur when there is a prolonged decrease in oxygen delivery to a region of cardiac muscle. The likelihood of an MI increases substantially when the lumen (channel of a blood vessel) of one or more of the coronary arteries (the three major arteries that supply blood to the heart muscle) is narrowed by 70% or more. Factors that increase the risk of a myocardial infarction include a history of angina, alcohol consumption, reduced pulmonary vital capacity, cigarette smoking, and atherosclerosis. Over one million heart attacks occur in the United States each year. Half live and half die. This is why so much emphasis is placed on prevention.

Various lifestyle modifications are recommended to reduce the risk of a myocardial infarction.

- Eliminate smoking.
- Reduce hypertension by diet, medication, or both.
- Exercise moderately at least three times weekly.
- Adjust calories to achieve ideal body weight.
- Decrease alcohol consumption.
- Control diabetes.
- Use aspirin therapy.
- Reduce dietary cholesterol/triglycerides.

Symptoms of a Heart Attack

Symptoms of a heart attack include oppressive or burning tightness or squeezing in the chest, a feeling of choking and indigestion-like expansion, a sense of "impending doom," and substernal pain with varying radiations to the neck, throat, jaw, shoulders, and one or both arms. The pain lasts 30 minutes to several hours and can be severe. It may occur at rest, does not subside with rest, and may not be relieved completely with nitroglycerin. Half of all patients experienced some of the following symptoms in the day or days before the attack: vague chest discomfort, weakness, fatigue, or sweating.

Treatment of Myocardial Infarction

Treatment for a myocardial infarction is aimed at allowing the heart to rest and undergo normal healing. Beta blockers combined with 81 mg of aspirin are frequently prescribed to reduce the risk of death or recurrence following an MI event. The beta blocker slows the action of the heart, thus reducing its workload. The aspirin prevents clot formation. Some prescribers may prefer or add on an ACE inhibitor.

Blood Clots

Blood clots transported in the blood, called thrombi (singular: **thrombus**), present a serious and potentially life-threatening problem. Thrombi develop from abnormalities in

- blood coagulation, resulting in hypercoagulability
- blood flow, leading to stasis
- platelet adhesiveness, resulting in hypercoagulability
- vessel walls (from damage or surgery)

Damage to tissue cells activates a pathway of coagulation, or **clotting cascade**, as shown in Figure 12.8. If any factor along the path is missing, blood will not clot, as occurs in people with hemophilia. Each step involves the activation of a factor, which then triggers the next step, until finally the fibrin clot is formed. However, vessel blockage can occur as the result of fat, air, and debris gaining entry into circulation.

Venous thrombi usually form in areas of low-velocity blood flow, surgical or other vein injury, or large venous sinuses (pockets formed by valves in deep veins). Symptoms include swelling, discoloration, and pain. A piece of the clot may break off and travel to the lung, causing a **pulmonary embolism (PE),** or sudden blocking of the pulmonary artery. A pulmonary embolism is very serious and may lead to death. Some patients have an undiagnosed deep vein thrombosis (DVT). A proximal (at or superior to the knee) DVT is the most serious and may be fatal.

Risk factors for DVT are

- age over 40 years
- bed rest for over four days
- estrogen combined with nicotine
- high-dose estrogen therapy
- major illness
- obesity
- pregnancy
- previous deep vein thrombosis

- surgery
- trauma
- varicose veins

Two classes of drugs—anticoagulants and antiplatelets—are used to reduce the risk of blood clots. An **anticoagulant** prevents clot formation by inhibiting clotting factors; an **antiplatelet** reduces the risk of clot formation by inhibiting platelet aggregation. Drugs in a third class, fibrinolytics, dissolve clots already formed.

Anticoagulant Agents

The therapy for deep vein thrombosis is either low-dose heparin, adjusted-dose heparin, low-molecular-weight heparin, or warfarin (Coumadin). The purpose is to prevent fatal blood clotting while ensuring adequate coagulation.

Patients on anticoagulant drug therapy should be monitored to prevent future embolisms and minimize risk of hemorrhage. The following are the most frequently used laboratory tests.

- **Partial thromboplastin time (PTT)** measures the function of the intrinsic and common pathways. (PTT is affected by heparin.)
- **Prothrombin time (PT)** assesses the function of the extrinsic and common pathways of the coagulation system; in particular, it measures the activity of the vitamin K–dependent factor. (PT is affected by warfarin.)
- The **International Normalized Ratio (INR)** standardizes the PT by comparing it to a standard index. This number will appear on the lab values. It is the most important indicator because it compensates for differences in laboratories that do the blood samples.
- **Hematocrit** is the proportion of the blood sample that is red blood cells.

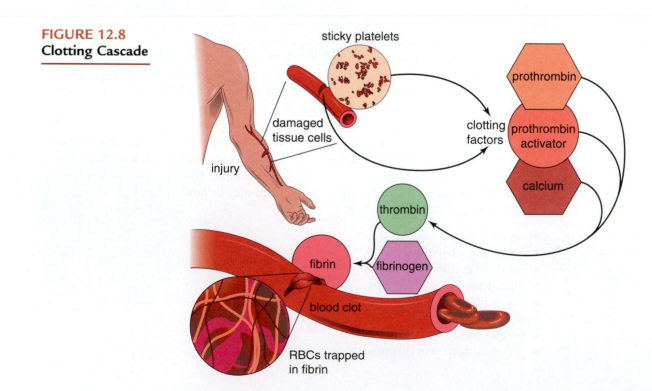

FIGURE 12.8
Clotting Cascade

A home monitor for "clotting time" has been approved. It is called CoaguChek.

Table 12.10 presents the most commonly used anticoagulant agents as well as antidotes for them. Anticoagulant therapy should be started with IV heparin, then overlapped a few days with warfarin, then switched to warfarin only. The warfarin dose is based on results of PT, INR, and hematocrit laboratory tests. The patient should take the dose without food, report any signs of bleeding, avoid hazardous activities, avoid foods high in vitamin K, use a soft toothbrush, and wear a Medi-Alert ID tag. The patient's urine may turn red-orange; the physician should be notified if urine turns dark brown or if red or tar-black stools occur, which is a possible indication of internal bleeding. Warfarin has a very large number of interactions with other drugs, so the technician should always check the patient's drug profile before dispensing the drug.

Types of Anticoagulant Drugs The most commonly prescribed anticoagulants are briefly described here.

Heparin is a naturally occuring circulatory anticoagulant produced in mast cells. *It does not dissolve a clot that has already formed.* Instead, heparin *inhibits thrombin formation,* thereby reducing the ability of blood to clot and preventing the formation of a new clot. Heparin and low molecular weight heparins are the only anticoagulants that can be used in pregnancy because they do not cross the placenta. Heparin should be used with caution, however, because hemorrhaging may easily occur. Some common side effects are bleeding from the gums and unexplained bruising. Heparin can be given only intravenously or subcutaneously, usually in the abdomen; it must never be administered intramuscularly, because an intramuscular injection will cause a hematoma (internal pooling of blood). Pharmacy technicians must be very careful to dispense needles with heparin that are only used to dose subcutaneous injections, such as needles used for insulin, allergy, or tuberculosis. If IM needles are dispensed

TABLE 12.10   Most Commonly Used Anticoagulant Agents and Antidotes

Generic Name	Pronunciation	Dosage Form	Brand Name	Dispensing Status
Anticoagulant Drugs				
bivalirudin	bye-VAL-i-roo-din	IV	Angiomax	Rx
fondaparinux	fon-da-PAIR-i-nux	injection	Arixtra	Rx
heparin	HEP-a-rin	injection, IV	(none)	Rx
lepirudin	lep-i-ROO-din	IV	Refludan	Rx
warfarin	WOR-far-in	tablet	Coumadin	Rx
Low-Molecular-Weight Heparins				
dalteparin	dal-TEP-a-rin	injection	Fragmin	Rx
enoxaparin	ee-nox-a-PAIR-in	injection	Lovenox	Rx
tinzaparin	tin-ZAP-a-rin	injection	Innohep	Rx
Antidote for Heparin				
protamine sulfate	PROE-ta-meen-SUL-fate	IV	none	Rx
Antidote for Warfarin				
phytonadione	fye-toe-na-DYE-one	Injection, IV	Mephyton, Vitamin K	Rx

for heparin, serious damage could occur. Commonly, a prescriber will write a prescription for syringes without specifying which type. Pharmacy personnel should know which drugs need which syringes. Heparin dosage should be titrated according to PTT results. Dosage of heparin is measured not in milligrams but in units based on biological activity; the pharmacy technician must convert units to milliliters to determine the correct amount. Low-dose heparin is used for prophylaxis of DVT or PE in postoperative patients, bedridden patients, obese patients, and patients with multiple bone fractures, hip prothesis insertion, MI, or gynecologic or abdominothoracic surgery (for surgery when the limbs are not moving to assist blood flow). Heparin flushes are dilute solutions used to keep IV lines open. They should not be confused with therapeutic doses of heparin.

Lepirudin (Refludan) is an alternative anticoagulant for patients who cannot tolerate heparin. This agent is a direct inhibitor of thrombin. As with all anticoagulants, excessive bleeding is the most important side effect. A concentration of 5 mg/mL is used for IV bolus, whereas solutions of 0.2 mg/mL or 0.4 mg/mL are recommended for continuous infusion.

Bivalirudin (Angiomax) is used in patients with unstable angina who are undergoing angioplasty. It is a specific and reversible thrombin inhibitor.

Fondaparinux (Arixtra) selectively inhibits a specific factor, called Xa, to inhibit thrombin formation. It is used to prevent DVT in patients having orthopedic surgery. It cannot be used in renal patients or patients weighing less than 50 kg (110 lb)—the same amount a patient must weigh in order to donate blood. A complete blood count (CBC), serum creatinine, and occult blood test are recommended periodically.

Warfarin (Coumadin) affects liver metabolism and prevents production of vitamin K–dependent clotting factors. Three to four days are necessary for warfarin to achieve an effect. It is a vitamin K antagonist and inhibits vitamin K–dependent clotting factors II, VII, IX, and X. The objective is to prevent future clots. As with heparin, warfarin has no effect on existing clots, but it can prevent clot formation, extension of formed clots, and secondary complications of thrombosis. Warfarin is rapidly and completely absorbed from the GI tract. Minor hemorrhaging (blood loss) may occur, but this is not an indication to stop warfarin therapy. Concomitant use with NSAIDs or aspirin increases the risk of bleeding due to impaired platelet function.

Low-Molecular-Weight Heparin Low-molecular-weight heparin (LMWH) presents less likelihood of bleeding. Drugs in this class are administered subcutaneously and are generally given 12 hours after surgery. There is no protein-binding problem as there is with regular heparin. These types of heparins have the following advantages:

- reduced bleeding
- reliable dose response
- longer plasma half-life
- no effect on platelets
- no need for anticoagulation monitoring
- manufactured in syringe with needle attached

Low-molecular-weight heparin products have become the standard of care for prophylaxis for abdominal surgery, duration of total hip replacement and total knee replacement recovery, some disease states, acute coronary syndrome, and treatment of deep vein thrombosis. These drugs are provided by the manufacturer in a syringe with an attached needle intended for subcutaneous injection. Although doses are fixed by the manufacturer, prescribers will sometimes use a dose based on body weight. In these latter cases, the person who administers the drug must use only part of the contents of a syringe and dispose of the rest of the drug. If a technician receives a prescription for a fraction of a dose, or of a mixed dose, it is prudent to check with the prescriber to ensure accuracy.

Enoxaparin (Lovenox) is used to prevent DVT after orthopedic surgery and is administered subcutaneously. It does not bind to heparin-binding proteins, and the half-life is two to four times that of heparin. The molecular weight of enoxaparin is approximately one-half that of heparin. At the recommended dose, single injections do not significantly influence platelet aggregation or affect clotting time. Platelet counts and the possibility of occult blood should be monitored, but it is not necessary to monitor PT or PTT. Side effects are hemorrhage and thrombocytopenia. In contrast to heparin and the other low-molecular-weight heparin products, dosage strengths for enoxaparin are stated in milligrams rather than units based on biological activity.

Dalteparin (Fragmin) is used to prevent DVT, which may lead to PE in patients undergoing abdominal surgery and who are at risk for thromboembolism complications. This group includes those 40 years of age and older, obese patients, patients with malignancy, those with a history of DVT or PE, and those undergoing surgical procedures requiring general anesthesia that lasts longer than 30 minutes.

Tinzaparin (Innohep), like other low-molecular-weight heparin products, uses a portion of the larger heparin molecule. Because of differences in dose, duration of action, and activity on various clotting factors, tinzaparin should not be interchanged with the other low-molecular-weight heparin agents. Tinzaparin is given once daily.

Antidote for Heparin **Protamine sulfate** is the antidote for heparin; 1 mg neutralizes 90 to 120 units of heparin (1 mg per 100 units of heparin).

Antidote for Warfarin **Phytonadione, vitamin K (Mephyton)** is an antagonist to warfarin. Charts are available to indicate the amount to administer based on the PTT. In severe hemorrhage, the patient is given fresh whole blood, which contains the clotting factors necessary to stop blood loss.

Antiplatelet Agents

Antiplatelet drugs interfere with the chemical reactions that cause platelets to be sticky. Table 12.11 presents the most commonly used antiplatelet agents.

TABLE 12.11   Most Commonly Used Antiplatelet Agents

Generic Name	Pronunciation	Dosage Form	Brand Name	Dispensing Status
General Antiplatelet Agents				
aspirin	AS-pir-in	oral liquid, tablet	(many)	OTC
clopidogrel	kloh-PID-oh-grel	tablet	Plavix	Rx
ticlopidine	tye-KLOE-pi-deen	tablet	Ticlid	Rx
Glycoprotein Antagonists				
abciximab	ab-SIKS-ih-mab	IV	ReoPro	Rx
eptifibatide	ep-ti-FIB-a-tide	IV	Integrilin	Rx
tirofiban	tye-roe-FYE-ban	IV	Aggrastat	Rx

General Antiplatelet Drugs Aspirin and several other drugs are commonly used as antiplatelet medications.

Aspirin works as an antiplatelet agent by inhibiting an enzyme that promotes clotting. Aspirin interferes with the enzyme cyclooxygenase and thereby disrupts production of thromboxane, prostacyclin, and prostaglandin. This action is irreversible, meaning clotting will be impaired until new platelets are circulating in the blood. Most patients with myocardial infarction, congestive heart failure, stroke, or other heart problems will be on low-dose aspirin daily. This is the "baby" aspirin, an 81 mg tablet that is enteric coated, which protects the lining of the stomach and is absorbed in the small intestine. However, in the presence of a MI, the patient should be given 325 mg *uncoated* aspirin tablet to chew immediately. It is very important to remember that uncoated aspirin is used when immediate absorption is needed, whereas enteric coated aspirin is used to protect the lining of the stomach in a nonemergency situation.

Aspirin has many side effects, especially GI symptoms. A patient with a history of peptic ulceration or other bleeding disorder should not take aspirin. The labeled use of aspirin for stroke is only for reduction of recurrent transient ischemic attack (TIAs), discussed later in the chapter, or for stroke in patients who have had transient ischemia of the brain due to fibrin platelet emboli.

Clopidogrel (Plavix) blocks the adenosine diphosphate (ADP, a chemical involved in energy transmission in biological systems) receptors and thus prevents fibrinogen binding and also reduces platelet adhesion and aggregation. Clopidogrel is approved to prevent the recurrence of atherosclerotic events such as MI and stroke. The major side effect of this drug is bleeding. Consequently, it should be discontinued 7 days before surgery. Platelet transfusion may be appropriate if rapid reversal of the pharmacologic effects of the drug is warranted. Clopidogrel can be taken without regard to food.

Ticlopidine (Ticlid) is chemically related to clopidogrel. It is used to reduce the risk of thrombotic stroke (fatal or nonfatal), both for patients who have had such as stroke and for those who have experienced stroke precursors. Because ticlopidine carries a risk of neutropenia and/or agranulocytosis, the drug should be reserved for patients who cannot tolerate aspirin. Ticlopidine therapy may begin as soon as the diagnosis of TIA or thrombotic stroke has been made and cerebral hemorrhage has been ruled out. The drug may be used indefinitely. Adverse effects may include neutropenia, thrombocytopenia, diarrhea, nausea, and rash. The established protocol includes routine monitoring of CBC and white cell differentials during the first 3 months of therapy. After that, CBCs need to be obtained only when signs or symptoms suggest infection.

Glycoprotein Antagonists A **glycoprotein antagonist** binds to a receptor on platelets, preventing platelet aggregation as well as the binding of fibrinogen and other adhesive molecules. The action of these antagonists is reversible. Glycoprotein antagonists are indicated for acute coronary syndrome and are administered during invasive procedures to prevent artery closure.

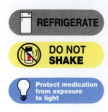

Abciximab (ReoPro) is a monoclonal antibody that is used to reduce acute cardiac complications in angioplasty patients at high risk for abrupt artery closure. The most common adverse effects are bleeding and thrombocytopenia. Abciximab is coadministered with aspirin after angioplasty; then heparin is infused and weight-adjusted to maintain a therapeutic bleeding time. Abciximab should be refrigerated and protected from light; it should not be shaken.

Eptifibatide (Integrilin) mimics native protein sequences in the platelet receptors. It blocks binding of the platelet glycoprotein, thereby preventing platelet aggregation and thrombosis. It is reversible within 2 hours after infusion, which makes it a

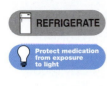

REFRIGERATE

Protect medication from exposure to light

Protect medication from exposure to light

very attractive agent for invasive procedures, which are the primary use of this drug. It is also used for acute coronary syndrome to prevent the blood from clotting. Eptifibatide is used in conjunction with heparin and aspirin. The primary side effects are bleeding and thrombocytopenia. It should be refrigerated and protected from light until dispensed.

Tirofiban (Aggrastat) is used for prophylaxis or treatment of thrombosis in adults with heparin-induced thrombocytopenia. It neutralizes clotting factor Xa and interrupts the blood coagulation cascade, thereby inhibiting thrombin formation. This drug must be protected from light.

Fibrinolytics Agents

A **fibrinolytic** dissolves clots by binding to the clot protein formed by fibrin. Table 12.12 lists the most commonly used fibrinolytic agents. All of them are supplied in the form of a powder to be dissolved in sterile water for injection or the diluent supplied with the drug for IV use only. When reconstituting the drug from the powder, the vial should be gently swirled, never shaken, because shaking can disturb the enzyme's molecular structure.

Alteplase (Activase) is a recombinant technology product. It is a tissue plasminogen activator that dissolves clots. Side effects include bleeding, arrhythmias associated with reperfusion, allergy, nausea, vomiting, hypotension, and fever. Alteplase is most effective when administered within the first 3 hours after a stroke or MI.

Reteplase (Retavase) is given in two injections of 10 mL separated by an interval of 30 minutes. The powder must be refrigerated and must remain sealed to protect it from light until it is to be used. No other medication should be added to the IV solution line. Bleeding is the most pronounced side effect.

Tenecteplase (TNKase) is another recombinant technology product that binds fibrin and converts plasminogen to plasmin. It is supplied as a powder to be dissolved in sterile water for injection, which is provided in an accompanying vial. This drug is incompatible with dextrose, so it should not be used in an IV line containing D_5W; the line should be flushed with saline before and after injection. Tenecteplase should not be shaken before or after reconstitution. A light foaming is normal when the diluent is added to the powder. After reconstitution it should be allowed to sit for a few minutes in order to prevent denaturing (modify the molecular structure) the solution.

Urokinase (formerly Abbokinase, renamed Kinlytic) is an enzyme obtained from a cultured fraction of fetal kidney cells that have been selected for their ability to break down fibrin clots. The clinical use of urokinase is for PE and MI.

TABLE 12.12   Most Commonly Used Fibrinolytic Agents

Generic Name	Pronunciation	Dosage Form	Brand Name	Dispensing Status
alteplase	AL-te-plase	IV	Activase	Rx
reteplase	REE-te-plase	IV	Retavase	Rx
tenecteplase	ten-EK-te-plase	IV	TNKase	Rx
urokinase	yoor-oh-KYE-nase	IV	Abbokinase, Kinlytic	Rx

Stroke

Under normal circumstances, the brain is one of the most oxygen-enriched organs in the human body. If cerebral circulation is abruptly stopped, the brain exhausts its supply of oxygen in approximately 10 seconds. Loss of consciousness quickly follows. The death of brain tissue is particularly tragic because the brain is incapable of cell regeneration.

Stroke is the result of an event that interrupts the oxygen supply to a localized area of the brain; a stroke by definition implies hypoxia. Stroke can be considered as a finite event, an ongoing event, or a series of protracted occurrences. A stroke may evolve over several hours, days, or months. In a **transient ischemic attack (TIA)**, an individual experiences temporary neurologic changes during a brief period of time. TIAs may be important warning signs and predictors of imminent stroke. A **reversible ischemic neurologic deficit (RIND)** is an event that reverses spontaneously but less rapidly than a TIA. RINDs last more than 24 hours and resolve in less than 21 days. In most cases, however, RINDs resolve (return to normal) within a matter of days, rather than weeks.

Causes of Stroke

A stroke may be caused by one of two primary events: (1) an **ischemic stroke** or cerebral infarction and (2) a **cerebral hemorrhage**. Ischemic stroke and cerebral hemorrhage differ significantly. Ischemic stroke is the result of obstruction to flow, whereas a hemorrhage involves primary rupture of a blood vessel. Ischemic strokes are by far the most common type of strokes.

Ischemic Stroke An ischemic stroke may occur after a newly formed thrombus becomes lodged at its site of origin in a cerebral blood vessel. As the lumen of the vessel narrows and becomes obstructed, blood flow through the vessel slows, diminishes, and, in some cases, even ceases. The reduced blood supply to the brain results in cerebral ischemia, and infarction with tissue necrosis may follow.

Emboli that move from one cerebral vessel to another are known as artery-to-artery emboli. Both cardiogenic and artery-to-artery emboli can ultimately lodge in distal vessels, causing TIAs or infarction. Regardless of the source of the ischemia, the diminished blood flow results in less oxygen reaching the cerebral tissues.

Cerebral Hemorrhage Hemorrhagic stroke may be marked by the sudden onset of severe headache, stiff neck, stupor, or a combination of these. Its effects are likely to be long lasting and irreversible. Cerebral hemorrhage is most likely to be due to hypertension, cerebral amyloid angiopathy, or arteriovenous malformation. Hypertensive hemorrhage and saccular ("berry") aneurysms occur in separate parts of the brain with such predictability that the location itself is helpful in differential diagnosis of the stroke. They are usually found in the thalamus, pons, cerebellum, or putamen. Saccular aneurysms are thin-walled dilations that protrude off one of the arteries or proximate branches. When one of these weakened sacs ruptures, blood flows into the subarachnoid space. These aneurysms carry a high risk of death.

Risk Factors for Stroke

Table 12.13 lists risk factors for stroke. Note that some can be changed by lifestyle modifications, whereas others cannot. Important risk factors include advanced age (risk doubles every 10 years after age 55), male sex (24% higher risk than for females),

TABLE 12.13   Stroke Risk Factors

Modifiable	Not Modifiable
Cigarette smoking	Age
Coronary artery disease	Gender
Diabetes	Genetic predisposition
Excesive alcohol intake	Prior stroke
Hyperlipidemia	Race
Hypertension	
Obesity	
Physical Inactivity	

hypertension, smoking, alcohol abuse, diabetes, and high cholesterol levels. In addition, oral contraceptive use by smokers, substance abuse, migraine headaches, and various cellular anomalies are responsible for 5% of ischemic strokes. Coronary artery disease appears to be the major cause of death among stroke survivors. Among the other important factors that contribute to the risk of a stroke are left ventricular hypertrophy and HF.

Several factors in a person's medical history are highly significant in the pathogenesis of cardiogenic embolic cerebrovascular accidents (CVAs)—strokes caused by heart disease. First is a history of nonrheumatic atrial fibrillations. These very rapid, disorganized contractions of cardiac muscle lead to incomplete emptying of the atria. The blood that remains pooled in the atria has a propensity to clot. A portion of the clot may leave the heart and move into the vessels of the head and neck. Other factors that may predispose to the occurrence of a CVA include rheumatic heart disease, acute MI, prosthetic heart valves, and left ventricular thrombi.

Stroke Management

In managing stroke, emphasis is on prevention. There are six major options in stroke management: antiplatelet therapy, anticoagulant therapy, fibrinolytic intervention, cerebrovascular surgery, nonpharmacologic therapy, and poststroke management. Pharmacologic treatment options for TIAs and prevention of initial strokes include antiplatelet and anticoagulant agents. Aspirin, as previously discussed, is extremely important. Some patients are prescribed enteric-coated 81 mg and others 325 mg. The prescriber must specify which.

In the aftermath of a stroke, determination of the cause is critical for establishing optimal poststroke therapy. Antiplatelets, anticoagulants, and fibrinolytic agents play important but very different roles in stroke management. For example, treating a hemorrhage with anticoagulant or fibrinolytic agents would be detrimental. Treatment goals should confirm the diagnosis of the cause of the stroke, evaluate the cause, stabilize the event, and then establish a plan to prevent further loss to the brain. Antiplatelet agents prevent platelet activation and formation of the platelet plug in one of two primary ways. First, these agents may interfere with the platelet aggregation induced by adenosine diphosphate (ADP). Second, antiplatelet agents may interfere with synthesis of thromboxane. For example, aspirin and dipyridamole (Persantine) interfere with thromboxane formation, whereas ticlopidine (Ticlid) and clopidogrel (Plavix) inhibit platelet aggregation through interference with ADP-induced platelet activity. Antiplatelet agents are most often used to prevent initial and recurrent thrombotic stroke.

Treatment options for acute thrombotic stroke include anticoagulant agents and fibrinolytic agents. Anticoagulant agents interfere with the synthesis or activation of the coagulation factors in the blood. Formed clots have the potential to continue to expand and cause greater neurologic damage; anticoagulant agents may prevent existing clots from expanding. Anticoagulant agents have been routinely used to treat acute cardiogenic stroke and are used for DVT and PE as well.

Fibrinolytic agents, also known as thrombolytic agents, differ from anticoagulant agents in one important aspect. Whereas anticoagulant agents can help prevent existing emboli and thrombi from expanding, fibrinolytic agents actually dissolve existing emboli and thrombi. Primary indications for fibrinolytic therapy include

- deep vein thrombosis
- acute peripheral occlusion
- acute myocardial infarction with embolization
- pulmonary embolism
- coronary embolus

The major fibrinolytic agents include tissue plasminogen activator (TPA) and urokinase described earlier in the section on blood clots.

Dissolution of the emboli and thrombi would appear to be clearly preferable to simple containment. Nevertheless, adoption of fibrinolytic agents as the pharmaceutical therapy of choice has been slow, even though clinical trials have demonstrated their efficacy in dissolving arterial and venous thrombosis.

Stroke and TIA prevention includes several pharmaceutical products that do not fall into previously discussed groups. These are listed in Table 12.14 and briefly mentioned here.

Aspirin-dipyridamole (Aggrenox) is approved to assist in preventing the recurrence of stroke or TIA. Each dose contains 25 mg of aspirin and 200 mg of extended-release dipyridamole and is taken twice daily. The daily dose falls short of the 75 mg of aspirin that is recommended to prevent heart attacks.

Dipyridamole (Persantine) inhibits platelet aggregation and may cause vasodilation. It maintains patency (ability to maintain open vessels) after surgical grafting procedures, including coronary artery bypass. It is used with warfarin to prevent other thromboembolic disorders. The primary side effect is dizziness. The technician should notify the physician or pharmacist if the patient is taking other medications that affect bleeding, such as NSAIDs or warfarin.

May cause DIZZINESS

Pentoxifylline (Trental) improves capillary blood flow by increasing erythrocyte flexibility and reducing blood viscosity. Tablets are time released, so it is important that the patient swallow them whole. They should be taken with food. Dizziness, headache, nausea, and vomiting are the primary side effects.

TABLE 12.14 TIA and Stroke Prevention Drugs

Generic Name	Pronunciation	Dosage Form	Brand Name	Dispensing Status
aspirin-dipyridamole	AS-pir-in dye-peer-ID-a-mole	capsule	Aggrenox	Rx
dipyridamole	dye-peer-ID-a-mole	tablet	Persantine	Rx
pentoxifylline	pen-tox-IF-i-leen	tablet	Trental	Rx

High Cholesterol and Related Diseases

As mentioned earlier in the chapter, high blood cholesterol is an important risk factor for heart attack and stroke. Consequently, drugs that can lower blood cholesterol levels have come to play an important part in efforts to prevent cardiovascular disease. An excessive amount of cholesterol in the blood is known as **hypercholesterolemia.** A related disease is **hyperlipidemia**, which is the condition in which the levels of one or more of the lipoproteins, discussed below, are elevated.

Causes and Treatment of Hyperlipidemia

Cholesterol itself is an odorless, white, waxlike, powdery substance that is present in all foods of animal origin but not in foods of plant origin. Some cholesterol is essential for good health. It circulates continuously in the blood for use by all body cells. For example, lymphocytes, adrenal cortical cells, muscle cells, and renal cells use cholesterol to make cell membranes and steroid hormones, and the liver uses it to make bile acids.

Hypercholesterolemia can be an inherited disorder, or it can develop as a result of environmental factors, in particular, a diet that contains high levels of fat. Food fats contain a mixture of three types of fatty acids: saturated, monounsaturated, and polyunsaturated. These terms refer to the chemical bonds that link carbon and hydrogen atoms in the fatty acid molecules. Saturated fatty acids contain as many hydrogen atoms as possible, and the molecules stick together densely. A monounsaturated fatty acid has two fewer hydrogen atoms, and two of the carbon atoms are connected to each other by a double bond; a polyunsaturated fatty acid contains more than one such double bond. Of these, saturated fats have the greatest effect on raising blood cholesterol levels.

In the body, the liver is responsible for making new cholesterol when needed and for processing cholesterol from food. The liver puts together packages containing triglycerides (the most common type of fat, in which a molecule of glycerin is bonded to three molecules of fatty acids), cholesterol, and carrier proteins and releases these molecules into the bloodstream. Because they consist of lipids bound to proteins, these packages are called **lipoproteins.** They are spherical particles with a core of triglycerides and cholesterol, in varying proportions, surrounded by a surface coat of phospholipids. Most of the blood lipoprotein consists of two types:

- **High-density lipoproteins (HDL)** carry 20 to 30% of the total serum cholesterol, these are referred to as "good cholesterol".
- **Low-density lipoproteins (LDL)** carry 60 to 70% of the total serum cholesterol and are known as the "bad choleterol".
- **Triglycerides** are neutral fats synthesized from carbohydrates for storage in adipose (fat) cells. They release free fatty acids in the blood.

As the lipoproteins circulate, the triglycerides are drawn off for energy or storage. As described above, the LDLs that remain continue circulating to bring needed cholesterol to the cells of the body. LDLs not used by cells may be deposited in artery walls, eventually clogging them as shown in Figure 12.9. The narrowing of the arteries due to deposits of cholesterol and fat on the inner surface of the vessel is known as **atherosclerosis.** Atherosclerosis can result in stroke, MI, or limbs lost to gangrene.

For hyperlipidemia, the greatest risk to human health is posed by elevated LDL levels. Because HDLs return cholesterol to the liver, high HDL levels lower the risk of atherosclerosis and the related threat of heart disease and stroke. For this reason,

FIGURE 12.9
**Cross Section of
Arteries**

(a) Normal artery (b)
Clogged artery

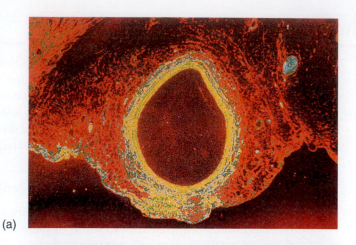
(a)

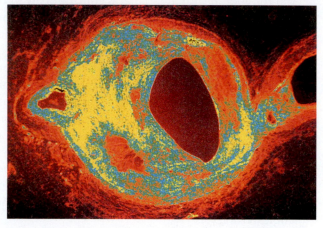
(b)

HDLs are sometimes called "good cholesterol," whereas LDLs are called "bad cholesterol." Considerable evidence collected over the last three decades has linked elevated LDLs and reduced HDLs to the development of coronary artery disease.

Premature atherosclerosis is the most common and significant consequence of hyperlipidemia. Both disorders are genetically determined but may be secondary to diabetes, obesity, alcoholism, hypothyroidism, liver disease, or kidney disease. In addition, in both men and women, total blood cholesterol increases throughout life. It enhances other risk factors for coronary artery disease.

Evidence now shows that lowering the blood lipid concentrations in a patient with atherosclerosis halts the process. Physicians recommend treatment for patients with hyperlipidemia because they are at increased risk and because the increased plasma lipid levels can be reduced somewhat by therapy with diet, drugs, or both. Most patients can achieve an average cholesterol reduction of 10% to 15% through diet. The major dietary recommendation is to reduce the amount of saturated fats in the diet and to ensure that the total fat intake does not exceed 30% of total calories. The treatment goals for cholesterol and LDL levels, in milligrams per 100 mL of blood, are as follows

- Total cholesterol: less than 200
- LDL cholesterol: less than 100
- HDL cholesterol: 60 or greater
- Triglyceride: less than 150

Lipid-Lowering Agents

Cholesterol-lowering drugs are always used as an adjunct to proper diet control. Table 12.15 presents the most commonly used hyperlipidemic agents. Physicians prescribe drugs based in part on lab values. Some medications work better to decrease LDLs, some to decrease triglycerides, and others to increase HDLs. Drugs from different classifications are often prescribed together because they are synergistic; for example, bile acids and niacin (Niacor), lovastatin (Altocor, Mevacor) and niacin (Niacor), and lovastatin (Altocor, Mevacor), and cholestyramine (Questran). However, interactions

TABLE 12.15   Most Commonly Used Lipid-Lowering Agents

Generic Name	Pronunciation	Dosage Form	Brand Name	Dispensing Status
HMG-CoA Reductase Inhibitors				
atorvastatin	a-tor-va-STAT-in	tablet	Lipitor	Rx
fluvastatin	floo-va-STAT-in	capsule	Lescol	Rx
lovastatin	loe-va-STAT-in	tablet	Altocor, Mevacor	Rx
pravastatin	prav-a-STAT-in	tablet	Pravachol	Rx
rosuvastatin	roe-soo-va-STAT-in	tablet	Crestor	Rx
simvastatin	sim-va-STAT-in	tablet	Zocor	Rx
Fibric Acid Derivatives				
clofibrate	kloe-FYE-brate	capsule	(none)	Rx
fenofibrate	fen-oh-FYE-brate	tablet	TriCor	Rx
gemfibrozil	jem-FYE-broe-zil	tablet	Lopid	Rx
Bile Acid Sequestrants				
cholestyramine	koe-les-TEER-a-meen	oral liquid	Questran	Rx
colesevelam	koh-le-SEV-a-lam	tablet	WelChol	Rx
colestipol	koe-LES-ti-pawl	oral liquid, tablet	Colestid	Rx
Other Cholesterol-Lowering Agents				
ezetimibe	ee-ZET-e-mib	tablet	Zetia	Rx
niacin	NYE-a-sin	tablet	Niacor	Rx
psyllium	SIL-ee-um	oral liquid	Fiberall, Metamucil	OTC
Omega–3 fatty acid		capsule	Lovaza	Rx
Combinations				
amlodipine-atorvastatin	am-LOE-di-peen a-tor-va-STAT-in	tablet	Caduet	Rx
ezetimibe-simvastatin	ee-ZET-e-mib sim-va-STAT-in	tablet	Vytorin	Rx
niacin-lovastatin	NYE-a-sin loe-va-STAT-in	tablet	Advicor	Rx
niacin (ER)-simvastatin	NYE-a-sin sim-va-STAT-in	tablet	Simcor	Rx
pravastatin–buffered aspirin	prav-a-STAT-in BUF-erd AS-per-in	tablet	Pravigard PAC	Rx

between these and other drugs can cause serious muscle problems. Any symptom of myalgia (muscle pain) should be reported to the physician immediately.

Some drugs increase cholesterol; obviously, patients with hyperlipidemia should avoid these medications. As in other situations, the advantages must be weighed against the disadvantages. For example, birth control pills increase cholesterol levels. More specifically, estrogen increases HDL, and progestin decreases HDL. Depending on the combination of these hormones in the birth control product, lipid profiles could change unfavorably. Estrogen given alone would have a favorable effect on the profile. Thiazide diuretics, loop diuretics, and glucocorticoids all increase the lipid profile unfavorably. In contrast, prazosin, clonidine, and calcium channel blockers increase HDL levels, so they would be good choices for someone with hyperlipidemia. Alli (orlistat) decreases LDLs. If a patient is taking a cholesterol-lowering drug, the technician should always check the profile for other drugs with interactions.

HMG-CoA Reductase Inhibitors An HMG-CoA reductase inhibitor, also known as a **statin** because the generic names of these drugs all end in "statin," inhibits the enzyme that catalyzes the rate-limiting step in cholesterol biosynthesis (HMG-CoA reductase is an abbreviated name for the enzyme). Side effects include GI upset and headache, which may dissipate with time. Any unexplained muscle pain or weakness, especially with fever, should be reported to the physician immediately. Liver enzymes should also be monitored regularly. Studies have shown that fluvastatin, lovastatin, and simvastatin have a greater cholesterol-lowering effect when taken at night because most cholesterol is produced at night. Patients taking statins should avoid drinking grapefruit juice within several hours of taking them, because grapefruit juice can inhibit intestinal metabolism of the statins and thus can significantly elevate serum levels. Some statins may need to be discontinued while the patient is on an antifungal or antibiotic. However, if the antifungal or antibiotic use is short-term, it is usually of no consequence. Most statins work better if taken in the evening.

Atorvastatin (Lipitor) is a potent lipid-lowering drug. It lowers LDLs significantly and also lowers triglycerides. Before atorvastatin appeared on the market, physicians had to resort to niacin or gemfibrozil to reduce triglyceride levels.

Lovastatin (Altocor, Mevacor) is an adjunct to dietary therapy to decrease elevated serum total and LDL concentration.

Rosuvastatin (Crestor) is very effective for lowering LDLs when it is combined with a healthy diet. It inhibits the synthesis of LDL. The most common side effects are muscle aches. It may be taken any time of the day with or without food.

Simvastatin (Zocor) acts on the enzyme that catalyzes the rate-limiting step in cholesterol biosynthesis. It should be taken at bedtime, and patients should report any muscle pain that is accompanied by fever. Simvastatin should be stored in well-sealed containers.

When required, a prescriber may switch a patient from one statin to another. The estimated equivalencies between the HMG-CoA reductase inhibitors are listed in Table 12.16. For example, 10 mg of rosuvastatin is equivalent to 80 mg of simvastatin. Patients should be monitored after a switch and doses adjusted as needed.

Fibric Acid Derivatives The exact mechanism of action for fibric acid derivatives is unknown. They increase the excretion of cholesterol in bile and therefore increase the risk of gallstones. If an oral anticoagulant is being taken concurrently, the dose of the anticoagulant should be decreased to maintain constant prothrombin time. When a fibric acid derivative is used in combination with a statin, there is risk of a reaction that destroys skeletal muscle and damages the kidney. As with statins, muscle pain should be reported to the physician.

TABLE 12.16   Statin Equivalency Chart

Generic Name	Brand Name	Equivalent Dose
atorvastatin	Lipitor	20 mg
rosuvastatin	Crestor	5 mg
fluvastatin	Lescol	160 mg
lovastatin	Altacor, Mevacor	80 mg
pravastatin	Pravachol	80 mg
simvastatin	Zocor	40 mg

Fenofibrate (TriCor) increases the catabolism (breakdown) of **VLDLs (very low-density lipoproteins)** by enhancing the synthesis of lipoprotein lipase. This drug is indicated as adjunctive therapy to dietary modification. If only marginal changes in total serum cholesterol and triglyceride concentrations are observed after 6 to 8 weeks of therapy, fenofibrate should be discontinued. The primary side effects of fenofibrate are mild GI disturbances such as gas, diarrhea, or constipation. It should be taken with food.

Clofibrate inhibits triglyceride synthesis in the liver and inhibits the breakdown of triglycerides in fat tissue. Adverse effects are headache, nausea, diarrhea, skin rash, and alteration of liver and kidney function.

Gemfibrozil (Lopid) lowers triglyceride and VLDL levels while increasing HDL levels by reducing liver triglyceride production. Adverse effects are GI symptoms (abdominal pain, diarrhea, nausea, vomiting), CNS symptoms (vertigo, headache), alteration in taste, and skin rash.

Bile Acid Sequestrants Bile acid sequestrants form a nonabsorbable complex with bile acids in the intestine. If a second medication is being used, it should be taken 1 hour before or 4 to 6 hours after the bile acid sequestrant. Constipation is the primary side effect.

Cholestyramine (Questran) stays in the intestines and combines with bile salts by combining with cholesterol and other fats, which are then removed in the feces. Adverse effects are nausea and vomiting due to the large doses required and pooling in the GI tract. Other effects are GI disturbances and binding to medication and fat-soluble vitamins (A, D, E, K). For this reason, vitamin supplementation may be necessary.

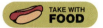

Colesevelam (WelChol) binds bile acids in the intestine, impeding their reabsorption and increasing the fecal loss of LDL. This drug should be taken with food.

Colestipol (Colestid) binds with bile acids to form an insoluble complex that is eliminated in the feces, thereby increasing fecal loss of LDL. This drug should be taken with water or fruit juice or sprinkled on food. After taking the granular form, the patient should rinse the glass with a full amount of liquid and drink the contents to ensure that the full dose is taken. Other drugs should be taken at least 1 hour before or 4 hours afterward. Side effects are primarily gastrointestinal, including constipation.

Other Cholesterol-Lowering Agents **Niacin (Niacor)** is vitamin B_3. It inhibits synthesis of VLDL by the liver and lowers triglyceride and LDL cholesterol levels. When first taken, it induces a strange phenomenon of extreme skin flushing. This is avoidable with aspirin prophylaxis 30 minutes before taking the drug, by taking it with food, and by increasing the dose very slowly. Other side effects are nausea, vomiting, diarrhea, and an increase in uric acid levels, which can produce symptoms of gout. Niacin is the most effective drug to increase HDL. The immediate-release type is preferred. Immediate-release and extended-release forms of this drug cannot be interchanged.

Niacin (Niaspan) should be taken at bedtime. It should not be crushed or halved. It raises HDL cholesterol and lowers LDL cholesterol. Flushing is the most common side effect. It is an extended-release form.

Psyllium (Fiberall, Metamucil) lowers cholesterol when used daily. It has the same effect as a high-fiber diet (as described in Chapter 10).

Ezetimibe (Zetia) lowers total cholesterol by inhibiting the absorption of cholesterol at the brush border of the small intestine, leading to a decreased delivery of cholesterol to the liver. It increases HDL.

Omega-3 Fatty Acids Elevated triglycerides may be treated with niacin, statins, or fibric acid derivatives as initial therapy. Omega-3 fatty acids in the form of fish oil supplements can be used as an alternative or adjunct in this treatment. If these supplements are purchased OTC it is important to verify that they are "USP" grade products. The omega-3 fatty acids in flaxseed and other products are different from the ones in fish. Diets high in these foods may decrease heart disease but not triglycerides. The fish oil supplements are the only ones that decrease triglyceride concentrations. There are also some claims by the health food industry that omega-3 fatty acids display some anti-inflammatory properties that may be beneficial for rheumatoid arthritis. Because some foods with omega-3 fatty acids have an unpleasant taste; refrigeration may improve their taste a little. The products should be destroyed when they get a strong rancid fishy taste or smell.

Omega-3 fatty acids **(Lovaza)**, derived from fish, interferes with the ability of the liver to synthesize triglycerides. It is indicated as an adjunct to diet. Lovaza is provided by the manufacturer as a soft gelatin capsule filled with light-yellow oil; bottles contain 120 capsules. It may be taken as a single dose of four capsules or as two capsules twice daily. The dose is 4 grams per day.

Combinations The combination **pravastatin–buffered aspirin (Pravigard PAC)** is approved to prevent heart attacks and strokes in patients with cardiovascular disease. The two drugs are both indicated to reduce the occurrence of cardiovascular events. Pravastatin lowers LDL and increases HDL. High cholesterol can lead to clogged vessels, which provide adhesion points for platelets. Buffered aspirin stops the clotting process and prevents the formation of clots in blood vessels, which can lead to MIs or strokes.

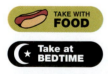

Niacin-lovastatin (Advicor) is an extended-release form of niacin along with an HMG-CoA reductase inhibitor. It is not intended for initial therapy. The statin will lower LDLs, and the niacin in turn lowers triglycerides and boosts HDLs with further lowering of the LDLs. It should be taken with food at bedtime.

Amlodipine-atorvastatin (Caduet) may be used to initiate treatment in patients with hyperlipidemia who have either hypertension or angina.

Chapter Terms

action potential the electrical signal that causes a muscle to contract

afterload arterial impedance, or the force against which cardiac muscle shortens; along with preload and contractility, determines cardiac output

angina pectoris spasmodic or suffocating chest pain caused by an imbalance between oxygen supply and oxygen demand

anticoagulant a drug that prevents clot formation by affecting clotting factors

antiplatelet a drug that reduces the risk of clot formation by inhibiting platelet aggregation

arrhythmia any variation from the normal heartbeat

ascites the accumulation of fluids in the abdominal organs and the lower extremities

atherosclerosis accumulation of lipoproteins and fats on the inner surfaces of arteries, eventually clogging the arteries and leading to MI, stroke, or gangrene

atrioventricular (AV) node part of the conduction system of the heart that carries the action potential from the atria to the ventricles with a delay

beta blocker a Class II antiarrhythmic drug that competitively blocks response to beta adrenergic stimulation and therefore lowers heart rate, myocardial contractility, blood pressure, and myocardial oxygen demand; used to treat arrhythmias, MIs, and angina

blood pressure (BP) the result of the heart forcing the blood through the capillaries; measured in millimeters of mercury, both when the heart is contracting and forcing the blood (systolic) and when the heart is relaxed and filling with blood (diastolic)

bradycardia abnormally slow heart rate (below 60 beats per minute)

calcium channel blocker a Class IV antiarrhythmic drug that prevents the movement of calcium ions through slow channels; used

for most supraventricular tachyarrhythmias and in angina

cardiomegaly enlargement of the heart due to overwork from overstimulation

cardiovascular (CV) pertaining to the heart and blood vessels

cerebral hemorrhage bleeding in the cerebellum

cholesterol an odorless, white, waxlike, powdery substance that is present in all foods of animal origin but not in foods of plant origin; circulates continuously in the blood for use by all body cells

clotting cascade a series of events that initiate blood clotting, or coagulation

congestive heart failure (CHF) a condition in which the heart can no longer pump adequate blood to the body's tissues; results in engorgement of the pulmonary vessels

contractility the cardiac muscle's capacity for becoming shorter in response to a stimulus; along with preload and afterload, determines cardiac output

depolarization reversal of the negative voltage across a heart or nerve cell membrane, caused by an inflow of positive ions

diastolic blood pressure the blood pressure measurement that measures the pressure during the dilation of the heart

ectopic pacemaker a pacemaker other than the SA node

fibrinolytic an agent that dissolves clots

glycoprotein antagonist an antiplatelet agent that binds to receptors on platelets, preventing platelet aggregation as well as the binding of fibrinogen and other adhesive molecules

high-density lipoproteins (HDLs) lipoproteins containing 5% triglyceride, 25% cholesterol, and 50% protein; "good cholesterol"

hypercholesterolemia excessive cholesterol in the blood

- **hyperlipidemia** elevation of the levels of one or more of the lipoproteins in the blood

- **hypertension** elevated blood pressure, where systolic blood pressure is greater than 140 mm Hg and diastolic pressure is greater than 90 mm Hg

International Normalized Ratio (INR) a method of standardizing the prothrombin time (PT) by comparing it to a standard index

ischemic stroke a cerebral infarction, in which a region of the brain is damaged by being deprived of oxygen

lipoprotein a spherical particle containing a core of triglycerides and cholesterol, in varying proportions, surrounded by a surface coat of phospholipids that enables it to remain in solution

low-density lipoproteins (LDLs) lipoproteins containing 6% triglycerides and 65% cholesterol; "bad cholesterol"

membrane stabilizing agent a Class I anti-arrhythmic drug that slows the movement of ions into cardiac cells, thus reducing the action potential and dampening abnormal rhythms and heartbeats

myocardial hypertrophy thickening of the heart muscle in response to overstimulation

- **myocardial infarction (MI)** a heart attack; occurs when a region of the heart muscle is deprived of oxygen

partial thromboplastin time (PTT) a test that measures the function of the intrinsic and common pathways in blood clotting; affected by heparin

preload the mechanical state of the heart at the end of diastole; along with afterload and contractility, determines cardiac output

prothrombin time (PT) a test that assesses the function of the extrinsic pathways of the coagulation system; affected by warfarin

pulmonary embolism (PE) sudden blocking of the pulmonary artery by a blood clot

repolarization restoration of the negative voltage across a heart or nerve cell membrane, caused by an outflow of positive ions

reversible ischemic neurologic deficit (RIND) a neurologic change, caused by a temporary shortage of oxygen, that reverses spontaneously but less rapidly than a TIA

- **sinoatrial (SA) node** the normal pacemaker area of the heart

stable angina a type of angina characterized by effort-induced chest pain from physical activity or emotional stress; usually predictable and reproducible

- **statin** an HMG-CoA reductase inhibitor, a drug that inhibits the rate-limiting step in cholesterol formation

stroke the result of an event (finite, ongoing, or protracted occurrences) that interrupts oxygen supply to an area of the brain; usually caused by cerebral infarction or cerebral hemorrhage

- **systolic blood pressure** a blood pressure measurement that measures the pressure during contraction of the heart

- **tachycardia** excessively fast heart rate

- **thrombus** blood clot

thrombocytopenia a decrease in the bone marrow production of blood platelets

transient ischemic attack (TIA) temporary neurologic change that occurs when part of the brain lacks sufficient blood supply over a brief period of time; may be a warning sign and predictor of imminent stroke

- **triglycerides** a neutral fat stored in animal adipose tissue which releases free fatty acids into the blood

unstable angina a type of angina characterized by chest pain that occurs with increasing frequency, diminishes the patient's ability to work, and has a decreasing response to treatment; may signal an oncoming MI

variant angina a type of angina characterized by chest pain due to coronary artery spasm; usually not stress induced

very-low-density lipoproteins (VLDLs) lipoproteins containing 60% triglycerides and 12% cholesterol

Chapter Summary

The Cardiovascular System and Causative Factors of Cardiovascular Disease

- The heart is a complicated organ. Many factors contribute to the development of heart disease. Some, such as heredity, gender, and age, are predetermined, but others can be influenced by lifestyle modification.
- Proper diet, exercise, and rest can do a lot to keep the heart functioning for a long time.

Angina

- Angina pectoris is an imbalance between oxygen supply to the heart and oxygen demand from the heart. The three types are stable, unstable, and variant.
- Drugs used to treat angina are beta blockers, nitrates, calcium channel blockers, and a metabolic modifier.
- Beta blockers may mask symptoms of hypoglycemia; therefore, diabetics should avoid them.
- Carvedilol (Coreg) is a beta blocker used for hypertension. It is nonselective and the only beta blocker approved for and used in heart failure.
- Sotalol (Betapace) is a beta blocker indicated for the treatment of arrhythmias that are life threatening.
- Nitrates are the drugs most used for angina; they dilate coronary vessels, leading to redistribution of blood flow to ischemic tissues. They reduce preload on the heart, which reduces cardiac workload.
- A transdermal nitroglycerin patch should be removed at night to avoid development of tolerance to the drug. The label should instruct the patient in this procedure.
- When patients begin using nitroglycerin, they commonly experience a severe headache.
- Nitroglycerin should be sold and stored in an amber glass container.
- Nitroglycerin should be replaced at least every 3 months; the patient should discard any remaining drug.
- Covera HS is a time-released verapamil tablet designed for bedtime dosing. It is approved for either angina or hypertension. The tablets do not release until about 4 to 5 hours after they have been swallowed. The drug is pumped out of two laser holes in the tablet. Patients may see a ghost tablet in their stool.
- Generic names of many beta blockers end in "lol."
- Generic names of many calcium channel blockers end in "ipine."

Arrhythmia

- Normal heart rhythm is generated by the sinoatrial (SA) node and propagated to the myocardium so that first the atria contract to fill the ventricles, then the ventricles contract to eject blood into the arteries.
- Heart rate abnormalities can be caused by ischemia, infarction, or alteration of chemical balances that allow heart cells other than the SA node to fire automatically and become ectopic pacemakers.
- Various types of arrhythmias show specific patterns on the ECG and are associated with different degrees of danger of sudden death.
- The various classes of antiarrhythmic drugs have characteristic electrophysiologic effects on the myocardium.
- The classes of drugs used to treat arrhythmias are grouped as Class I (membrane-stabilizing agents), Class II (beta blockers), Class III (potassium channel blockers), Class IV (calcium channel blockers), and others.
- Phenytoin (Dilantin) is an antiarrhythmic drug that is also used to control seizures.
- Digoxin (Lanoxicaps, Lanoxin) is an important drug in managing atrial flutter, fibrillation, and congestive heart failure. It increases the force of contraction, the refractory

period, and stimulation due to ion imbalance. The three primary signs of digtoxity are nausea, vomiting, and arrhythmias.

- Atropine is used for bradycardia, or heart rates less than 60 beats per minute. It is also used preoperatively to inhibit salivation and secretions.

Congestive Heart Failure

- Congestive heart failure (CHF) occurs when the pumping ability of the heart can no longer sustain the blood flow required to meet the metabolic needs of the body.
- In CHF, blood accumulates in the heart and circulation to other parts of the body is reduced; the kidney responds to the reduced blood flow by retaining water, causing fluid to accumulate in the body tissues.
- Fluid accumulates in the lungs when the left side of the heart fails. Fluid accumulates in the abdomen and lower extremities when the right side of the heart fails.
- Medications to treat the effects of heart failure include vasodilators, angiotensin-converting enzyme (ACE) inhibitors, and human B-type natriuretic peptide. These medications counteract contraction of small blood vessels (thus reducing the stress on the heart) and retention of fluids.
- Generic names of most ACE inhibitors end in "pril."

Hypertension

- Cardiac output, which is the product of heart rate and stroke volume, is determined by preload, afterload, and contractility.
- Hypertension is treated in stepwise fashion.
  Step 1. Change lifestyle.
  Step 2. Add a first-line drug.
  Step 3. Add a diuretic if not given in step 2.
  Step 4. Add a third drug that is synergistic with the others.
- High blood pressure should be treated with salt restriction, weight control, regular exercise, reduction of alcohol consumption, cessation of smoking, stress control, and medicine as prescribed.

- The first-line drug for hypertension can be a diuretic, a beta blocker, an ACE inhibitor, or a calcium channel blocker.
- ACE inhibitors reduce blood pressure by competitive inhibition of angiotensin-converting enzyme (ACE), preventing the conversion of angiotensin I to angiotensin II, a potent vasoconstrictor.
- Angiotensin receptor blockers (ARBs) reduce blood pressure by blocking angiotensin II at its receptors. Bound antiotensin II is not able to exert its effects. ARBs lead to less coughing and angioedema than ACEIs do because ACE, which breaks down bradykinin, is not inhibited.
- Generic names of most ARBs end in "artan."
- Calcium channel blockers reduce blood pressure by arteriolar dilation, which leads to reduced peripheral resistance.
- Beta blockers, calcium channel blockers and Ace inhibitors are all equally effective drugs used in the treatment of hypertension.
- Clonidine is the only antihypertensive that has a transdermal delivery system.
- Minoxidil (Loniten, Rogaine) reduces blood pressure and stimulates hair growth.
- Combination drugs have additive effects to relax blood vessels and lower pressure. Two low doses of different drugs usually cause fewer side effects than pushing the dose of either drug.

Myocardial Infarction (MI)

- Myocardial infarction (MI) occurs when there is a prolonged decrease in oxygen delivery to a region of cardiac muscle, which dies.
- MI is the leading cause of death in industrialized nations.
- Symptoms include oppressive or burning tightness or squeezing in the chest, a feeling of choking and indigestion-like expansion, a sense of "impending doom," and substernal pain, which may radiate to the neck, throat, jaw, shoulders, and one or both arms.
- Beta blockers and low-dose aspirin are prescribed for reducing the risk of death or recurrence following an MI.

Blood Clots

- Blood clots in the bloodstream (thrombi) can cause life-threatening pulmonary embolism and other serious damage.
- Anticoagulants prevent clot formation by affecting clotting factors; antiplatelets reduce the risk of clot formation by inhibiting platelet aggregation.
- The therapy for deep vein thrombosis (DVT) is either low-dose heparin, adjusted-dose heparin, or low-molecular-weight heparin, and warfarin (Coumadin). The purpose is to prevent fatal blood clotting while ensuring adequate coagulation.
- Partial thromboplastin time (PTT) measures the function of the intrinsic and common pathways; it is affected by heparin.
- Heparin inhibits thrombin formation, thereby reducing clot formation; it does not dissolve a clot that has already formed.
- Lepirudin (Refludan) is an alternative anticoagulant for patients who cannot tolerate heparin.
- Protamine sulfate is the antidote for heparin.
- Phytonadione, vitamin K (Mephyton) is an antidote for warfarin.
- Low-molecular-weight heparins are given 12 hours after surgery. The advantages of these heparins are reduced bleeding, reliable dose response, longer plasma half-life, and no effect on platelets.
- Tinzaparin (Innohep) should not be interchanged with the other low-molecular-weight heparins.
- Aspirin is prescribed to prevent strokes and MIs
- Glycoprotein antagonists are administered during invasive procedures to prevent artery closure.
- Eptifibatide (Integrilin) mimics native protein sequences in the platelet receptors. It is used in conjunction with heparin and aspirin.
- Fibrinolytic agents dissolve clots. They are used for massive PE and MI.

Stroke

- A stroke may be caused by one of two primary events: cerebral hemorrhage and cerebral infarction.
- A TIA is a very strong predictor of an impending stroke.
- Risk factors for stroke include advanced age, male gender, hypertension, smoking, alcohol abuse, diabetes, and high cholesterol levels.
- Emphasis should be on stroke prevention.
- Antiplatelet agents prevent platelet activation and formation of the platelet plug.
- Anticoagulant agents are used for deep vein thrombosis and pulmonary emboli and in prevention of stroke.

High Cholesterol and Related Diseases

- Food fats contain a mixture of three fatty acids: saturated, monounsaturated, and polyunsaturated.
- The liver packages triglycerides, cholesterol, and carrier proteins in spherical particles called lipoproteins, which circulate in the blood.
- LDLs (low-density lipoproteins) not used by the cells may be deposited in artery walls, eventually clogging them.
- HDLs (high-density lipoproteins) may prevent cholesterol buildup in arteries.
- Triglycerides release free fatty acids in the blood to be stored in adipose cells.
- Drugs are used as an adjunct to proper diet to prevent buildup of LDLs.
- Some combinations of these drugs are synergistic; others can be dangerous. Any symptom of muscle pain should be reported to the physician immediately.
- Thiazide diuretics, loop diuretics, and glucocorticoids all increase the lipid profile unfavorably.
- Simvastatin (Zocor) acts on the enzyme that catalyzes the rate-limiting step in cholesterol biosynthesis.

- Atorvastatin (Lipitor) is a potent lipid-lowering drug. It lowers LDLs significantly and also lowers triglycerides. Before this drug, physicians had to resort to niacin or gemfibrozil to reduce triglyceride levels.
- Statins are HMG-CoA reductase inhibitors and the generic name ends in "statin."
- Fenofibrate (TriCor) increases the catabolism of VLDLs.

- Ezetimibe (Zetia) decreases cholesterol by inhibiting the absorption of cholesterol at the brush border of the small intestine.
- Manufacturers have combined drugs with synergistic mechanisms of action to lower cholesterol.

Drug List

The following drugs were discussed in this chapter. Each generic drug name is followed in parentheses by one or more brand names.

Antianginal Drugs

Beta Blockers
- acebutolol (Sectral)
- atenolol* (Tenormin)
- betaxolol (Kerlone)
- bisoprolol (Zebeta)
- carvedilol (Coreg)*
- esmolol (Brevibloc)
- labetalol (Normodyne, Trandate)
- metoprolol* (Lopressor, Toprol-XL)
- nadolol (Corgard)
- nebivolol (Bystolic)
- pindolol (Visken)
- propranolol (Inderal)*
- sotalol (Betapace)
- timolol (Blocadren)

Nitrates
- isosorbide dinitrate (Dilatrate SR, Isordil)
- isosorbide mononitrate (Imdur, Ismo)
- nitroglycerin* (Minitran, Nitrolingual, Nitrostat, NitroDur)

Calcium Channel Blockers
- amlodipine* (Norvasc)
- diltiazem (Cardizem, Dilacor XR)*
- felodipine (Plendil)
- isradipine (DynaCirc)
- nicardipine (Cardene)
- nifedipine* (Procardia)

- nisoldipine (Sular)*
- verapamil* (Calan, Covera HS, Isoptin, Verelan)

Metabolic Modifier
- ranolozine (Ranexa)

Antiarrhythmic Agents

Membrane-Stabilizing Agents
- disopyramide (Norpace)
- flecainide (Tambocor)
- lidocaine (Xylocaine)
- mexiletine (Mexitil)
- moricizine (Ethmozine)
- phenytoin (Dilantin)*
- procainamide (Procanbid, Pronestyl)
- propafenone (Rythmol)
- quinidine
- tocainide (Tonocard)

Potassium Channel Blockers
- amiodarone (Cordarone)
- dofetilide (Tikosyn)

Other Antiarrhythmic Agents
- atropine
- digoxin* (Lanoxicaps, Lanoxin)
- isoproterenol (Isuprel)

Antidote for Digoxin Toxicity
- digoxin immune Fab (Digibind)

ACE Inhibitors
- benazepril* (Lotensin)
- captopril (Capoten)
- enalapril (Vasotec)*
- fosinopril (Monopril)
- lisinopril* (Prinivil, Zestril)
- moexipril (Univasc)
- perindopril (Aceon)
- quinapril* (Accupril)
- ramipril (Altace)*
- trandolapril (Mavik)

Human B-type Natriuretic Peptide
- nesiritide (Natrecor)

Vasodilators
- epoprostenol (Flolan)
- fenoldopam (Corlopam)
- hydralazine (Apresoline)
- isoproterenol (Isuprel)
- isosorbide-hydralazine (BiDil)*
- milrinone (Primacor)
- minoxidil (Loniten, Rogaine)
- nitroprusside (Nitropress)
- sildenafil (Revatio, Viagra)*
- treprostinil (Remodulin)

Drugs for Treating Hypertension

Angiotensin II Receptor Antagonists (ARBs)
- candesartan (Atacand)*
- eprosartan (Teveten)
- irbesartan (Avapro)*
- losartan (Cozaar)*
- olmesartan (Benicar)*
- telmisartan (Micardis)*
- valsartan (Diovan)*

CNS Agents
- clonidine (Catapres, Catapres-TTS, Duraclon)*
- guanfacine (Tenex)
- methyldopa (Aldomet)

Peripheral Acting Agents (Alpha Blockers)
- alfuzosin (Uroxatral)*
- doxazosin (Cardura)
- phentolamine (Regitine)
- prazosin (Minipress)
- terazosin (Hytrin)*

Direct Renin Inhibitors
- aliskiren (Tekturna)

Combinations
- amlodipine-benazepril (Lotrel)*
- amlodipine-valsartan (Exforge)
- atenolol-hydrochlorothiazide (Tenorectic)*
- benazepril-hydrochlorothiazide (Lotensin HCT)
- bisoprolol-hydrochlorothiazide (Ziac)*
- enalapril-diltiazem (Teczem)
- enalapril-hydrochlorothiazide (Vaseretic)
- irbesartan-hydrochlorothiazide (Avalide)*
- lisinopril-hydrochlorothiazide (Zestoretic)*
- losartan-hydrochlorothiazide (Hyzaar)*
- trandolapril-verapamil (Tarka)*
- valsartan-hydrochlorothiazide (Diovan HCT)*

Anticoagulants
- bivalirudin (Angiomax)
- fondaparinux (Arixtra)
- heparin
- lepirudin (Refludan)
- warfarin (Coumadin)*

Low-Molecular-Weight Heparins
- dalteparin (Fragmin)
- enoxaparin (Lovenox)
- tinzaparin (Innohep)

Antidote for Heparin
- protamine sulfate

Antidote for Warfarin
- phytonadione, vitamin K (Mephyton)

Antiplatelet Agents
- aspirin*
- clopidogrel (Plavix)*
- ticlopidine (Ticlid)

Glycoprotein Antagonists
- abciximab (ReoPro)
- eptifibatide (Integrilin)
- tirofiban (Aggrastat)

Fibrinolytic Agents
- alteplase (Activase)
- reteplase (Retavase)
- tenecteplase (TNKase)
- urokinase (Abbokinase)

Stroke Prevention
aspirin-dipyridamole (Aggrenox)*
dipyridamole (Persantine)
pentoxifylline (Trental)

Lipid-Lowering Agents

HMG-CoA Reductase Inhibitors (Statins)
atorvastatin (Lipitor)*
fluvastatin (Lescol)
lovastatin (Altocor, Mevacor)
pravastatin (Pravachol)*
rosuvastatin (Crestor)*
simvastatin (Zocor)*

Fibric Acid Derivatives
clofibrate
fenofibrate (TriCor)*
gemfibrozil (Lopid)*

Bile Acid Sequestrants
cholestyramine (Questran)
colesevelam (WelChol)
colestipol (Colestid)

Miscellaneous Cholesterol-Lowering Drugs
ezetimibe (Zetia)*
niacin (Niacor)
Omega-3 fatty acid (Lovaza)
psyllium (Fiberall, Metamucil)

Combinations
amlodipine-atorvastatin (Caduet)*
ezetimibe-simvastatin (Vytorin)*
niacin-lovastatin (Advicor)
niacin ER-simvastatin (Simcor)
pravastatin–buffered aspirin (Pravigard PAC)

Chapter Review

Pharmaceuticals and Body Functions

Select the best answer from the choices given.

1. Which drug is sold in an amber glass container and should not be repackaged?
   a. Ticlid
   b. Lopid
   c. nitroglycerin
   d. lisinopril

2. Which syringe would *not* be appropriate to dispense with heparin?
   a. IM syringes
   b. TB syringes
   c. allergy syringes
   d. insulin syringes

3. Which drug causes flushing when the patient begins taking it?
   a. lidocaine
   b. niacin
   c. Dilantin
   d. tocainide

4. Which is the "bad" cholesterol?
   a. HDLs
   b. lymphocytes
   c. LDLs
   d. bile acids

5. Which beta blocker is preferred for the heart?
   a. beta-1
   b. beta-2
   c. nonselective
   d. all of the above

6. Which over-the-counter diet drug will lower cholesterol?
   a. Cordarone
   b. Alli
   c. Procanbid
   d. all of the above

7. Which drug class is a good first-step prescription for hypertension?
   a. beta blockers
   b. calcium channel blockers
   c. diuretics
   d. all of the above

8. The leading cause of death in industrialized nations is
   a. cancer.
   b. MI.
   c. stroke.
   d. a and b.

9. Which factor(s) increase risk of heart attack?
   a. proper diet
   b. appropriate rest
   c. cigarette smoking
   d. all of the above

10. A beta blocker is given after an MI to
    a. speed heart action.
    b. reduce risk of death.
    c. prevent stroke.
    d. improve breathing.

The following statements are true or false. If the answer is false, rewrite the statement so it is true.

_____ 1. The drug of choice for acute angina attacks is Lanoxin.

_____ 2. A nitroglycerin patch should be left on for 24 hours.

_____ 3. Drug combinations usually improve compliance but increase side effects.

_____ 4. Heparin inhibits thrombin formation and dissolves a clot after it has formed.

_____ 5. Nutrition guidelines indicate that the total intake of fat should not exceed 65% of the diet.

_____ 6. Cerebral hemorrhage differs significantly from ischemia. Ischemia is the result of obstruction to flow; hemorrhage involves primary rupture of a blood vessel.

_____ 7. Lidocaine is never used as an antiarrhythmic agent.

_____ 8. The advantages of low-molecular-weight heparins are reduced bleeding, reliable dose response, elimination of the need for monitoring, and longer plasma half-life.

_____ 9. Vessel blockage can be of several types: fat, air, and accumulation of debris.

_____ 10. Captopril directly inhibits angiotensin II.

Place the correct letter in each blank.

a. ACE inhibitor

b. beta blocker

c. calcium channel blocker

_____ 1. Inderal

_____ 2. nifedipine

_____ 3. Calan

_____ 4. DynaCirc

_____ 5. Betapace

_____ 6. captopril

_____ 7. Lotensin

_____ 8. Visken

_____ 9. Vasotec

_____ 10. Accupril

_____ 11. Toprol XL

_____ 12. Normodyne

_____ 13. Altace

_____ 14. acebutolol

_____ 15. propranolol

_____ 16. amlodipine

_____ 17. lisinopril

_____ 18. quinapril

_____ 19. verapamil

_____ 20. metoprolol

Diseases and Drug Therapies

1. Identify four types of drugs used to treat arrhythmias. List two drugs per group.

2. Discuss the stepwise treatment of hypertension.

3. What is the difference between anticoagulants and fibrinolytics? List the ones discussed and designate their class.

4. Classify the lipid-lowering drugs, using the brand name.

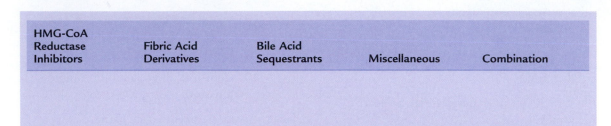

HMG-CoA Reductase Inhibitors	Fibric Acid Derivatives	Bile Acid Sequestrants	Miscellaneous	Combination

Dispensing Medications

1. Mr. Bob Day receives Pravachol 40 mg po daily to lower his cholesterol levels.

   How many doses would be dispensed for a 90 day supply?

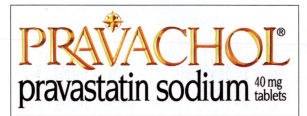

2. The intern sent the following orders down:

   Mr. Brown, 50 mg protamine sulfate STAT.

   You check Mr. Brown's chart, and he received 3,000 units of heparin. What would be the correct dosage for the protamine sulfate?

3. Mrs. Jones brings in the following prescription. Is this a good combination? Why or why not?

Rx

MT. HOPE MEDICAL PARK
ST. PAUL, MN (651) 555-3591

DEA# _____

Pt. name __Bill Jones__ Date __Aug 5, 07__

Address _____

Mevacor twenty (20) mg with
*   evening meal # thirty (30)*

Questran four (4) g bid # sixty (60)

_____ Dispense as written

_____ Fills _____ times (no refill unless indicated)

_____ *J. Cruns* _____ M.D.

Internet Research

Use the Internet to complete the following assignments.

1. Locate statistics on heart disease. What is the yearly incidence of myocardial infarction in the United States? How many individuals are currently living with congestive heart failure? Coronary artery disease? Make sure to include the date associated with your data source(s). List your Internet sources.

2. Research low-molecular-weight heparins. Create a table explaining their use.

What Would you do?

1. The patient complains that the blood pressure medication only makes him feel worse and it is expensive, so stopping the drug is just the best thing to do. What would you do?

Drugs for Muscle and Joint Disease and Pain

13

Learning Objectives

- Define muscle relaxants.
- Identify muscle relaxants and their various mechanisms of action.
- Identify the nonnarcotic analgesics, and describe their uses and mechanisms of action.

- Understand an autoimmune disease.
- Identify agents used to treat arthritis, rheumatoid arthritis, and gout, and discuss their usage and side effects.

Preview chapter terms and definitions.

M uscle relaxants are used to reduce spasticity in multiple sclerosis, cerebral palsy, skeletal muscle injuries, orthopedic surgery, postoperative recovery, and spinal cord injury. Other problems that involve muscles and joints are treated with nonsteroidal anti-inflammatory drugs (NSAIDs). Many NSAIDs are achieving OTC status. This means that more NSAIDs will be used by patients for self-medication. The pharmacy technician must be aware of the side effects and proper use of these drugs.

Muscles and Joints

Bones of the skeletal system, which provides the framework of the human body, are connected at joints. A joint is the place of union or junction between two or more bones of the skeleton. Joints allow the rigid skeleton flexibility. The work of movement at joints is performed by skeletal muscles, which are contractile tissues. That is, joints and muscles work together to allow the body to move. Any injury or illness that seriously affects a joint or muscle impedes movement of that part of the body and can have a devastating effect on the quality of life. Even relatively minor injuries, stiffness, or minor but persistent pain can be very annoying.

The human body contains a wide variety of joints. The anatomy of a typical joint is shown in Figure 13.1. In addition to the components shown in Figure 13.1, ligaments (noncontractile connective tissue that ties one bone to another bone) are essential to maintaining the bones in correct alignment and forming the

FIGURE 13.1
Anatomy of a Joint

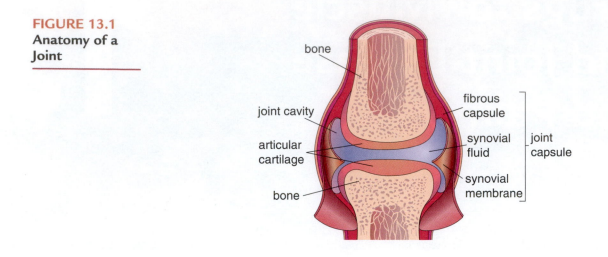

fibrous capsule that encloses the moving parts. Joints can be classified in a number of ways. One method of classification is joint structure. Joints can be classified by their structure into the following types:

- Cartilaginous—articulating bone surfaces are covered with cartilage
- Fibrous—articulating bone surfaces are attached by fibrous connective tissue
- Synovial—articulating surface is covered by a fluid-filled, fibrous sac

Furthermore, joints can be classified based on whether they permit no movement, a slight degree of movement, or a variety of types of movement. Figure 13.2 presents a variety of joint types.

A muscle is an organ that produces movement by contracting (shortening itself). Muscles are connected to bones by tough cordlike tissues called tendons. Figure 13.3 shows involvement of bones, muscles, and tendon to produce movement at the elbow joint. In addition to skeletal movement, muscle contraction pumps blood, facilitates motility in the gastrointestinal tract, and produces uterine contraction during birth. Muscles are typically grouped into the following three types:

- Skeletal—striated muscle in which contraction is voluntary; contraction is used for locomotion and maintaining posture
- Smooth—muscle in which contraction is involuntary; occurs in the lining of various organs such as the stomach, esophagus, uterus, and bladder
- Cardiac—heart muscle; involuntary, but the texture of the muscle is striated

These three types of muscles are illustrated in Figure 13.4.

Muscle Relaxants

Skeletal muscles are voluntarily controlled by impulses originating in the central nervous system (CNS). Electrical impulses are conducted through the spinal cord by somatic neurons that eventually communicate with the muscle at the neuromuscular junction (illustrated in Figure 8.3). The neurotransmitter **acetylcholine** (ACh) is released to bind with nicotinic receptors on the muscle cell membrane. When the neurotransmitter binds to the receptor, calcium is released, causing a contraction in the muscle fibers. Relaxation occurs when ACh is broken down by acetylcholinesterase. Skeletal muscle contractions can be either voluntary (movement) or involuntary (tone, posture).

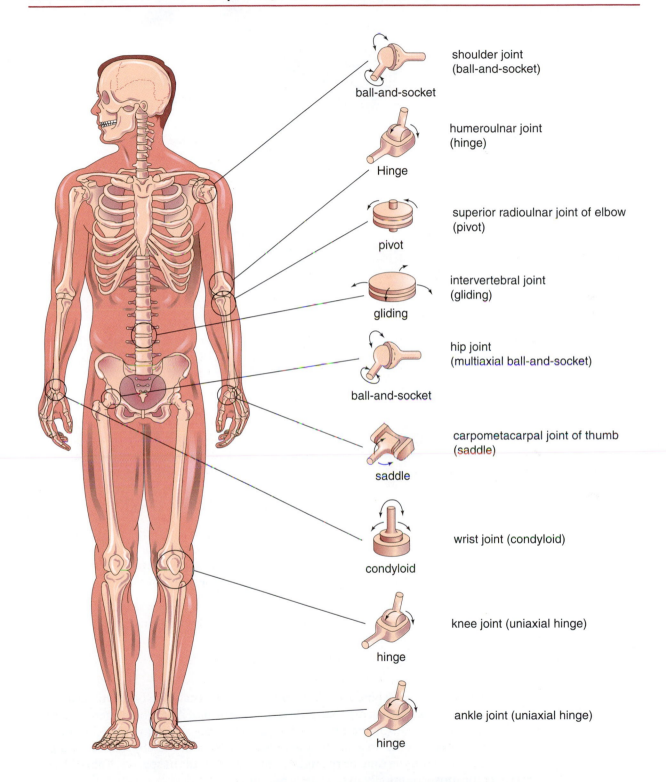

ball-and-socket

shoulder joint
(ball-and-socket)

Hinge

humeroulnar joint
(hinge)

pivot

superior radioulnar joint of elbow
(pivot)

gliding

intervertebral joint
(gliding)

ball-and-socket

hip joint
(multiaxial ball-and-socket)

saddle

carpometacarpal joint of thumb
(saddle)

condyloid

wrist joint (condyloid)

hinge

knee joint (uniaxial hinge)

hinge

ankle joint (uniaxial hinge)

FIGURE 13.3
Involvement of
Bones, Muscles,
and Tendon
to Produce
Movement at the
Elbow Joint

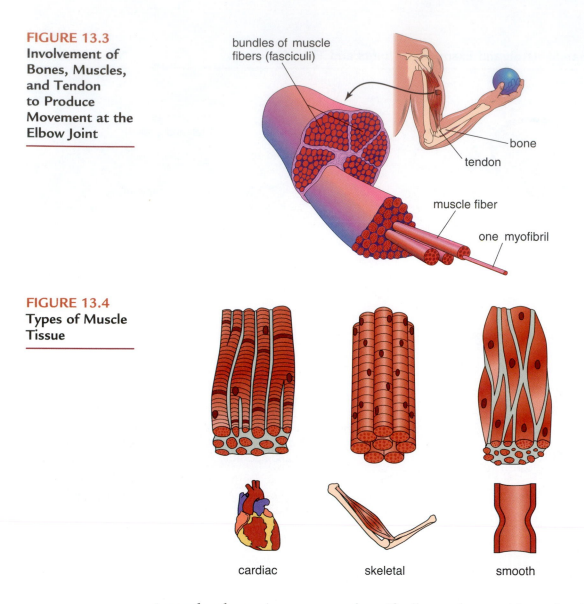

bundles of muscle
fibers (fasciculi)

bone

tendon

muscle fiber

one myofibril

FIGURE 13.4
Types of Muscle
Tissue

cardiac   skeletal   smooth

A **muscle relaxant** is an agent used specifically to reduce muscle tension. These substances act on motor neurons or at the neuromuscular junction. These agents block normal muscle function by one of the following mechanisms:

- blocking release of ACh
- preventing destruction of ACh at nicotinic receptors (continuous depolarization leads to paralysis by fatigue)
- preventing ACh from reaching nicotinic receptors (competitive nondepolarizing inhibitors)

Agents that continuously bind to ACh nicotinic receptors can also block normal muscle function; like the agents that prevent destruction of ACh, these agents act as depolarizing agents, causing paralysis by fatigue. Centrally acting muscle relaxants do not directly relax muscles. Instead, they depress the CNS and thereby reduce the anxiety that increases muscle tone or the reflex signals that result in spasms. Table 13.1 presents the most commonly used muscle relaxants.

Muscle relaxants are used to reduce spasticity in multiple sclerosis, cerebral palsy, skeletal muscle injuries, orthopedic surgery, postoperative recovery, and spinal cord

TABLE 13.1   Most Commonly Used Muscle Relaxants

Generic Name	Pronunciation	Dosage Form	Brand Name	Dispensing Status	Control Schedule
baclofen	BAK-loe-fen	injection, tablet	Lioresal	Rx	
carisoprodol	kar-eye-soe-PROE-dawl	tablet	Soma	Rx	C-IV*
chlorzoxazone	klor-ZOX-a-zone	capsule, tablet	Paraflex, Parafon Forte DSC	Rx	
cyclobenzaprine	sye-kloe-BEN-za-preen	tablet	Flexeril	Rx	
dantrolene	DAN-troe-leen	capsule, IV	Dantrium	Rx	
diazepam	dye-AZ-e-pam	IV, tablet	Valium	Rx	C-IV
metaxalone	me-TAX-a-lone	tablet	Skelaxin	Rx	
methocarbamol	meth-oh-KAR-ba-mawl	injection, IV, tablet	Robaxin	Rx	
orphenadrine	or-FEN-a-dreen	injection, IV, tablet	Norflex	Rx	

*in some states

injury. Some dispensing issues are common among the muscle relaxants. To avoid possible drug interactions, a drug history should be done on a patient before administering any of these drugs. The pharmacy technician will often obtain this history. The sedative properties of these drugs cause the patient to relax, which in turn reduces reflex impulse conduction. Side effects of the muscle relaxants are sedation, reduced mental alertness, reduced motor abilities, and GI upset. Patients taking these drugs should avoid alcohol.

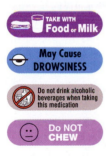

Baclofen (Lioresal) is a centrally acting muscle relaxant. That is, it does not directly act on the muscle or neuromuscular junction but inhibits transmission of monosynaptic and polysynaptic reflexes at the spinal cord level to relieve **muscle spasticity**, a condition whereby muscle fibers are in a state of continuous, involuntary contraction as a result of reflex impulses. It is used for treating reversible spasticity resulting from spinal cord lesions or multiple sclerosis. Its mode of action may be hyperpolarization of the terminals of the fibers that carry the initial stimulus signal that initiates the reflex. It also has a number of unlabeled uses including hiccups and bladder spasticity. Baclofen should be taken with food or milk and may impair coordination and judgment. Abrupt withdrawal after prolonged use may cause hallucinations, tachycardia, or spasticity.

Carisoprodol (Soma) is a centrally acting skeletal muscle relaxant that is sometimes subject to abuse. Once the drug is ingested, the molecules are cleaved to the active metabolite: meprobamate, a Schedule IV controlled substance that relieves anxiety leading to muscle tension. Because of the abuse potential, carisoprodol is a scheduled substance in many states. It causes drowsiness and dizziness. Use with alcohol and other CNS depressants increases the risk of toxicity; it also interacts with clindamycin, phenothiazines, and monoamine oxidase inhibitors (MAOIs).

Chlorzoxazone (Paraflex, Parafon Forte DSC) is indicated for symptomatic treatment of muscle spasms and pain associated with acute musculoskeletal conditions. It does not directly affect the muscle or the neuromuscular junction but is believed to act, like baclofen, on the spinal cord by depressing polysynaptic reflexes. It may cause drowsiness and dizziness. Alcohol consumption should be avoided while taking this medication.

Cyclobenzaprine (Flexeril) is indicated for treating muscle spasms associated with acute painful musculoskeletal conditions and for supportive therapy in tetanus.

It is a centrally acting skeletal muscle relaxant that is pharmacologically related to tricyclic antidepressants. It reduces tonic somatic motor activity influencing both alpha and gamma motor neurons. Onset of action is usually within 1 hour. The drug should not be used for more than 2 to 3 weeks. It may impair ability to perform hazardous activities requiring physical coordination.

Dantrolene (Dantrium) acts on skeletal muscle beyond the neuromuscular junctions. It reduces muscle responsiveness to stimulation and decreases the force of contraction by reducing the amount of calcium released from the sacs of the T tubules. It is used in treating spasticity related to spinal cord injuries, stroke, cerebral palsy, and multiple sclerosis. The side effects are malaise, weakness, fatigue, possible liver toxicity, and photosensitivity. Alcohol and other CNS depressants should be avoided. Dantrolene is also given before surgery to patients susceptible to malignant hyperthermia; this use was discussed in greater detail in Chapter 6.

Diazepam (Valium), a benzodiazepine, relieves anxiety causing muscle contraction. Some authorities consider it to be the best muscle relaxer, but it has significant abuse potential. It should not be discontinued abruptly after prolonged use.

Metaxalone (Skelaxin) is available in 800 mg scored tablets. The drug has no direct action on muscle, endplate, or fiber. It probably relaxes muscles through general CNS depression and may cause drowsiness. The patient should notify the physician if a skin rash or yellowish discoloration of the skin and/or eyes occurs.

Methocarbamol (Robaxin) is used to treat muscle spasms associated with acute painful musculoskeletal conditions and as supportive therapy in tetanus. It causes skeletal muscle relaxation by reducing the transmission of impulses from the spinal cord to skeletal muscles. Methocarbamol may cause drowsiness or impair judgment or coordination. Patients should avoid alcohol or other CNS depressants and should notify the physician of rash, itching, or nasal congestion. The drug may turn urine brown, black, or green.

Orphenadrine (Norflex) is indicated to treat muscle spasms and to provide supportive therapy in tetanus. It is an indirect skeletal muscle relaxant thought to work by central atropine-like effects; it has some euphorigenic (induces a state of euphoria) and analgesic properties. Orphenadrine may cause drowsiness. The tablet should be swallowed whole, not crushed or chewed. The patient should avoid alcohol, because orphenadrine also may impair coordination and judgment.

Inflammation and Swelling

An **analgesic** is any medication taken to relieve pain. A **nonnarcotic analgesic** is used for mild to moderate pain, inflammation, and fever. Pain may be either dull, throbbing **somatic pain** from skin, muscle, and bone or sharp, stabbing **visceral pain** from organs. Figure 13.5 shows the pathway by which inflammation, pain, and fever develop when a tissue is injured. The nonnarcotic analgesics are believed to relieve pain by interrupting the pathway. They inhibit the enzyme cyclooxygenase and thereby decrease the conversion of arachidonic acid to prostaglandins (PGs), thromboxane A_2, and prostacyclin. Because the body cannot store PGs, they must be newly synthesized to be released during inflammation. Thus, the inhibition of cyclooxygenase reduces the synthesis of PGs and thereby reduces their influence at sites of inflammation and tissue damage.

Similarly, decreasing the synthesis of PGs can reduce a fever. Fever is a response by the body's temperature-regulating center, the hypothalamus, to substances called endogenous pyrogens, which are produced in response to bacterial or viral infections. The subsequent release of PGs from the brain causes the body "thermostat" to reset at a higher temperature—a fever.

FIGURE 13.5
Pain Pathway in Tissue Injury

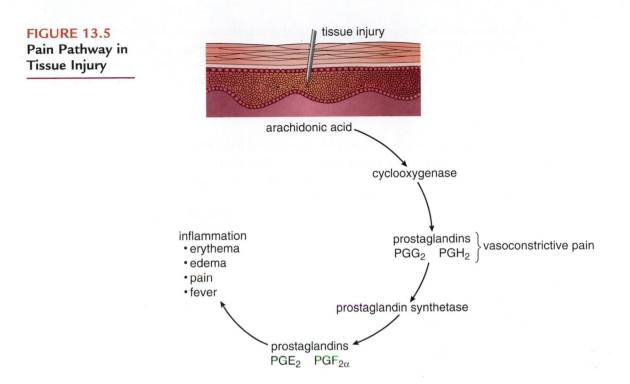

tissue injury

arachidonic acid

cyclooxygenase

prostaglandins
PGG$_2$ PGH$_2$ } vasoconstrictive pain

prostaglandin synthetase

prostaglandins
PGE$_2$ PGF$_{2\alpha}$

inflammation
• erythema
• edema
• pain
• fever

Although nonnarcotic analgesics offer benefits, adverse gastrointestinal (GI) effects may limit their use, because PGs promote mucosal production in the stomach, protecting the gastric lining from autodigestion by acids. By preventing the production of PGs, nonnarcotic analgesics risk exposing the stomach to ulceration. These products also elevate serum concentrations of hepatic enzymes, promote water and electrolyte retention, and can cause acute renal insufficiency. In addition, some nonnarcotic analgesics can displace oral anticoagulants, sulfonylureas, phenytoin, and sulfonamides from binding to plasma proteins. Table 13.2 lists the most commonly

TABLE 13.2	Most Commonly Used Nonnarcotic Analgesics			
Generic Name	**Pronunciation**	**Dosage Form**	**Brand Name**	**Dispensing Status**
Salicylates				
aspirin (acetylsalicylic acid)	AS-pir-in	capsule, gum, oral liquid, suppository	(many)	OTC
buffered aspirin	BUF-erd AS-pir-in	tablet	Ascriptin, Bufferin	OTC
choline magnesium trisalicylate	KOE-leen-mag-NEE-zhum-trye-sa-LIS-il-ate	liquid, tablet	Trilisate	Rx
salsalate	SAL-sa-late	tablet	Amigesic	Rx
Antipyretic Analgesic				
acetaminophen	a-seat-a-MIN-oh-fen	oral liquid, suppository, tablet	Tylenol	OTC
Acetaminophen Antidote				
acetylcysteine	a-set-il-SIS-teen	oral, IV	Mucomyst, Acetadote	Rx

used nonnarcotic analgesics. Nonsteroidal anti-inflammatory drugs (NSAIDs) are a class of drugs that are analgesic, **antipyretic** (fever reducing), and anti-inflammatory. The prototype NSAID is aspirin (salicylate). Acetaminophen, which is both analgesic and antipyretic, is not an NSAID, because it has little if any effect on inflammation.

Salicylates

Salicylates were initially discovered and isolated from the bark of the white willow tree and were first used for rheumatic fever. They have both analgesic (pain-relieving) and antipyretic (fever-reducing) as well as anti-inflammatory properties. The primary analgesic action is peripheral rather than central. In contrast, the primary antipyretic action is central, presumably in the hypothalamus. Salicylates reduce fever by increasing blood flow to the skin and inhibiting PG synthesis.

Salicylates are indicated for

- arthritis
- inflammation of arthritis and rheumatism
- menstrual cramps
- muscular aches and pains
- pain and fever of influenza or other infections
- simple headache (headache other than migraine)

Salicylates should be avoided after surgery or tooth extraction, in hemophiliac patients (because they can interfere with normal clotting), and in patients with asthma, nasal polyps, chronic sinusitis, and bleeding ulcers (because salicylates may trigger an allergic-like hypersensitivity reaction).

Low dosages (300 mg to 900 mg per day) of salicylate can be taken safely. More than 4 g per day can cause problems; 10 g per day can be lethal. It is not uncommon, however, for a patient with rheumatoid arthritis to take 3 g to 6 g per day under a physician's supervision.

If used during pregnancy, salicylates may result in anemia, prolonged pregnancy and labor, and excessive bleeding before, during, and after delivery. They can also contribute to birth defects. Use of salicylates in the last trimester may result in prematurity, stillbirth, newborn death, low birth weight, and bleeding into the fetal brain. Salicylates can also cause closure of the ductus arteriosus, causing premature distribution of blood to the lungs. Moreover, the gastric irritation caused by salicylates and other NSAIDs must not be treated with misoprostol (Cytotec), a PG analog, in pregnant patients, because PGs stimulate uterine contraction. Healthcare workers who are pregnant should wear gloves when dispensing misoprostol.

Patients taking probenecid or sulfinpyrazone should not take a salicylate, which can prevent the excretion of uric acid and precipitate an attack of gout. Salicylates should not be taken with methotrexate because they can increase methotrexate levels to a life-threatening toxic range. If a patient taking warfarin (Coumadin) is also taking aspirin, the pharmacy technician should alert the pharmacist. Some prescribers are using the two drugs in combination, but this does increase bleeding times.

The side effects of salicylates include GI upset, tinnitus (ringing in the ears), and platelet changes. The nonionized portion of the acetylsalicylic acid is lipid soluble and is easily absorbed into the gastric mucosal cells, which in turn causes further damage that can actually disrupt the integrity of the gastric mucosal barrier. This is why pharmacy data bases provide the pharmacy technician warnings when these drugs are dispensed and also why the FDA stipulates that they be accompanied by a Medication Guide.

Aspirin has some serious side effects that are often overlooked. **Salicylism**, mild salicylate intoxication, is characterized by tinnitus (ringing in the ears), dizziness, headache, and mental confusion. Severe intoxication is characterized by hyperpnea (abnormal increase in the depth of breathing), nausea, vomiting, acid-base disturbances, petechial hemorrhages, hyperthermia, delirium, convulsions, and coma. The lethal dose for aspirin is usually over 10 g for an adult. The advent of childproof caps for medicine has reduced the incidence of pediatric intoxication.

Aspirin should not be given to children. **Reye syndrome** can develop in children who have been given aspirin after having been exposed to chickenpox or other viral infections. This syndrome includes a range of mental changes (mild amnesia, lethargy, disorientation, and agitation) that can culminate in coma and progressive unresponsiveness, seizures, relaxed muscles, dilated pupils, and respiratory failure.

Low-dose (81 mg to 325 mg) aspirin taken daily has been shown to reduce the risk of heart attacks and strokes in patients with a prior history of cardiovascular disease (heart attack, stroke, bypass surgery). At low doses, aspirin appears to irreversibly inhibit the formation of thromboxane A_2, a prostaglandin molecule that facilitates platelet aggregation in blood vessels. Aspirin taken on a daily basis should be enteric coated to protect the lining of the stomach. Aspirin taken for a myocardial infarction (MI) must be plain, however, so that it can more quickly enter the bloodstream to prevent clot formation.

Choline magnesium trisalicylate (Trilisate) is approved for the treatment of arthritis. It must be taken with food, but it does not cause as many stomach problems as other drugs in this class. It acts on the hypothalamus to reduce fever and block pain impulses. Much lower doses of choline magnesium trisalicylate are necessary to have an antipyretic effect than is needed to inhibit pain. The liquid form may be mixed with fruit juices, but one needs to remain in an upright position for 30 minutes after taking it.

Salsalate (Amigesic) is approved for minor pain or fever and arthritis. It does not appear to inhibit platelet aggregation and causes less stomach problems than other drugs in this class. Salsalate should be taken with food. The fact that it will not "thin" the blood makes it a very important member of this drug class.

Antipyretic Analgesic

Acetaminophen (Tylenol) is an effective analgesic and antipyretic without the anti-inflammatory, antirheumatic, or uric acid excretory effects of aspirin. The mechanism and site of action have not been established, but they appear to involve central PG inhibition. Like salicylates, acetaminophen acts centrally to cause antipyresis. Acetaminophen has a very limited side effect profile and therefore is perhaps the safest drug to recommend. Furthermore, acetaminophen may be taken in pregnancy. However, if overingested it can be lethal, and because it is in so many pain medications an overdose can happen without prescribers realizing it. Pharmacy technicians need to be aware of the maximum acetaminophen dose when dispensing combination narcotics. Most prescribers do not take this into consideration. If the prescription allows the patient to take more than 4 grams/day, the prescriber must be notified. Acetaminophen is still a first-line medication for mild to moderate pain.

Acetaminophen is given in the same doses as aspirin and is equipotent to aspirin as an antipyretic or for simple analgesia. It can be especially useful in patients

- with peptic ulcer
- taking a uricosuric agent for gout
- taking oral anticoagulants
- with clotting disorders

- at risk for Reye syndrome
- intolerant to aspirin (still a 6% chance of cross-intolerance)
- with post-surgical pain

Acetaminophen does not cause GI irritation, bleeding, alteration of platelet adhesiveness, or potentiation of oral anticoagulants. There are few interactions. However, it should be taken with caution and under medical supervision if a patient has severe liver disease or is an alcoholic. At a dosage of over 4 g per day, liver damage can occur. This risk increases if the patient is fasting or is ingesting alcohol.

Acetylcysteine (Mucomyst, Acetadote) is the only antidote for an acetaminophen overdose; it is also approved for some bronchial diseases. It acts as an alternate substrate and conjugates with the acetaminophen, detoxifying the active metabolite. Acetylcysteine has a strong, rotten egg-like smell, which limits its use. The IV form is primarily used because of the convenience. For bronchial conditions it comes in a form that can be inhaled, through a vaporizer, and an oral dose form. If the oral dose is used for overdose, it must be given in a loading dose and then followed by 17 subsequent doses. The IV dose also is loaded, but a loading dose is given three times followed by a maintenance dose, then followed by two other doses given over a 21 hour period. This administration may vary depending upon acetaminophen levels. Acetylcysteine should be administered as soon as possible, preferably within 4 hours of ingestion, but it can be effective in patients treated up to 8 to 10 hours after ingestion.

Mixed Analgesics

A mixed analgesic is a drug containing both a narcotic and an NSAID or acetaminophen. Chronic use of mixed analgesics can lead to kidney failure because these drugs have additive toxic effects on the kidneys. Furthermore, many of the OTC analgesics can cause problems for persons who drink alcohol daily. The FDA wants manufacturers to put an alcohol warning on the labels of all OTC analgesics. For acetaminophen, the problem is liver toxicity; for ibuprofen, an NSAID, it is increased GI bleeding.

Mixed analgesics containing a narcotic combined with aspirin, ibuprofen or acetaminophen are often prescribed with more concern for the narcotic than for the nonnarcotic dose. The pharmacy technician can play a critical role here. When a prescription for any of these drugs is received, it would be prudent to calculate the dose of the nonnarcotic to see whether it exceeds the toxicity dosage.

Arthritis and Related Disorders

The word **arthritis** is derived from the Greek word for joint, *arthron*, and it literally means joint inflammation. Arthritis can take many forms, but the most common complaint of arthritis patients is persistent pain. This pain is caused by functional problems of the joints.

Forms of Arthritis

The three most common forms of arthritis are osteoarthritis, bursitis, and rheumatoid arthritis.

Osteoarthritis is a degenerative joint disease in which cartilage in joints becomes thinner and less elastic, eventually causing bone to wear and become deformed. It is a common age-related condition of synovial joints. The most

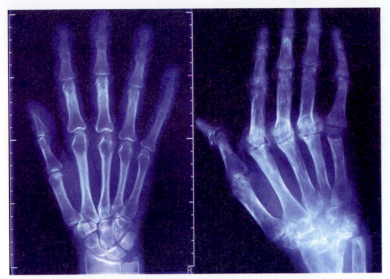

X-ray images of a healthy wrist and hand (left) and a wrist and hand affected by rheumatoid arthritis (right)

commonly affected joints are the sternoclavicular joint, spine, hips, knees, fingers, and big toes. Joints carrying large loads (knees) and those under stress (fingers) are especially likely to be affected. Osteoarthritis generally appears after age 40. The disease is characterized by progressive pain, stiffness, limitation of motion, and deformed joints. Stiffness in the morning is the most prevalent complaint; it is also common after inactivity such as sitting.

Bursitis is inflammation of a bursa, a saclike pouch filled with synovial fluid and located at a site of friction, such as the point where a muscle or tendon passes over bone. The cause of bursitis is usually unknown, although trauma, overuse, chronic infection, arthritis, or gout may be involved.

Rheumatoid arthritis (RA) is an **autoimmune disease** in which the body's immune system attacks and destroys its own connective tissue. In order to treat rheumatoid arthritis, drugs must be administered that turn off the immune system. This makes the body very susceptible to infections, cancer, and other diseases. That is why infection and malignancies are the primary side effects of the drugs. Unlike osteoarthritis, which affects cartilage, rheumatoid arthritis is characterized by inflammation of the joint's synovial membrane. The synovium (see Figure 13.1) swells and thickens. Fingerlike projections grow from the synovium into cartilage, bone, tendon, and joint spaces, causing reabsorption of bone and cartilage. As the disease progresses, bone-to-bone contact occurs, with eventual joint fusion. Most destruction occurs close to the inflamed synovial membrane.

Because cartilage has no nerves, pain originates from the surrounding joint structures, such as bone, tendon, ligament, and muscle. Morning stiffness is usually symmetric and lasts longer than 60 minutes. The same joints on both sides are affected approximately 70% of the time. The small joints of the hand are usually affected first, followed by the feet, ankles, knees, wrists, elbows, shoulders, temporomandibular joints, and vertebral column. Patients are prone to cold and feel changes in barometric pressure.

Laboratory tests for rheumatoid arthritis are the erythrocyte sedimentation rate (ESR), which indicates the presence of inflammation, and the rheumatoid factor (RF), for which 80% of arthritis patients have a positive result. Criteria for a diagnosis of rheumatoid arthritis include the following:

- joint tenderness or pain on motion
- morning stiffness
- presence of RF
- soft-tissue swelling in a first joint, followed within three months by swelling in a second joint
- sterile, turbid synovial fluid
- X-ray changes showing erosions

Therapy is aimed at relieving pain, maintaining or improving mobility, and minimizing disability. It may include medication, physical therapy, and patient education. Heat or cold, depending on which relieves pain, for 15 to 20 minutes before exercise should reduce pain and stiffness. Because there is no cure, the goals of treatment are to slow the progress of the disease.

Nonsteroidal Anti-Inflammatory Drugs

The **nonsteroidal anti-inflammatory drug (NSAID)** category (including aspirin) are the predominant drugs used to treat arthritis, but they have many other uses as well. Like salicylates, other NSAIDs have anti-inflammatory, analgesic, and antipyretic properties. They work to relieve inflammation and swelling, which in turn reduces pain. They may take longer to reduce fever than other agents, but the effects last longer. In addition to being used for the pain and inflammation of arthritis and rheumatism, NSAIDs are used for headache, menstrual cramps, backache, muscle aches, flu, and fever. NSAIDs may not be the only drug the patient is taking to treat arthritis. Although they decrease joint pain and swelling, they do not reduce joint destruction.

NSAIDs work by inhibiting prostaglandin (PG) synthesis in tissues, thereby preventing the sensitization of pain receptors to other mediators of inflammation. Thus, they generally act in the affected tissues and not centrally, as opiates do. Any central actions that NSAIDs do exhibit are usually unwanted side effects, with the exception of lowered body temperature. It is unlikely, though, that all NSAIDs act only on PGs and by only one mechanism.

The action of NSAIDs in inhibiting PG synthesis explains their primary side effect: GI upset. PGs perform three protective functions in the GI tract: increasing mucosal blood flow, increasing mucus production, and decreasing free acid production. Thus, by inhibiting PG synthesis, NSAIDs also inhibit the protective effect of PGs on the gastric mucosa. Not surprisingly, then, one in five chronic NSAID users develops some type of GI gastropathy. This drug class should always be taken with food, be administered in the lowest dose for the shortest period of time possible, and must have a medication guide dispensed with it. Nausea, abdominal cramps, heartburn, ulcers, and indigestion are all associated with NSAID use. For this reason, proton pump inhibitors to be administered with these agents may be indicated in selected patients. NSAIDs can also increase heart or circulation problems, and this effect must be taken into consideration.

The next most common side effect of NSAID use is kidney damage. Acute renal failure, fluid retention, hypertension, hyperkalemia, interstitial nephritis, and papillary necrosis can all be attributed to NSAID use. Other side effects include liver abnormalities, blood clotting irregularities, bone marrow depression, tinnitus, jaundice, dizziness, drowsiness, rash, and dry mouth.

NSAIDs can interact with the following drugs:

- other NSAIDs, including aspirin
- beta blockers
- cyclosporine
- digoxin
- diuretics
- methotrexate
- oral hypoglycemics
- warfarin

Because NSAIDs are protein-bound, they can be displaced from protein by other drugs such as aspirin; the result is decreased plasma concentration and increased clearance of the NSAIDs. Consequently, concurrent use of the two should be discouraged, as the combination may lead to additive or synergistic toxicity rather than increased efficacy. Also, other NSAIDs may interefere with the cardioprotective effects of low-dose (81 mg to 325 mg) aspirin.

Because the NSAIDs (and acetaminophen) work peripherally and opiates primarily work centrally, there is synergy between them when they are combined. Therefore, the nonnarcotic analgesics are often combined with opiates in mixed drugs (e.g., hydrocodone-acetaminophen). The combinations often provide better analgesia than either type of agent alone, with a lowered opiate requirement.

Table 13.3 lists some commonsense tips for NSAID users, and Table 13.4 presents the most commonly used NSAIDs. All NSAIDs should be administered with food. Sufficient time, usually two to three weeks, must be allowed with one agent before changing to another. A Medication Guide must be dispensed with all NSAIDs. Many problems that involve muscles and joints are treated with NSAIDs. Many NSAIDs are achieving OTC status. This means they will be used to self-medicate. The pharmacy technician must be aware of the side effects and proper use of these drugs.

It is most important to realize that although all NSAIDs have similar mechanisms of action, patients' responses to these drugs vary widely. Clinical trials have not shown any of these agents to be superior to the others for managing rheumatoid arthritis. Given the wide variation in patients' reactions, inadequate response or loss of response to one NSAID does not imply inefficacy of others. If one drug does not achieve the desired results, treatment with another NSAID is appropriate before considering adding other agents. Rotating these agents is common, and patients seem to get better results when this is done.

Conventional NSAIDs Several NSAIDs are available as OTC drugs, and others will probably become available in the future. The only NSAIDs with parenteral forms are indomethacin and ketorolac, and these are for short-term use only.

Diclofenac (Arthrotec, Cataflam, Solaraze, Voltaren, Flector) can induce signs and symptoms of hepatotoxicity: nausea, fatigue, pruritus, jaundice, upper-right-quadrant tenderness, and flu-like symptoms. Therefore, regular liver function tests are important. The patient should report any blood in the stool to the prescriber. Cataflam has a more rapid onset of action than does the sodium salt, Voltaren, because it is absorbed in the stomach rather than the duodenum. Topical forms are Solaraze (3%) and Voltaren Topical (1%). These forms are dispensed with dosing cards, which patients should use to measure the amount to be applied. The prescribed amount should be

---

TABLE 13.3   Tips for NSAID Users

- Take with food.
- Use antacids.
- Do not use gastric irritants such as alcohol.
- Stop the NSAID before any elective surgical procedure (7 days with aspirin, 1–2 days with other NSAIDs).
- Use the lowest possible dose.
- Be aware of the side effects.
- Take sufficient fluids.
- If sensitive to aspirin, avoid NSAIDs.

TABLE 13.4 Most Commonly Used Drugs for Arthritis and Related Disorders

Generic Name	Pronunciation	Dosage Form	Brand Name	Dispensing Status
Conventional NSAIDs				
diclofenac	dye-KLOE-fen-ak	patch, tablet, topical	Cataflam, Flector Solaraze, Voltaren	Rx
diclofenac-misoprostol	dye-KLOE-fen-ak mye-soe-PROST-awl	tablet	Arthrotec	Rx
diflunisal	dye-FLOO-ni-sal	tablet	Dolobid	Rx
etodolac	ee-TOE-doe-lak	capsule, tablet	Lodine	Rx
fenoprofen	fen-oh-PROE-fen	capsule, tablet	Nalfon	Rx
flurbiprofen	flure-bi-PROE-fen	tablet, ophthalmic	Ansaid, Ocufen	Rx
ibuprofen	eye-byoo-PROE-fen	capsule, oral liquid, tablet	Advil, Motrin	OTC, Rx
indomethacin	in-doe-METH-a-sin	capsule, IV, oral liquid, suppository	Indocin	Rx
ketoprofen	kee-toe-PROE-fen	capsule, tablet	Orudis, Oruvail	Rx
ketorolac	kee-toe-ROLE-ak	injection, IV, tablet	Toradol	Rx
meclofenamate	me-kloe-FEN-am-ate	capsule	(none)	Rx
mefenamic acid	me-fe-NAM-ik AS-id	capsule	Ponstel	Rx
meloxicam	mel-OX-i-kam	oral liquid, tablet	Mobic	Rx
nabumetone	na-BYOO-me-tone	tablet	Relafen	Rx
naproxen	na-PROX-en	oral suspension, tablet	Aleve	OTC
			Anaprox, Naprosyn	Rx
oxaprozin	ox-a-PROE-zin	tablet	Daypro	Rx
piroxicam	peer-OX-i-kam	capsule	Feldene	Rx
sulindac	sul-IN-dak	tablet	Clinoril	Rx
tolmetin	TOLE-met-in	capsule, tablet	Tolectin	Rx
COX-2 Inhibitors				
celecoxib	sel-a-KOX-ib	capsule	Celebrex	Rx
Other				
tramadol	TRA-ma-dawl	tablet	Ultram	Rx
tramadol-acetaminophen	TRA-ma-dawl a-seat-a-MIN-oh-fen	tablet	Ultracet	Rx

massaged into the area that is painful, and the area where the drug is applied should not be washed for at least an hour. Flector is the patch. It should be applied to the most painful area and changed every 12 hours. It must be kept dry. Arthrotec is diclofenac combined with misoprostel; it protects the stomach from NSAID-induced ulcers.

Etodolac (Lodine) dosage should not exceed 1,200 mg per day. Patients should be told not to crush the tablets and to report any blood in the stool to the prescriber. A black stool usually indicates blood of gastric origin. Bright red blood in the stool is usually from rectal origin and indicates hemorrhoids.

Flurbiprofen (Ansaid) is used to treat arthritis and **(Ocufen)** treats ocular inflammation. For best results, Ansaid should be taken three to four times a day, not to exceed 300 mg per day. An eye drop is used to lessen problems that can occur during surgery. It should be instilled into the eye 1–2 hours before the surgery. Flurbiprofen also relieves inflammation and itching of the eye.

Ibuprofen (Advil, Motrin) comes in liquid dosage forms and is the first OTC analgesic for children since acetaminophen. It controls fever well and can be alternated with acetaminophen. Ibuprofen has a slower onset of action than acetaminophen but a longer duration. Consequently, alternating ibuprofen and acetaminophen works well. The adult formulations are also available OTC in strengths of 200 mg per tablet, caplet, or capsule. However, the patient can easily take more than one tablet at a time and attain the 400 mg, 600 mg, or 800 mg prescription formulation. Unless recommended by the physician, this could be very dangerous. If the patient is taking OTC agents, the physician should be notified if a fever lasts more than 3 days or pain longer than 10 days.

Indomethacin (Indocin) has been the prototype NSAID for comparison with other such drugs. Its potency is believed to be mediated by PGs, and it has more adverse effects than the newer agents. Because of its side effect profile, indomethacin is not used as frequently as the other NSAIDs for arthritis. Indomethacin is the only NSAID available as a suppository. The primary use is in the treatment of gout, but it is also used in neonates. Normally, the ductus arteriosus constricts during the first day after birth, resulting in functional closure. Intravenously administered indomethacin is used in neonates to promote closure of the patent ductus arteriosus and to alleviate the associated symptoms of cardiac failure. It should be administered over 20 to 30 minutes at a concentration of 0.5 to 1.0 mg/mL in preservative-free sterile water for injection. The IV formula should be reconstituted just before administration and any unused portion discarded. The latter is especially important in a neonatal unit.

Ketorolac (Toradol) is indicated for short-term use (less than 5 days) in moderate-to-severe pain. It acts peripherally to inhibit PG synthesis. It is useful in patients who cannot tolerate narcotics. When injected, a dose of 30 mg provides the analgesia comparable to 12 mg of morphine or 100 mg of meperidine. Side effects include nausea, dyspepsia (abdominal discomfort, heartburn), GI pain, and drowsiness.

Mefenamic acid (Ponstel) should not be used for more than 4 to 7 days because it can cause blood dyscrasias, an abnormal condition of the blood or bone marrow. It is used primarily for dysmenorrhea (menstrual cramps).

Meloxicam (Mobic) appears to cause less GI toxicity than most NSAIDs. For that reason it has become a very popular drug for arthritis. It can be dosed once or twice daily.

Nabumetone (Relafen) should be taken in the morning with food. The lowest effective dose should be used for chronic treatment. As with other NSAIDs, alcohol should be avoided because it may add to the irritant action of the drug in the stomach.

Naproxen (Naprosyn, Aleve) is the least risky NSAID for cardiovascular events, which is partly why it is prescribed frequently. It should be used in the lowest effective dose for the least amount of possible time. Aleve is available as an OTC product.

Piroxicam (Feldene) has the advantage of once-a-day dosing. It is for acute or long-term therapy of arthritis. Therapeutic effects are evident early in treatment, and the response increases over several weeks. As with other NSAIDs, the patient needs to take the drug for at least 2 weeks before discontinuing it to allow the drug sufficient time to reach its therapeutic effectiveness.

Warning

Toradol and tramadol may look alike.

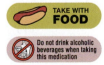

TAKE WITH FOOD

Do not drink alcoholic beverages when taking this medication

Sulindac (Clinoril) is a renal-sparing drug metabolized in the liver. It must be metabolized to the active form. In other words, it is a prodrug. The active metabolite inhibits cyclooxygenase and is structurally similar to indomethacin. Both sulindac and indomethacin have more side effects than the newer agents.

COX-2 Inhibitors Two enzymes have been found to play a critical role in the inflammation process. These are **cyclooxygenase-1 (COX-1)** and **cyclooxygenase-2 (COX-2)**. Both are present in the synovial fluid of patients with arthritis. COX-2 is associated with pain and inflammation, whereas COX-1 has a more extensive role in the body, including protection of the gastrointestinal lining. This difference is the basis for a new class of NSAIDs called COX-2 inhibitors, which offer other options for treating arthritis. Whereas traditional NSAIDs nonselectively block both the COX-1 and the COX-2 enzymes, COX-2 inhibitors block only the COX-2 enzyme, which is induced during inflammation. Inhibition of COX-2 alone has been shown to decrease pain with a much lower risk of adverse GI events. COX-2 inhibitors are prescribed for rheumatoid arthritis, osteoarthritis, menstrual cramps, and acute pain.

Celecoxib (Celebrex) was the first COX-2 inhibitor to be approved by the FDA. Although GI upset is less than with the older NSAIDs, it remains the primary side effect. Fluid retention is another significant side effect with this drug. Celecoxib has the potential for cross-reactivity in patients who are allergic to sulfonamides, and it may increase cardiovascular risk. A label should be attached when dispensing this drug to instruct patients to take it with food. At the time of this writing, celecoxib is the only COX-2 still on the market, because all of the others have been recalled by the FDA.

Other Drugs Used to Treat Rheumatoid Arthritis **Tramadol (Ultram)** is a totally synthetic agent that acts centrally. It binds to opiate receptors and inhibits reuptake of norepinephrine and serotonin. It is used for moderate to severe pain. The most common side effects include dizziness, vertigo, nausea, constipation, and headache. Recent data suggest that tramadol has a higher abuse potential than originally thought and is a controlled substance in some states. Tramadol has a slow onset of action, but once it begins to act, it gives good pain control.

Disease-Modifying Antirheumatic Drugs

The existing treatments for rheumatoid arthritis are divided into two categories:

1. agents that provide only symptomatic relief
2. agents that can potentially modify disease progression

The former category includes NSAIDs, which were discussed above, and corticosteroids, which will be discussed in other chapters. The latter category includes a variety of agents that are collectively referred to as **disease-modifying antirheumatic drugs (DMARDs)**. The latest evidence shows that early, mild rheumatoid arthritis should be treated with more than NSAIDs because joint damage occurs earlier than previously thought. The newer therapeutic approaches to the treatment of rheumatoid arthritis focus on the use of novel biologic response modifiers with the ability to inhibit lymphocytes and cytokine activity. DMARDs are considered to be second-line agents. Even though they may slow the progression of the disease, side effects limit their use. Table 13.5 gives an overview of the most commonly used DMARDs.

Abatacept (Orencia) inhibits T-cell activation. T-cells play a key role in the inflammatory process. It is approved for rheumatoid arthritis (RA) patients who have failed

TABLE 13.5   Most Commonly Used DMARDs

Generic Name	Pronunciation	Dosage Form	Brand Name	Dispensing Status
abatacept	ab-a-TA-cept	IV	Orencia	Rx
adalimumab	a-da-LIM-yoo-mab	injection	Humira	Rx
anakinra	an-a-KIN-ra	injection	Kineret	Rx
auranofin	aw-RAY-noh-fin	capsule	Ridaura	Rx
aurothioglucose	aw-roh-thye-oh-GLOO-kose	injection	Solganal	Rx
azathioprine	az-a-THYE-oh-preen	tablet	Imuran	Rx
cyclophosphamide	sye-kloe-FOSS-fa-mide	injection, IV, tablet	Cytoxan	Rx
etanercept	et-a-NER-cept	injection	Enbrel	Rx
hydroxychloroquine	hye-drox-ee-KLOR-oh-kwin	tablet	Plaquenil	Rx
infliximab	in-FLIX-i-mab	IV	Remicade	Rx
leflunomide	le-FLOO-noe-mide	tablet	Arava	Rx
methotrexate	meth-oh-TREX-ate	injection, IV, tablet	Rheumatrex	Rx
penicillamine	pen-i-SIL-a-meen	capsule	Cuprimine	Rx

TNF (tumor necrosis factor) inhibitors. It can be used alone or in combination with other drugs but should never be used with TNF inhibitors. Abatacept is packaged as a powder in a silicone-free disposable syringe that must be reconstituted with 20 mL of sterile water, then further diluted with NS. It is stored in the refrigerator. Abatacept is administered as a 30 minute infusion. It is given at 2 and 4 weeks after the first infusion, then every 4 weeks. As with all of the DMARDs, the primary side effects are infections and malignancies, because abatacept acts on the immune system.

Adalimumab (Humira) is a biologic response modifier that blocks tumor necrosis factor. It is administered subcutaneously every week. Adalimunab increases the risk of infections and cancer. It is approved for RA, but only for patients who have failed other DMARDs. Adalimunab is preservative free and is dispensed in a carton that has two dose trays, each containing a 1 mL prefilled glass syringe, and it must be stored in the refrigerator. It is administered every other week as a subcutaneous injection. Other drugs do not need to be discontinued. Adalimumab increases the risk of infections and malignancies. It is stored in the refrigerator.

Anakinra (Kineret) is an interleukin receptor antagonist used for arthritis. The primary side effect is redness, rash, and itching at the injection site.

Azathioprine (Imuran) depresses bone marrow, thereby increasing the potential for infection. Other side effects are liver toxicity and GI upset. Response in rheumatoid arthritis may not occur for up to 3 months.

Cyclophosphamide (Cytoxan) depresses the bone marrow, increasing the potential for infection. Other side effects are GI upset and ulcers, liver toxicity, reproductive organ failure, and hair loss. Patients must remain well hydrated during use of this drug. Without proper hydration, the drug can cause irreparable damage to the urinary bladder. The patient should force fluids up to 2 L per day.

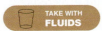
TAKE WITH FLUIDS

Etanercept (Enbrel) is a biologically engineered protein that inhibits the action of tumor necrosis factor (TNF). (Growing evidence suggests that TNF plays a key role in the pathogenesis of rheumatoid arthritis.) Etanercept was the first biologically engineered product approved for the treatment of rheumatoid arthritis. This drug is indicated in the treatment of moderate to severe RA in patients who have experienced an inadequate response to one or more of the other arthritis drugs. Etanercept can be used in combination with methotrexate in patients who do not respond adequately to methotrexate alone. Etanercept must be stored in the refrigerator. The drug is diluted with bacteriostatic water prior to injection and must not be mixed with any other dilutent. The solution should be administered as soon as possible after reconstitution; it should not be stored for more than 6 hours. Injection site reactions are the primary side effect.

Hydroxychloroquine (Plaquenil) is used to suppress acute attacks of malaria and for treatment of systemic lupus and rheumatoid arthritis. It can cause corneal deposits, retinal changes, GI upset, and skin rash. The patient should always wear sunglasses in bright sunlight and watch for vision changes, ringing in the ears, or hearing loss.

Infliximab (Remicade) was initially approved for Crohn disease and has been more recently approved for rheumatoid arthritis. It is given intravenously every 8 weeks.

Leflunomide (Arava) is a pyrimidine synthesis inhibitor that interferes with the proliferation of lymphocytes. Leflunomide retards the progression of rheumatoid arthritis, reduces pain and joint swelling, and improves functional ability. Evidence suggests that this drug exhibits an additive effect when combined with methotrexate. Side effects of leflunomide include diarrhea, rash, and alopecia (hair loss). It is also associated with elevations in liver enzymes. In the event of overdose or toxicity, cholestyramine should be administered. The tablets should be protected from light. There is a possibility of a serious interaction with warfarin. The International Normalized Ratio (INR) should be checked a few days after beginning therapy and then on a regular basis. Leflunomide tends to increase infections. It has a very long half-life. Eliminating the active metabolite can take up to 2 years.

Methotrexate (Rheumatrex) is an antineoplastic agent used to treat metastasis, arthritic conditions, and psoriasis. It should be taken on an empty stomach. Exposure to sunlight should be avoided. Side effects include nausea, vomiting, and hair loss. For prolonged use, especially in rheumatoid arthritis and psoriasis, a baseline liver function panel should be performed and repeated on a regular basis.

Penicillamine (Cuprimine) is a chelating agent used to treat lead, mercury, copper, and gold poisoning. It lowers the rheumatoid factor (RF) level and selectively inhibits T lymphocytes. Side effects are bone marrow depression (with increased risk of infection), proteinuria, rash, and drug-induced autoimmune disease (lupus erythematosus). Cross-sensitivity with penicillin is possible. Loss of taste may also occur. Cuprimine should be taken on an empty stomach.

Steroids are believed to relieve symptoms and slow joint damage. It is very important that a patient on steroids take calcium and vitamin D. Hormone replacement therapy has been shown to have a positive effect on osteoarthritis because it helps calcium enter the bones.

Drugs for Gouty Arthritis

Gouty arthritis, often referred to merely as gout, usually affects single joints, causing a **tophus** (a deposit of sodium urate) to form around the joint. Tophi may form in tissues, joint cartilage, ear lobes, and metatarsals. Typically, the first joint affected is the big toe; it becomes painful, swollen, and red. The disease is related to the patient's metabolism of uric acid, which is normally excreted by the kidneys. The affected

Warning

A prescription written for penicillamine can be misread as penicillin.

patient overproduces or has improper excretion of uric acid, so aspirin is contraindicated, because it competes with uric acid for kidney excretion. The condition is usually inherited. Persons prone to gout should also avoid the following drugs, which could precipitate an attack.

- cytotoxic agents
- diuretics
- ethanol
- nicotinic acid
- salicylates

Table 13.6 presents the most commonly used agents for gouty arthritis.

Allopurinol (Zyloprim) is a xanthine oxidase inhibitor used to prevent attacks of gouty arthritis. Uric acid forms primarily from metabolism of purine bases, guanine, and adenine. Side effects are rash and hepatotoxicity. The prescriber should monitor liver function and complete blood counts before initiating therapy and during therapy. Allopurinol should be used with caution in patients taking diuretics.

Colchicine is the drug of choice for acute gout attacks. It interferes with leukocytes, reducing their mobility and joint phagocytosis, and also reduces uric acid production. The oral dose is one to two tablets of 0.5 mg or 0.6 mg strength, then one tablet every hour (not more than 10 to 15 tablets) until pain is relieved or GI side effects (nausea, vomiting, diarrhea) occur. The IV dose is 2 mg to 3 mg, diluted in 30 mL of normal saline and given slowly over 5 minutes; it may be repeated in 6 to 8 hours. There is a high potential for phlebitis (inflammation of a vein).

Indomethacin (Indocin) is the NSAID most used for gouty arthritis.

Probenecid-colchicine (Col-Probenecid) dissolves tophi, reduces serum urate levels, and increases uric acid excretion in urine. Risk of kidney stone formation increases as more uric acid passes through the kidney. Although probenecid-colchicine is not useful in acute attacks, it is used in the treatment of chronic gouty arthritis complicated by frequent, recurrent acute attacks.

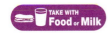

Sulfinpyrazone (Anturane) prevents tubule reabsorption of uric acid in the kidney and therefore is used in the treatment of chronic gouty arthritis. It also has antithrombotic and antiplatelet activity. Side effects are rash and GI disorders. This drug should be taken with food or milk to avoid aggravation or reactivation of ulcers.

TABLE 13.6	Most Commonly Used Drugs for Gouty Arthritis			
Generic Name	**Pronunciation**	**Dosage Form**	**Brand Name**	**Dispensing Status**
Acute Attack Therapy				
colchicine	KOL-chi-seen	injection, IV, tablet	(none)	Rx
Chronic Therapy				
allopurinol	al-oh-PURE-i-nawl	tablet	Zyloprim	Rx
indomethacin	in-doe-METH-a-sin	capsule, IV, oral liquid, suppository	Indocin	Rx
probenecid-colchicine	proe-BEN-e-sid KOL-chi-seen	tablet	Col-Probenecid	Rx
sulfinpyrazone	sul-fin-PEER-a-zone	capsule, tablet	Anturane	Rx

Chapter Terms

acetylcholine (ACh) a neurotransmitter that binds to ACh receptors on the membranes of muscle cells, beginning a process that ultimately results in muscle contraction

analgesic pain relieving

antipyretic fever reducing

arthritis joint inflammation; persistent pain due to functional problems of the joints

autoimmune disease illness in which the immune system attacks and destroys healthy tissue within the body

bursitis inflammation of a bursa

cyclooxygenase-1 (COX-1) an enzyme that is present in most body tissues and produces protective prostaglandins to regulate physiological processes such as GI mucosal integrity

cyclooxygenase-2 (COX-2) an enzyme that is present in the synovial fluid of arthritis patients and is associated with the pain and inflammation of arthritis

disease-modifying antirheumatic drugs (DMARDs) agents that can modify the progression of rheumatoid arthritis

gouty arthritis a disease resulting from the improper excretion of uric acid; also called gout

muscle relaxant a drug that reduces or prevents skeletal muscle contraction

muscle spasticity a condition whereby muscle fibers are in a state of involuntary, continuous contraction that causes pain

nonnarcotic analgesic a drug used for pain, inflammation, and fever that is not a controlled substance

nonsteroidal anti-inflammatory drugs (NSAIDs) anti-inflammatory, analgesic, and antipyretic drugs that are not controlled substances or steroids; used to treat arthritis and for other indications such as pain and inflammation

osteoarthritis a degenerative joint disease resulting in loss of cartilage, elasticity, and thickness

Reye syndrome a condition that can develop in children who have been exposed to chicken pox or other viral infections and are given aspirin; characterized by amnesia, lethargy, disorientation, and agitation that can culminate in coma and respiratory failure

rheumatoid arthritis (RA) an autoimmune disease in which the body's immune system attacks its own connective tissue; characterized by inflammation of the synovial membrane of the joints

salicylates a class of nonnarcotic analgesics that have both pain-relieving and antipyretic (fever-reducing) properties

salicylism mild salicylate intoxication, characterized by ringing in the ears, dizziness, headache, and mental confusion

somatic pain dull, throbbing pain from skin, muscle, and bone

tophus a deposit of sodium urate around a joint

visceral pain sharp, stabbing pain from the organs

Chapter Summary

Muscle Relaxants

- The side effects of muscle relaxants are sedation, reduced mental alertness, reduced motor abilities, and GI upset. Patients taking these drugs should avoid alcohol.
- Diazepam (Valium), a benzodiazepine, is a highly effective muscle relaxer, but its abuse potential restricts its use.
- Methocarbamol (Robaxin) causes skeletal muscle relaxation by reducing the transmission of impulses from the spinal cord to skeletal muscles.
- Orphenadrine (Norflex) is an indirect skeletal muscle relaxant thought to work by central atropine-like effects. The tablet should be swallowed whole, not crushed or chewed.
- Carisoprodol (Soma) is subject to abuse. Once the drug is ingested, the molecules are cleaved to the major metabolite, meprobamate, which is a controlled substance. Soma is a controlled substance in many states.
- Chlorzoxazone (Paraflex, Parafon Forte DSC) is for symptomatic treatment of muscle spasms and pain associated with acute musculoskeletal conditions. It acts on the spinal cord and subcortical levels by depressing polysynaptic reflexes.
- Cyclobenzaprine (Flexeril) is a centrally acting skeletal muscle relaxant that is pharmacologically related to tricyclic antidepressants. Onset of action is usually within one hour, and the drug should not be used for more than two to three weeks.
- Baclofen (Lioresal) is used for treating reversible spasticity, spinal cord lesions, and multiple sclerosis and is sometimes used for hiccups. It should be taken with food or milk.

Inflammation and Swelling

- Analgesics are used for mild-to-moderate pain, inflammation, and fever. A widely accepted mechanism for many of their actions is their ability to inhibit the enzyme cyclooxygenase and thereby decrease the conversion of arachidonic acid to prostaglandins (PGs), thromboxane A_2, or prostacyclin.
- Somatic pain (from injury to skin, muscle, and bone) is dull and throbbing, while visceral pain (from the organs) is sharp and stabbing.
- Fever is a response by the body's temperature-regulating center (the hypothalamus) to substances called endogenous pyrogens produced as a result of bacterial or viral infections. The subsequent release of PGs from the brain causes the body "thermostat" to reset at a higher temperature.
- Adverse GI effects may limit the use of nonnarcotic analgesics.
- Aspirin, salicylate, is the prototype NSAID.
- Salicylates have analgesic (pain-relieving), anti-inflammatory, and antipyretic (fever-reducing) properties.
- The primary analgesic actions of salicylates are peripheral rather than central. Their primary antipyretic action is central and presumed to be in the hypothalamus.
- Salicylates are indicated for simple headache, arthritis, pain and fever with influenza, muscular aches and pains, menstrual cramps, and inflammation.
- Salicylates cause gastrointestinal ulceration. They should be avoided by patients with asthma, nasal polyps, chronic sinusitis, bleeding ulcers, and hemophilia. They should not be taken after surgery or tooth extraction.
- More than 4 g of aspirin per day can cause problems; 10 g can be lethal.
- Mild salicylate intoxication is characterized by ringing in the ears (tinnitus), dizziness, headache, and mental confusion.
- Acetaminophen acts centrally to cause antipyresis. It is an effective analgesic and antipyretic without the anti-inflammatory, antirheumatic, or uric acid excretory effects of aspirin.

- A patient with severe liver disease or alcoholism should not take acetaminophen.
- At a dose of above 4 g of acetaminophen per day, liver damage can occur.
- Alcohol can cause a problem with OTC analgesics, according to the FDA. For acetaminophen, the problem is liver toxicity; for NSAIDs, it is increased GI bleeding.

Arthritis and Related Disorders

- The most common complaint from arthritis patients is persistent pain. Because cartilage has no nerves, pain originates from surrounding joint structures, such as bone, tendon, ligament, and muscle.
- Therapy for arthritis is aimed at relieving pain, maintaining or improving mobility, and minimizing disability. It may include medication, physical therapy, and patient education.
- NSAIDs take longer to reduce fever than other products, but the effect lasts longer.
- NSAIDs are used for headache, menstrual cramps, backache, muscle aches, flu, fever, and the pain and inflammation of arthritis, rheumatism, and gouty arthritis.
- NSAIDs inhibit PG synthesis in inflamed tissues, thereby preventing the sensitization of pain receptors to mediators of inflammation. Thus, they generally act peripherally rather than centrally as other pain killers do.
- PGs perform three protective functions in the GI tract: increased mucosal blood flow, increased mucus production, and decreased free acid production.
- Side effects of NSAIDs are GI upset, nausea, abdominal cramps, heartburn, indigestion, ringing in the ears, ulcers, jaundice, dizziness, and rash. Gastropathy develops in one in five chronic NSAID users.
- Many patients will need to take a proton pump inhibitor with NSAIDs.
- Concurrent use of multiple NSAIDs (including aspirin) should be discouraged, as the combination may lead to additive or synergistic toxicity rather than increased efficacy. However, some research indicates that the use of NSAIDs and opiates may be synergistic.

- Clinical trials have not shown the superiority of any NSAIDs over the others for the management of rheumatoid arthritis.
- Inadequate response or loss of response to one NSAID does not imply that the others would be ineffective. There is considerable patient-to-patient variability in response. Usually, after 2 to 3 weeks, if the patient is not responding to one NSAID, a change can be made to another one.
- All NSAIDs should be administered with food and dispensed with a Medication Guide.
- Ketorolac (Toradol), when injected, has shown pain relief equal to narcotics. It is for short-term use only.
- Sulindac (Clinoril) is a renal-sparing drug that is metabolized in the liver.
- Nabumetone (Relafen) should be taken in the morning with food.
- Naproxen (Naprosyn) is the least risky NSAID for cardiovascular events.
- Tramadol (Ultram) acts centrally to bind to opiate receptors. It is used for moderate to severe pain. Its onset is slow, but once it begins to act, pain control appears to be equivalent to that provided by narcotics.
- DMARDs are disease-modifying antirheumatic drugs that are second-line agents for rheumatoid arthritis. Even though these drugs may slow the progression of the disease, the side effects limit their use.
- Mild rheumatoid arthritis should be treated with more than NSAIDs because joint damage occurs earlier than thought.
- Methotrexate (Rheumatrex) should be taken on an empty stomach, and exposure to the sun should be avoided. Methotrexate is an antineoplastic agent commonly used to treat arthritic conditions.
- Hydroxychloroquine (Plaquenil) is an antimalarial drug also used to treat arthritis.
- Aspirin should not be given to a patient with gout; it competes with uric acid for kidney excretion.
- Cytotoxic agents, diuretics, ethanol, nicotinic acid, and salicylates can precipitate a gout attack.

- Colchicine is the drug of choice for an acute gout attack.

- Colchicine, probenecid-colchicine, indomethacin, allopurinol, and sulfinpyrazone are all used for gout.

Drug List

The following drugs were discussed in this chapter. Each generic drug name is followed in parentheses by one or more brand names.

Muscle Relaxants
baclofen (Lioresal)
carisoprodol* (Soma)
chlorzoxazone (Paraflex, Parafon Forte DSC)
cyclobenzaprine* (Flexeril)
dantrolene (Dantrium)
diazepam (Valium)
metaxalone (Skelaxin)*
methocarbamol (Robaxin)
orphenadrine (Norflex)

Salicylates
aspirin
buffered aspirin (Ascriptin, Bufferin)
choline magnesium trisalicylate (Trilisate)
salsalate (Amigesic)

Antipyretic Analgesic
acetaminophen (Tylenol)*

Antidote to Acetaminophen
Acetyleysteine (Mucomyst, Acetadote)

Nonsteroidal Anti-inflammatory Drugs (NSAIDS)
diclofenac (Cataflam, Flector, Solaraze, Voltaren)*
diclofenac-misoprostol (Arthrotec)
diflunisal (Dolobid)
etodolac (Lodine)
fenoprofen (Nalfon)
flurbiprofen (Ansaid, Ocufen)
ibuprofen (Advil, Motrin)*
indomethacin (Indocin)
ketoprofen (Orudis, Oruvail)
ketorolac (Toradol)
meclofenamate
mefenamic acid (Ponstel)
meloxicam (Mobic)*
nabumetone (Relafen)
naproxen (Aleve, Anaprox, Naprosyn)*
oxaprozin (Daypro)
piroxicam (Feldene)
sulindac (Clinoril)
tolmetin (Tolectin)

COX-2 Inhibitors
celecoxib (Celebrex)*

Other
tramadol (Ultram)
tramadol-acetaminophen (Ultracet)

Disease-Modifying Antirheumatic Drugs (DMARDs)
abatacept (Orencia)
adalimumab (Humira)
anakinra (Kineret)
auranofin (Ridaura)
aurothioglucose (Solganal)
azathioprine (Imuran)
cyclophosphamide (Cytoxan)
etanercept (Enbrel)
hydroxychloroquine (Plaquenil)
infliximab (Remicade)
leflunomide (Arava)
methotrexate (Rheumatrex)
penicillamine (Cuprimine)

Drugs to Treat Gout
allopurinol* (Zyloprim)
colchicine
indomethacin (Indocin)
probenecid-colchicine (Col-Probenecid)
sulfinpyrazone (Anturane)

Chapter Review

Pharmaceuticals and Body Functions

Select the best answer from the choices given.

1. Which drug, even though it is <u>not</u> a controlled substance in all states, is subject to much abuse?
   a. Valium
   b. Flexeril
   c. Soma
   d. Robaxin

2. Which drug is biologically engineered and inhibits tumor necrosis factor?
   a. Robaxin
   b. Flexeril
   c. Lioresal
   d. Enbrel

3. Which muscle relaxer is also used to prevent hyperthermia?
   a. Soma
   b. Dantrium
   c. Valium
   d. Robaxin

4. Which drug class/es must be dispensed with a medication guide?
   a. NSAIDs
   b. antidepressants
   c. both A and B
   d. None of the above

5. Which drug is sometimes used to control hiccups?
   a. Lioresal
   b. Skelaxin
   c. Flexeril
   d. Paraflex

6. Which sticker should be put on all NSAIDs?
   a. Take with FOOD
   b. Avoid sun exposure
   c. Be sure to take all medication
   d. REFRIGERATE

7. Mild salicylate intoxication is characterized by all of the following *except*
   a. ringing in the ears.
   b. headache.
   c. dizziness.
   d. throbbing pain.

8. The problem with combining alcohol and acetaminophen is
   a. GI bleeding.
   b. liver toxicity.
   c. urinary tract infection.
   d. salicylate toxicity.

9. Centrally acting muscle relaxants do <u>not</u>
   a. directly relax muscles.
   b. depress the CNS.
   c. reduce anxiety that increases muscle tone.
   d. cause sedation.

10. Which NSAID has an IM dosage form?
    a. ketorolac
    b. piroxicam
    c. sulindac
    d. naproxen

The following statements are true or false. If the answer is false, rewrite the statement so it is true.

1. Clinical trials have shown the superiority of certain NSAIDs over others for the management of rheumatoid arthritis.

2. Salicylates can actually precipitate an attack of gout.

3. Ketorolac injection is for long-term use.

4. The only NSAIDs available in parenteral forms are Nalfon and Motrin.

5. The drug of choice for an acute gout attack is Anturane.

6. Voltaren is a nonnarcotic pain reliever that primarily acts centrally.

7. Criteria for rheumatoid arthritis are morning stiffness, joint tenderness or pain on motion, and presence of rheumatoid factor.

8. Salicylates are indicated for simple headache, arthritis, and pain and fever with flu.

9. An acceptable dose of Lodine would be 2000 mg per day.

10. Two NSAIDs that come as ophthalmics are ketoprofen and indomethacin.

Diseases and Drug Therapies

1. List four ways to block normal muscle function.

2. Why is Soma such a potentially addictive substance?

3. Complete the chart by putting an X if the heading applies to the drug.

4. Which of the drugs in the chart come in these forms?

   Suppository _____

   Patch _____

   IM _____

   Topical _____

5. Explain how Ultram works.

6. List the criteria for rheumatoid arthritis.

NSAIDs	Ophthalmic	OTC	IV
diclofenac			
etodolac			
fenoprofen			
flurbiprofen			
ibuprofen			
indomethacin			
ketoprofen			
ketorolac			
meclofenamate			
mefenamic acid			
nabumetone			
naproxen			
oxaprozin			
piroxicam			
sulindac			
tolmetin			

Dispensing Medications

1. List six classes of patients who come to the pharmacy needing an OTC analgesic for whom you would recommend use of acetaminophen.

2. What would you dispense? Give the brand name and route of administration.
   a. diclofenac: Instill one drop into the affected eye four times daily beginning 24 hours after cataract surgery and continuing 2 weeks.
   b. flurbiprofen: 100 mg tid #30
   c. indomethacin: 0.2 mg/kg over 20 to 30 minutes at 6 A.M. and 6 P.M.
   d. indomethacin: 50 mg rectally tid
   e. ketorolac: 30 mg q2h to q4h

3. How do you mix IV indomethacin?

Internet Research

Use the Internet to complete the following assignments.

1. OTC analgesics are used widely. Find a source of information that would be useful to a patient trying to select from among the commonly sold analgesics. Make a chart comparing aspirin, acetaminophen, and ibuprofen. List indications, contraindications, and side effects for each. List your Internet sources.

2. Locate information related to ongoing clinical trials aimed at the development of new treatments for rheumatoid arthritis. Create a table listing at least three experimental therapies. Indicate the phase (one through three) of testing currently under way and where (institution and country) the trials are taking place. List your Internet sources.

What Would You Do?

1. The pharmacist continues to forget to attach the medication guide to the NSAIDs. Should you go ahead and do it?

Hormonal Disorders and Their Treatment

14

Learning Objectives

- Explain the concept of hormones and how they regulate the body.
- Discuss thyroid replacement therapy.
- Discuss adrenal sex hormones and male dysfunction.
- Understand the concept of hormone replacement therapy.
- Understand the formulation of oral contraceptives.
- Recognize the urgent need for drugs used at delivery.
- Describe the diseases of the genital systems and how to avoid them.
- Discuss corticosteroids.
- Understand diabetes and the proper treatment and care of patients.
- Know the applications for growth hormone.

Preview chapter terms and definitions.

The endocrine system regulates a number of functions to keep the body in balance as well as to control complicated processes such as those involved in reproduction. The hormones that trigger the activity are also used in treatment. The pharmacologic agents used in these treatments include thyroid preparations, calcium, oral contraceptives, pregnancy tests, drugs used at delivery, corticosteroids, drugs used in treatment of diabetes, and growth hormone.

The Endocrine System

The **endocrine system**, illustrated in Figure 14.1, consists of glands and other structures that elaborate, or produce, secretions called hormones and release them directly into the circulatory system. The various hormones are responsible for specific regulatory effects on organs and other tissues of the body. The tissue affected by a hormone is called its **target**. Through the work of hormones, the endocrine system maintains homeostasis of the body by regulating the physiologic functions involved in normal daily living and in stress.

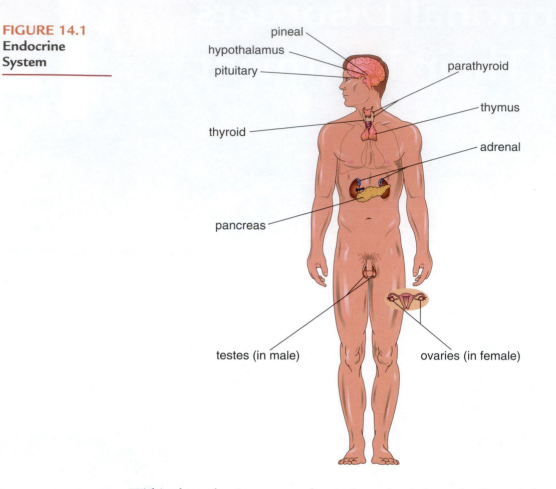

FIGURE 14.1
Endocrine
System

pineal
hypothalamus
pituitary
parathyroid
thymus
thyroid
adrenal
pancreas
testes (in male)
ovaries (in female)

Within the endocrine system, the pituitary gland plays a leading role because its hormones regulate several other endocrine glands, as well as a number of body activities, as shown in Figure 14.2. Regulation of hormone synthesis by a particular gland is achieved via an intricate negative feedback mechanism involving that gland, the hypothalamic-pituitary axis, and autoregulation. In a **feedback mechanism**, some of the output signals of a system return as input so as to exert some control over the process. Physiologic factors such as dopamine and stress can also influence the hypothalamic-pituitary axis and autoregulation.

Thyroid Disorders

The **thyroid gland**, shown in Figure 14.3, produces hormones that stimulate various body tissues to increase their metabolic activity. These hormones, triiodothyronine (T_3) and thyroxine (T_4), are both stored as thyroglobulin, which the thyroid cells must break down before it can be released into the bloodstream. Both T_3 and T_4 are generally bound to protein molecules. Activity occurs when the hormones are not bound, but T_3 is more potent than T_4. The feedback mechanism that controls the thyroid is the hypothalamic-pituitary axis, which produces thyroid-stimulating hormone (TSH), which in turn stimulates the thyroid to produce T_3 and T_4 (see Figure 14.4). These hormones build up in circulating blood and slow the pituitary's activity in producing and releasing TSH. In response to rising levels of T_3 and T_4, the hypothalamic-pituitary axis produces less TSH. For a patient with signs of

FIGURE 14.2   Pituitary Hormones

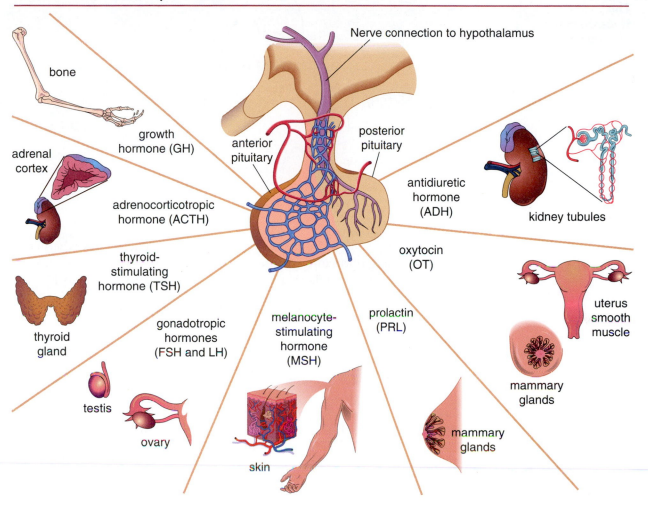

bone

growth
hormone (GH)

adrenal
cortex

adrenocorticotropic
hormone (ACTH)

thyroid-
stimulating
hormone (TSH)

thyroid
gland

gonadotropic
hormones
(FSH and LH)

testis

ovary

melanocyte-
stimulating
hormone
(MSH)

skin

Nerve connection to hypothalamus

anterior
pituitary

posterior
pituitary

antidiuretic
hormone
(ADH)

kidney tubules

oxytocin
(OT)

prolactin
(PRL)

uterus
smooth
muscle

mammary
glands

mammary
glands

FIGURE 14.3
Thyroid Gland

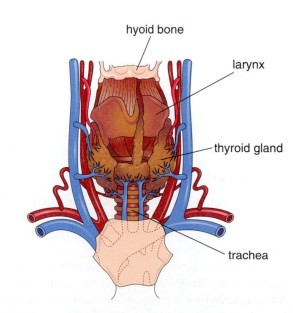

hyoid bone

larynx

thyroid gland

trachea

FIGURE 14.4
The Hypothalamic-Pituitary Axis

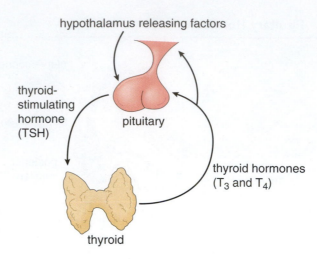

hypothalamus releasing factors

thyroid-stimulating hormone (TSH)

pituitary

thyroid hormones (T$_3$ and T$_4$)

thyroid

hormonal imbalance, measuring the amount of serum TSH can determine whether the thyroid is functioning normally; if it is, another level of control may be involved. It is also important to note, though, that some peripheral conversion of T$_4$ to T$_3$ occurs in the tissues.

Hypothyroidism

Hypothyroidism (also called myxedema) refers to conditions in which the production of thyroid hormones is below normal. Cretinism arises in children as a result of congenital (at birth) hypothyroidism, often caused by an iodine deficiency in the mother's diet during pregnancy. It can cause severe mental retardation and is marked by a thick tongue, lethargy, lack of response to commands, and short stature. It can be corrected if treated within the first 6 to 12 months of life. Symptoms include

- apathy
- constipation
- decreased heart rate
- depression
- dry skin, nails, and scalp
- easy fatiguing
- enlarged thyroid
- lowered voice pitch
- myxedema (accumulation of gel-like substances in skin and connective tissue)
- puffy face
- reduced mental acuity
- swelling of eyelids
- tongue enlarged and thickened
- weight gain

The causes of hypothyroidism include a defect in the function of the thyroid due to autoimmune destruction of the gland, radioactive iodine therapy, or surgical removal of the thyroid. Pituitary dysfunction or an abnormality in the hypothalamus can also cause thyroid failure.

Thyroid replacement therapy is indicated for hypothyroid states and thyroid cancer. In the absence of natural hormones, thyroid hormone replacement is required. Although thyroid hormone increases metabolism replacement therapy should not be used to treat obesity. Drugs commonly used to treat hypothyroidism are listed in

Table 14.1. Hypothyroidism causes increased sensitivity to numerous drugs. Correction may increase requirements for other drugs because of increases in their metabolism and conversion.

Warning

Levothyroxine and levofloxacin (an antibiotic) can be misread for each other.

Levothyroxine (Levothroid, Levoxyl, Synthroid) is synthetic T_4. It is recommended for chronic therapy. Levothyroxine can be very cardiotoxic, so the patient should immediately report any chest pain, increased pulse, palpitations, heat intolerance, or excessive sweating to the physician. In overdose, it can cause "too rapid" a correction and, therefore, a risk of cardiotoxicity and hyperthyroidism. Levothyroxine alters the protein binding of other drugs, so the technician should check the patient profile for drugs currently being taken. Levothyroxine also increases liver metabolism of phenytoin and phenobarbital.

Generic levothyroxine products and Synthroid are therapeutically equivalent, and they are now **AB rated** according to the FDA (that is, shown by studies to be bioequivalent, as a generic should be to the corresponding brand name drug). One clinical study showed that switching products does not cause problems, but it is usually undesirable to switch brands once a patient has become stable. Some prescribers are concerned that the small FDA-allowable compositional differences between Synthroid and generic levothyroxine brands could affect blood levels. All thyroid patients should undergo TSH tests periodically and approximately 6 weeks after changes in dosage or brands. Once the patient is stable on a brand, the prescriber should write **Dispense As Written (DAW)** and write the prescription for that brand name only. Most pharmacy computer programs will automatically switch all drugs to a generic brand; when the switch happens with this drug, the technician may frequently need to switch the drug back to the brand.

Hyperthyroidism

Hyperthyroidism, also called thyrotoxicosis, is due to excessive thyroid hormone. The most common cause of hyperthyroidism is Graves disease, a condition in which the production of the thyroid hormone is increased. The other causes of hyperthyroidism include

- excessive endogenous iodine from intake of thyroid hormones
- thyroid nodules (Plummer disease) or surgical removal of nodules
- a tumor in the pituitary causing overproduction of TSH or a tumor causing excessive TSH releasing factor in the hypothalamus

Symptoms of hyperthyroidism include

- decreased menses
- diarrhea

TABLE 14.1   Most Commonly Used Agents for Hypothyroidism

Generic Name	Pronunciation	Dosage Form	Brand Name	Dispensing Status
levothyroxine, T_4	lee-voe-thye-ROX-een	injection, tablet	Levothroid, Levoxyl, Synthroid	Rx
thyroid	THYE-roid	tablet	Armour Thyroid	Rx

- exophthalmos (a condition in which fat collects behind the eyeball, and eyelids do not close; also, due to a lack of lubrication in the eye, corneal ulceration can result; see Figure 14.5)
- flushing of skin
- heat intolerance
- nervousness
- perspiration
- tachycardia
- weight loss

Adults with hyperthyroidism may have heart problems. This effect is due to prolonged hyperactivity, which is caused by the excessive hormone levels.

For children, hyperthyroidism is managed with surgery and hormone replacement therapy. In adults, surgery is indicated for malignant lesions, esophageal obstruction, failure of thyroid therapy, or large multinodular goiter.

Thyroid storm presents with clinical features similar to thyrotoxicosis, but the features are more exaggerated. It is a life-threatening medical emergency. Thyroid storm commonly lasts approximately 3 days, although symptoms may persist for an additional 8 days. Treatment includes IV fluids, antipyretics, cooling blankets, and sedation. Antithyroid drugs are given in large doses.

Table 14.2 presents the most commonly used agents for hyperthyroidism.

Methimazole (Tapazole) is used in the palliative treatment of hyperthyroidism to return the hyperthyroid patient to a normal metabolic state before a thyroidectomy and to control thyrotoxic crisis that may accompany surgery. Methimazole is also used in preparation for radiation therapy of the thyroid. The patient should be monitored for hypothyroidism, hyperthyroidism, T_3 and T_4 levels, CBC (complete blood count) with differential, and liver function (baseline and as needed).

In preparation for a thyroidectomy, both propylthiouracil and methimazole inhibit synthesis of thyroid hormone and produce a state of euthyroid (normal thyroid function), reducing surgical problems during the procedure. As a result, mortality in thyroidectomy is low.

Both propylthiouracil and methimazole cause altered taste and mild **alopecia** (hair loss). Bone marrow depression with fever, sore throat, and malaise can occur and can be serious. An autoimmune reaction and a Coumadin-like anticoagulant reaction can also occur.

Propylthiouracil, PTU, blocks the synthesis of T_3 and T_4 and the conversion of T_4 to T_3. This drug is used for palliative (affording relief) treatment of hyperthyroidism, as adjunctive therapy to ameliorate hyperthyroidism in preparation for surgical treat-

FIGURE 14.5
Symptom of Hyperthyroidism

Protrusion of the eyeballs, known as exophthalmos, is a symptom of hyperthyroidism.

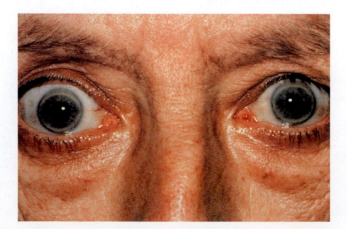

TABLE 14.2　Most Commonly Used Agents for Hyperthyroidism

Generic Name	Pronunciation	Dosage Form	Brand Name	Dispensing Status
methimazole	meth-IM-a-zole	tablet	Tapazole	Rx
propylthiouracil, PTU	proe-pil-thye-oh-YOOR-a-sil	tablet	(none)	Rx
radioactive iodine, ^{131}I	RAY-dee-oh-act-ive EYE-oh-dine	capsule, oral solution	(none)	Rx

ment or ^{131}I (a radioactive isotope of iodine with an atomic mass of 131) therapy, and management of thyroid storm. The recommended dose should not be exceeded. Patients should notify the physician or pharmacist in the event of fever, sore throat, unusual bleeding or bruising, headache, or general malaise. If the patient is taking chronic therapy, the following parameters should be monitored: CBC with differential, prothrombin time (PT), liver function tests, thyroid function tests (T_4, T_3, and TSH), and periodic blood cell counts. Administration of propylthiouracil is preferred over methimazole in thyroid storm.

Radioactive iodine, ^{131}I, is selectively absorbed by the thyroid tissue, where it destroys thyroid cells. It is indicated for elderly and other patients unable to tolerate other therapy or surgery. It is used only when the patient is unresponsive to other therapy. Radioactive iodine therapy should also be used cautiously in children because of its carcinogenic potential and the hypothyroid effect on growth. An adverse effect can be hypothyroidism, and the patient must then receive thyroid hormones. Radiation burns may also injure tissue. Symptoms of radioactive iodine therapy can last up to one year.

Male Hormones and Impotence

The sex hormones are controlled by pituitary hormones, particularly follicle-stimulating hormone (FSH) and luteinizing hormone (LH).

An **androgen** is a hormone that promotes development and maintenance of male physical characteristics. In males, androgens are produced by the testes. They are also produced by the ovaries in females (in whom they are largely converted into female hormones, discussed in the following section); in both males and females, they are also produced in the adrenal glands and the peripheral fat tissue. The most important male hormone is **testosterone**, which is produced by the testes. The pituitary hormones travel in the bloodstream to the testes, where they stimulate the Leydig cells to produce testosterone and release it into the blood. Through a feedback mechanism, the increased testosterone levels then slow the secretion of the releasing factors by the hypothalamus.

Testosterone is responsible for initiating sperm production and for behavioral characteristics (e.g., normal aggressiveness), libido, and sexual potency. It is required during adulthood for the maintenance of libido, sexual potency, fertility (sperm production), muscle mass and strength, fat distribution, bone mass, erythropoiesis (red blood cell production), and prevention of baldness.

In **hypogonadism**—deficient sex hormone production and secretion—the androgens must be replaced. This may cause **virilization** (the development of male characteristics), **anabolic treatment** (muscle building), and stimulation of red blood cell production. Therefore, androgens are used to treat anemia. They are also used in breast cancer and for endometriosis, although they are not the drug of choice for these disorders. Preliminary data suggest that androgen therapy may decrease abdominal fat mass and increase muscle mass in elderly men.

Androgens can cause a number of side effects including virilization, **hirsutism** (abnormal hairiness, especially in women), and acne. Hepatoxicity and abnormally high levels of red blood cells are also problems. Other adverse effects from androgen therapy include oily skin, ankle edema, **priapism** (frequent or prolonged, painful penile erections), and, ironically, **gynecomastia** (breast enlargement in males with or without tenderness). Use of a low initial dosage in nonvirilized men (i.e., those lacking male secondary sex characteristics) mimics the natural increase in serum testosterone concentration during puberty. It produces virilization gradually, which minimizes adverse effects, especially priapism. Gynecomastia is the result of the conversion of testosterone to estradiol (E_2) through peripheral pathways. Men with hepatic cirrhosis are predisposed to gynecomastia.

When administered orally, testosterone undergoes extensive first-pass metabolism in the gastrointestinal tract and liver. To overcome this problem, various testosterone derivatives (e.g., fluoxymesterone and methyltestosterone) have been developed for oral administration. In the past, most men with hypogonadism received biweekly deep intramuscular injections of testosterone.

Scrotal transdermal systems overcome some of the drawbacks associated with oral and intramuscular administration. Applying a transdermal testosterone patch to the scrotal skin in the morning provides a serum testosterone concentration that mimics the natural **circadian** (on a 24 hour cycle) secretion of the hormone in young, healthy men. Because scrotal skin is at least five times more permeable to testosterone than skin at other sites, an inadequate serum testosterone concentration results if a scrotal patch is applied to other areas of the body. To optimize contact, the scrotal skin should be dry-shaved before the patch is applied. Many men prefer scrotal transdermal systems to intramuscular testosterone injections because the patch avoids the pain and discomfort of injections and is easy to apply. Other patients find it embarrassing to explain the transdermal patch to their sex partners. Testosterone patches, like other testosterone dosage forms, are classified as Schedule III controlled substances because of the abuse potential as an anabolic steroid.

Male **impotence** (failure to initiate or to maintain an erection until ejaculation) may have many causes, including testosterone deficiency, alcoholism, cigarette smoking, psychological factors, and medications. Table 14.3 lists drugs that may cause impotence. Alcohol is a primary reason for male dysfunction or impotence. Table 14.4 presents the most commonly used agents for male impotence.

Testosterone (Androderm, AndroGel, Testoderm) is delivered through transdermal systems or patches. Androderm and AndroGel are not applied to the genitals. Instead, these are applied to a fleshy area of the back, abdomen, upper arm, or thigh. In contrast, Testoderm is applied to the scrotum. The usual starting dosage for Androderm is two patches applied every evening (approximately every 24 hours). Patients should be cautioned not to use the same site more than once every 7 days. The system may be worn while taking a shower or bath. Virilization of a female sex partner is unlikely, because the occlusive outer film prevents the partner from coming in contact with the drug. These drugs increase libido and sexual potency within weeks or months and also improve the patient's sense of well-being. AndroGel should be applied once daily, preferably in the morning, to clean, dry, intact skin. The application site should be allowed to dry before dressing. Hands should be washed with soap and water after handling this drug.

TABLE 14.3   Drugs That May Cause Impotence

alcohol (the most significant)	H2 blockers
amphetamines	haloperidol
antihypertensives	lithium
corticosteroids	opiates
estrogens	some antidepressants

Striant, another brand name for testosterone, is a buccal (under the tongue) system.

Alprostadil (Edex, Muse, Caverject) is available under three brand names to treat impotence. Edex is a penile injection. Muse (Medicated Urethral System for Erection) is a urethral suppository for impotence. It comes with a small plastic applicator that inserts a micropellet of alprostadil into the urethra. Muse works quickly, usually within 10 minutes. The side effects are penile pain and urethral burning. High doses can cause hypotension and dizziness. Muse can also affect the female partner, causing vaginal burning and itching. It should be refrigerated unless it is going to be used within fourteen days. **Caverject** is the first drug specifically approved for impotence; it is in the form of an injection to be made into the corpora cavernosa on the sides of the penis, hence the name. The manufacturer provides Caverject as a kit that contains six syringes and single-dose vials of freeze-dried powder for reconstitution and administration. The vials should be refrigerated until dispensed, but they may be kept at room temperature for up to 3 months. In **Caverject Impulse**, the powder and the water are

TABLE 14.4   Most Commonly Used Agents for Male Impotence

Generic Name	Pronunciation	Dosage Form	Brand Name	Dispensing Status	Control Schedule
alprostadil	al-PROS-ta-dil	injection, suppository	Caverject, Caverject Impulse, Edex, Muse	Rx	
danazol	DA-na-zawl	capsule	Danocrine	Rx	
methyltestosterone	meth-il-tes-TOS-te-rone	capsule, tablet	Android, Testred	Rx	C-III
oxymetholone	ox-i-METH-oh-lone	tablet	Anadrol	Rx	
papaverine	pa-PAV-er-een	capsule, injection	(none)	Rx	
testosterone	tes-TOS-te-rone	gel, injection, tablet, transdermal patch	Androderm (nonscrotal), AndroGel, Striant, Testoderm (scrotal)	Rx	C-III
Phosphodiesterase Inhibitors					
sildenafil	sil-DEN-a-fil	tablet	Viagra	Rx	
tadalafil	tah-DAL-a-fil	tablet	Cialis	Rx	
vardenafil	var-DEN-a-fil	tablet	Levitra	Rx	

stored in separate chambers in the prefilled syringe. Turning the plunger before injection mixes the powder and water and dials the specified dose.

Phosphodiesterase inhibitors, which are among the best-selling current drugs, have replaced other drugs used for male impotence. These drugs produce smooth muscle relaxation and inflow of blood into the penis in response to sexual stimulation. They have many interactions with other drugs, however, particularly a potentially lethal interaction with nitrates (nitroglycerine, isosorbide dinitrate, and isosorbide mononitrate) used to treat ischemic heart disease, as described in Chapter 12.

Sildenafil (Viagra), the first oral therapy for impotence, enhances the relaxant effect of nitric oxide released in response to sexual stimulation. This allows an erection to occur naturally. It should be taken at least 1 hour before sexual activity. Pharmacy technicians must watch the interaction profile carefully, because sildenafil has several interactions. Its interaction with nitrates is potentially lethal. Other interactions to watch for are erythromycin and antifungal medications. Sildenafil can cause temporary vision disturbances, headache, and indigestion. It will decrease blood pressure for several hours.

◁▷◁▷ **May cause BLURRED VISION**

Vardenafil (Levitra) has the same side effect profile as sildenafil, but is often used in sildenafil nonresponders. Patients should be discouraged from smoking or drinking alcohol for a few hours before sexual activity.

Tadalafil (Cialis) is sometimes called the "weekender" because it is effective for 36 hours. Peak plasma levels are obtained in 2 hours. It has a faster onset and longer duration than the other phosphodiesterase inhibitors. Tadalafil has the same interactions with nitrates and other drugs as sildenafil and vardenafil, but it has a significantly different chemical structure.

Female Hormones

Exogenously administered female hormones can prevent conception, ease the symptoms of menopause, and help prevent osteoporosis. Currently, however, there is much debate regarding the proper use of these drugs. Two of the most important female hormones are estrogen and progesterone. **Estrogen** stimulates the development of female secondary sex characteristics and promotes the growth and maintenance of the female reproductive system. **Progesterone** is responsible for controlling the preparation of the uterus for a fertilized ovum.

Estrogen

Estrogen is a group of hormones that are formed in the ovaries from androgenic precursors. When the hypothalamic-pituitary axis releases FSH to the ovaries, it stimulates estrogen production for 1 to 14 days and progesterone production for 14 to 28 days. As both hormones build up in the bloodstream, a feedback mechanism reduces the activity of the hypothalamus in producing and releasing the gonadotropin-releasing hormone (GnRH).

Estrogen compounds are the growth hormones of reproductive tissue in females. In addition, they share some actions of androgens on the skeleton and other tissues. Estrogen produces endometrial growth, increased cervical mucus, cornification (thickening and maturing) of vaginal mucosa, growth of breast tissue (ducts and fat deposit), increased epiphyseal closure, sodium retention, carbohydrate metabolism, and calcium utilization.

Estrogen is used for birth control formulations, relief of menopausal symptoms, reduction of osteoporosis in combination with other drugs (e.g., bisphosphonates), gonadal failure, and prostatic cancer. Symptoms of estrogen deficiency include irregular bleeding and irregular cycles. **Vasomotor** symptoms, which affect the blood vessels, may also appear. Commonly known as "hot flashes," vasomotor instability starts in the face and moves down over the body; the severity is related to the rate of estrogen decline. Other symptoms may include atrophic vulvovaginitis, characterized by excessive vaginal dryness; **dyspareunia** (painful intercourse); and infections (because fewer of the lactobacilli that produce protective acidity are present because of the dryness, which is due to the reduced estrogen level). Estrogen depletion also leads to a reduction in the amount of glycogen to be metabolized, raised pH of the vaginal area, and loss of lubrication, causing urethral and bladder atrophy. **Hormone therapy (HT)** relieves the symptoms of estrogen deficiency.

The rate of estrogen production declines with the onset of menopause, which is defined as the cessation of menses for 1 year; it is accompanied by a change in the site, amount, and pattern of estrogen production. The **climacteric** (the syndrome of endocrine, somatic, and psychological changes that occur at the end of the female reproductive period) is characterized by gradual loss of ovarian function and irregular bleeding before the termination of menses. With decreased estrogen production at menopause, estrogen-responsive tissues atrophy. Menopausal symptoms may include vasomotor instability (hot flashes), drying and atrophy of the vaginal mucosa, insomnia, irritability, and other mood changes. A certain amount of depression is also related to menopause.

As ovarian function declines with age, androstenedione, produced in the adrenal cortex, becomes the primary source of estrogen, and estrone becomes the dominant circulating estrogen. Because the naturally occurring concentration of androstenedione and the efficiency of its conversion may vary considerably among women, HT is often provided to ease the transition into menopause. A small amount of estrogen continues to be produced through the metabolism of adrenal steroids to estradiol in peripheral fat tissue. Depending on body fat, some women may not need estrogen. Estrogen is also effective in preventing bone loss, lowering cholesterol levels, and improving the color and turgor of skin.

Progestins

Progestin, which is a group of synthetic forms of progesterone, simulates the effect of progesterone. Both progesterone and estrogen prevent ovulation. Progesterone achieves this by inhibiting the secretion of luteinizing hormone (LH), whereas estrogen suppresses the secretion of follicle-stimulating hormone (FSH), thereby blocking follicular development and ovulation.

Progestin is used primarily in birth control pills and to prevent uterine cancer in postmenopausal women who take hormone replacement therapy. Another important use is to treat menstrual dysfunction such as irregular cycles, protracted uterine bleeding, dysmenorrhea, amenorrhea, and endometriosis. It is believed that poorly cycling estrogens may promote hypertrophy of the endometrium. Treatment with a progestin lowers the incidence of endometrial hyperplasia. Progestin alone does not promote menstrual bleeding, but in patients who either have endogenous estrogen or are treated first with estrogen, cyclic treatment with progestin helps to restore normal cycling. Table 14.5 lists the most commonly used types of progestin.

Hormone Therapy

Table 14.5 presents the most commonly used estrogen supplements for hormone therapy for the symptoms of menopause. It is important for the technician to know that even if these medications have the exact same ingredients, they cannot be interchanged. The doses will differ slightly in each.

It is especially important to remind patients taking any form of estrogen, whether it is birth control pills or hormone therapy, that smoking is associated with greater morbidity, especially in patients over 35 years of age. Estrogen plus nicotine increases the risk of blood clots, which increases the risk of deep vein thrombosis (discussed in Chapter 12).

Research is constantly revealing new information about hormone therapy's risks and benefits. Some studies recommend that it be used only to manage the vasomotor symptoms of menopause and that use should be limited to the shortest duration possible. Hormone therapy is also associated with some risk of breast cancer. For this reason, some practitioners do not prescribe estrogen to patients who have had breast cancer or who have a family history of breast cancer. For many women, the benefits of HT in reducing the symptoms of menopause and especially decreasing bone loss far outweigh the risk of breast cancer.

Whether or not to use HT is a decision for a woman and her physician. The advantages and disadvantages will be different for each woman depending on her family history and her physical condition. If a woman who has been on HT for a long time chooses not to continue, however, hormones should be tapered.

Estrogen-Only Hormone Therapy Products **Conjugated estrogens** include **Cenestin**, **Enjuvia**, and **Premarin**, each a little different from the other. Cenestin and Enjuvia are derived from plants. Premarin is made from pregnant mares' urine, hence the name. Cenestin contains nine of the types of estrogen that occurs in Premarin and 10 of the types included in Enjuvia.

Estradiol (Alora, Climara, Elestrin, Esclim, Estrace, Estraderm, Estrasorb, Estring, Evamist, Femring, Menostar, Vivelle, Vivelle Dot) is bioidentical to human hormones. It is produced in many shapes and forms, none of which are interchangeable. Topical estrogen may be a little safer than pills, because it avoids first pass through the liver. **Femring** is supplied on a ring inserted into the vagina for 30 days. **Vivelle Dot**, a small patch, is placed on the abdomen for 3½ days (according to the manufacturer's recommendation, though for most patients this will actually mean 3 days). **Elestrin** is a gel that is contained in a pump and should be applied over the entire upper arm and shoulder area.

Estring and **Femring** contain the medication in a ring to be inserted in the vagina. The ring releases an initial burst of estradiol, followed by a tapered low dose for a 90 day period. Insertion of the ring is similar to using a diaphragm. If removed, the ring should be rinsed in lukewarm water before being reinserted. This drug relieves symptoms of urogenital atrophy without releasing appreciable systemic concentrations of estradiol. Therefore, it is not used for vasomotor symptoms or for the prevention of osteoporosis. If the patient has an intact uterus, she will also need a progestin so as to prevent endometrial hyperplasia. **Estrasorb** is an estrogen cream form of this drug. Because it is topical and does not go through the liver, it is safer than oral tablets. Two foil packets should be applied each day, one to each leg. One packet should be rubbed to the top of one thigh and on the the calf. The procedure is repeated on the other leg. The patient should exercise care in skin-to-skin contact with another person such as a sexual partner. If the patient has an intact uterus, a progestin should be added to the regimen.

TABLE 14.5   Most Commonly Used Estrogen Supplements

Generic Name	Pronunciation	Dosage Form	Brand Name	Dispensing Status
Estrogen Only				
conjugated estrogen	CON-ju-gate-ed ES-troe-jen	cream, injection, IV, tablet	Cenestin, Enjuvia, Premarin	Rx
estradiol	es-tra-DYE-awl	cream, injection, patch, ring to insert, tablet	Alora, Climara, Elestrin, Esclim, Estrace, Estraderm, Estrasorb, Estring, Evamist, Femring, Menostar, Vivelle, Vivelle Dot	Rx
estropipate	es-troe-PIP-ate	cream, tablet	Ogen	Rx
ethinyl estradiol	ETH-in-il es-tra-DYE-awl	tablet	Estinyl	Rx
Estrogen-Progestin				
conjugated estrogen–medroxyprogesterone	CON-ju-gate-ed ES-troe-jen me-DROX-ee-proe-JES-te-rone	tablet	Premphase, Prempro	Rx
estradiol-levonorgestrel	es-tra-DYE-awl lee-voe-nor-JES-trel	patch	Climara Pro	Rx
estradiol-norethindrone	es-tra-DYE-awl nor-eth-IN-drone	patch, tablet	Activella, CombiPatch	Rx
estradiol-norgestimate	es-tra-DYE-awl nor-JES-ti-mate	tablet	Ortho-Prefest	Rx
ethinyl estradiol–norethindrone	ETH-in-il es-tra-DYE-awl nor-eth-IN-drone	tablet	femhrt	Rx

Evamist is a topical estrogen spray in a metered dose pump. The initial dose is one spray per day, which is titrated to relief of symptoms not to exceed two or three sprays. It is applied to the inside of the forearm at the same time each day. The spray should be allowed to dry for a few minutes. Sun screen should be applied before the spray; if applied after, it decreases the effectiveness of the spray. Topical estrogens can be administered in lower doses than oral estrogens because they bypass the liver.

Estrogen-Progestin Hormone Therapy Products Combination therapy with an estrogen product and a progestin is necessary only for women with an intact uterus. In the normal cycle, high levels of estrogen before ovulation cause cells in the uterine lining to multiply. Estrogen can cause the same effect when given for HT, leading to endometrial hyperplasia, which may progress to uterine cancer. A progestin counteracts these effects. Therefore, women with an intact uterus should receive both an estrogen and a progestin. If progestin therapy can be avoided, however, the risk of side effects from HT medication decreases tremendously.

Conjugated estrogen–medroxyprogesterone (Premphase, Prempro) contains the same conjugated estrogens as the estrogen-only product Premarin, discussed previously, but also a progestin. Each Prempro tablet contains both estrogen and progestin. Premphase is a course of 28 daily tablets, of which the maroon tablets to be taken during the first 14 days contain only estrogen and the blue tablets to be taken during the second 14 days contain both estrogen and progestin, simulating the natural cycle.

Ethinyl estradiol–norethindrone (femhrt) contains a combination of hormones commonly used in oral contraceptives, but at a much lower dosage: 1 mg norethindrone acetate (progestin) and 5 mg ethinyl estradiol (estrogen) in femhrt 1/5, or half those amounts in Low-Dose Femhrt 0.5/2.5, the lowest effective dose approved by the FDA. It provides many health benefits (such as prevention of bone loss and lowered risk of ovarian and endometrial cancer) in addition to estrogen replacement.

Estradiol-levonorgestrel (Climara Pro) is indicated for menopausal symptoms and is provided by the manufacturer as a patch. It decreases the intensity and number of hot flashes, night sweats, and vaginal dryness associated with menopause. The patch is stored at room temperature and is applied once weekly.

Estradiol-norethindrone (CombiPatch) is a matrix transdermal in which the drugs are incorporated within the adhesive matrix layer and released continuously. The patch should be applied twice weekly to a smooth, fold-free area of dry skin on the abdomen and should be worn continuously. It should be stored in the refrigerator before dispensing. **Activella** is the tablet form of this drug combination. Activella is indicated for symptoms of menopause, vulvar atrophy, and the prevention of osteoporosis. It also decreases total cholesterol but at the expense of decreased HDL. It is derived from soy and a synthetic progestin. Activella is used to control moderate-to-severe vasomotor symptoms of menopause.

Contraceptives

Prescription contraceptives, typically **oral contraceptives (OCs)**, famous as "the pill," are among the most frequently prescribed pharmaceutical agents in the United States. For these products to be optimally effective with the lowest frequency of side effects, patients should be well informed as to their proper use.

The advantages of OCs include ease of use, high efficacy rate, and relative safety. Most OCs prescribed today are a combination of estrogen and a progestin. These combination pills suppress ovulation by interfering with the production of the hormones that regulate the menstrual cycle. High levels of estrogen, as occur after ovulation, suppress the production of follicle-stimulating hormone (FSH) so that eggs do not mature. The progestin suppresses the production of luteinizing hormone (LH) so that eggs are not released. The progestin also alters the cervical mucus from a watery, nonviscous secretion to a viscous, cellular secretion that forms a physical barrier that prevents the penetration of sperm. In addition, the progestin changes the composition of the **endometrium** to make it unsuitable for implantation. Some progestin-only forms of "the pill" are also available, and their mechanism relies on the effects of progestin on the cervical mucus and endometrium.

Combination OCs provide both estrogen and progestin in the same pill for each of 21 consecutive days, which may be followed by 7 days of inert pills during the interval when menstruation takes place. Progestin-only OCs are usually taken once a day, every day, without a pill-free interval. In addition to preventing pregnancy, oral contraceptives have several noncontraceptive benefits. Many women who take an OC experience more regular menstrual cycles, reduced menstrual flow, and less severe menstrual pain and cramps. Epidemiologic evidence shows that OCs may protect against ovarian and endometrial cancer, benign breast disease, ectopic pregnancy, and ovarian cysts. They may also reduce the risk of pelvic inflammatory disease.

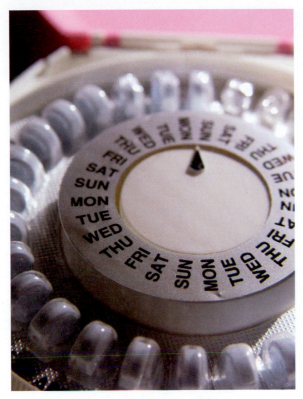
A variety of birth control pills are available

The most serious adverse effect of OCs is the development of cardiovascular complications, such as heart attack, stroke, or other forms of thromboembolic disease. The OCs currently available contain much lower amounts of estrogen and progestin than those first introduced in the 1960s, and the frequency of adverse cardiovascular effects has been reduced.

Tricycling is the practice of taking OCs on three 21 day cycles without a pill-free interval. Evidence suggests that because the OC suppresses endometrial thickening, menstrual cycles (i.e., the cyclic sloughing off of this layer) can be safely extended to 3 months. The benefits of tricycling include less menstrual pain and lower incidences of premenstrual syndrome (PMS), headaches, and endometriosis.

Most Commonly Prescribed Oral Contraceptives

Table 14.6 presents the most commonly used contraceptive agents. Most OCs available today contain ethinyl estradiol as estrogen and norethindrone or levonorgestrel as progestin. The classic side effects associated with birth control pills (nausea, weight gain, and breast tenderness) result from the levels of the progestin necessary for effectiveness. Women who smoke are at increased risk for thromboembolic complications, and those who are prescribed oral contraceptives should not smoke. The combination of nicotine and estrogen is associated with increased frequency of blood clots. Oral contraceptives should be taken at the same time each day to attain maximum effectiveness. Taking the medication at bedtime reduces the nausea. Antibiotics may interfere with the efficacy of this form of contraception, so backup measures should always be used in patients on antibiotics.

Estradiol cypionate–medroxyprogesterone (Lunelle) is given once a month and is an injectable contraceptive. In addition to progestin, it has an estrogen component. Patients who use estradiol cypionate–medroxyprogesterone generally have irregular periods or none. After injections are discontinued, normal fertility may not resume for as long as 13 months. For states in which pharmacists are permitted to administer injections, this drug may be given in some pharmacies. (Withdrawn from market.)

Estradiol-drospirenone (Angeliq) has the spironolactone analog drospirenone. Drospirenone also has mineralocorticoid activity as well as progestin activity, so it works as a potassium-sparing diuretic, thus reducing the risk of sodium and fluid retention and weight gain. Estradiol-drospirenone increases triglycerides and HDLs, but lowers LDLs, and reduces blood pressure.

Ethinyl estradiol–desogestrel (Cyclessa, Desogen, Kariva, Mircette, Ortho-Cept) suppresses gonadotropins, which results in inhibition of ovulation. The regimen includes 2 days of placebo tablets, followed by 5 days of low-dose estrogen. The lower estrogen dose is possibly associated with less effect on the coagulation and fibrinolytic systems than contraceptives that contain greater amounts of estrogen, so it may be less risky for smokers.

TABLE 14.6   Most Commonly Used Contraceptive Agents

Generic Name	Pronunciation	Dosage Form	Brand Name	Dispensing Status
Combination Oral Contraceptives				
estradiol cypionate–medroxyprogesterone*	es-tra-DYE-awl sip-EYE-on-ate me-DROX-ee-proe-JES-te-rone	injection	Lunelle*	Rx
estradiol-drospirenone	es-tra-DYE-awl-droh-SPYE-re-none	tablet	Angeliq	Rx
ethinyl estradiol–desogestrel	ETH-in-il es-tra-DYE-awl des-oh-JES-trel	tablet	Cyclessa, Desogen, Kariva, Mircette, Ortho-Cept	Rx
ethinyl estradiol–drospirenone	ETH-in-il es-tra-DYE-awl droh-SPYE-re-none	tablet	Yasmin, Yaz	Rx
ethinyl estradiol–ethynodiol diacetate	ETH-in-il es-tra-DYE-awl e-thye-noe-DYE-awl dye-AS-e-tate	tablet	Demulen	Rx
ethinyl estradiol–etonogestrel	ETH-in-il es-tra-DYE-awle ee-toe-noe-JES-trel	ring	NuvaRing	Rx
ethinyl estradiol–levonorgestrel	ETH-in-il es-tra-DYE-awl LEE-voe-nor-jes-trel	tablet	Aviane, Levlen, Lybrel, Nordette, Seasonale, Seasonique, Tri-Levlen, Triphasil, Trivora-28	Rx
ethinyl estradiol–norelgestromin	ETH-in-il es-tra-DYE-awl nor-el-JES-troe-min	patch	Ortho Evra	Rx
ethinyl estradiol–norethindrone	ETH-in-il es-tra-DYE-awl nor-eth-IN-drone	tablet	Estrostep Fe, Loestrin Fe, Loestrin 24 Fe, Ovcon	Rx
ethinyl estradiol–norgestimate	ETH-in-il es-tra-DYE-awl nor-JES-ti-mate	tablet	Ortho Tri-Cyclen, Ortho Tri-Cyclen Lo	Rx
ethinyl estradiol–norgestrel	ETH-in-il es-tra-DYE-awl nor-JES-trel	tablet	Lo/Ovral, Low-Ogestrel, Ovral	Rx
Progestin-Only Contraceptives				
levonorgestrel	LEE-voe-nor-jes-trel	implant	Norplant II	Rx
medroxyprogeste-rone	me-DROX-ee-proe-JES-te-rone	injection, tablet	Depo-Provera, Provera	Rx
norethindrone	nor-eth-IN-drone	tablet	Micronor	Rx
Emergency Contraceptives				
levonorgestrel	LEE-voe-nor-jes-trel	tablet	Plan B	OTC
norgestrel	nor-JES-trel	tablet	Ovrette	Rx

* Withdrawn from Market

Ethinyl estradiol–drospirenone (Yasmine, Yaz) reduces bloating; Yaz has also been approved for the treatment of acne. Because of the low dose of progestin in this pill, Yaz may not be as effective in women who weigh more than approximately 154 pounds. Yasmine maintains a 28 day cycle, Yaz provides a shorter period because it has only four inactive tablets. Ethinyl estradiol–drospirenone, like estradiol–drospirenone, uses drospirenone, a spironolactone analog that has mineralocorticoid activity, as its progestin component. There is less bloating and less weight gain with this drug than with other OCs, but the serum potassium may increase. A patient may actually experience weight loss—an effect that has made this drug very popular. However, the weight loss is due to the diuretic activity of drospirenone.

Ethinyl estradiol–etonogestrel (NuvaRing) is a vaginal ring. A new ring is inserted once a month. The ring remains in for 3 weeks and is then removed for 1 week. If it is accidentally expelled or removed for some reason, it can be washed off and reinserted. If the ring is out for more than 3 hours, a backup contraceptive should be used for 7 days. It is stored in the refrigerator before dispensing, but it may be stored at room temperature for as long as 4 months.

Ethinyl estradiol–levonorgestrel (Levlen, Lybrel, Nordette, Seasonale, Seasonique, Tri-Levlen, Triphasil, Trivora-28) is available in many combinations of these two drugs. This drug works by preventing the ovaries from releasing an egg, increasing the thickness of mucus at the opening of the uterus, and increasing the thickness of the endometrial lining so that the egg cannot attach. The primary side effects are headache, nausea, and breast tenderness. Like other birth control pills, it should be taken the same time each day. Seasonique contains 7 days of estrogen. Seasonale and Seasonique are taken for 3 months, and women on these drugs have only 3 periods per year. There will be more breakthrough bleeding with these pills than with the traditional 28 day cycle pills, but it will decrease with use. Seasonale has a 7 day pill-free interval period, whereas Seasonique has no pill-free interval, but rather a 7 day low-dose estrogen period. Lybrel is approved for continuous use; thus, women on this OC will have no periods at all. Lybrel should provide a lower incidence of PMS, headaches, and anemia than other forms of birth control. While on this group of pills, the endometrial thickening is suppressed, so monthly bleeding is not necessary to slough it off.

Ethinyl estradiol–norelgestromin (Ortho Evra) is a transdermal contraceptive patch with three layers. The back layer provides structural support and protects the middle adhesive layer, which contains the drugs. The third layer is a transparent release liner and is removed just prior to application. Ethinyl estradiol–norelgestromin prevents pregnancy through suppression of gonadotropins. A new patch is applied every 7 days for 3 weeks. Then a week is skipped. The next patch should be applied during the first 24 hours of the menstrual cycle. If it is not applied within this period, a backup form of contraception such as a spermicide, condom, or diaphragm should be used for the first 7 days. Occasionally there is a problem with skin irritation or with the patch becoming loose and falling off. It must be reattached even if it is just partly attached. Ethinyl estradiol–norelgestromin is not as effective for women who weigh more than 198 pounds than it is for lighter-weight women.

Ethinyl estradiol–norethindrone (Estrostep Fe, Loestrin, Loestrin 24 Fe, Ovcon) should be taken for at least 3 months. Loestrin, Loestrin 24 Fe, and Estrostep Fe are also approved for the treatment of acne, as is Ortho Tri-Cyclen Lo. Sebum, an oily substance produced by sebaceous glands, contributes to acne, and estrogens decrease sebum production. Therefore, theoretically, all oral contraceptives should improve acne. An additional feature of Estrostep Fe and Loestrin 24 Fe is an iron supplement to replace iron lost in menstruation. Loestrin 24 Fe has 24 hormone tablets and 4 iron tablets and extends the hormone period by 3 days while maintaining the 28 day cycle. Women taking Loestrin 24 Fe will experience shorter periods.

Progestin-Only Contraceptives As mentioned in the discussion of combination oral contraceptives, progestins act to prevent pregnancy by inhibiting the secretion of LH, which causes egg release; causing thickening of the cervical mucus to impede the entry of sperm; and altering the uterine lining to prevent implantation of a blastocyst. Therefore, progestins can be used as contraceptives by themselves without additional estrogens. In addition to tablets such as **norgestrel (Micronor)**, long-term parenteral applications are available, including **medroxyprogesterone (Depo-Provera)**, an intramuscular injection that prevents pregnancy for 3 months at a time.

Levonorgestrel (Norplant II) comes in matchstick-sized, flexible, closed capsules. The capsules are implanted under local anesthesia through a single incision in the subcutaneous tissue of the upper arm, where the hormone is released and easily diffused into the bloodstream. The implants maintain their effectiveness for as long as five years and must be removed surgically by the end of the fifth year of use.

Many of the side effects associated with progestins—and oral contraceptives—are similar to the symptoms of pregnancy. The effects generally attributed to the progestational component include weight gain, depression, fatigue, acne, and hirsutism (abnormal hairiness, especially in women).

Interactions with Oral Contraceptives Oral contraceptives interact with many drugs. The technician should carefully check the patient profile for drugs listed in Table 14.7. The drug classes are the important element to watch in this list. If a contraceptive interacts with any drug in a class, there is an excellent chance it will react with all the drugs in that class.

Emergency Contraceptives In the event of unprotected sex, administration of an emergency contraceptive may prevent pregnancy if medications are taken quickly enough (usually within 24 hours). There is a great demand for emergency forms of contraception, and many patients want them to be available without prescription. They point out that by the time an appointment can be made with a physician and a prescription is written, it is too late for medication to be effective. Emergency contraception is a controversial topic.

Norgestrel (Ovrette) is an oral progestin that is supplied in 75 mcg tablets for use as a regular contraceptive, one tablet daily. For a contraceptive emergency (most often in the ER for rape victims), 40 tablets are taken at once. Norgestrel is available only by prescription.

Levonorgestrel (Plan B) is used to prevent pregnancy following unprotected intercourse or a known or suspected contraceptive failure. It prevents ovulation or fertilization by altering the tubal transportation of the sperm or ova. If implantation has already occurred, levonorgestrel is not effective. It is a two dose regimen. Nausea is a predominant side effect. Plan B is provided by the manufacturer in blister packages that contain two large doses of levonorgestrol of 0.75 mg each. The first dose should be taken within 72 hours of intercourse. The second tablet is taken 12 hours after the first tablet. If the patient vomits within one hour of taking either dose, that dose must be repeated. The most common side effects are nausea and abdominal pain, headache, fatigue, and menstrual changes.

Plan B is designed to prevent pregnancy after unprotected sex, condom or diaphragm failure, or sexual assault. It should not be used as a routine form of birth control and is not effective at terminating pregnancies (i.e., post-implantation).

Plan B is available without a prescription, but is kept behind the counter because the pharmacy technicians must check identification to ensure that the purchaser is at least 18 years of age.

TABLE 14.7   Oral Contraceptive Interactions

Class	Drugs	Type of Interaction
antibiotics	erythromycin, griseofulvin, penicillins, rifampin, tetracyclines	May decrease OC effectiveness; interfere with enterohepatic cycling and recycling of estrogen, which can cause a fluctuation in hormone levels.
anticonvulsants	carbamazepine, felbamate, phenobarbital, phenytoin, primidone	Decrease OC action through increased metabolism of hormones.
antifungals	fluconazole, itraconazole, ketoconazole	May decrease OC action (see *antibiotics*).
benzodiazepines	alprazolam, chlordiazepoxide, diazepam, flurazepam, triazolam	Metabolism of benzodiazepines that undergo oxidation may be decreased, increasing central nervous system (CNS) effects.
bronchodilator	theophylline	Theophylline metabolism may be decreased, increasing side effects.
corticosteroids	hydrocortisone, methylprednisolone, prednisolone, prednisone	Effects may be increased owing to inhibition of metabolism by OC.
lipid-lowering agents	clofibrate	Metabolism of clofibrate may be increased, decreasing OC effect.
tricyclic antidepressants (TCAs)	amitriptyline, imipramine	TCA metabolism may be decreased, increasing the side effects.

Pregnancy Tests and Pregnancy

Detecting a pregnancy early allows a woman to make informed lifestyle decisions and seek appropriate healthcare resources for an optimal outcome. Critical organ systems develop during the first month of embryogenesis; these systems are affected by the mother's diet (e.g., vitamins, caffeine), environment (e.g., smoking), medications, and consumption of alcoholic beverages. Early confirmation of pregnancy allows for earlier prenatal care, earlier detection of an ectopic pregnancy (a potentially life-threatening condition), and more time for counseling and consideration of alternatives.

Pregnancy tests are based on detecting the hormone human chorionic gonadotropin (hCG), a glycoprotein produced by trophoblastic cells (the outer cells of the blastocyst) and their descendants in the placenta. Because hCG levels can be measured as early as 6 to 8 days after conception, a woman can test for pregnancy after the first day of a missed menstrual period (depending on the test used). All currently marketed tests detect hCG with monoclonal antibodies (MCAs) specific for the hormone. A chromogen-reactive enzyme linked to one of the antibodies changes color in the presence of hCG, indicating pregnancy. MCA tests provide results in 1 to 5 minutes. These tests differ in the time and number of steps required to complete the test, the clarity of instructions, and the ease with which the test results can be determined. Consumers generally achieve better than 95% accuracy with home pregnancy tests. The tests currently on the market include Life Sign, One Step, e.p.t., Fact Plus, Accu-Clear, Clearblue, and Baby Check.

To use a kit properly, these steps should be followed.

1. Check the expiration date.
2. Read the instructions twice.

3. Wait the recommended number of days after the menstrual period.
4. Collect the sample from the first morning urine.
5. Collect the urine in a clean container; do not use a plastic cup.
6. If the test cannot be done immediately, refrigerate the urine. Be sure to set out the continer with the urine 20 to 30 minutes before the test is performed.
7. If the test is positive, make an appointment to see a doctor.
8. If the test is negative, wait 3 to 5 days. If menstruation does not begin, perform the test again. If the second test is negative and menstruation has not started, see a doctor.

False-negative test results can be due to chilled urine, chilled test reagents, diluted urine, or high-dose pancreatic enzyme replacement. False-positive results can be due to collecting the urine in a waxed paper cup, an undetected or recent abortion, or elevated levels of hCG (e.g., in tumor).

Sexually active women should make sure they get the daily requirements of folic acid, iron, and calcium. Pregnancy commonly occurs without the mother even being aware that she is pregnant, and these three substances are very important in the formation of the fetus. Folic acid prevents tubular defects; iron prevents anemia, preterm delivery, and low birth weight in infants; calcium is important for bone development.

There are very few OTC drugs that a pregnant woman can take. Acetaminophen (Tylenol) is one of the few drugs available that appear completely safe (but see Chapter 13).

Drugs Used During Childbirth

For almost the entire history of human beings, women delivered babies naturally, without medical intervention or drugs. Childbirth is fraught with dangers to both the mother and child, and death or serious injury is not uncommon. Even during relatively uncomplicated deliveries, childbirth is extremely painful for the mother. With the advent of modern medicine and pharmaceutical products, women and their physicians have numerous tools at their disposal. For relatively simple deliveries, women may choose not to use drugs, though they are available to ameliorate pain. For emergency situations, however, drugs are necessary. If labor ceases, utilization of a drug that induces labor could prevent the need for a Caesarean section (C-section). If a C-section is performed, then certainly drugs are involved. Also, if uncontrolled bleeding occurs, drugs are probably indicated. Table 14.8 lists the drugs most commonly used at birth.

TABLE 14.8   Most Commonly Used Drugs at Birth

Generic Name	Pronunciation	Dosage Form	Brand Name	Dispensing Status
dinoprostone	dye-noe-PROST-one	gel, suppository	Cervidil, Prepidil, Prostin E	Rx
magnesium sulfate	mag-NEE-zhum-SUL-fate	IV	none	Rx
methylergonovine	meth-il-er-goe-NOE-veen	injection, IV	Methergine	Rx
misoprostol	mye-soe-PROS-tawl	tablet	Cytotec	Rx
nifedipine	nye-FED-i-peen	capsule	Procardia	Rx
oxytocin	ox-i-TOE-sin	injection, IV	Pitocin	Rx

Dinoprostone (Cervidil, Prepidil, Prostin E) promotes cervical ripening (softening to permit delivery) in patients at or near term in whom there is medical or obstetrical indication for the induction of labor. Prepidil is a gel that is packaged in a syringe. Prostin E is a suppository in a foil wrapper. Carvidil is a vaginal insert with a string attached so that it can be removed at the appropriate time.

Methylergonovine (Methergine) is used for the prevention and treatment of hemorrhage when the uterus fails to contract to its original size following delivery because of muscle failure (atony) or because of infection or retention of placental fragments (subinvolution). Methylergonovine stops the bleeding by causing constriction of blood vessels, primarily in the uterus.

Misoprostol (Cytotec) is used for cervical ripening. It is a prostaglandin E analog and is also used for induction. The tablets are usually cut into halves or fourths and inserted into the vagina. Pregnant women should not touch misoprostol because it can induce premature labor.

Oxytocin (Pitocin) is a synthetic duplicate of a natural hormone, secreted by the posterior lobe of the pituitary, that stimulates contraction of uterine smooth muscle at term, when uterine muscle is most sensitive to the hormone. Such a drug is called an **oxytocic agent**. Side effects for the mother may include vomiting, irregular heart rate, tachycardia, and postpartum bleeding. The child may experience bradycardia, arrhythmias, and jaundice. This drug should be used as a last resort.

Drugs Used for Premature Labor A drug used to slow labor is called a **tocolytic agent**. Very few tocolytic agents are available.

Magnesium sulfate is used to prevent seizures in pre-eclampsia or eclampsia (caused by hypertension) during pregnancy. This drug has severe consequences when used in error. It is a high-alert drug, so special care needs to be taken when dispensing this intravenous drug. It has a tocolytic effect (slows uterine contraction) and is also used frequently for this purpose.

Nifedipine (Procardia) is a calcium channel blocker (see Chapter 12) used as a tocolytic. It relaxes smooth muscle. The soft capsule contains 10 or 20 mg of nifedipine. The capsule is punctured and placed under the tongue so that the laboring patient will have faster absorption.

Drugs Used for Pain Control during Labor and Delivery The use of drugs for pain control during labor and delivery can produce some difficult decisions for the attending physician. On the one hand, one goal is to keep the mother comfortable. On the other hand, however, the baby needs to be alert and ready to take the first breath on its own. Narcotics most frequently used for pain control are butorphanol, fentanyl, and morphine. Meperidine is not a good choice, because if the baby is delivered 60 minutes or more after administration, the metabolite, normeperidine can accumulate in the infant. Local anesthetics are a good choice and are given as an epidural or spinal injection. Also, local anesthetics, such as lidocaine, are used for local infiltration of the perineum and vagina before, and during repair of, an episiotomy. When general anesthesia is used, nitrous oxide combined with oxygen is the most common agent. Sodium pentothal is also used as a general anesthetic.

For all use of medications, the goal is always to strike a balance between obtaining a desired therapeutic effect for the mother and avoiding toxicity and other deleterious side effects for the baby. During childbirth, reaching this goal is complicated because there are two patients involved.

Sexually Transmitted Diseases

Most genital system diseases are transmitted by sexual activity and are, therefore, called sexually transmitted diseases (STDs), formerly known as venereal diseases. The best way to avoid STDs is to abstain from sexual contact or to be in a long-term, mutually monogamous relationship with a partner who has been tested and is known to be uninfected. Figure 14.6 shows the structural anatomy of the male and female genital systems. One of the most severe STDs, acquired immunodeficiency syndrome (AIDS), caused by human immunodeficiency virus (HIV), was discussed in Chapter 5. Other important STDs are discussed in the following sections.

Chlamydia

If untreated, an infection by *Chlamydia trachomatis* can progress to serious reproductive and other health problems with both short-term and long-term consequences. Chlamydia is known as the "silent" disease, because many people with chlamydia have no symptoms. It can occur in the rectum from anal intercourse and in the throat from oral sex. Chlamydial infections frequently occur with gonorrhea. Partners are frequently reinfected if their sex partners are not treated. It can be easily treated and cured with antibiotics.

Gonorrhea

Gonorrhea was described by the Greek physician Galen in 150 A.D. It is caused by *Neisseria gonorrhoeae.* The organism attaches to mucosal cells in the oropharyngeal area, eye, joints, rectum, and male and female genitalia. Infection sets up inflammation, with leukocytes moving into the area and resultant pus production. Incubation is several days. Males experience painful urination and pus discharge. Complications can cause urethral scarring with partial blockage of the urethra. Blockage of the ductus deferens results in sterility. The female disease is more insidious. It may cause abdominal pain due to pelvic inflammatory disease (PID), which involves extensive infection of the uterus, cervix, fallopian tubes, and ovaries. Scarring in the fallopian tubes may block movement of the ovum; if the blockage is total, an ectopic pregnancy or sterility may result.

In either sex, untreated disease can cause a systemic infection involving the heart, meninges, eyes, pharynx, and joints (arthritis). The eyes of newborns can become infected and blindness can result. In most states, erythromycin or silver nitrate solution is applied to the eyes of newborns as a prophylactic. If the mother is known to be infected, the infant is given penicillin intramuscularly.

Gonorrhea infection can be acquired at any point of sexual contact, including the pharynx and anus. Recovery does not confer immunity, and reinfection is possible. Penicillin has been effective against gonorrhea for many years, although higher doses are now needed because the organism has developed some resistance. The *Chlamydia trachomatis* microorganism is commonly found with gonorrhea.

Syphilis

Syphilis, which first appeared in Europe in the fifteenth century, is caused by the spirochete *Treponema pallidum,* a kind of bacterium that moves with a corkscrew-like action. A long incubation time allows sexual partners to be traced and treated before

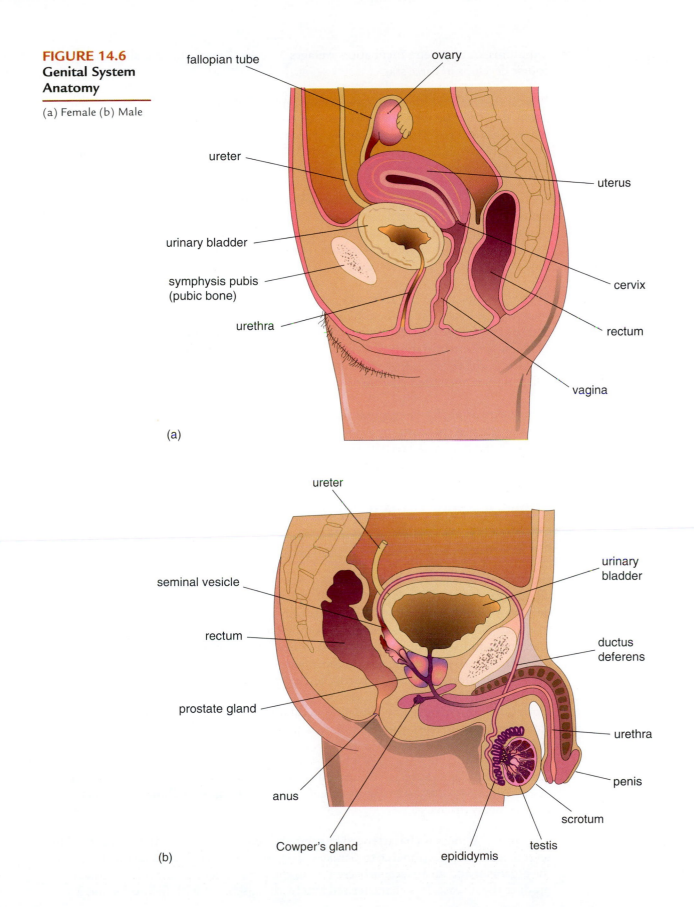

FIGURE 14.6
Genital System Anatomy

(a) Female (b) Male

fallopian tube

ovary

ureter

uterus

urinary bladder

symphysis pubis (pubic bone)

cervix

urethra

rectum

vagina

(a)

ureter

seminal vesicle

urinary bladder

rectum

ductus deferens

prostate gland

urethra

penis

anus

scrotum

Cowper's gland

epididymis

testis

(b)

symptoms are apparent. Incubation averages 3 weeks (2 weeks to several months). The course develops in three stages.

Primary-Stage Infection A primary-stage syphilis infection produces a small, hard-based, usually painless ulcer known as a **chancre** at the site of infection. Usually, the lesion heals in a few weeks. Females may be unaware of the infection if the chancre is on the cervix. In males, the chancre may be in the urethra. Fluids from the sore are highly infectious. Bacteria enter the bloodstream and lymphatic system.

Secondary-Stage Infection A secondary-stage syphilis infection produces skin rashes, patchy hair loss, malaise, and mild fever. Lesions on mucous membranes contain organisms and are highly infectious. Symptoms subside after a few weeks, and the disease becomes latent. After two to four years of latency, the disease is usually no longer infectious.

Tertiary-Stage Infection A tertiary-stage syphilis infection usually occurs after an interval of at least 10 years. Lesions appear as a rubbery mass of tissue in many organs and sometimes the skin. There may be extensive damage, including deafness, blindness, CNS lesions, or perforation of the roof of the mouth resulting from a hyperimmune reaction to the remaining spirochetes. Because symptoms in the first two stages are not disabling, patients often enter the latent period without receiving medical attention.

Congenital Syphilis Congenital syphilis occurs in newborns as a result of infection crossing the placenta into the fetus. Neurologic damage to the fetus results if pregnancy occurs during the tertiary stage. Pregnancy during the primary or secondary stage is likely to produce a stillborn child.

Other Sexually Transmitted Diseases

Several other sexually transmitted diseases play a major role in public health and are briefly discussed here.

Genital Herpes Genital herpes is caused by the herpes simplex virus. Lesions appear after approximately a week of incubation and cause a burning sensation. Vesicles develop, with infectious fluid, and then heal in approximately 2 weeks. The virus goes into a latent period in nerve cells and reappears in response to emotional stress, menstruation, illness, or scratching of the infected area. A pregnant mother may deliver by Caesarean section so that the infant will not contract the virus in the birth canal. If infection occurs in the uterus, birth defects may occur.

Nongonococcal Urethritis Nongonococcal urethritis (NGU) may be caused by catheters or chemical agents; some of the cases are acquired sexually. Symptoms are often mild in males, but serious in females.

Candidiasis Candidiasis is a disease caused by the yeastlike fungus *Candida albicans*, usually as an opportunistic overgrowth of yeast cells. It causes itching and a thick, yellow, cheesy discharge.

Vaginitis Vaginitis is characterized by vaginal discharge and odor. It can be caused by several bacteria. Infection due to *Gardnerella vaginitis* results from interaction between the organism and an anaerobic bacterium in the vagina, neither of which alone can produce the disease. It is characterized by a frothy discharge with fishy odor and a vaginal pH of 5 to 6. Vaginitis may also be caused by *Trichomonas vaginalis*, an organism normally found in both sexes. *T. vaginalis* causes an infection if vaginal acidity is disturbed. Leukocytes infiltrate the site and result in a profuse, yellowish or light cream-colored discharge with a disagreeable odor. It causes irritation and itching.

Agents for Treating Sexually Transmitted Diseases

Table 14.9 presents the most commonly used agents for sexually transmitted diseases. Many of these medications were also discussed in Chapters 4 and 5.

Azithromycin (Zithromax) is provided by the manufacturer in several forms. The powdered form is approved to be administered as a one-time dose to treat some sexually transmitted bacterial infections. For chancroid (syphilis lesion) in men and chlamydia in women, a 1 g dose is used. For gonococcal infections in either sex, a one-time dose of 2 g is administered.

TABLE 14.9   Most Commonly Used Agents for Sexually Transmitted Diseases

Generic Name	Pronunciation	Dosage Form	Brand Name	Dispensing Status
Antibacterial				
azithromycin	az-ith-roe-MYE-sin	injection, IV, oral liquid, tablet	Zithromax	Rx
ceftriaxone	sef-trye-AX-one	injection, IV	Rocephin	Rx
doxycycline	dox-i-SYE-kleen	capsule, IV, oral liquid	Doryx, Vibramycin	Rx
erythromycin	er-ith-roe-MYE-sin	capsule, IV, oral liquid, tablet, topical	(many salts)	Rx
metronidazole	me-troe-NYE-da-zole	capsule, injection, IV, oral liquid	Flagyl	Rx
penicillin G benzathine	pen-i-SIL-in G BENZ-a-theen	injection	Bicillin L-A	Rx
spectinomycin	spek-ti-noe-MYE-sin	injection	Trobicin	Rx
tetracycline	te-tra-SYE-kleen	capsule, oral liquid, tablet, topical	Sumycin	Rx
Antifungal				
clotrimazole	kloe-TRIM-a-zole	cream, solution, tablet, troche	GyneLotrimin, Mycelex	OTC, Rx
fluconazole	floo-KOE-na-zole	IV, oral liquid, tablet	Diflucan	Rx
ketoconazole	kee-toe-KON-a-zole	tablet, shampoo	Nizoral	OTC
miconazole	mi-KON-a-zole	cream, suppository	Monistat	OTC
tioconazole	tye-o-KON-a-zole	cream	Vagistat-1	OTC
Antiviral				
acyclovir	ay-SYE-kloe-veer	capsule, oral liquid, ointment, tablet	Zovirax	Rx
valacyclovir	val-ay-SYE-kloe-veer	tablet	Valtrex	Rx

Ceftriaxone (Rocephin) is used frequently, especially against penicillinase-producing bacteria. **Spectinomycin (Trobicin)** is an alternate drug in cases of resistance to ceftriaxone. **Tetracycline (Sumycin)** is commonly used to control *Chlamydia trachomatis*, which frequently occurs with gonorrhea. Tetracycline and **erythromycin** are both effective against chlamydia.

Penicillin G benzathine (Bicillin L-A) is used to treat syphilis. It is especially effective during the primary stage, and it is the only agent active against growing bacteria. Penicillin is administered in low concentration, but it is appropriate treatment because the spirochete grows slowly. It is effective for approximately 2 weeks.

Doxycycline (Doryx, Vibramycin*)*** is used to treat lymphogranuloma venereum.

Metronidazole (Flagyl) is used to treat *Gardnerella vaginitis* (formerly called *Haemophilus vaginalis*) infections. It is important that the patient complete the full course of treatment.

Acyclovir (Zovirax) and **valacyclovir (Valtrex)** are commonly used to treat genital herpes. These medications interfere with DNA synthesis of the virus and lessen severity of outbreaks, shorten healing time, and reduce the frequency of attacks.

Miconazole (Monistat) and **clotrimazole (GyneLotrimin, Mycelex)** are used to treat *Candida albicans* infections.

Ketoconazole (Nizoral) and **fluconazole (Diflucan)** are also frequently used to treat candidiasis.

Drug Therapy for Bone Disease

Bone is a living tissue that is continuously being replaced as a result of the balance between **osteoclast** (a cell that resorbs bone) and **osteoblast** (a cell that forms bone) activity. In normal, healthy bone (see Figure 14.7), the opposing activities of osteoclasts and osteoblasts are balanced. As adults age, however, resorption of bone tissue exceeds the deposit of new bone. Furthermore, newly formed bone is less dense and more fragile than original bone. Reduction or weakening of bone mass increases the risk of bone fracture. For adults over age 50, these processes occur at a faster rate for women than for men. The condition of reduced bone mineral density, disrupted microarchitecture of bone structure, and increased likelihood of fracture is known as **osteoporosis**. Osteoporosis occurs as a result of deficiency in estrogen, calcium, and vitamin D. The reduction in bone mass is accelerated and more severe in women who have had an early hysterectomy because without a uterus a woman's body produces less estrogen. With less estrogen, lower amounts of calcium are utilized by bony tissue. Daily calcium with vitamin D daily is essential to the prevention of bone loss.

Risk factors for osteoporosis can be divided into those that are not modifiable and those that may be modifiable. Gender, race, heredity, and age are risk factors that cannot be modified. Risk factors that are potentially modifiable include calcium intake, cigarette smoking, alcohol abuse, and weight-bearing exercise—all of which involve lifestyle choices. Modification of osteoporosis risk factors benefits all patients, regardless of gender, age, or type of osteoporosis.

Weight-bearing exercise contributes to developing and maintaining bone mass, provided that calcium intake is adequate. Walking, jogging, weightlifting, and dancing are examples of weight-bearing exercise. Elderly persons may benefit from careful exercise because it improves muscle function and agility, which reduces the risk of falls.

Hormone therapy (HT) with estrogen, with or without progestin, has been recommended for some postmenopausal women at risk of osteoporosis. HT reduces the rate of bone loss in women with estrogen deficiency. In women with established

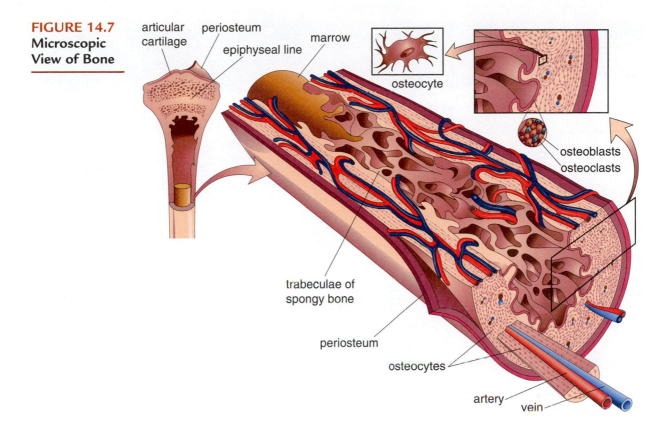

FIGURE 14.7
Microscopic View of Bone

articular cartilage

periosteum

epiphyseal line

marrow

osteocyte

osteoblasts
osteoclasts

trabeculae of spongy bone

periosteum

osteocytes

artery
vein

osteoporosis, HT maintains or increases bone density at all skeletal sites and decreases the risk of hip fracture. As mentioned earlier, however, HT also presents some risks. A 1% increase in the risk of breast cancer, myocardial infarction, and stroke among postmenopausal women has been associated with long-term HT. For women with no history or family history of breast cancer, heart disease, vascular problems, or stroke, though, the benefits of HT may outweigh the risks, especially if there is a history or family history of osteoporosis. Use of estrogen alone increases the risk of endometrial hyperplasia and cancer in women with an intact uterus. These women should receive progestin with the estrogen. Women who have undergone a hysterectomy may take estrogen alone, but they should also take calcium and vitamin D.

Table 14.10 lists the most commonly used agents for the prevention and treatment of osteoporosis other than HT products, which were listed in Table 14.5.

Bisphosphonates

Many drugs for osteoporosis belong to the bisphosphonate group. These drugs bind to hydroxyapatite (the mineral component of bone) and interfere with the resorption of bone by osteoclasts. Bisphosphonates should be taken before the first meal of the day, with 6 to 8 ounces of water to prevent esophageal burning, and the patient should remain upright after taking the drug. These difficulties can lead to compliance problems; some of these products, however, can be taken weekly or even monthly rather than daily. Pain in the jaw is a common side effect and should be monitored most closely.

Alendronate (Fosamax) is a bisphosphonate compound approved by the FDA for treating osteoporosis. In addition to its use in preventing osteoporosis, alendronate is used in hypercalcemia of malignancy and in Paget's bone disease, a disorder of

TABLE 14.10 Most Commonly Used Agents for Osteoporosis

Generic Name	Pronunciation	Dosage Form	Brand Name	Dispensing Status
Bisphosphonates				
alendronate	a-LEN-droe-nate	tablet	Fosamax, Fosamax Plus D	Rx
etidronate	eh-tih-DROE-nate	tablet	Didronel	Rx
ibandronate	eye-BAN-droh-nate	tablet, IV	Boniva	Rx
risedronate	ris-ED-roe-nate	tablet	Actonel	Rx
tiludronate	tye-LOO-droe-nate	tablet	Skelid	Rx
zoledronic acid	zo-le-DROE-nik AS-id	IV	Zometa, Reclast	Rx
Other Drugs for Osteoporosis				
calcitonin-salmon	kal-si-TOE-nin SAM-en	injection, nasal spray	Miacalcin	Rx
calcium	KAL-see-um	chewable, oral liquid, tablet	Caltrate, Os-Cal, Tums, Viactiv	OTC
raloxifene	ral-OX-i-feen	tablet	Evista	Rx
teriparatide	ter-i-PAR-a-tide	injection	Forteo	Rx

unknown cause that affects the middle-aged and elderly population and results in excess bone destruction and unorganized bone repair.

Alendronate must be taken at least 30 minutes before the first food, beverage, or medication of the day. In order to avoid esophageal burning, the patient should drink 6 to 8 ounces of water while swallowing the alendronate tablet and should avoid lying down for 30 minutes. Also, absorption is enhanced if the patient waits at least 30 minutes before eating. Alendronate is dosed once a day.

Take on an empty stomach

Ibandronate (Boniva) is also a bisphosphonate approved for the treatment of osteoporosis. It is manufactured in a once-a-month tablet or IV formulation administerd every 3 months. The IV form is associated with more side effects than the oral form. Oral ibandronate is cumbersome to take, because it must be taken 60 minutes before the first food or drink of the day, with 6 to 8 ounces of plain water, and the patient must remain upright for 60 minutes. This often leads to noncompliance. For patients who may have problems remembering to take a monthly pill, the manufacturer offers a reminder. Patients can enroll in the "My Boniva" program, where they will receive notifications by email, phone, or regular mail that it is time to take their pill.

Risedronate (Actonel) is a bisphosphonate that inhibits bone resorption by actions on osteoclasts or on osteoclast precursors. It is indicated for the treatment and prevention of osteoporosis in post-menopausal women and in Paget Disease for both men and women. Risedronate is approved for once-a-week dosing.

Tiludronate (Skelid) is a bisphosphonate approved for Paget's disease. It should be taken with 6 to 8 ounces of water. Tiludronate should not be taken within 2 hours of eating or taking other medications. Patients should maintain calcium and vitamin D intake. At least 3 months are needed to assess the patient's response to tiludronate.

Zoledronic acid (Zometa, Reclast) is a bisphosphonate for IV infusion. It is indicated for hypercalcemia. A dose should not exceed 4 mg and should not be administered in less than 15 minutes. It may have a quicker onset and a longer duration of action than other drugs used to treat hypercalcemia.

Other Osteoporosis Medications

Teriparatide (Forteo) is a human parathyroid hormone used for treating osteoporosis. It stimulates bone formation and resorption by regulating calcium and phosphate metabolism with bony tissue. Whereas other drugs only slow osteoporosis, teriparatide actually stimulates new bone growth. It is indicated for postmenopausal women with osteoporosis who are at high risk for fracture. Teriparatide is pen-injected subcutaneously and must be refrigerated while stored. This drug is not for long-term use. Once patients finish a course of treatment, they should be started on a bisphosphonate or calcitonin. The patient must also be on a calcium and vitamin D supplement.

Calcitonin-salmon (Miacalcin) is a peptide hormone that suppresses the activity of osteoclasts. A synthetic replica of the calcitonin produced by salmon is used because this molecule is more potent than the calcitonin produced by the human thyroid gland. Calcitonin-salmon in nasal spray form should be reserved for women who refuse or cannot tolerate HT, or for whom HT is contraindicated. The spray should be applied to a different nostril each day. The medication may be used at any time of day. The pump must be activated before the first dose. Most adverse effects are local, involving the nose.

Raloxifene (Evista) is a selective estrogen receptor modulator that acts to prevent bone loss in the same manner as estrogen does. Because raloxifene actually inhibits some estrogen receptors, this drug has the potential to block some estrogen effects such as those associated with an increased risk of breast and uterine cancer. It represents an alternative preventative therapy for osteoporosis for women who should not take HT. It has estrogen agonist effects in bone and lipids. Women who are taking raloxifene should also be on calcium and vitamin D to increase bone mineral density in the vertebral column.

Calcium (Caltrate, Os-Cal, Tums, Viactiv) should be taken daily. The recommended dose is 1,000 to 1,500 mg (the highest dose is prescribed for postmenopausal women) plus dietary supplements. This treatment prevents a negative calcium balance that may contribute to osteoporosis. Calcium carbonate is probably better absorbed when taken orally. Tums is an inexpensive way to get one's daily supply of calcium. A problem with Tums is that it lacks vitamin D. Without vitamin D, the calcium is not absorbed into bone tissue. Viactiv is an excellent way to get calcium. Three of these soft, milk chocolate, chewable candies provide 1,500 mg. The patient needs to be sure to take them three times a day. Eating all three at one time does not allow full absorption, because the body can only absorb approximately 600 mg of calcium at one time.

Adrenal Gland Disorders and Corticosteroid Therapy

The adrenal glands are located on the top of the kidneys. The medulla, or inner portion, functions like the sympathetic nervous system and produces catecholamines such as epinephrine (adrenaline). The cortex, or outer portion, produces several types of steroid hormones. Each such hormone, known as a **corticosteroid**, has its own combination of **glucocorticoid** (involved in cholesterol, fat, and protein metabolism) and **mineralocorticoid** (involved in regulating electrolyte and water balance) activity. The principal adrenal steroid hormone is cortisol. It is responsible for **gluconeogenesis** (conversion of fatty acids and proteins to glucose), protein catabolism, anti-inflammatory reactions, stimulation of fat deposition, and sodium and water retention (steroids are necessary for mineral retention). The adrenal cortex also produces various sex hormones.

As with the other hormones discussed earlier, the production of cortisol and other steroids begins in the hypothalamic-pituitary axis. The hypothalamus produces corticotropin releasing factor (CRF), which stimulates the pituitary to produce adrenocorticotropic hormone (ACTH), which in turn enters the bloodstream and travels to the adrenal cortex, where it stimulates the release of cortisol into the blood. Through a feedback mechanism, the rising cortisol levels slow the action of the hypothalamus in producing and releasing CRF. Steroid production follows a **circadian rhythm** (regular recurrence in cycles of 24 hours). As Figure 14.8 shows, it peaks in the morning, and the low point occurs close to midnight.

When the corticosteroid cortisol (hydrocortisone) was isolated, a milestone in medicine was reached. Results of clinical trials in rheumatoid arthritis were dramatic, and soon cortisone, another corticosteroid, was found to cause symptomatic improvement in an amazing number of disease states. Further research led to the development of other corticosteroids—prednisone, methylprednisolone, triamcinolone, and dexamethasone—that had greater anti-inflammatory potency (glucocorticoid) and less effect on renal sodium resorption (mineralocorticoid). These drugs are used as anti-inflammatory or immunosuppressive agents in treating a variety of diseases, including those of hematologic, allergic, inflammatory, neoplastic, and autoimmune origin.

Addison disease is a life-threatening deficiency of glucocorticoids and mineralocorticoids that is treated with daily administration of corticosteroid. The symptoms of Addison disease include

- debilitating weakness (may have respiratory failure)
- hyperkalemia
- bronze color of skin, produced by excessive melanin production, typically on the nipples, at creases, and on the lips and inside the mouth
- low levels of serum sodium and glucose
- reduced blood pressure
- weight loss

Cushing disease is caused by an overproduction of steroids; it can also result from excessive administration of corticosteroids over an extended period. Patients have a protruding abdomen; a round, puffy face; and fat deposits above the shoulder blades. The fat distribution may not change even with cessation of the drug.

The major reason for using corticosteroids is to inhibit inflammation. Corticosteroids cause leukocytes to be sluggish; lessen their ability to destroy infection; decrease fever, redness, and swelling; and may help an infection to spread. These drugs

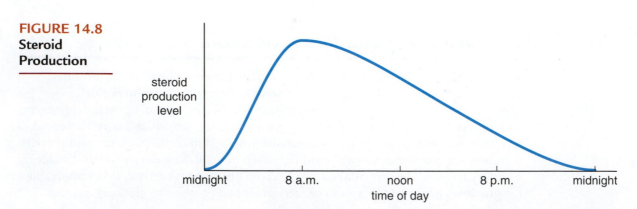

FIGURE 14.8
Steroid Production

steroid production level

midnight   8 a.m.   noon   8 p.m.   midnight
time of day

play a significant role in treating asthma, rashes, and skin disorders. A patient taking a corticosteroid within the last 12 to 18 months who is going into a stressful situation (e.g., surgery or tooth extraction) may need steroid supplementation.

Corticosteroids are available in many dosage forms: tablets, syrups, injections, inhalants, nose drops, IV, creams, ointments, lotions, and suppositories, and others. They are commonly packed in dose packs. For example, the Medrol Dosepak contains 21 tablets of 4 mg. On the first day, the patient takes a loading dose; then the dose decreases each day thereafter, as described on the package.

Long-term use of corticosteroids may have several side effects. Table 14.11 lists the adverse effects of glucocorticoids. Caution should be used in patients with diabetes mellitus, uncontrolled hypertension, tendency to congestive heart failure, severe infection or altered immunity, or peptic ulcer disease with active gastrointestinal bleeding. Glucocorticoids can also cause hypothalamic-pituitary axis suppression related to the dose and duration. If the drugs are given for a week or longer, there is a risk of adrenal insufficiency. If this happens, the corticosteroid should be tapered off and discontinued. If steroids are stopped suddenly, the glands may stop working completely, so it is important to taper off the dosage.

Steroid withdrawal can cause anorexia, nausea, and vomiting; myalgia and arthralgia; lethargy, headache, and sluggishness; weight loss; postural hypotension; fever; and depression.

TABLE 14.11	Adverse Effects of Glucocorticoids Related to Dose and Duration
Type of Effect	**Side Effect**
cardiovascular	hypertension due to sodium retention
dermatologic	impaired wound healing, striae, and thinning of skin (thin facial skin; veins may be visible)
	petechiae and purpura
gastrointestinal	precipitation of peptic ulcer disease (irritating to the gastrointestinal tract)
	pancreatitis
immune system	suppression of skin test (reduces inflammation)
	reduction of white blood cell function (suppression of white blood cells in bone marrow)
	increased occurrence of and susceptibility to infections
metabolic	redistribution of fat deposits (truncal obesity, moon facies, buffalo hump)
	acne, hirsutism, menstrual irregularities
	growth suppression (children)
	hyperglycemia (diabetogenic)
	hypokalemia
	sodium and water retention leading to swelling and edema
musculoskeletal	osteoporosis, vertebral compression (bone resorption)
	spontaneous fractures
	aseptic necrosis of bone (death of bone, generally in the heads of long bones)
neuropsychiatric	alterations in mood and/or schizophrenic tendencies
	rebound of psychosis when drug is discontinued
	manic-depressive, suicidal, or schizophrenic tendencies
ophthalmic	cataracts due to precipitation with long-term use
	increased intraocular pressure, thus a potential for glaucoma

TABLE 14.12   Corticosteroid Preparations and Adrenal Cortex Hydrocortisone Daily Equivalents*

Corticosteroid	Brand Name	Equivalency (mg)*	Anti-Inflammatory Potency
cortisone acetate	(none)	25.0	0.8
hydrocortisone	(many)	20.0	1.0
prednisone	Deltasone	5.0	3.0
prednisolone	Pediapred	5.0	4.0
methylprednisolone	Medrol, Solu-Medrol	4.0	5.0
triamcinolone	Aristocort	4.0	5.0
betamethasone	Celestone	0.6	25.0
dexamethasone	Decadron	0.75	30.0

*Quantity is equivalent to 20 mg of hydrocortisone.

Corticosteroids are usually administered in the morning to minimize the hypothalamic-pituitary axis suppression and side effects and to better mimic the natural circadian body rhythm. Frequently, every-other-day dosing is employed.

The adrenal cortex produces hydrocortisone at a rate of approximately 20 mg per day. Table 14.12 lists corticosteroid preparations in relation to the average daily secretion of hydrocortisone. This table lists the quantity of a synthetic hormone that is equivalent to 20 mg of hydrocortisone.

Diabetes

Diabetes is a serious disease that affects millions of people. It is characterized by high blood sugar, which is due to insufficient levels of the critically important hormone insulin. If left untreated, diabetes can cause a range of serious conditions and eventually death.

The pancreas contains specialized cells, called the islets of Langerhans, that produce insulin. Insulin helps cells burn glucose for energy, combines with membrane receptors to allow glucose uptake, enhances transport and incorporation of amino acids into protein, increases ion transport into tissues, and inhibits fat breakdown. Thus, insulin is critical in maintaining blood glucose levels, as well as having other metabolic roles.

In persons with diabetes, either the secretion or the utilization of insulin is inadequate, which leads to excessive blood glucose levels. The normal blood glucose level is around 100 mg/dL. At elevated levels the kidneys will not be able to reabsorb the excess, and glucose will spill into the urine. Levels consistently above 140 to 160 mg/dL are associated with long-term effects of diabetes. An elevated blood sugar level is known as **hyperglycemia**.

Diabetes is a devastating disorder that can damage all major organ systems. Over time, diabetes can destroy eyesight, kidneys, and peripheral circulation. The results are blindness, a need for dialysis, and amputation of limbs. Although approximately 20% of persons older than 60 years have diabetes, some estimates suggest that only half of the diabetics in the United States are diagnosed. Furthermore, many diabetics do not properly manage their disease.

Types of Diabetes

Type I diabetes occurs most commonly in children and young adults, but it may occur at any age. The average age of diagnosis is 11 or 12 years. These patients are insulin dependent; that is, they have no ability to produce insulin. They may produce antibodies to islet cells in an autoimmune response. This group comprises 5 to 10% of the diabetic population.

Type II diabetes comprises 80% to 90% of diabetic cases. Most patients are over 40 years of age, with the majority being female. Patients with type II diabetes may have a relative insulin insufficiency (impaired insulin secretion); however, insulin receptor resistance on cells may be the primary culprit. The peripheral target tissues are resistant to insulin produced. Glucose is not absorbed because the cells do not respond to insulin. Most type II diabetics are overweight, and the best treatment is to lose weight.

Gestational diabetes occurs during pregnancy and increases the risk of fetal morbidity and death. The onset occurs during the second and third trimesters. Gestational diabetes can be treated with diet, exercise, and insulin. Usually, it disappears after the birth of the baby, but 30 to 40% of women who have gestational diabetes will develop type II diabetes in 5 to 10 years. Oral contraceptives raise blood glucose levels, especially in these women, so whether they should use this type of birth control is debatable.

Secondary diabetes is caused by drugs. Among these drugs are oral contraceptives, beta blockers, diuretics, calcium channel blockers, glucocorticoids, and phenytoin. Secondary diabetes may return to normal when the drug is discontinued.

Symptoms and Complications of Diabetes

Symptoms of diabetes include

- frequent infections
- glycosuria (presence of glucose in the urine)
- hunger
- increased urination (polyuria) and nocturia (excessive urination at night)
- numbness and tingling
- slow wound healing (hyperglycemia inhibits activity of neutrophils, a type of white blood cell)
- thirst
- visual changes
- vomiting
- weight loss, easy fatigability, irritability, nausea, and ketoacidosis.

Although acute **hypoglycemia**, in which blood glucose levels fall below 70 mg/dL, is the more dangerous condition, chronic hyperglycemia, if unchecked, can result in long-term complications that can destroy the quality of life. If diabetes goes unchecked, the diabetic runs the risk of developing the following complications.

- Retinopathy is the leading cause of blindness in the United States. The vessels become damaged, resulting in insufficient blood supply; rupture causes loss of sight.
- Neuropathy is the result of a lack of blood flow to nerves, leaving them unable to function. Symptoms are dull aching to sharp stabbing pains.
- Vascular problems lead to atherosclerosis of peripheral coronary and cerebrovascular vessels. The decreased blood flow causes neuropathy and slows healing, especially in the feet and legs. Wounds that fail to heal can lead to amputation.

- Dermatologic involvement is often expressed as boils, acne, or fungal infections.
- Nephropathy, or kidney damage, occurs in 10 to 21% of diabetics and is the primary cause of end-stage renal disease.

Treating Diabetes

The goal of treatment of diabetes is to approximate nondiabetic physiology as closely as possible. The treatment consists of diet, exercise, and medications. Blood glucose monitoring is very important to prevent both acute and long-term complications and to guide treatment for reaching target fasting blood glucose goals. To avoid long-term complications, diabetes should be controlled to maintain fasting blood glucose levels between 80 and 120 mg/dL. Patients with Type I diabetes must receive insulin. Those with Type II diabetes may be able to control the disease through diet and exercise alone, but commonly they have to add a drug and eventually may need insulin. Cases of diabetes that are difficult to control are referred to as "brittle."

Treatment for type II diabetes follows a stepwise approach as follows:

1. lifestyle changes
2. oral monotherapy
3. combination oral therapy
4. oral drug plus insulin
5. insulin only

To help avoid complications, the American Diabetes Association recommends the following treatment for the type II patient.

- behavioral therapy for 3 months
- an ACE inhibitor (unless the blood pressure is under 130/80) to control blood pressure and also to help with neuropathies
- a statin (unless the LDL is less than 100 and the HDL is greater than 40)
- an enteric-coated aspirin

General treatment guidelines for a patient with any type of diabetes include the following:

- attention to diet
- blood pressure control
- compliance with the medication regimen
- control of hyperlipidemia
- daily foot inspections
- increased physical activity
- learning to recognize hypoglycemia
- monitoring progress at home through blood glucose testing
- monitoring progress at the doctor's office through measurement of glycosylated hemoglobin (HbA1C)
- patient education
- prompt treatment of all infections
- setting individual goals

Diet is very important. Eating approximately the same amount of food on a consistent schedule every day makes it easier to keep insulin and food working together. When buying prepared food or an OTC drug, the diabetic should always read the list of ingredients on the label. Many of these preparations contain sugars. Exercise is equally important. The diabetic should exercise regularly unless the blood glucose level is above 240 mg/dL or below 100 mg/dL. It is best to exercise about the same time each day.

Diabetics must also take very good care of their feet, which are particularly vulnerable to infections. Diabetic ulcers (open wounds that are typically slow to heal) are the leading cause of foot and leg amputation and the leading reason for hospital admissions among diabetics. Patients should be instructed to avoid the use of OTC foot products, unless directed by the physician. They should be instructed to moisturize their feet daily to prevent the skin from cracking. They should also keep nails trimmed to avoid ingrown toenails. It is very common for diabetics to have neuropathies of the legs. This sensation can be very painful or there can be total numbness in the extremities, both of which are very troublesome. With numbness, patients can injure their foot and not even be aware of it, which in turn can lead to serious infections.

Becaplermin gel (Regranex), listed in Table 14.13, is a recombinant human platelet-derived growth factor that speeds the healing of lower-extremity diabetic ulcers. Some studies have shown that this drug, which acts locally and has very little systemic effect, can actually increase the incidence of complete healing of diabetic foot ulcers. If the wound does not decrease by 30% in 10 weeks or heal in 20 weeks, use of this drug should be reassessed.

Insulin

Human insulin is composed of two short, linked protein chains. The first, chain A, has 21 amino acids and produces an acidic solution when dissolved. The second, chain B, has 30 amino acids and produces a basic solution. The two protein chains are joined by disulfide linking. Because insulin is a protein, it is enzymatically degraded in the GI tract. For this reason, insulin cannot be administered orally; rather it is administered subcutaneously.

Based on the time of their pharmacological action, insulin products are classified as rapid-acting, short-acting, intermediate-acting, or long-acting. The differences are related to the molecular structure of insulin. Regular insulin molecules have a strong attraction to each other and clump together in groups of six, called hexamers. Clumping delays absorption of insulin by 30 to 60 minutes as the clumps slowly dissociate, or break up.

Short-acting insulin has one amino acid on the protein chain either replaced or in a different position, which modifies the structure of the insulin molecule to prevent hexamer formation. The result is faster onset of action (15 to 30 minutes) and shorter time to peak action for a dose (30 to 90 minutes), but the duration of action is also shorter. Short-acting insulin needs to be injected 15 minutes before to 20 minutes after eating.

Most diabetic patients require a combination of shorter-acting insulin to cover postmeal glucose elevations and longer-acting insulin to maintain basal levels throughout the day. Insulin needs may vary every 6 to 8 hours. More insulin may be

Warning

It is very easy to grab the wrong type of insulin from the refrigerator. Always double-check insulin, because they look exactly alike. All types of insulin are designated as high-alert medication by the Institute of Safe Medication Practices.

TABLE 14.13 Most Commonly Used Drug for Lower-Extremity Diabetic Ulcers

Generic Name	Pronunciation	Dosage Form	Brand Name	Dispensing Status
becaplermin gel	be-KAP-ler-min	gel, topical	Regranex	Rx

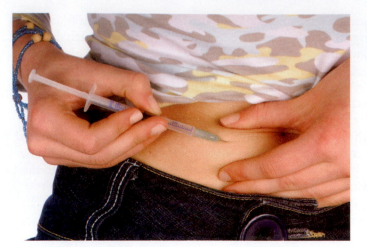
Patient injecting self with insulin.

required during stress, infection, and pregnancy. Table 14.14 lists the types of insulin available and the duration of action for each type.

Insulin should not be injected into an area of the body that will receive a rigorous workout. The injection site should be rotated frequently because decreased subcutaneous fat can lead to lipoatrophy at the injection site. Figure 14.9 illustrates the method of rotating insulin administration sites. Insulin enters blood best from the abdomen, then the arms and legs, and last the buttocks.

Every diabetic should be aware of the risk of hypoglycemia (blood glucose <70 mg/dL). Hypoglycemia can be caused by any of several factors: skipping or not finishing meals, too much exercise, a poorly adjusted medication regimen, or certain drugs (anabolic steroids, beta blockers, disopyramide, ethanol, pentamidine, salicylates, sulfonamides, phenobarbital, and quinine). Signs and symptoms of hypoglycemia are

- confusion
- double vision
- headache
- hunger
- nervousness
- numbness and tingling in mouth and lips
- palpitations
- sweating
- thirst
- visual disturbances
- weakness

Treatment of hypoglycemia necessitates giving the patient additional sugars. Milk or sugars in any form (fruit juices, soft drinks, or candy) are highly effective. Glucose tablets are available, and type I diabetics should have glucagon on hand (which requires a prescription).

TABLE 14.14	Duration of Action for Insulin Products
Type	**Onset and Duration of Action**
Humalog (lispro), NovoLog (aspart), Apidra (glulisine)	**Rapid-Acting:** Onset is 10 to 30 minutes, duration is 3 to 5 hours
Humulin-R, Novolin R (regular)	**Short-Acting:** Onset is 30–60 minutes, duration is 6 to 10 hours
Novolin N (NPH)	**Intermediate-Acting:** Onset is 1–3 hours and duration is 16 to 24 hours
Lantus (glargine), Levemir (detemir)	**Long-Acting:** Onset is 1 hour and duration is 24 to 28 hours (no peak of action; more closely mimics natural insulin release)
mixed	quick onset, longer duration—these are short-acting insulins mixed with intermediate-acting insulins and are dosed twice daily

FIGURE 14.9
Rotation of Administration Sites for Insulin

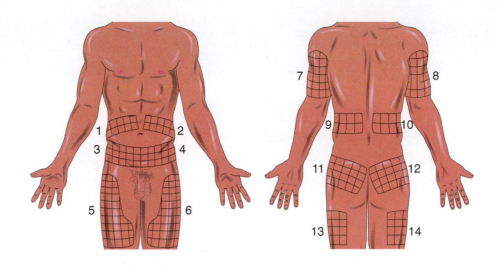

Dispensing Issues of Insulin Dispensing insulin has some inherent problems, including:

- The different types of insulin are packaged in similar-appearing boxes and all contain 10 mL vials, which can cause confusion.
- There are 100 Units of insulin per mL, which means one bottle of insulin has 1000 Units. Remember that insulin is dispensed in milliliters, but administered in Units, and the pharmacy technician must determine how long the insulin will last for each patient. Furthermore, doses must be correct for insurance reimbursement.
- A new dose of 500 Units per mL is available—pharmacy technicians should make sure that this is not given to patients in place of the 100 Units per mL dose, as this mistake could be fatal.

Most Commonly Used Insulin Types Table 14.15 lists the most commonly used types of insulin. In an emergency situation, insulin does not require a prescription (however, the 500 Units per mL type as well as some of the new insulins do need a prescription), but the person dispensing this drug will need documentation in order to make sure the correct insulin is dispensed. Some states require a prescription for a syringe and most definitely require proof of need. Regular and short-acting insulin are clear; all others are cloudy. When two types of insulin are combined, a longer-acting insulin is paired with an insulin of rapid onset, causing the insulin to take effect quicker and last longer. When mixing two types of insulin, the regular type should be drawn up first. Glargine (Lantus) should not be mixed with any other type of insulin.

Manufacturers have developed pens for the easy administration of insulin. The pen consists of a disposable needle and a syringe of insulin. They are available in various shapes and forms and most are very easy to use. Examples include the Flex Pen, Novo Nordisk, and the OptiClik. The latter must be dispensed by the physician; if the physician fails to dispense the pen, the patient can call 1-800-207-8049.

Regular insulin (Humulin R) may be administered subcutaneously, intramuscularly, or intravenously. This is the only type of insulin that may be administered intravenously.

Insulin lispro (Humalog) is a rapid-onset insulin, so patients can inject it immediately before or after meals. In this way, the dose can be adjusted depending on the amounts and types of foods eaten. In addition, blood glucose can be tested, and then

TABLE 14.15   Most Commonly Used Human Insulin Products

Generic Name	Pronunciation	Dosage Form	Brand Name
NPH isophane insulin	NPH EYE-so-fayn IN-soo-lin	injection	Humulin N
insulin aspart	IN-soo-lin AS-part	injection	NovoLog
insulin detemir	IN-soo-lin-DET-e-meer	injection	Levemir
insulin glargine	IN-soo-lin GLAR-jeen	injection	Lantus
insulin glulisine	IN-soo-lin-GLOO-lis-een	injection	Apidra
insulin lispro	IN-soo-lin LYE-sproe	injection	Humalog
regular insulin	RE-gyoo-lar IN-soo-lin	injection, IV	Humulin R, Novolin R
Mixtures			
insulin aspart with protamine–insulin aspart	IN-soo-lin AS-part with PROE-ta-mine IN-soo-lin AS-part	injection	NovoLog Mix 70/30
insulin lispro with protamine–insulin lispro	IN-soo-lin LYE-sproe with PROE-ta-mine IN-soo-lin LYE-sproe	injection	Humalog Mix 75/25
NPH–regular insulin	NPH REG-yoo-lar IN-soo-lin	injection	Humulin 70/30

the drug can be dosed accordingly. It may be used with a pump to maintain proper blood glucose levels.

Insulin aspart (NovoLog) is a rapid-acting insulin analog. It is made by substituting aspartic acid for one of the amino acids in insulin. It is similar to Humalog, but Humalog uses the amino acid lysine. NovoLog may also be used with a pump. Each dose should be injected before meals. In order to maintain glucose levels, a longer-acting insulin may be needed.

Insulin glargine (Lantus) is a synthetic type of long-acting insulin. It differs from human insulin by three amino acids. Insulin glargine is associated with less nocturnal hypoglycemia and weight gain than conventional insulin. Because it precipitates when injected in subcutaneous tissue, insulin glargine may cause pain at the injection site. The precipitation causes the insulin to be absorbed slowly and to maintain a relatively constant blood level over 24 hours. There is no noticeable peak in action, and insulin glargine more closely approximates physiologic insulin release than other insulin. It cannot be mixed with any other insulin.

Warning

Lispro and Lantus are often confused.

Noninsulin Injections

Several types of noninsulin medications for diabetes are also administered as injections. These are listed in Table 14.16.

Exenatide (Byetta) is an incretin mimetic. That is, it mimics a hormone secreted by the intestines in response to the presence of food that induce the beta cells to produce insulin. Natural incretins could not be used for therapy because they are too quickly broken down. Exenatide is a synthetic version of an incretin analog originally found in the saliva of the Gila monster. Exenatide stimulates the production of insulin and slows the rate of gastric emptying. Therefore it is approved only for type II diabetes, because the body must be able to produce some insulin for exenatide to work. It does cause some mild to moderate nausea, which improves with time. The slower gastric emptying and nausea reduces hunger. Exenatide is most effective when

TABLE 14.16   Types of Noninsulin Injections for Diabetes Treatment

Generic Name	Pronunciation	Dosage Form	Brand Name	Dispensing Status
exenatide	ex-EN-a-tide	injection	Byetta	Rx
pramlintide	PRAM-lin-tide	injection	Symlin	Rx

used in combination with another diabetes drug. It not only improves blood sugar control, but leads to weight loss.

Pramlintide (Symlin) is an analog of amylin, a peptide hormone that is normally secreted along with insulin and that works to control blood glucose along with insulin after a meal. Pramlintide also modulates gastric emptying. Pramlintide improves glucose control in patients who use insulin and allows patients to lower their insulin dose. Pramlintide, which is approved for both Type I and Type II diabetes, is not used as a first-line drug because it can cause severe hypoglycemia. It is dispensed in a disposable pen and is available in two strengths of 60mg and 120mg.

Oral Hypoglycemic Agents

Oral hypoglycemic agents cause the pancreas to release stored insulin. They are not effective in type I diabetes because there is no insulin available for the body to release. Table 14.17 presents the most commonly used oral hypoglycemic agents. The goal of therapy is to maintain an **HbA1C (glycosylated hemoglobin)** level of less than 7%. The HbA1C is an average of the blood glucose levels over a period of time. Insulin can always be added to therapy for the type II diabetic.

First-Generation Sulfonylureas First-generation sulfonylurea drugs increase insulin release. They are older drugs with more side effects than more recent agents. They are now rarely used.

Second-Generation Sulfonylurea Second-generation sulfonylureas allow better glycemic control than the first generation. However, these are also now being replaced with newer drugs. As more people are diagnosed with diabetes, there is much more interest in its control and therefore more research is being conducted in pursuit of additional products.

Glipizide (Glucotrol, Glucotrol XL) is taken with food at breakfast time. If Glucotrol is switched to the XL form, it should be given in the same total daily dose. Glipizide promotes release of insulin from beta cells in the pancreas, increases insulin sensitivity at peripheral sites, and lowers blood glucose concentration.

Glyburide (DiaBeta, Glynase, Micronase) is supplied in micronized dosage forms. It is an adjunct to diet and exercise in the management of diabetes.

Glimepiride (Amaryl) causes a lesser degree of hypoglycemia than glyburide. It should be taken with breakfast or the first main meal.

Enzyme Inhibitors Enzyme inhibitors block the conversion of saccharides into glucose, thereby lowering postprandial (after a meal) hyperglycemia. Carbohydrate absorption in the small intestine is slowed through inhibition of intestinal wall enzymes.

Acarbose (Precose) lowers blood glucose by delaying the hydrolysis of ingested complex carbohydrates and disaccharides and the absorption of glucose. For hypoglycemia, patients should use oral glucose tablets while taking this drug, because it

TABLE 14.17 Most Commonly Used Oral Hypoglycemic Agents

Generic Name	Pronunciation	Dosage Form	Brand Name	Dispensing Status
First-Generation Sulfonylureas				
chlorpropamide	klor-PROE-pa-mide	tablet	Diabinese	Rx
tolbutamide	tole-BYOO-ta-mide	tablet	(none)	Rx
Second-Generation Sulfonylureas				
glimepiride	GLYE-me-pye-ride	tablet	Amaryl	Rx
glipizide	GLIP-i-zide	tablet	Glucotrol, Glucotrol XL	Rx
glyburide	GLYE-byoo-ride	tablet	DiaBeta, Glynase, Micronase	Rx
Enzyme Inhibitors				
acarbose	ay-KAR-bose	tablet	Precose	Rx
miglitol	MIG-li-tawl	tablet	Glyset	Rx
Biguanide				
metformin	met-FOR-min	oral liquid, tablet	Glucophage, Riomet	Rx
Glitazones/Thiazolidinediones				
pioglitazone	pye-oh-GLIT-a-zone	tablet	Actos	Rx
rosiglitazone	roe-see-GLIT-a-zone	tablet	Avandia	Rx
Meglitinides				
nateglinide	na-TEG-li-nide	tablet	Starlix	Rx
repaglinide	re-PAG-lin-ide	tablet	Prandin	Rx
Gliptins				
sitagliptin	sit-a-GLIP-tin	tablet	Januvia	Rx
Combinations				
glipizide-metformin	GLIP-i-zide met-FOR-min	tablet	Metaglip	Rx
glyburide-metformin	GLYE-byoo-ride met-FOR-min	tablet	Glucovance	Rx
pioglitazone-metformin	pye-oh-GLIT-a-zone met-FOR-min	tablet	Actoplus Met	Rx
rosiglitazone-glimepride	roe-see-GLIT-a-zone GLYE-me-pye-ride	tablet	Avandryl	Rx
rosiglitazone-metformin	roe-see-GLIT-a-zone met-FOR-min	tablet	Avandamet	Rx
sitagliptin-metformin	si-ta-GLIP-tin/met-FOR-min	tablet	Janumet	Rx

inhibits the conversion of sucrose and other sugars to glucose. The primary side effects of acarbose are abdominal pain, diarrhea, and flatulence (gas), which may be due to undigested carbohydrates undergoing digestion by bacteria in the large intestine. The drug is contraindicated in the presence of cirrhosis, inflammatory bowel disease, colon ulceration, and intestinal obstruction.

Miglitol (Glyset), like acarbose, reduces hyperglycemia by slowing carbohydrate absorption in the small intestine. Side effects are similar to those of acarbose. Miglitol is indicated in the treatment of type II diabetes and is prescribed either as a first-line monotherapy or in combination with other medications.

Biguanides Biguanides decrease intestinal absorption of glucose and improve insulin sensitivity. One of these compounds, **Metformin (Glucophage, Riomet)**, rarely causes hypoglycemia and has a favorable effect on serum lipids. It should be used with caution in patients with liver, heart, or lung disease. The dose should be increased over several weeks, and it should be taken with food. Metformin is withheld for 18 hours before testing with iodinated material. It interacts with cimetidine, vitamin B_{12}, and folic acid. Metformin is synergistic with sulfonylureas. Side effects are nausea, metallic aftertaste, and weight loss. The best candidates are overweight diabetics with a high lipid profile. Metformin decreases triglyceride levels and blood pressure. Lactic acidosis is a rare, but possible, sequela (aftereffect). Pharmacy technicians need to remember that metformin is provided as XL and plain, with the tablets of these two being very similar in appearance. A dispensing error could cause very serious consequences.

Thiazolidinediones Thiazolidinediones (sometimes referred to as glitazones) lower blood glucose by improving cellular response to insulin. Patients on these drugs need to be aware of macular edema, which has emerged as a side effect.

Pioglitazone (Actos) depends on the presence of insulin. Liver enzymes should be carefully monitored for elevated enzyme levels every 2 months for the first 12 months. Side effects include elevated HDL levels, lowered triglyceride levels, weight gain, anemia, and edema. Pioglitazone may be taken without regard to food. Patients taking this drug must avoid alcohol.

Rosiglitazone (Avandia) increases insulin sensitivity in muscle and adipose tissue. It is indicated in the treatment of hyperglycemia and is prescribed alone or as an adjunct to metformin. The side effects are similar to those for pioglitazone. Rosiglitazone can be taken without regard to food.

Meglitinides Meglitinides stimulate insulin release from the pancreatic cells. Patients using this drug class must be type II (have a working pancreas) for the medication to be effective.

Repaglinide (Prandin) and **nateglinide (Starlix)** should be taken 15 minutes before a meal. If a meal is skipped, then that dose should be skipped. If a meal or large snack is added, then the drug should be taken 15 minutes prior to it. The dosing of these drugs is very dependent on the eating habits of the patient.

Gliptins This class of diabetes medication enhances the incretin system in the body. When a meal arrives in the intestine, cells in the intestine secrete incretins, which stimulate beta pancreas cells to release insulin and signal the liver to cease glucagon production.

Sitagliptin (Januvia) can be given alone or in conjunction with other hypoglycemic agents; it works best when used with other agents. Sitagliptin causes less hypoglycemia and weight gain than most diabetic drugs; in part this is because it does not lower the HbA1C as well as other agents. It can be taken with or without food.

Combinations Combinations of various medications are used as diabetes progresses. Because of the complexity of the disease, it is often necessary to combine therapies. Agents used to treat the disease include those that increase pancreatic insulin secretion (sulfonylureas); reduce hepatic glucose production (biguanides); and delay intestinal carbohydrate absorption, increase glucose uptake, and decrease lipolysis (thiazolidin-ediones). It is commonly necessary for patients to transition from monotherapy to the use of multiple antidiabetic medications that target different metabolic functions. The combination drugs listed in Table 14.17 do this. They usually cost less than if the drugs were dosed separately.

Peripheral Neuropathy

Many diabetic patients have some form of peripheral neuropathy. It can manifest as numbness, insensitivity to pain or temperature, or as tingling in the arms or (more commonly) legs. Therapy should first deal with the underlying cause (hyperglycemia). Next, symptom relief should be sought. Drugs that help with pain management include anticonvulsants (see Chapter 8) such as pregabalin (Lyrica) and antidepressants (see Chapter 7) such as duloxetine (Cymbalta), which are approved for neuropathic pain. Gabapentin (Neurontin), another anticonvulsant, is an excellent drug that is well tolerated for this pain. Although diabetes is the major cause of peripheral neuropathy, there are other causes. At this time there are very few medications with which to treat it.

Growth Disorders

From childhood to adulthood, **growth hormone (GH)** plays a fundamental role in metabolism. Measurements of height and weight over time serve as an index of physical and emotional health. Growth failure is a well-recognized disorder of childhood. In many children, a deficiency of endogenous growth hormone causes retardation of growth, which may be treated with exogenous hormone replacement.

Growth rates vary by sex and age throughout childhood. Growth delay may be caused by various factors including family growth patterns, genetic disorders, malnutrition, systemic or chronic illness, psychosocial stress, or a combination of these. In addition, growth delay may be due to an endocrine deficiency. Thyroxine, cortisol, insulin, and GH all affect skeletal and somatic growth.

Nonendocrine-related disorders that can cause growth delay include intrauterine growth retardation, chromosomal defects, abnormal growth of cartilage or bone, poor nutrition, and a variety of systemic diseases. Some patients show a variation from normal growth (constitutional growth delay); these patients include those who are small for their age and those who have delay in skeletal growth, in the onset of puberty, and in adolescent development. Another type of growth delay is a family trait (i.e., it is genetically inherited). These patients are shorter than their peers, but are comparable in height with other family members and grow at a parallel rate. Puberty occurs at the expected time and progresses as usual. However, adult height is short (less than 5 feet 4 inches for men and less than 4 feet 11 inches for women).

Growth hormone is a mixture of peptides (essentially short protein molecules) from the anterior pituitary gland released in response to **growth hormone releasing factor (GHRF)**. The major component is the peptide somatotropin. The pituitary releases GH in response to stimulation by GHRF, which is secreted by the hypothalamus. GH release occurs irregularly throughout the day and during sleep stages III and IV (the deepest stages of non-REM sleep). GH stimulates the growth of skeletal muscle and connective tissue. It increases the rate of protein synthesis and fatty acid mobilization from adipose tissue and decreases the rate of glucose utilization. It is inhibited by glucocorticoids, obesity, depression, progesterone, hypokalemia, and altered thyroid function.

Growth hormone deficiency occurs in one in 5,000 children in a male-to-female ratio of 4 to 1. Among the known causes are intracranial infection (from tuberculosis and meningitis), skull fracture, radiation, and cancer. It can be treated by the administration of somatropin or other growth promotion agents.

Originally, somatotropin (as it is called when produced naturally by the human body) was recovered from the pituitaries of human cadavers, a process that required 20 to 30 cadavers to obtain sufficient hormone to treat one patient. Today, the drug is supplied through recombinant DNA technology. Genetic material from the human cell is inserted into microorganisms, which then reproduce with the genes and produce the hormone. The hormone is recovered, purified, and packaged. We will return to this process in Chapter 16. Table 14.18 presents the synthetic human growth hormones most commonly used as growth-promotion agents. Somatropin is identical to naturally produced somatotropin; somatrem has an additional amino acid.

Growth hormone replacement therapy is most successful when begun at a young age. That is, the younger the patient at the time of GH treatment, the greater the height that may be achieved through replacement. Bone age and the extent of epiphyseal fusion at the time of treatment also influence the eventual response to GH. Growth hormone treatment is minimally effective if employed after ages 15 to 16 years in boys or 14 to 15 years in girls. Approximately 80 to 90% of patients who receive GH experience "catch-up" growth. Maximum increases in growth occur within the first 6 to 12 months of therapy, with a decline in response after that. Growth hormone therapy should be continued throughout childhood and adolescence to avoid slowing of growth velocity. When epiphyseal closure has occurred, little further response occurs. Treatment duration usually ranges from 2 to 10 years. Growth hormone has not been effective for patients under the following conditions: families of short stature; growth retardation associated with psychosocial dwarfism; steroid-induced short stature; Down syndrome; bone and cartilage disorders; or renal, GI, or cardiac disease.

Hypothyroidism has been observed in less than 5% of treated patients. Thyroid supplementation is unnecessary, however, unless the patient has thyroid deficiency during treatment. The hypothyroidism appears to be more a change in the conversion of thyroxine or thyroid-controlling hormone than a true deficiency. However, glucose intolerance may develop. In addition, transient immune changes may reduce beta-lymphocyte numbers with variations in T helper and T suppressor numbers. There may be some pain and pruritus at the injection site.

TABLE 14.18   Most Commonly Used Synthetic Human Growth Hormones

Generic Name	Pronunciation	Dosage Form	Brand Name	Dispensing Status
somatrem	SOE-ma-trem	injection	Protropin	Rx
somatropin	soe-ma-TROE-pin	injection	Humatrope	Rx

Chapter Terms

AB rated of a generic drug, rated as bioequivalent to the branded drug by the FDA as shown by an experimental study

Addison disease a life-threatening deficiency of glucocorticoids and mineralocorticoids that is treated with the daily administration of corticosteroid

alopecia hair loss

anabolic treatment muscle building

androgen hormone that promotes development and maintenance of male characteristics

blastocyst the stage in development at which a fertilized egg has divided into 70–100 cells and is ready to implant, consisting of the inner embryoblast and an outer layer that will become the placenta

chancre small, usually painless, highly infectious ulcer; the primary lesion of syphilis

circadian regularly recurring on a cycle of 24 hours

climacteric the syndrome of endocrine, somatic, and psychic changes occurring at the end of the reproductive period in females

corticosteroid steroid hormone produced by the adrenal cortex

Cushing disease a disease caused by overproduction of steroids or by excessive administration of corticosteroids over an extended period

Dispense As Written (DAW) instruction in a prescription to prevent substitution of generic drugs for the branded drug

dyspareunia a condition of the female in which normal intercourse is painful

endocrine system glands and other structures that elaborate internal secretions, called hormones, that are released directly into the circulatory system

endometrium the lining of the uterus, which grows in the early part of the menstrual cycle to be ready to receive a fertilized egg and breaks down at the end of the cycle, leading to menstruation

estrogen one of the group of hormones that stimulate the growth of reproductive tissue in females

feedback mechanism the return of some of the output of a system as input so as to exert some control on the process

gestational diabetes diabetes that occurs during pregnancy when insufficient insulin is produced

glucocorticoid corticosteroid involved in metabolism and immune system regulation

growth hormone (GH) a fundamental hormone that affects metabolism, skeletal growth, and somatic growth; deficiency causes growth retardation

growth hormone releasing factor (GHRF) a neuropeptide secreted by the hypothalamus that stimulates the secretion of growth hormone by the pituitary

gynecomastia excessive development of the male mammary glands, with or without tenderness

HbA1C glycosylated hemoglobin (Hb stands for hemoglobin), an "average" of the sugar measured in blood glucose over a period of time

hirsutism abnormal hairiness, especially in women

hormone therapy (HT) replacement of deficient hormones such as estrogen

hyperglycemia elevated blood sugar level

hyperthyroidism a condition caused by excessive thyroid hormone and marked by increased metabolic rate; also called thyrotoxicosis

hypoglycemia low blood glucose level (less than 70 mg/dL)

hypogonadism a deficiency of hormone production and secretion

hypothyroidism a deficiency of thyroid activity that results in a decreased metabolic rate, tiredness, and lethargy in adults and causes cretinism in children

impotence failure of the male to initiate or to maintain an erection until ejaculation

mineralocorticoid corticosteroid involved in electrolyte and water balance

oral contraceptive (OCs) a combination of one or more hormonal compounds taken orally to prevent the occurrence of pregnancy

osteoblast a cell that forms bone

osteoclast a cell that resorbs bone

osteoporosis the condition of reduced bone mineral density, disrupted microarchitecture of bone structure, and increased likelihood of fracture

oxytocic agent a drug that promotes contraction of uterine muscle at term of pregnancy

priapism frequent or prolonged, painful penile erections

progestin a synthetic hormone that emulates the effects of progesterone

progesterone the hormone that prepares the uterus for the reception and development of the fertilized ovum

secondary diabetes diabetes caused by drugs

target a cell, tissue, or organ that is affected by a particular hormone

testosterone a hormone that is responsible for sperm production, sexual potency, and the maintenance of muscle mass and strength, among other functions

thyroid gland a gland that produces hormones that stimulate various body tissues to increase their activity level

thyroid storm a life-threatening medical emergency with the symptoms of thyrotoxicosis, but more exaggerated

tocolytic agent a drug that slows labor in pregnancy, used to treat premature labor

type I diabetes insulin-dependent diabetes, in which the pancreas has no ability to produce insulin

type II diabetes a type of diabetes characterized by insulin insufficiency or by the resistance of the target tissues to the insulin produced

vasomotor affecting constriction and dilation of blood vessels

virilization the development of male characteristics

Chapter Summary

The Endocrine System

- The endocrine system maintains the body's homeostasis by regulating physiologic functions involved in normal daily living and stress. The tissue affected by a hormone is called the target.
- Regulation of hormone synthesis is achieved via an intricate negative feedback mechanism involving the gland, the hypothalamic-pituitary axis, and autoregulation.

Thyroid Disorders

- The thyroid gland produces hormones that stimulate various body tissues to increase the level of activity.
- Thyroid replacement therapy should not be used to treat obesity.
- Hypothyroidism is treated with levothyroxine (Levoxyl, Synthroid) or thyroid extract (Armour Thyroid).

- Hyperthyroidism is treated with propylthiouracil and methimazole (Tapazole); both drugs cause altered taste and mild alopecia. Radioactive ^{131}I is also used.

Male Hormones and Impotence

- Testosterone undergoes extensive first-pass metabolism in the gastrointestinal tract and liver after oral administration. To overcome this problem, various testosterone derivatives have been developed, as well as innovative dosage forms.
- The testosterone patch not only increases libido and sexual potency, but also improves the patient's sense of well-being.
- Testosterone substances are classified as Schedule III.
- Impotence may have many causes, including testosterone deficiency, alcoholism, cigarette smoking, medications, and psychological factors.
- The following drugs may cause impotence: alcohol, amphetamines, antidepressants, antihypertensives, corticosteroids, estrogens, H_2 blockers, haloperidol, lithium, and opiates.
- Alcohol is a primary reason for male dysfunction.
- Male impotence is treated primarily with phosphodiesterase inhibitors sildenafil (Viagra), tadalafil (Cialis), and vardenafil (Levitra).

Female Hormones

- Progestins are used primarily in birth control pills and to prevent uterine cancer in postmenopausal women on hormone replacement therapy (HT).
- The side effects of progestin are weight gain, depression, fatigue, acne, and hirsutism.
- HT prevents bone loss and relieves the symptoms of menopause.
- The adverse effects of estrogen are nausea, fluid retention, breast tenderness, vomiting, weight gain, and breakthrough bleeding. Hypercoagulability is also attributed to estrogen use, especially if combined with nicotine.
- HT is a personal decision between a woman and her physician. The advantages must be weighed against the disadvantages. The risks and benefits are different for each woman, depending on her family history and her own physical condition.
- The advantages of oral contraceptives include ease of use, high efficacy rate, and relative safety. Most are a combination of estrogen and progestin. They suppress ovulation by interfering with the production of hormones that regulate the menstrual cycle. They also alter the cervical mucus to prevent penetration of sperm and change the composition of the endometrium to inhibit implantation. The progestin-only pills rely on the effects of progestin on the cervical mucus and endometrium.
- Many women taking "the pill" experience more regular menstrual cycles, reduced menstrual flow, and less severe menstrual pain and cramps. There is evidence that oral contraceptives may protect against ovarian and endometrial cancer, benign breast disease, ectopic pregnancy, fibroadenomas, and ovarian cysts. They may also reduce the risk of pelvic inflammatory disease. Lybrel, a new birth control pill, when taken continuously, will prevent the woman from having a period.
- Some studies indicate that birth control pills should not be prescribed to women who have hypertension, diabetes mellitus, or elevated cholesterol. Women should not smoke while taking birth control pills.
- Many forms of contraceptives are on the market. They are available in pill form, creams, patches, rings, and implants.
- "The pill" should be taken at the same time every day. Taking it at bedtime reduces the possibility of nausea and skin discoloration.
- Lunelle is an injectable contraceptive that in some states may be administered in the pharmacy by the pharmacist. (withdrawn)
- There is a big push for emergency contraceptives and for them to be available over the counter.

- Oral contraceptives can interact with the following classes of drugs: antibiotics, anticonvulsants, antifungals, benzodiazepines, bronchodilators, corticosteroids, lipid-lowering agents, and tricyclic antidepressants (TCAs).
- Pregnancy tests are based on detecting the hormone human chorionic gonadotropin (hCG). The home pregnancy tests on the market are very simple to use.
- Not many drugs are used at delivery, but two that can be very important are oxytocin (Pitocin) and methylergonovine (Methergine).

Sexually Transmitted Diseases

- Most diseases of the genital system are transmitted by sexual activity and are, therefore, called sexually transmitted diseases (STDs).
- A long-acting penicillin (penicillin G benzathine) should be used to treat syphilis.

Drug Therapy for Bone Disease

- Lifestyle changes to decrease bone loss include increasing calcium intake, ceasing cigarette smoking and alcohol abuse, and engaging in weight-bearing exercises.
- Biphosphonates are the drug class most used to treat osteoporosis. They should be taken on a weekly or monthly basis 30 minutes before the first meal of the day with 6 to 8 ounces of water, and the patient should remain upright for at least 30 minutes.
- Alendronate (Fosamax) is a bisphosphonate approved by the FDA for the treatment of osteoporosis. It should be taken 30 minutes before the first meal of the day with a full glass of water; the patient must not lie down for 30 minutes after taking it and should wait at least 30 minutes before eating.
- Calcitonin-salmon (Miacalcin) should be reserved for women who are not on HT.
- Calcium carbonate (Tums) is an inexpensive way to get the daily supply of calcium. However, it must be supplemented with vitamin D and should be taken throughout the day, not all at once because the body can only absorb a certain amount of calcium at one time, around 600 mg. Calcium supplements prevent a negative calcium balance, a factor in osteoporosis.

Adrenal Gland Disorders and Corticosteroid Therapy

- Corticosteroids are used as anti-inflammatories and immunosuppressants and in treating diseases of hematologic, allergic, neoplastic, and autoimmune origin.
- The major reason for using corticosteroids is to inhibit inflammation.
- Addison disease is a deficiency of glucocorticoids and mineralocorticoids; Cushing disease is caused by an overproduction or excessive administration of steroids over an extended period.
- Corticosteroids have adverse effects with metabolic, cardiovascular, gastrointestinal, immunologic, dermatologic, musculoskeletal, ophthalmic, and neuropsychiatric implications. They should be used with great caution in diabetes, hypertension, congestive heart failure, severe infections, and peptic ulcer disease. Suppression of the hypothalamic-pituitary axis is dose related. If possible, patients should take the dose in the morning to minimize hypothalamic-pituitary axis suppression and side effects. This more closely mimics the circadian rhythm of the body's release of corticosteroids.

Diabetes

- Scattered throughout the pancreas are islets of specialized cells. Alpha cells produce glucagon, which raises blood sugar levels; beta cells produce insulin, which lowers blood sugar levels.
- The four types of diabetes are type I, type II, gestational, and secondary.
- Type I diabetics must have insulin. Type II may be able to control the disease through diet and exercise, but often have to add a drug or even insulin. Gestational diabetes usually returns to normal after the baby's birth, but the mother is at high risk of

developing type II diabetes. Secondary (drug-induced) diabetes can return to normal when the drug is discontinued.

- Short-term hypoglycemia is more dangerous, but long-term hyperglycemia has devastating complications. Retinopathy, neuropathy, nephropathy, and vascular and dermatologic complications can affect the quality and length of life.
- In an emergency situation, insulin may not require a prescription, but the 500 Units per mL always requires a prescription, as well as some of the newer insulins. Some states require a prescription for needles.
- Insulin lispro (Humalog) is a rapid-onset insulin, so patients can inject it immediately before or after meals.
- Insulin glargine (Lantus) is a long-acting insulin that provides a constant concentra-

tion level over 24 hours. It more closely approximates physiologic insulin release.
- There are nine classes of diabetes drugs other than insulins.

Growth Hormone

- Measurement of height and weight over time serves as an index of physical and emotional health. A deficiency of growth hormone causes growth failure.
- Human growth hormone is supplied through recombinant DNA technology.
- Once epiphyseal closure has occurred, little further response to GH treatment can be expected.

Drug List

The following drugs were discussed in this chapter. Each generic drug name is followed in parentheses by one or more brand names.

Thyroid Preparations
levothyroxine, T_4 (Levothroid, Levoxyl, Synthroid)*
methimazole (Tapazole)
propylthiouracil, PTU
radioactive iodine, ^{131}I
thyroid (Armour Thyroid)

Drugs to Treat Male Impotence
alprostadil (Caverject, Edex, Muse)
danazol (Danocrine)
methyltestosterone (Android, Testred)
oxymetholone (Anadrol)
papaverine
sildenafil (Viagra)*
tadalafil (Cialis)*
testosterone (Androderm, AndroGel, Striant, Testoderm)
vardenafil (Levitra)

Hormone Therapy Products

Estrogen-Only Hormone Therapy Products
conjugated estrogen (Cenestin, Enjuvia, Premarin)*
estradiol (Alora, Climara, Elestrin, Esclim, Estrace, Estraderm, Estrasorb, Estring, Evamist, Femring, Menostar, Vivelle, Vivelle Dot)*
estropipate (Ogen)
ethinyl estradiol (Estinyl)

Estrogen-Progestin Hormone Therapy Products
conjugated estrogen–medroxyprogesterone (Premphase, Prempro)*
estradiol-levonorgestrel (Climara Pro)*
estradiol-norethindrone (Activella, CombiPatch)
estradiol-norgestimate (Ortho-Prefest)
ethinyl estradiol–norethindrone (femhrt)

Contraceptives

Combination Oral Contraceptives
estradiol cypionate–medroxyprogesterone (Lunelle) (withdrawn)
estradiol drospirenone (Angeliq)
ethinyl estradiol–desogestrel (Cyclessa*, Desogen, Kariva, Mircette, Ortho-Cept)
ethinyl estradiol–drospirenone (Yasmin, Yaz)*
ethinyl estradiol–ethynodiol diacetate (Demulen)
ethinyl estradiol–etonogestrel (NuvaRing)
ethinyl estradiol–levonorgestrel (Aviane, Levlen, Lybrel, Nordette, Seasonale, Tri-Levlen, Triphasil, Trivora-28)*
ethinyl estradiol–norelgestromin (Ortho Evra)*
ethinyl estradiol–norethindrone (Estrostep Fe*, Loestrin Fe, Loestrin Fe 24, Ovcon)
ethinyl estradiol–norgestimate (Ortho Tri-Cyclen, Ortho Tri-Cyclen Lo)*
ethinyl estradiol–norgestrel (Lo/Ovral, Low-Ogestrel, Ovral)*

Progestin-Only Contraceptives
levonorgestrel (Norplant II)
medroxyprogesterone (Depo-Provera, Provera)
norethindrone (Micronor)

Emergency Contraceptives
levonorgestrel (Plan B)
norgestrel (Ovrette)

Drugs Used at Birth
dinoprostone (Cervidil, Prepidil, Prostin E)
magnesium sulfate
misoprostol (Cytotec)
methylergonovine (Methergine)
nifedipine (Procardia)
oxytocin (Pitocin)

Agents for Sexually Transmitted Diseases

Antibacterial
azithromycin (Zithromax)
ceftriaxone (Rocephin)
doxycycline (Doryx, Vibramycin)
erythromycin
metronidazole (Flagyl)
penicillin G benzathine (Bicillin L-A)
spectinomycin (Trobicin)
tetracycline (Sumycin)

Antifungal
clotrimazole (GyneLotrimin, Mycelex)
fluconazole (Diflucan)
ketoconazole (Nizoral)
miconazole (Monistat)
tioconazole (Vagistat-1)

Antiviral
acyclovir (Zovirax)
valacyclovir (Valtrex)

Agents for Bone Diseases

Bisphosphonates
alendronate (Fosamax, Fosamax Plus D)*
ibandronate (Boniva)
risedronate (Actonel)*
tiludronate (Skelid)
zoledronic acid (Zometa, Reclast)

Other Drugs for Osteoporosis
calcitonin-salmon (Miacalcin)*
calcium (Caltrate, Os-Cal, Tums, Viactiv)
raloxifene (Evista)*
teriparatide (Forteo)

Corticosteroids
betamethasone (Celestone)
cortisone acetate
dexamethasone (Decadron)
hydrocortisone
methylprednisolone (Medrol, Solu-Medrol)*
prednisolone (Pediapred)
prednisone* (Deltasone)
triamcinolone (Aristocort)

Agent for Diabetic Ulcers
becaplermin gel (Regranex)

Insulins
NPH isophane insulin (Humulin N)
insulin glulisine (Apidra)
insulin aspart (NovoLog)
insulin detemir (Levemir)
insulin glargine (Lantus)*
insulin lispro (Humalog)*
regular insulin* (Humulin R, Novolin R)

Mixtures

insulin aspart with protamine–insulin aspart (NovoLog Mix 70/30)

insulin lispro with protamine–insulin lispro (Humalog Mix 75/25)

NPH–regular insulin (Humulin 70/30)

Noninsulin Injections for Diabetes

exenatide (Byetta)

pramlintide (Symlin)

Oral Hypoglycemics

First-Generation Sulfonylureas

chlorpropamide (Diabinese)

tolbutamide

Second-Generation Sulfonylureas

glimepiride (Amaryl)*

glipizide (Glucotrol, Glucotrol XL)*

glyburide (DiaBeta, Glynase, Micronase)*

Enzyme Inhibitors

acarbose (Precose)

miglitol (Glyset)

Biguanide

metformin (Glucophage, Riomet)*

Glitazones/Thiazolidinediones

pioglitazone (Actos)*

rosiglitazone (Avandia)*

Meglitinides

nateglinide (Starlix)

repaglinide (Prandin)

Gliptins

sitagliptin (Januvia)

Combinations

glipizide-metformin (Metaglip)

glyburide-metformin (Glucovance)*

metformin-sitagliptin (Janumet)

pioglitazone-metformin (Actoplus Met)

rosiglitazone-glimepride (Avandryl)

rosiglitazone-metformin (Avandamet)

sitagliptin-metformin (Janumet)

Synthetic Human Growth Hormones

somatrem (Protropin)

somatropin (Humatrope)

Chapter Review

Pharmaceuticals and Body Functions

Select the best answer from the choices given.

1. The thyroid hormones T_3 and T_4 are both formed from
   a. serotonin.
   b. thyroglobulin.
   c. acetylcholine.
   d. norepinephrine.

2. The most frequently prescribed thyroid agent is
   a. Synthroid.
   b. Thyrolar.
   c. Cytomel.
   d. all of the above

3. Hydrocortisone has the same activity as
   a. cortisol.
   b. prednisolone.
   c. prednisone.
   d. methylprednisolone.

4. Oral contraceptives may interact with all the listed drugs *except*
   a. antifungals.
   b. antibiotics.
   c. NSAIDs.
   d. TCAs.

5. All the listed drugs can cause secondary diabetes *except*
   a. beta blockers.
   b. birth control pills.
   c. glucocorticoids.
   d. NSAIDs.

6. Which drug decreases intestinal enzyme conversion of sugars into glucose?
   a. Glucophage
   b. Regranex
   c. Precose
   d. Glucotrol

7. For which type of diabetes is insulin always indicated?
   a. type I
   b. type II
   c. gestational
   d. all of the above

8. The steroid with the most anti-inflammatory potency is
   a. hydrocortisone.
   b. prednisone.
   c. dexamethasone.
   d. triamcinolone.

9. Which drug is used for osteoporosis?
   a. Fosamax
   b. Glucophage
   c. Flagyl
   d. Protropin

10. Most diseases of the genital system are transmitted by
    a. using public bathrooms.
    b. not going to the bathroom when one really needs to.
    c. uncleanliness.
    d. sexual activity.

The following statements are true or false. If the answer is false, rewrite the statement so it is true.

_____ 1. Steroids are frequently dosed every other day to avoid hypothalamic-pituitary axis involvement.

_____ 2. Treatment of the diabetic includes diet, exercise, and medication.

_____ 3. Caution should be used in treating patients with corticosteroids if they have diabetes, severe infection, or peptic ulcer disease.

_____ 4. There is considerable evidence that oral birth control pills protect against ovarian cancer.

_____ 5. Pregnancy tests are based on detecting the hormone HPA.

_____ 6. Steroid levels are highest at 7 P.M. to 8 P.M.

_____ 7. The major reason for using corticosteroids is to inhibit inflammation.

_____ 8. Acutely, hyperglycemia poses a greater risk, but hypoglycemia poses a greater long-term risk.

_____ 9. Androgens do not have a feedback control.

_____ 10. Androderm is a system that should be applied to the scrotum.

Diseases and Drug Therapies

1. List the positive effects and side effects of estrogen.

2. List the symptoms of diabetes.

3. List the conditions in which estrogen is contraindicated.

4. List and identify the differences in the thyroid medications.

5. What are some causes for growth delay?

Match the following adjectives with the listed drugs.

   a. first generation
   b. second generation
   c. enzyme inhibitor
   d. biguanide

6. Glucophage

7. Precose

8. glyburide

9. chlorpropamide

10. tolbutamide

Match the following two diseases with the listed symptoms.

    a. Addison disease
    b. Cushing disease

11. deficiency of glucocorticoids _____

12. overproduction or excessive administration of steroids over an extended period _____

13. round, puffy face _____

14. weakness (respiratory failure) _____

Dispensing Medications

1. Mrs. Jones is picking up the following prescription. What definite instructions should she be given?

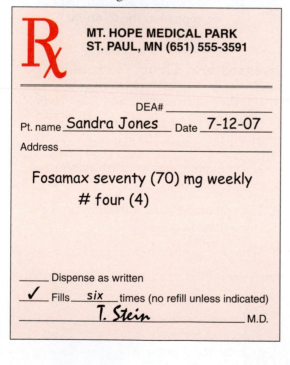

2. Betty Sue Jones brings in the following prescriptions. Identify the problem areas.

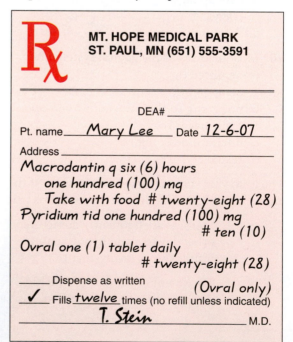

3. Mary Lee delivered an 11 pound boy. She is doing well and is ready to return to work. She has a urinary tract infection and brings in the following prescription. Check her profile and identify the problem areas.

Patient Profile

Patient name __Mary Lee__
Address __7243 Sandpiper Cove__
Age __28__   Sex __F__   Race __Cau__   Height __5'6"__   Weight __130__
Allergies __none__

DIAGNOSES

__gestational diabetes__

MEDICATIONS

Date	No.	Prescriber	Drug and Strength	Quantity	Sig	Refills
6/07	103	T. Stein	Prenatal vitamins	30	qd	6
10/07	1002	T. Stein	Humalog	2	prn	prn

Internet Research

Use the Internet to complete the following activities.

1. Osteoporosis is the most common bone disease affecting the Western world. Use the Internet to find out who is at risk for this disease and how it is diagnosed. Who should be screened? List your Internet sources.

2. Patient education is an important part of managing diabetes. Find three Internet sites that help address this need. Create a table comparing and contrasting the sites. For each site list its strengths and weakness in two separate columns.

What Would You Do?

1. Every Friday night a teenage diabetic comes in to get needles. He has a prescription with PRN refills. Often the insurance company will not pay for them, so he pays with cash.

Topical, Ophthalmic, and Otic Medications

15

Learning Objectives

- Describe the skin as an organ.
- Understand the physiology of the skin.
- Know the topical drugs and the conditions they treat.
- Explain the action of the topical corticosteroids and their application.
- Recognize the classes of antiseptics and disinfectants.
- Recognize the ophthalmic and otic agents and their uses.

Preview chapter terms and definitions.

Topical, ophthalmic, and otic medications are used to treat a variety of conditions, such as skin disorders, allergic and inflammatory reactions, infections, infestations, glaucoma, conjunctivitis, and otalgia. These classes of drugs range from mild agents to stronger forms of antibiotics, antiseptics, disinfectants, and corticosteroids.

Skin Ailments and Their Treatment

The skin is a major organ that accounts for 10% of body weight. It is equipped to deal with microbial, chemical, and physical assaults on the body. It is an important source of sensory input and is the main organ involved in temperature regulation. Correction of skin defects may be indicated, even when they do not pose a hazard to health, because of the mental attitude of the affected person or of society.

Figure 15.1 illustrates the anatomy of the skin. The **epidermis** is the top layer of the skin and is derived from embryonic ectoderm. It continually forms new cells in a basal layer; sheds old, dead cells; and also produces nails, hair, and glands. Pressure or friction on any part of the body stimulates skin growth, resulting in a thickening called a callus. Melanocytes, cells that produce the pigment melanin, are interspersed throughout the epidermis, mostly just slightly below the basal layer.

The **dermis,** which is below the epidermis, is composed of connective tissue with upward projections into the epidermis. It is supplied with capillaries and

FIGURE 15.1
Anatomy of the Skin

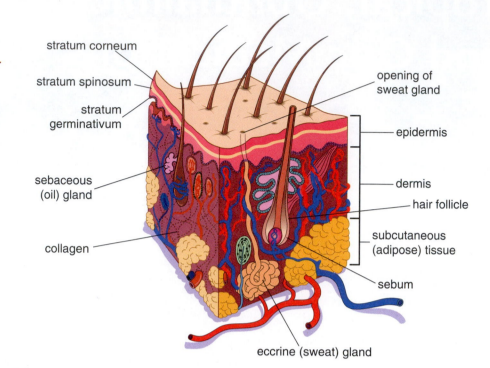

stratum corneum

stratum spinosum

stratum germinativum

opening of sweat gland

epidermis

dermis

hair follicle

sebaceous (oil) gland

subcutaneous (adipose) tissue

collagen

sebum

eccrine (sweat) gland

sensory nerve terminals that do not penetrate the epidermis. The dermis contains smooth muscle at hair follicles (arrector pili), in sheets in the areola of the nipple, and in the scrotum, where the muscle action causes wrinkled skin.

Two types of glands are widely distributed in the skin: sebaceous glands and sweat glands. Sebaceous glands secrete sebum, a substance that oils the skin and hair, preventing them from drying, and that is also toxic to certain types of bacteria. Most sebaceous glands develop from hair follicles and empty their secretions into the follicles. The other sebaceous glands empty their secretions directly onto the surface of the epidermis. The product of most of the body's sweat glands (called eccrine sweat glands) consists of water and salts. The larger, deeper sweat glands of the axillary, perineal, and genital regions (called apocrine sweat glands) produce sweat containing various organic materials, which produce an offensive odor when broken down by bacteria on the skin. The apocrine glands in the skin of the external ear canal produce cerumen (earwax), which has antibacterial and antifungal activity; it also contains squamous cells and dust.

In the treatment of skin ailments, most physicians generally prescribe creams more frequently than ointments. Dermatologists, however, prescribe ointments more frequently than creams because they are usually treating more troublesome skin problems. Creams and ointments should not be considered interchangeable. As a general rule, a dry skin problem is treated with an ointment, and a wet, oozing lesion is treated with a cream. Substituting a cream for an ointment on a dermatologist's prescription could produce a failed treatment.

Ultraviolet Radiation, Photoxicity, and Photosensitivity

Energy from the sun reaches the earth as electromagnetic radiation. Familiar examples of electromagnetic radiation are radio waves, microwaves, visible light, ultraviolet light, and x-rays. The energy from the sun not only enables us to see but also warms the planet, provides energy as food (beginning with photosynthesis), and plays a critical role in climate and weather patterns. The energy also interacts with our skin and produces suntans.

In contemporary Western culture, many people consider suntans attractive. Unfortunately, the rays of the sun that produce suntans are also very damaging to skin. Even with minimal sun exposure, skin will eventually show some signs of photoaging. With prolonged exposure, the skin undergoes hypermelanization and hyperkeratosis. The best way to prevent sun-damaged skin is to avoid excessive exposure to the sun and, while spending time outdoors, to protect the skin with sunscreen. To be effective, sunscreen should contain a rating of at least SPF (sunburn protection factor) of 15.

The rays responsible for suntans and sunburns are ultraviolet (UV) radiation. Ultraviolet radiation is higher in energy than visible light. Humans cannot see UV radiation, but this energy does interact with the atoms in the cells of our epidermis. Ultraviolet-A (UV-A) radiation is informally referred to as the suntan region, and UV-B as the sunburn region. To be effective, a sunscreen must protect against both UV-A and UV-B rays; it should contain a combination of oxybenzone and para-aminobenzoic acid or combinations of other agents that block both UV-A and UV-B rays. Avobenzone, titanium dioxide, or zinc oxide provide protection against dangerous UV wavelengths. **Phototoxicity** is the property of some chemicals whereby the substance becomes toxic to a cell upon exposure to light. Topical agents that cause phototoxicity occur in medications, suntan preparations, scents, cosmetics, certain dyes, and industrial products.

Photosensitivity is an abnormal sensitivity to light, especially of the eyes, but it can also include increased sensitivity of the skin to sunlight. Photosensitivity can increase the patient's susceptibility to phototoxicity. Many drugs in certain classes cause photosensitivity through biochemical interactions in the body, so it is important to alert a patient to this side effect when dispensing such a drug. The following classes have drugs that may cause photosensitivity: antihistamines, antibiotics, antifungals, antiretrovirals, antimalarials, antivirals, antineoplastics (chemotherapeutic agents), antiplatelets, diuretics, ACE inhibitors, statins, anticonvulsants, antipsychotics, antidepressants, sedatives, hypnotics, analgesics, NSAIDs, hormones, antidiabetic agents, topicals, and vitamins. Table 15.1 lists some of the drugs that cause photosensitivity. The technician will need to watch for the computer prompts or whatever system the pharmacy has in place to know whether a particular drug will need a sticker to warn the patient to avoid exposure to sunlight while taking the medication. Because photosensitivity is common and occurs in various ways, individual patients may react differently to a particular drug.

Even though sun exposure deleteriously affects everyone's skin, skin pigment will affect the reactions of skin to sun exposure. Fair-skinned persons are more likely to have atrophy and scaling of the epidermis than dark-skinned persons. Skin cancer is also more prevalent in lightly pigmented persons than in those with dark skin. For all skin cancer victims, tumor growth is more common in areas exposed to the sun than in covered or shaded areas of the body.

Several categories of skin cancer are recognized as follow:

- **Actinic keratosis:** a precancerous condition resulting from overexposure to sunlight
- **Basal cell carcinoma:** a slow-growing tumor that usually forms polyps and rarely metastasizes
- **Keratoacanthoma:** an epithelial tumor that first grows rapidly but usually regresses and heals
- **Melanoma:** a highly malignant cancer that forms from melanocytes; sunburn greatly increases the risk of this skin disorder

TABLE 15.1 Some Drugs That Cause Photosensitivity

Drug Class	Drug Example	Drug Class	Drug Example
ACE inhibitors	all agents	chemotherapeutic agents	dacarbazine
antibiotics	griseofulvin		fluorouracil, 5-FU
	quinolones		methotrexate
	sulfas		procarbazine
	tetracyclines		vinblastine
antidepressants	clomipramine	diuretics	acetazolamide
	maprotiline		furosemide
	sertraline		metolazone
	tricyclic antidepressants (TCAs)		thiazides
antihistamines	cyproheptadine	hypoglycemics	sulfonylureas
	diphenhydramine	NSAIDs	all agents
antipsychotics	haloperidol		
	phenothiazines		
cardiovascular drugs	amiodarone		
	diltiazem		
	quinidine		
	simvastatin		
	sotalol		

- **Squamous cell carcinoma:** a type of cancer that grows more rapidly than basal cell carcinoma; cells tend to keratinize; metastasis is uncommon

Pharmacologic treatment can help improve the condition of sun-damaged skin (see Table 15.2). **Retinoid** compounds (which are related to vitamin A and regulate skin cell growth) are also used to treat this condition. Some patients will find initiation of therapy difficult because of the intense erythema (redness of the skin due to an excess of capillaries) and peeling that occur at the beginning of these treatments. After three months, however, a rapid improvement is seen in the skin. Topical preparations of vitamins A, C, and E are also used. The alpha hydroxy acids are promoted as over-the-counter methods to improve the appearance of skin. They work by removing dead skin cells lying on the surface of the skin. For severe sunburn, corticosteroids are usually used. Aspirin can reduce irritation, pain, and edema.

Aloe gel has soothing and wound-healing properties. It inhibits bradykinin, a pain-producing agent, and the synthesis of thromboxane, which may speed the healing of burns. Aloe gel also has antibacterial and antifungal properties. When combined with lidocaine, aloe gel is especially soothing.

Benzocaine (Dermoplast) and **lidocaine (Solarcaine)** are topical anesthetics that provide temporary relief of sunburn pain. These should be used only on intact skin for short periods of time.

Hydrocortisone (Anusol-HC, Cortaid) can also be used on intact skin to decrease inflammation and accelerate healing. It will also help with pain relief.

Mequinol-tretinoin (Solagé) combines the synergestic action of two agents, mequinol (2%) and tretinoin (0.01%). Tretinoin, a retinoid, competitively inhibits the formation of melanin precursors. Mequinol is a substrate for the enzyme tyrosinase. Solagé inhibits melanogenesis and oxidizes free radicals that damage melanocytes. Combined, these drugs treat solar lentigines (commonly called liver spots; the singular is *lentigo*), which are pigmented, regularly shaped lesions. These areas result from chronic sun exposure. Mequinol-tretinoin, along with sun avoidance, application of effective sunscreens, and the wearing of protective clothing, can minimize damage to these areas. It should be applied only to the darkened areas and not to any skin that is undamaged. Improvement occurs gradually. This combination drug is also prescribed for the treatment of freckles. Photosensitizing drugs and sunlight must be avoided when using mequinol-tretinoin. Patients should also be instructed not to bathe or shower for at least 6 hours following application and not to apply makeup until at least 30 minutes have passed. The application of Solagé may induce minor stinging or burning. Some freckles may reappear after the drug is discontinued. Solagé is highly flammable and therefore should be kept away from open flames or high temperatures.

Warning

Stickers warning patients to apply drugs appropriately should be placed on all topical drugs, especially the liquids. It is not uncommon for someone to ingest a topical. This can be very dangerous.

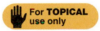

Skin Disorders and Their Pharmaceutical Treatment

Skin disorders may present as a variety of conditions. Diagnosis of abnormalities may be based on characteristics such as size, color, shape, location of the problem, and other symptoms. A biopsy may be undertaken for microscopic examination, which can further reveal the exact nature and extent of the skin problem. The condition may be confined to the skin or may reveal disease processes affecting the entire body. Table 15.3 lists the drugs most commonly used for skin diseases and disorders discussed in this section. Many of these may overlap and are used to treat more than one skin disease. As with other body systems, one drug can be used for several ailments. In Table 15.3, however, they are for the most part listed only under the primary use of the drug.

TABLE 15.2	Most Commonly Used Drugs to Treat Sun-Damaged Skin			
Generic Name	**Pronunciation**	**Dosage Form**	**Brand Name**	**Dispensing Status**
aloe gel		gel	(many)	OTC
aspirin	AS-pir-in	oral liquid, tablet	(many)	OTC
benzocaine	BEN-zoe-kayn	aerosol, cream, gel, liquid, lozenge, ointment, swab, wax	Dermoplast	OTC
hydrcortisone	hye-droe-KOR-ti-sone	aerosol, cream, gel, injection, lotion, ointment, solution, suppository, tablet	Anusol-HC, Cortaid, Solu-Cortef	OTC, Rx
lidocaine	LYE-doe-kayn	cream, gel, injection, jelly, liquid, ointment, solution, spray	Solarcaine	OTC
mequinol-tretinoin	MEK-win-awl tret-i-NOE-in	topical solution	Solagé	Rx
vitamin A	VYE-ta-min A	capsule, injection, tablet	(many)	OTC, Rx
vitamin C	VYE-ta-min C	capsule, injection, IV, tablet	(many)	OTC
vitamin E	VYE-ta-min E	capsule, oral liquid, tablet, topical	(many)	OTC

TABLE 15.3 Most Commonly Used Agents for Skin Diseases and Disorders

Generic Name	Pronunciation	Dosage Form	Brand Name	Dispensing Status
Acne Vulgaris				
adapalene	a-DAP-a-leen	cream, gel, topical solution	Differin	Rx
azelaic acid	ay-ze-LAY-ik AS-id	cream	Azelex	Rx
azithromycin	az-ith-roe-MYE-sin	injection, oral liquid, tablet	Zithromax	Rx
benzoyl peroxide	BEN-zoe-il per-OX-ide	cream, lotion, soap	Brevoxyl, Zoderm	OTC
clindamycin–benzoyl peroxide	klin-da-MYE-sin BEN-zoe-il per-OX-ide	gel	BenzaClin	Rx
isotretinoin	eye-soe-tret-i-NOE-in	capsule	Accutane, Claravis	Rx
tazarotene	ta-ZAR-oh-teen	cream, gel	Avage, Tazorac	Rx
tetracycline	tet-ra-SYE-kleen	capsule, suspension, tablet	none	Rx
tretinoin	tret-i-NOE-in	capsule, cream, gel, topical solution	Retin-A, Vesanoid	Rx
Wrinkles				
botulinum toxin type A	bot-yoo-LYE-num TOX-in TIPE A	injection	Botox	Rx
tretinoin	tret-i-NOE-in	cream	Renova	Rx
Psoriasis and Eczema				
acitretin	a-si-TRET-in	capsule	Soriatane	Rx
alefacept	a-LEF-a-sept	injection	Amevive	Rx
calcipotriene	kal-si-poe-TRY-een	cream, ointment, topical solution	Dovonex	Rx
coal tar	KOLE TAR	gel, lotion, shampoo	Cutar, Tarsum	OTC
cyclosporine	sye-kloe-SPOR-een	capsule, oral liquid	Neoral	Rx
doxepin	DOX-e-pin	cream	Zonalon	Rx
efalizumab	e-fa-li-ZOO-mab	injection	Raptiva	Rx
methotrexate	meth-o-TREX-ate	injection, IV, tablet	Rheumatrex, Trexall	Rx
pimecrolimus	pim-e-KROE-li-mus	cream	Elidel	Rx
tacrolimus	ta-KROE-li-mus	ointment	Protopic	Rx
tazarotene	ta-ZAR-o-teen	cream, gel	Tazorac	Rx
urea	you-REE-ah	cream, lotion	Carmol, Keralac	OTC
Viral Infections				
acyclovir	a-SYE-kloe-veer	cream	Zovirax	Rx
diethyl ether	dye-ETH-il EE-ther	spray	Wartner	OTC
docosanol	doe-KOE-san-awl	cream	Abreva	OTC
imiquimod	i-MIK-wi-mod	cream	Aldara	Rx
penciclovir	pen-SYE-kloe-veer	cream	Denavir	Rx

Generic Name	Pronunciation	Dosage Form	Brand Name	Dispensing Status
Dandruff				
selenium sulfide	se-LEE-nee-um SUL-fide	shampoo	Head & Shoulders Intensive Treatment, Selsun Blue	OTC
Unwanted Facial Hair				
eflornithine	ee-FLOR-nith-een	cream	Vaniqa	Rx
Actinic Keratosis				
aminolevulinic acid	a-mee-noe-LEV-yoo-lin-ik AS-id	topical solution	Levulan	Rx
diclofenac	di-KLOE-fen-ak	gel	Solaraze	Rx
fluorouracil	flor-oh-YOOR-a-sil	cream, topical solution	Efudex	Rx
imiquimod	i-MIK-wi-mod	cream	Aldara	Rx
Fungal Infections				
amphotericin B	am-foe-TAIR-i-sin B	cream, IV, lotion	Fungizone	Rx
butenafine	byoo-TEN-a-feen	cream	Lotrimin Ultra	OTC
			Mentax	Rx
ciclopirox	sye-kloe-PEER-ox	cream, lotion, nail lacquer	Loprox, Penlac	Rx
clotrimazole	kloe-TRIM-a-zole	cream, lotion, tablet, topical solution, troche, vaginal	Gyne-Lotrimin, Lotrimin AF cream, Mycelex	OTC
clotrimazole–betamethasone	kloe-TRIM-a-zole bay-ta-METH-a-sone	cream, lotion	Lotrisone	Rx
econazole	e-KON-a-zole	cream	Spectazole	Rx
griseofulvin	gris-ee-oh-FUL-vin	oral suspension, tablet	Fulvicin-U/F, Grifulvin V	Rx
itraconazole	it-ra-KON-a-zole	capsule, IV, oral liquid	Sporanox	Rx
ketoconazole	kee-toe-KON-a-zole	gel	Xolegel, Nizoral	OTC, Rx
miconazole	mye-KON-a-zole	lotion, ointment, spray, vaginal cream, vaginal suppository	Monistat, Lotrimin AF powder and sprays	OTC, Rx
miconazole–zinc oxide–petrolatum	mye-KON-a-zole zink OK-syde pet-roe-LAY-tum	ointment	Vusion	Rx
nystatin	nye-STAT-in	cream, ointment, oral liquid, powder, tablet, troche	Mycostatin, Nilstat	Rx
oxiconazole	ox-i-KON-a-zole	cream, lotion	Oxistat	Rx
sertaconazole	ser-tah-KON-a-zole	cream	Ertaczo	Rx
sulconazole	sul-KON-a-zole	cream	Exelderm	Rx
terbinafine	ter-BIN-a-feen	cream, gel, tablet	Lamisil	Rx
			Lamisil AT	OTC
tolnaftate	tole-NAF-tayt	cream, powder, solution	Tinactin Antifungal	OTC

seborrhea and acne vulgaris, two common skin disorders.

Seborrhea is a skin condition caused by excessive secretion, which gives the skin an oily appearance, especially in areas where the glands are most active. This condition can fluctuate in severity as a result of stress.

Acne vulgaris results from increased glandular activity at puberty, when the sebaceous glands enlarge and become more productive. It is characterized by elevated sebum secretion. Acne usually resolves in early adulthood, but chronic forms or severe exacerbations may last into adult life. Lesions are most common on the head and neck. They begin when the terminal of a sebaceous duct becomes plugged, forming a blackhead. The gland and hair follicle then become engorged with sebum and form a papule. If the contents of the papule become infected, it turns into a pustule surrounded by an inflamed area. Maintaining free-flowing sebum is the aim of treatment. Most cases respond to ultraviolet light. Washing with soap and water also has a drying effect. Systemic treatment with antibiotics (tetracycline and, to a lesser extent, erythromycin or clindamycin) has been helpful in moderate-to-severe acne. Treatment may have to be continued for long periods.

Adapalene (Differin) is a retinoid for acne treatment that is less likely to cause skin irritation than tretinoin because it is water-based, whereas tretinoin contains alcohol. It is applied at night or as a sunscreen during the day.

Azithromycin (Zithromax) has been shown to be as effective as other antibiotics for treatment of acne vulgaris. Systemic antibiotics reduce the proliferation of acne. The antibiotic must be lipid soluble to penetrate the follicle. The big advantage of azithromycin is its long half-life, which allows for once-a-day dosing.

Benzoyl peroxide (Brevoxyl, Zoderm) has antibacterial and mild drying effects, which help remove excess oils. It is used to treat acne.

Clindamycin–benzoyl peroxide (BenzaClin) is a topical gel for acne. The strengths are 1% for clindamycin and 5% for benzoyl peroxide. It is probably more economical for the patient to have these medications prescribed separately because, once the gel is mixed, it is good for only 7 days. So the **beyond-use date** (the date after which a compounded preparation should not be used) for this drug would be 7 days after it is mixed, and that date should be put on the package at some point.

Isotretinoin (Accutane), a retinoid, should be used as a treatment of last resort for severe acne. The danger of isotretinoin is that it is very **teratogenic** (causes birth defects). For isotretinoin to be used by a patient, participation in a special program called iPLEDGE is mandated by the FDA. A patient must sign an agreement to use birth control (both males and females) and undergo pregnancy testing while receiving isotretinoin. The prescriber must register the person with the iPLEDGE program, and then the patient must go online and register. Finally, the dispensing pharmacy must re-register the person online. Failure of any of the parties to follow protocol will halt the dispensing of the drug by the pharmacist. In the pharmacy, a pharmacy technician is responsible for setting up the iPLEDGE program. A patient must have his or her iPLEDGE card in order to receive their prescription. Furthermore, if a patient has any form of mental illness, he or she will most likely not be accepted in the program. A depressed mood is a major side effect of this drug. Isotretinoin must always be taken with a full glass of water to prevent the capsule from melting in the esophagus.

Tretinoin (Retin-A, Vesanoid), a retinoid, is a topical medication approved for treatment of acne. It is also used to treat photodamaged skin and some skin cancers. The epidermal cells in the sebaceous follicle become less adherent, which allows for easy removal. Tretinoin removes keratinocytes in the sebaceous follicle and loosens the keratic (thickening) cells at the mouth of the duct, causing easy sloughing and sebum discharge. Thus, the drug helps the skin to renew itself more quickly and improves its texture and appearance. Patients should avoid direct sunlight when using this drug.

Tazarotene (Avage, Tazorac), a synthetic retinoid, has been approved for acne and psoriasis treatment. It modulates epithelial tissue and exerts some anti-inflammatory and immunological activity. A thin layer should be applied in the evening to very dry skin. It will make the skin very sensitive to sunlight. Tazarotene is a prodrug that is converted to its active form, tazarotenic acid, by de-esterification There is some systemic absorption. Because of the prolonged retention of tazarotene within the body, the therapeutic effects can last up to 3 months after discontinuation.

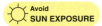

Some birth control pills, discussed in Chapter 14 (see Table 14.6), decrease testosterone and sebum production, thus improving acne. Examples of this activity include ethinyl estradiol–norgestimate (Ortho Tri-Cyclen) and ethinyl estradiol–norethindrone (Estrostep Fe). The lowest dose possible should be used.

Wrinkles Renova is a lower dosage form of tretinoin (Retin-A) that has been approved for use in eliminating wrinkles. It is provided by the manufacturer in one strength. Renova is an emollient cream base that is more moisturizing than Retin-A. Its sloughing action allows new tissue to form that does not have the wrinkled appearance of older tissue. Although this medication may cause a mild inflammatory reaction in normal skin, it does help to reduce some effects of too much sun exposure, fine wrinkles, rough skin, and brown spots. Wrinkles reappear when the drug is discontinued. The hands should be thoroughly washed after each application. Patients should avoid the sun and should not exceed the prescribed dose, as severe irritation can result.

Botulinum toxin type A (Botox) is a neuromuscular blocking agent that is used to temporarily improve lines and wrinkles of the face. It is a neurotoxin produced by *Clostridium botulinum* that affects only the presynaptic membrane of the neuromuscular junction. Botulinum toxin type A produces a state of denervation, which means that affected muscles cannot move until new fibrils grow from the nerve and form a junction. Effects of a single treatment last for approximately 3 months; treatments are very expensive.

Although used primarily for acne vulgaris, **tazarotene (Avage, Tazorac)** can also be used to reduce the appearance of fine wrinkles, mottled light and dark skin patches, and benign facial lentigines (noncancerous freckles). Patients should cleanse the skin thoroughly and let it dry before applying the medication. Application will cause a passing sensation of stinging or burning.

Allergic and Inflammatory Reactions Pruritus (itching) is associated with a number of skin disorders, such as urticaria (hives or systemic itching wheals), rash, infections, or irritation from chemical substances. Several systemic diseases, including liver disease, uremia, Hodgkin disease, diabetes, and thyroid disorders, may cause itching. Pregnancy, senility, and various psychological and psychiatric disorders may also cause excessive itching. Treatments to relieve itching may include topically applied baths containing starch, sodium bicarbonate, magnesium sulfate (Epsom salts), colloidal oatmeal, or potassium permanganate. Camphor in liniments and ointments has a cooling, antipruritic effect. Antihistamines are also commonly used to relieve itching. If someone is allergic to a drug, a rash is the most common reaction. Drug rashes typically start on the trunk and spread to the limbs. Patients who react to a drug with a rash should stop taking the drug immediately. A pharmacy technician, upon hearing of a drug-caused rash, should notify the pharmacist immediately.

Eczema, also referred to as dermatitis, is a hot, itchy, red, oozing condition characteristic of an acute stage of inflammation. Typically, eczema is classified as either atopic or contact. Patients with eczema should avoid the sun. Corticosteroids may be used to treat eczema.

Atopic eczema, also called atopic dermatitis, is a chronic pruritic eruption of unknown cause; allergic, hereditary, and psychogenic factors appear to be involved. Figure 15.2 shows an example of atopic eczema. It is treated with **doxepin (Zonalon)**, a topical formulation of a drug otherwise used for depression. Doxepin is prescribed for itching because it has strong antihistaminic effects. It is a stronger histamine blocker than diphenhydramine or hydroxyzine. A thin film should be applied four times a day with an interval of at least 3 to 4 hours between applications. Like oral doxepin (Chapter 7), Zonalon may cause drug interactions. Patients can get significant absorption, especially if they are using it on a fairly large area. Direct sun exposure and alcohol should be avoided.

Contact dermatitis is an inflammatory reaction produced by contact with an irritating agent. Figure 15.3 shows an example of contact dermatitis. The itching associated with contact dermatitis may be relieved by antihistamines and the other treatments mentioned at the beginning of this section. Specifically, it is treated with **doxepin (Zonalon).**

To treat poison oak, poison ivy, and most other forms of contact dermatitis, hydrocortisone is employed. A 1% formulation is recommended for adults, whereas the 0.5% formulation is intended for children. Hydrocortisone soothes skin and significantly decreases itching, which therefore decreases the desire of the patient to scratch, so healing accelerates. These are OTC medications. If hydrocortisone is inef-

FIGURE 15.2
Atopic Eczema

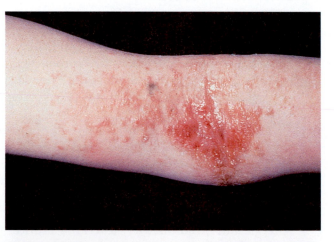

FIGURE 15.3
Contact Dermatitis

This allergic reaction occurred in response to the leather components of a wristwatch band.

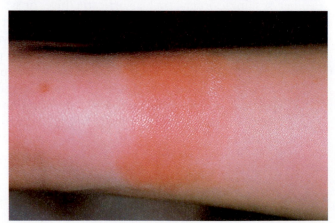

fective, then the patient should see a physician, who might prescribe oral or injected steroids.

Pimecrolimus (Elidel), a drug that is similar to antirejection drugs, is approved for the treatment of eczema. An immunosuppressant, it reduces itching and inflammation by suppressing the release of cytokines from the T cells. The patient should apply a thin layer to all areas of the skin diagnosed as having eczema. The drug should not be applied to areas that do not have eczema. Other skin products should not be applied to the areas with eczema.

Tacrolimus (Protopic) is also similar to antirejection drugs or a topical immuno-modulators (TIM). The advantage of this drug over a steroid is that tacrolimus will not cause thinning of the skin or other side effects of long-term steroid use. Tacrolimus may be used anywhere on the body, even the face. It is approved for use by children between 2 to 15 years of age in the 0.03% concentration and by adults in the 0.1% concentration.

Psoriasis **Psoriasis** is a chronic noncontagious condition in which epidermis cells multiply and die at excessive rates, producing patches of red, scaly skin (called plaques) that are slightly raised with defined margins. Plaques usually occur on the elbows and knees, but any part of the body may be affected (see Figure 15.4). A tendency to develop these lesions is genetically determined, but usually they do not occur until adulthood. Attacks are precipitated by illness, injury, or emotional stress. The immune system, particularly the T cells, is involved as well, and psoriasis is complicated by arthritis in 10 to 20% of patients. Psoriasis has no cure. Treatment is based on severity and individual requirements. Three types of treatment are used: topical therapy, phototherapy, and systemic therapy. Sometimes they are combined.

Alefacept (Amevive) is administered intramuscularly for 12 weeks to patients with psoriasis who do not respond sufficiently well to a topical treatment. Alefacept interferes with lymphocyte or white blood cell activation and proliferation. It is specifically designed to attack T cells rather than the entire immune system. The injection sites should be rotated; a subsequent site should be more than 1 inch (2.5 cm) from the previous injection or from any skin that is red, tender, bruised, or hard. When taking this drug, the patient should have periodic blood tests. A second course of therapy may be considered after the patient has been agent-free for 12 weeks. Alefacept has the same side effects as immunosuppressants.

Acitretin (Soriatane) is a retinoic acid analog. It has demonstrated significant clearing of psoriasis when administered as monotherapy and total clearing in some patients when used in combination with UV-B and UV-A therapy. It may allow lower

FIGURE 15.4
Psoriasis

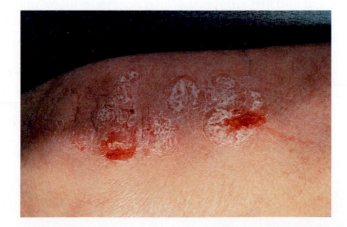

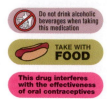

doses of phototherapy. The dose must be individualized. When the patient first begins acitretin therapy, the psoriasis may worsen. However, conditions should improve with time. Acitretin is a known teratogen, and a consent form for female patients is included in the package. This drug can also interfere with oral contraceptives. Alcohol must be avoided while on this drug. It should be taken with food. The patient should be advised not to donate blood while on treatment and for 3 years after discontinuation.

Coal tar (Cutar, Tarsum) is commonly prescribed, in combination with a topical steroid, to control the inflammation, itching, redness, and scaling of psoriasis. The drug is also referred to as LCD, which stands for liquor carbonis detergens, a synonym for coal tar.

Calcipotriene (Dovonex) is a topical treatment for psoriasis. It is a synthetic analog of vitamin D that regulates skin cell production and proliferation. It should not be used on the face because the face is especially sensitive to the skin irritation, stinging, redness, and peeling caused by this drug. Patients should wash their hands after each application. Watch to make sure that patients do not use more than 100 g of ointment per week, because absorption of the vitamin D might cause serum calcium levels to become too high.

Efalizumab (Raptiva) is a monoclonal antibody approved to treat psoriasis. It is a sterile powder for subcutaneous injection. Because this drug is an immunosupressant, it increases the risk of infection and latent infections. Efalizumab increases the risk of malignancy and decreases platelet count. Vaccines should be avoided while on this drug. Efalizumab is injected subcutaneously once per week.

Methotrexate (Rheumatrex, Trexall) is used in oral or injectable forms to treat psoriasis. It may inhibit normal cell growth of bone marrow tissues.

Neoral is the brand of **cyclosporine** used to treat severe psoriasis.

Urea (Carmol, Keralac) promotes hydration and removal of excess keratin. It should not be used near the eyes or on broken or inflamed skin. The moisturizing effect is enhanced by applying it to the skin while it is still damp after washing or bathing.

Viral Infections Viral infections can cause several skin disorders, including shingles, cold sores, and warts. Herpes zoster (shingles) is caused by the same virus that causes chickenpox. Vesicles appear with erythema and edema. The distribution is usually unilateral and confined to one **dermatome** (area of the skin associated with a pair of dorsal nerve roots that emerge horizontally from the spinal cord) or a few dermatomes. Pain in the area may precede the outbreak and linger afterward. The virus resides in dorsal root ganglions until immunity wanes, and then it erupts. Treatment is palliative; it affords relief but does not cure, although antivirals such as acyclovir (see Chapter 5), if initiated early enough, may prevent recurrent outbreaks.

Another herpes virus, herpes simplex 1, causes cold sores. Figure 15.5 shows an example of a cold sore caused by the herpes simplex 1 virus.

Docosanol (Abreva) is an OTC topical indicated for the treatment of cold sores. It blocks the virus from invading the cells and is most effective when administered at the first sign of an outbreak. It must be applied five times a day in order to be effective.

A **wart** is a virally caused epidermal tumor. Remission is due to developing immunity, but the virus may lie dormant and later cause reinfection. Genital warts are transmitted by sexual contact. Warts can be removed by surgery or destroyed by local freezing. Some OTC products may be effective if the wart is small. Most agents contain salicylic acid as an active ingredient.

Diethyl ether (Wartner), an OTC cryotherapy, is an aerosol spray that contains

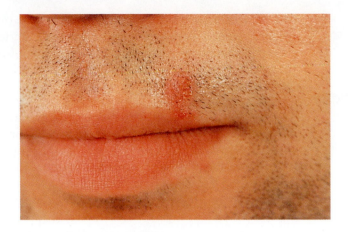

Figure 15.5
A Cold Sore Caused by the Herpes Simplex 1 Virus

propane. It is sprayed onto an applicator, the applicator cools and is applied to the wart, and the wart freezes. This treatment is as effective as the liquid nitrogen used in physicians' offices. Usually only one application is needed, but if the wart does not fall off within 10 days, the medication can be applied again.

Imiquimod (Aldara) stimulates the immune process at the site of the lesions. It should be used for 3 weeks at bedtime at the site of the lesions. Imiquimod is approved for the treatment of external and genital and perianal warts. It also has FDA approval for psoriasis.

Dandruff Dandruff is shedding of scales from the scalp that is more rapid than in other parts of the body. When entrapped by hair, these scales become more noticeable. Dandruff is a cosmetic problem rather than a medical one. **Selenium sulfide (Head & Shoulders Intensive Treatment, Selsun Blue)** has a direct effect on epidermal cells. If it is used daily, dandruff should be controlled.

Unwanted Facial Hair **Eflornithine (Vaniqa)** decreases unwanted facial hair and is approved to be used only by women. It slows the rate of hair growth by blocking cell division and other functions necessary for hair growth. Eflornithine may cause temporary redness, stinging, or rash on the skin where it is applied. In medical trials, adverse effects were mild and resolved without medical treatment. A thin layer should be applied twice daily at least 8 hours apart. There are no known interactions with this drug.

Actinic Keratosis Actinic keratosis is a scaly skin lesion that is caused by excessive sun exposure and can lead to skin cancer. **Fluorouracil (Efudex)** is used topically for management of multiple actinic keratoses and superficial basal cell carcinomas. Fluorouracil is an antimetabolite. Procedures for proper handling and disposal of chemotherapy agents (antineoplastic drugs, drugs that inhibit tumor development and growth) should be followed when working with this drug. Patients may experience nausea, vomiting, and hair loss, and direct sunlight should be avoided. Fluorouracil may cause permanent sterility.

Aminolevulinic acid (Levulan) is a topical compound indicated for the treatment of actinic keratosis. The drug undergoes a photodynamic reaction upon exposure to light of the appropriate wavelength. Aminolevulinic acid must be applied by a health professional and followed by a blue light treatment. It is important that application of aminolevulinic acid be limited to the lesion. Patients undergoing photodynamic treatment must be instructed to avoid sunlight and tanning beds during the course of their treatment. Aminolevulinic acid must be used immediately after it is compounded.

Diclofenac is a nonsteroidal anti-inflammatory drug (NSAID) that is approved for topical treatment of actinic keratosis as Solaraze (3%) or Voltaren Topical (1%). The mechanism of action for this use is unknown. Patients should be warned to avoid sunlight when using this product. The gel should be applied to the lesions twice a day for 60 to 90 days. The area should not be covered, and other lotions should not be applied to it.

Fungal Infections Skin and nails are susceptible to various fungal infections described here. **Candidiasis** is an infection by the fungus *Candida albicans* that usually causes lesions in the mouth (where it is called thrush) and vagina. It may be treated with agents such as clotrimazole and miconazole. Swish-and-swallow nystatin is frequently used if the mouth is involved.

Ringworm (tinea) is caused by a microscopic fungus that infects the horny (scaly) layer of the skin or the nails. The infection spreads outward as the center heals, leaving a ring. Ringworm responds to topical antifungal agents. All forms can be controlled by the oral antifungal **griseofulvin (Fulvicin-U/F, Grifulvin V)**, which accumulates in keratin. Topical **butenafine (Lotrimin Ultra, Mentax)** and **terbinafine (Lamisil AT)** are also used to treat ringworm. Butenafine and terbinafine are more effective because they kill the fungus, whereas the other antifungal agents only terminate fungal growth. Lotrimin Ultra or Lamisil AT should be used for athlete's foot, jock itch, and ringworm.

Butenafine (Lotrimin Ultra, Mentax) is used to treat athlete's foot (see Figure 15.6), ringworm, and jock itch. It is applied once daily for 4 weeks. After the last application, the drug may maintain its effect for an additional 4 weeks. This is why it is considered the drug of choice for athlete's foot and ringworm. Lotrimin Ultra OTC is identical to the prescription drug Mentax. It also remains active after the patient stops using it. It is important to read the generic names of these drugs. Only Lotrimin Ultra is butenafine; Lotrimin AF cream is clotrimazole, and Lotrimin AF sprays and powder are miconazole.

Ciclopirox (Penlac, Loprox) is probably the most effective topical for nail fungus. Nail fungus (onychomycosis) is extremely difficult to treat. The aging population in the United States is very prone to this infection. It can cause the nail to thicken, which in turn can cause foot problems. Itraconazole (Sporanox) and terbinafine (Lamisil) are the first-line drugs for nail fungus infections. Nail fungus infections are difficult to treat topically because it is so difficult to penetrate the nail or get the medicine under the nail so as to treat the fungus directly. Because of this, these infections are commonly treated with oral medications.

Clotrimazole (Lotrimin AF cream) is a topical, OTC version of this drug, which

FIGURE 15.6
Athlete's Foot

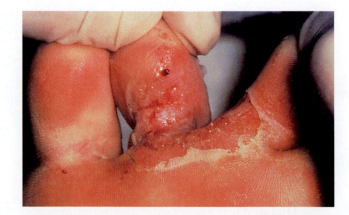

is also used in the prescription oral lozenge Mycelex (see Chapter 5). "AF" simply means "Anti-fungal." Again, it is necessary to pay attention to the generic names. Lotrimin AF *spray* or *powder* is miconazole.

Itraconazole (Sporanox) is especially useful for fungal nail infections and comes in capsule, oral liquid, and intravenous dosage forms. Pulse dosing (discussed in Chapter 5) is commonly used with this drug. Pulse dosing is an effective way to administer antifungal medications for finger and toenail infections. It is effective and less expensive than other forms.

Ketoconazole (Xolegel) is a 2% gel indicated for seborrheic dermatitis for persons 12 years and older. Seborrheic dermatitis is characterized by red, flaking, scaly skin on the face and trunk; on the scalp it is called dandruff. **Ketoconazole (Nizoral)** is available as a shampoo for patients with fungal infections of the scalp. It is used daily for 2 weeks. Patients should wait 20 minutes after application before using sunscreen or makeup on the affected areas.

Miconazole (Monistat, Lotrimin AF) is available as a powder or liquid spray. Note that Lotrimin AF spray or powder is miconazole, whereas Lotrimin AF cream is clotrimazole.

Miconazole–zinc oxide–petrolatum (Vusion) is a new therapy approved for diaper dermatitis (diaper rash) when accompanied by a proven fungal infection with *Candida albicans*. It is an ointment that contains miconazole for the fungal infection and zinc oxide and petrolatum (petroleum jelly) for the diaper rash. Vusion should be applied in a thin layer to the affected area. The child should be at least 4 weeks of age before it is used.

Sertaconazole (Ertaczo) is an imidazole antifungal agent. It is believed to inhibit the synthesis of ergosterol, which is a key component of the cell membrane of fungi. Sertaconazole is approved to treat ringworm that affects the scalp, feet, hands, groin, or toenails and also for athlete's foot. These infections are generally transmitted through close human contact or by indirect contact. Because the infections are superficial, topical therapy is generally sufficient. Sertaconazole is applied to the affected area twice daily for 4 weeks. The most common side effect is contact dermatitis.

Terbinafine (Lamisil) is a topical cream or tablet that may be used to treat fungi. It inhibits the biosynthesis of fungal membrane sterols. For athlete's foot, it should be applied twice daily and for ringworm and jock itch four times daily. The treatment course takes only 1 week, as opposed to 4 weeks for other antifungal agents. Systemic absorption of the topical medication is also low. Terbinafine remains active for 1 week or longer after patient use ceases.

Tolnaftate (Tinactin Antifungal) is an OTC drug recommended for treatment of jock itch. It is not recommended for nail infections and should not be used around the eyes. Side effects are pruritus, contact dermatitis, irritation, and stinging. If skin irritation develops, infection worsens, or there is no improvement within 10 days, the patient should consult a physician.

Skin Infections

Skin infections are common. Although most can be managed with nonprescription topical antimicrobial products, some do not respond to ordinary products, necessitating treatment with a prescription drug. The severity of a skin infection depends on the extent to which the skin and its structures are involved. There can be drainage, swelling, fever, and malaise.

Common Skin Infections   **Impetigo** is a superficial, but highly contagious, skin infection that is common in early childhood, particularly in warm, humid climates and where hygiene is poor. It is uncommon in adults, but it may be seen, particularly in elderly and immunocompromised patients. An example is shown in Figure 15.7. Impetigo is caused by *Staphylococcus* or *Streptococcus* and is characterized by bullae (blisters) and encrustations. Impetigo is treated with mupirocin (Bactroban) cream or ointment. For disseminated involvement with multiple lesions, systemic therapy with an antibiotic is recommended.

Erysipelas, a form of cellulitis, is characterized by redness and warmth, local pain, edematous plaque with sharply established borders, chills, malaise, and fever. The infection spreads progressively and rapidly through the superficial layers of the skin. Facial involvement may assume a butterfly distribution. Erysipelas usually responds well to oral antibiotics. However, if systemic toxicity (high fever with elevated white blood cell count) results, parenteral antibiotics should be administered.

Folliculitis is an inflammation of a hair follicle by a minute, red, pustulated nodule without involvement of the surrounding tissues. There is little pain. It commonly occurs in men on the bearded part of the face.

A **furuncle** (boil) is a staphylococcal infection beginning in a sebaceous gland and the associated hair follicle. The follicular infection is more extensive and deeper than in folliculitis. It begins with itching, local tenderness, and erythema, followed by swelling, marked local pain, and pus formation within the lesion. A **carbuncle** is a coalescent mass of infected follicles with deeper penetration than in furuncles. Pain, erythema, swelling, purulent drainage, fever, and systemic toxicity are common.

Other Skin Conditions Treated with Antimicrobials Burns are especially difficult to treat. The use of effective topical antimicrobial agents has been associated with a reduction in mortality.

Rosacea is a chronic dermatologic disorder with an inflammatory-vascular component (erythema, papules, and pustules), which may become infected, as well as a sebaceous and ocular component. It is characterized by flushing, erythema, papules, and pustules. Triggers of rosacea include stress, temperature, hot drinks, exercise, spicy food, alcohol, or any topical product that would irritate the skin. Sunlight exposure is a major exacerbating factor of rosacea. Before drug thereapy is initiated, the specific triggers should be identified so as to be avoided. Because the disorder is not curable, only its symptoms are treated with antibiotics. Topical agents used for treatment are Metro Gel, Azelex, Sulfacet R, and Finacea. Oracea is an oral medication.

Antibiotic Treatment of Skin Infections Table 15.4 presents the most commonly

FIGURE 15.7
An Impetigo Infection

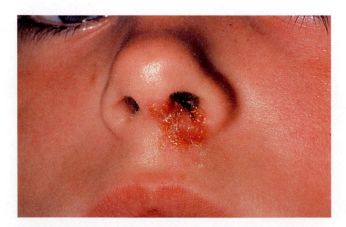

used antibiotic drugs that are used to treat skin infections.

Azelaic acid (Azelex) is a topical treatment for mild-to-moderate inflammatory acne vulgaris. After the skin is washed and patted dry, a thin film of cream should be gently rubbed into the affected area twice daily. Hands should be washed after each application. Improvement usually occurs within 4 weeks.

Bacitracin–neomycin–polymyxin B (Triple Antibiotic, Neosporin, Mycitracin) is used to prevent or treat minor skin infections.

Clindamycin (Cleocin T) is considered to be an effective topical antibiotic for acne.

Mafenide (Sulfamylon) is used primarily to treat burns. The major problem with this drug is the pain upon application. Infections can occur despite adequate topical treatment. Routine use of prophylactic antibiotics is recommended.

Mupirocin (Bactroban) is a much-used, topical treatment for impetigo caused by *Staphylococcus aureus* or *Streptococcus pyogenes*. It should not be applied to the eye; use should be discontinued if rash, itching, or irritation occurs or if there is no improvement within five days. Mupirocin is applied three times a day for 12 days.

Retapamulin (Altabax) is an ointment approved for the topical treatment of impetigo for both adults and children. The active ingredient is derived from an edible mushroom. Retapamulin should be used twice a day for 5 days. It is the only topical prescription antibacterial agent with a 5 day twice a day dosing, which is an advantage of this drug. Retapamulin is slower acting than the other topical used for impetigo, mupirocin. Retapamulin is one of several drugs from a new class of antibiotics. This class of antibiotics, the pleuromutilins, inhibits bacterial protein synthesis in the same way as mupirocin, but binds at different sites.

Silver sulfadiazine (Silvadene) is a cream that is extensively used. It works on the

TABLE 15.4   Most Commonly Used Antibiotic Agents Used in the Treatments of Skin Infections

Generic Name	Pronunciation	Dosage Form	Brand Name	Dispensing Status
azelaic acid	a-zeh-LAY-ik-AS-id	cream, gel	Finacea	Rx
bacitracin–neomycin–polymyxin B	bas-i-TRAY-sin nee-oh-MYE-sin pol-ee-MIX-in B	ointment	Triple Antibiotic, Neosporin, Mycitracin	OTC
clindamycin	klin-da-MYE-sin	gel, lotion, topical solution	Cleocin T	Rx
erythromycin	er-ith-roe-MYE-sin	swab, topical solution	EryDerm, T-Stat	Rx
mafenide	MA-fe-nide	cream, topical solution	Sulfamylon	Rx
metronidazole	met-troe-NYE-da-zole	gel	MetroGel	Rx
mupirocin	myoo-PEER-oe-sin	cream, ointment	Bactroban	Rx
neomycin–polymyxin B	nee-oe-MYE-sin pol-i-MIX-in B	irrigation solution, ointment	Neosporin G.U. Irrigant	Rx
retapamulin	ret-a-PAM-yoo-lin	ointment	Altabax	Rx
silver sulfadiazine	SIL-ver sul-fa-DYE-a-zeen	cream	Silvadene	Rx
sulfur-sulfacetamide	SUL-fer sul-fa-SEE-ta-mide	cream, lotion	Rosac, Rosula	Rx

bacterial cell wall and cell membrane. Silver sulfadiazine frequently darkens in its container, a jar, or after being applied to the skin, but this color change does not interfere with its antimicrobial properties. Hypersensitivity to this drug is rare, and it is painless upon application. Mafenide is more effective and has better penetration than silver sulfadiazine in treating some bacterial infections.

Use of the **sulfur-sulfacetamide (Rosac, Rosula)** combination for rosacea has been limited because of the inability of the delivery system to mask the sulfur odor. Improved formulations are now available. Rosac not only contains antibiotics, it also contains sunscreen, which helps to decrease the triggering of rosacea by sun exposure.

Topical Corticosteroids

When corticosteroids are applied to inflamed skin, they suppress the immune response, thereby relieving the redness, swelling, and itching. Table 15.5 lists the most commonly used topical steroids. Topical corticosteroids should be applied as a very thin film and used sparingly. Because they can penetrate the skin, they may be absorbed to significant levels in the systemic circulation; thus, they have the ability to suppress the hypothalamus-pituitary axis. Local effects can be skin eruptions, burning sensation, atropic striae (streaks and lines), and **petechiae** (minute red spots on the skin due to the escape of a small amount of blood).

The 0.5% and the 1.0% formulations of hydrocortisone are available as OTC medications. Both strengths can be effective and are the drugs of choice for poison ivy. Severe poison ivy may require short-term treatment with oral corticosteroids. Hydrocortisone is also effective in cases of severe diaper rash. Because the stronger formulation can easily penetrate children's tender skin, leading to a greater potential for systemic absorption with adverse effects, only the 0.5% formulation should be used with children.

Topical corticosteroids vary greatly in potency and delivery system. It is common for manufacturers to provide a drug at different levels of potency. Generally, products are available as creams or ointments and sometimes as gels. As a rule, ointment formulations are more potent than creams, with the gel form generally in between. Exceptions occur when manufacturers alter the delivery system of a cream or gel to enhance penetration, thereby delivering more drug to the lower skin layer. These variations produce a range of products, including superpotent topical steroids. Table 15.6 lists the three strongest classes of the superpotent topical steroidal agents. Topical steroids are used for a variety of dermatological conditions. The more potent ones can cause adrenal suppression, so they must be used with caution.

The potency of topical corticosteroids is determined by the location and seriousness of the condition to be treated. Only low-potency agents should be used on the face, genitals, and armpits. Medium-potency products are usually used on the trunk, arms, and legs. High-potency steroids should be reserved for skin conditions that are resistant to the lower-dosage drugs. Also, high-dose steroids that are used intermittently (pulse-dosed) have been shown to be more effective than a low-potency agent used on a daily basis. Generally, high-potency steroids should not exceed 2 weeks or 50 g per week.

Warning

Creams and ointments should not be considered interchangeable.

Most superpotent topical steroids have restrictions that limit their use to 2 consecutive weeks of treatment and/or a maximum of 45 g to 50 g in any one week, because of systemic absorption. An exception is diflorasone diacetate, 0.05% ointment (Psorcon), which is not restricted to two-weeks or in the quantity of its prescription. Psorcon is also the only superpotent topical steroid approved for use under occlusive dressings when enhanced penetration is required.

TABLE 15.5   Most Commonly Used Topical Corticosteroids

Generic Name	Pronunciation	Dosage Form	Brand Name	Dispensing Status
alclometasone	al-kloe-MET-a-sone	cream, ointment	Aclovate	Rx
amcinonide	am-SIN-oh-nide	cream, lotion, ointment	Cyclocort	Rx
betamethasone	bay-ta-METH-a-sone	cream, foam, lotion, ointment	Beta-Val, Diprolene, Diprosone, Luxiq	Rx
clobetasol	kloe-BAY-ta-sawl	cream, ointment	Clobex, Olux, Temovate	Rx
clocortolone	kloe-KOR-toe-lone	cream	Cloderm	Rx
desoximetasone	des-ox-i-MET-a-sone	cream, gel, ointment	Topicort	Rx
diflorasone	dye-FLOR-a-sone	cream, ointment	Florone, Psorcon	Rx
fluocinolone	floo-oh-SIN-oh-lone	cream, ointment	Capex, Synalar	Rx
fluocinonide	floo-oh-SIN-oh-nide	cream, gel, ointment	Lidex	Rx
fluticasone	floo-TIK-a-sone	cream, lotion, ointment, spray	Cutivate	Rx
halcinonide	hal-SIN-oh-nide	cream, ointment	Halog	Rx
halobetasol	hal-oh-BAY-ta-sawl	cream, ointment	Ultravate	Rx
hydrocortisone	hye-droe-KOR-ti-sone	cream, gel, ointment, solution, shampoo	Scalpicin	OTC
hydrocortisone butyrate	hye-droe-KOR-ti-sone byoo-TEER-ate	cream, ointment, solution	Locoid	Rx
hydrocortisone-lidocaine	hye-droe-KOR-ti-sone LYE-do-kayn	cream	Lida-Mantle HC	Rx
hydrocortisone valerate	hye-droe-KOR-ti-sone va-LAIR-ate	cream, ointment	Westcort	Rx
mometasone furoate	moe-MET-a-sone FYOOR-oh-ate	cream, ointment	Elocon	Rx
triamcinolone	trye-am-SIN-oe-lone	cream, lotion, ointment	Kenalog	Rx

External Parasites

Two types of external parasites use the human body as a host: lice and scabies mites. Lice spend their entire life cycle on the skin surface, hair, and clothing fibers of their host. An infestation of lice is called **pediculosis.** The mites that cause scabies may spend part of their life cycle on the skin surface and the remainder in burrows in the host's skin.

Human Lice Lice are wingless insects that live parasitically on various animals, including most mammals. Human lice exist in all climate zones, from arctic conditions to the tropics, and may infest persons of any walk of life. They live up to 45 days, but may die prematurely because of scratching, combing, or disease. Injured or weak lice fall off the host. Human blood is the only source of nourishment. Lice are spread

TABLE 15.6 Potency Comparison of Superpotent Topical Steroids

Generic Name	Dosage Form	Brand Name	Percent
Very High Potency			
augmented betamethasone dipropionate	ointment	Diprolene	0.05
clobetasol propionate	cream, ointment	Clobex, Olux, Temovate	0.05
halobetasol propionate	cream, ointment	Ultravate	0.05
High Potency			
amcinonide	cream, ointment	Cyclocort	0.1
betamethasone dipropionate	cream, lotion, ointment	Diprolene AF, Diprosone	0.05
betamethasone valerate	ointment	Beta-Val	0.1
desoximetasone	cream, ointment	Topicort	0.25
diflorasone	cream, ointment	Florone, Psorcon	0.05
fluocinolone	cream	Synalar	0.2
fluocinonide	cream, gel, ointment	Lidex	0.05
halcinonide	cream, ointment	Halog	0.1
triamcinolone	cream	Kenalog	0.5
Intermediate Potency			
betamethasone dipropionate	lotion	Diprosone	0.05
betamethasone valerate	cream	Beta-Val	0.1
	foam	Luxiq	0.12
clocortolone	cream	Cloderm	0.1
desoximetasone	gel	Topicort	0.05
fluocinolone	cream	Synalar	0.05
flurandrenolide	cream, lotion	Cordran, Cordran SP	0.05
fluticasone propionate	cream	Cutivate	0.05
hydrocortisone butyrate	ointment, solution	Locoid	0.1
hydrocortisone valerate	cream, ointment	Westcort	0.2
hydrocortisone-lidocaine	cream	Lida-Mantle HC	0.5
mometasone fuorate	cream, ointment	Elocon	0.1
triamcinolone	cream, lotion, ointment	Kenalog	0.025, 0.1
Low Potency			
alcometasone	cream, ointment	Aclovate	0.05%
desonide	cream, lotion	DesOwen	0.05%
fluocinolone	cream, gel, solution	Synalar	0.01%
hydrocortisone	cream, ointment	Cortizone-5	0.05
hydrocortisone	cream, lotion, ointment	Cortizone-10, Preparation H	1%
hydrocortisone	cream, ointment, lotion, solution	Anusol HC	2.5%

by direct contact with the infested person's head, body, or personal items such as hats, hairbrushes, combs, or bedding. The symptom of an infestation of lice is itching.

Humans can be infested by three types of lice: body lice, head lice, and pubic lice. DNA studies suggest that body lice evolved from head lice, possibly when *Homo sapiens* first began to wear clothing (possibly 70,000 years ago). In contrast, pubic lice are more closely related to lice that live on nonhuman primates, such as gorillas, than to human head or body lice.

Body lice are 2 to 4 mm long and live in clothing and moist areas of the body such as the waistline and armpits. Body lice do not always require treatment with drugs. Instead, they can often be treated by removing clothing, bathing the patient, and putting on clean bedding and clothes. Body lice are sensitive to heat, so washing clothes in hot water or using a clothes dryer can eliminate both adult lice and eggs.

The head louse, *Pediculus humanus capitis,* is 1 to 2 mm long and lives on the scalp and hair, but not on eyebrows or lashes. Head lice infestation is one of the most common contagious diseases in the United States. Children are the age group at greatest risk because they play in close contact and often share possessions.

Head lice are not generally believed to transmit any viral or bacterial diseases. They feed on blood from the scalp, which produces the intense pruritus. A female head louse has a life span of 40 days, during which she lays approximately ten eggs (nits) per day. These nits are cemented to hair shafts close to the scalp and take advantage of body heat, which helps them to hatch in approximately 8 days. This is why the treatment must be repeated. The nits are best seen by shining a bright light on the scalp. They appear white and look like dandruff. They cannot be shaken off. Figure 15.8 shows an adult head louse and a nit. Head lice are transmitted by direct contact.

Pubic, or crab, lice are 0.8 to 1.2 mm long and live in the pubic area. The infestation may resemble dermatitis and be very itchy; corticosteroids worsen this condition. Pubic lice are transmitted by sexual contact and should be treated so as to eliminate the parasite. In rare cases, pubic lice may inhabit the scalp.

Table 15.7 presents the most commonly used agents for lice. The OTC drugs available are as effective as the prescription drugs for treating lice.

FIGURE 15.8
Human Head Louse

(a) Adult on hair (b) Nit on hair shaft

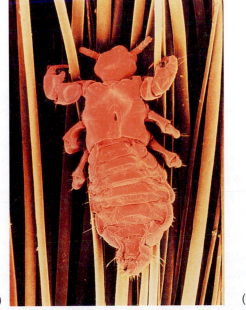

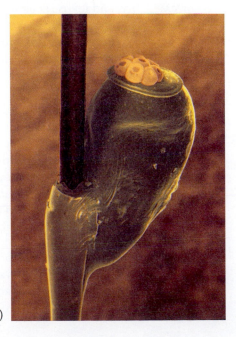

(a)

(b)

TABLE 15.7   Most Commonly Used Agents for Lice

Generic Name	Pronunciation	Dosage Form	Brand Name	Dispensing Status
crotamiton	kroe-TAM-i-ton	cream, lotion	Eurax	Rx
lindane	LIN-dane	lotion, shampoo	(none)	Rx
permethrin	per-METH-rin	cream, lotion	Elimite	Rx
			Nix	OTC
pyrethrins	pye-REE-thrins	shampoo, spray	Rid Mousse	OTC

Instructions to the patient vary with the type of lice infestation.

- **Body Lice:** Shower or bathe and apply 20 g to 30 g of cream or lotion to the whole body from the neck down; then wash off in 24 hours. Repeat in one week.
- **Head Lice:** Massage 2 ounces or less of cream or lotion into premoistened hair for 4 minutes, and rinse out. Repeat after 1 week. The repetition is important so as to eliminate eggs.
- **Pubic Lice:** Apply a thin layer of cream or lotion that extends to the thighs, trunk, and axillary regions; wash off within 24 hours. Repeat in 1 week.

For both head and pubic lice, it is important to comb the hair with a clean, fine-toothed comb to remove the nits.

Lindane is used for treating head, body, and pubic lice. It is directly absorbed by the parasites and ova through the exoskeleton; it stimulates their nervous systems, causing seizures and death. This drug requires a prescription and is for topical use only. Very specific instructions come with the product. Clothing and bedding should be washed in hot water or dry-cleaned. Combs and brushes may be washed with lindane shampoo and then thoroughly rinsed with water. This drug should be used as a second-line effort after first trying an OTC medication. Lindane can cause neurotoxicity, and its use is banned in some states. Preparations can be irritating to the eyes, mucous membranes, and skin. Overuse may cause dermatitis.

Pyrethrin (Rid Mousse), which is extracted from chrysanthemum seeds, is an OTC drug usually used for head lice. The mechanism of action involves disruption of lice neuronal transmission and is similar to the action of the now-banned insecticide DDT. Pyrethrin and lindane are similarly efficacious, but pyrethrin is less toxic. Pyrethrin must be applied to premoistened hair and scalp for 10 minutes and then rinsed off; treatment is repeated in 1 week. Patients sensitive to ragweed may be sensitive to impurities in pyrethrins.

Permethrin (Elimite, Nix) is at least as effective as lindane, with the advantage that, unlike lindane, it produces virtually no effects on the central nervous system (CNS). A 1% concentration is the drug of choice for treating head lice. It has residual action lasting up to 14 days that continues to kill any lice hatched after the initial application. It is available as an OTC drug.

Scabies Scabies is produced by small (0.2–0.4 mm long), eyeless, white-colored, flattened mites with an oval shape (Figure 15.9). Along with spiders and ticks, mites belong to the class of animals called arachnids (similar to insects, but having eight legs rather than six).

FIGURE 15.9
Scabies Mite

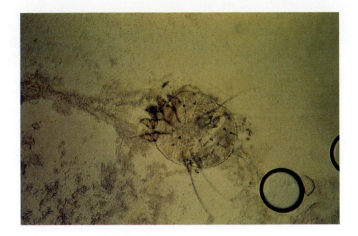

The female mite burrows into the epidermis and secretes substances that disintegrate the skin; she then digests the skin and sucks the intercellular fluid. No blood is consumed, because the capillaries are below the epidermis. The mite deposits fecal pellets that probably cause the intense itch.

When infected, the patient experiences an intense itching that worsens at night after the bed is warmed by body heat. This intense itching may be due to increased activity, feeding, and excretion of the mites. Lesions appear as very small, wavy, thread-like, slightly elevated, grayish-white burrows, most often in the finger webs. Burrows usually are from 1 mm to 10 mm long. Figure 15.10 shows the common sites of scabies infestation.

Some of the products used for lice infestation are also effective for treating scabies. The common treatment consists of a 25% benzoyl benzoate cream or lotion that is spread over the entire skin from the neck down at bedtime. The application should be repeated in the morning. Repeated treatment is rarely needed. Persistent inflammation and itching may be due to scratching, contact dermatitis, or a secondary infection rather than the mite infestation. Additional applications could cause dermatitis. A 5 to 10% sulfur ointment should be used for infants under 2 years of age. This is preferred because of potential absorption of gamma benzene hexachloride with neurological toxicity.

FIGURE 15.10
Sites of Scabies
Infestation

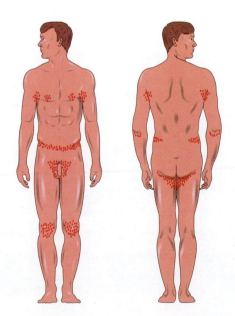

Antiseptics and Disinfectants

Chemicals have long been used to control **suppuration** (formation or discharge of pus), to control the spread of disease, and to preserve food. Investigators such as Robert Koch and Louis Pasteur in the middle of the nineteenth century showed that infection and putrefaction were due to microorganisms. Nevertheless, it was only after Joseph Lister, in the 1860s and 1870s, developed techniques for antiseptic surgery and the control of postoperative sepsis that physicians began to appreciate the importance of disinfecting the skin of the patient undergoing surgery, the hands of the surgeon, the instruments, and the operating theater.

A variety of agents, listed in Table 15.8, are used as antiseptics and disinfectants. These chemicals have specific actions.

The most desirable property of a germicide is its ability to destroy microorganisms rapidly and completely. No single germicide is equally effective against all types of organisms. Furthermore, many agents that rapidly destroy organisms may be too toxic to be applied to human or animal tissue cells. Esthetic factors, such as odor, taste, and staining quality, may also influence germicide selection. If a germicide is used in or around the mouth, bad odor or taste may reduce patient compliance. Patients may also object to materials that stain the oral mucosa, skin, or clothing.

Antiseptics and disinfectants have two uses. They are used to disinfect instruments and to treat accessible infections in the oral cavity and on body surfaces. The ideal antiseptic must possess the ability to inhibit all forms of infectious organisms without being toxic to the patient or inducing sensitization of human tissues. It should be capable of penetrating tissues and of acting in the presence of body fluids (i.e., serum, pus, and mucus). It should be soluble in water, stable, noncorrosive, and inexpensive. No agent meets all these requirements. If an antiseptic is to be used to clean instruments or to maintain sterility in a clean room, it is always best to use two separate agents with different mechanisms of action. Table 15.9 lists the most commonly used antiseptics and disinfectants. The oral cavity is very difficult to disinfect. Very few drugs will adhere to the mucosal lining long enough to overcome bacteria or ease pain.

Heavy metal compounds, in concentrations as low as one part per million, inhibit microorganisms. These ions have a strong affinity for proteins. Activity is reduced in the presence of organic matter (mucus). These compounds are irritating and astringent (causing constriction or drawing together). They do not consistently kill bacteria.

TABLE 15.8   Actions of Antiseptics and Disinfectants

Agent	Action
antiseptic	a substance that inhibits growth and development of microorganisms, but does not necessarily kill them
disinfectant	a chemical applied to objects to free them from pathogenic organisms or render such organisms inert
fungicide	a substance that destroys fungi
germicide	a substance that destroys bacteria, but not necessarily spores
preservative	an agent that prevents decomposition by either chemical or physical means
sanitizer	an agent that reduces the number of bacterial contaminants to a safe level
sporicide	a substance that destroys spores

TABLE 15.9   Most Commonly Used Antiseptics and Disinfectants

Generic Name	Pronunciation	Dosage Form	Brand Name	Dispensing Status
hexachlorophene	hex-a-KLOR-oh-feen	liquid antiseptic	pHisoHex	OTC
isopropyl alcohol	eye-so-PROE-pil AL-koe-hawl	liquid disinfectant	(many)	OTC
povidone-iodine	POE-vi-done EYE-oh-dyne	aerosol, antiseptic, cream, douche, foam, gel, ointment, shampoo, solution, suppository	Betadine	OTC
sodium hypochlorite	SOE-dee-um hye-poe-KLOR-ite	liquid disinfectant	Clorox	OTC
Heavy Metal Compounds				
zinc oxide	ZINK OX-ide	ointment	Desitin Creamy	OTC
Orals				
benzocaine	BEN-zoe-kayn	gel, paste, spray	Hurricaine	Rx
			Orabase-B	OTC
carbamide peroxide	KAR-ba-mide per-OX-ide	solution	Gly-Oxide Oral	OTC
chlorhexidine gluconate	klor-HEX-i-deen GLOO-koe-nate	oral liquid antiseptic	Hibiclens	OTC
clove oil	KLOVE OIL	oil	Eugenol	OTC
Others				
benzalkonium chloride	benz-al-KOE-nee-um KLOR-ide	solution	Zephiran	OTC
hydrogen peroxide	HYE-droe-jen per-OX-ide	solution	(many)	OTC
phenytoin	fen-i-TOE-in	capsule	Dilantin	Rx

Since the advent of new chemicals with better properties, heavy metal compounds are infrequently used as antiseptics or disinfectants.

Isopropyl alcohol is supplied in 70% or 90% concentrations. This alcohol is inexpensive, spreads well, dries slowly, and does not extract cutaneous fats. It primarily removes bacteria, but can also kill some bacteria. Isopropyl alcohol denatures proteins and produces a marked stinging reaction when applied to cuts or abrasions. To be effective, alcohol must dry and be left on the wound being administered to for at least 2 minutes.

Sodium hypochlorite (Clorox) disinfects and deodorizes by killing most germs and their odors. It is a common laundry and household product (chlorine bleach) that is used in cleaning and stain removal.

Hexachlorophene (pHisoHex) is a surgical scrub and bacteriostatic skin cleanser that is especially effective if gram-positive infection is present. It should not be left on skin for long periods of time.

Povidone-iodine (Betadine) is an aqueous solution that does not stain and causes little discomfort when applied to an open wound. It is among the most effective disinfectants available. It has a broad microbicidal spectrum against bacteria, fungi, viruses, protozoa, and yeasts.

Zinc oxide is a mild antiseptic and astringent used for some conjunctival and skin diseases. It is the main ingredient in calamine lotion. The oxide salt, a zinc salt, is combined with a petroleum jelly and a waxy lanolin base for use in treating diaper rash and other minor skin irritations.

Benzalkonium chloride (Zephiran) is used as a preoperative skin disinfectant and for storing instruments and hospital utensils.

Hydrogen peroxide is a strongly disinfecting, cleansing, and bleaching agent. It is used to prepare dental surfaces before filling and to clean wounds. The release of oxygen provides the antiseptic action.

Phenytoin (Dilantin) can be used as a topical for wound healing. It speeds the process by stimulating the growth of collagen fibroblasts through its side effects. The same process that causes gingival hyperplasia causes the wound to heal. (Open a 100 mg capsule and sprinkle the contents in 5 mL of sterile saline. Soak gauze in it and place the gauze over the wound.) There are no systemic effects.

Chlorhexidine gluconate (Hibiclens) is a skin cleanser for surgical scrub, skin wounds, germicidal hand rinse, and antibacterial dental rinse. It is active against gram-positive and gram-negative organisms and yeast. Studies show that patients on ventilators who have scheduled mouth cleansings throughout the day with chlorhexidine gluconate have significantly decreased incidences of pneumonia.

Clove oil (Eugenol) is an antiseptic used on exposed dentin. Mixed with zinc oxide or zinc acetate, it is used as dental applications in temporary fillings and cements and in periodontal and intra-alveolar packs.

Carbamide peroxide (Gly-Oxide Oral) releases oxygen on contact with oral tissues and reduces inflammation, inhibits odor-forming bacteria, and relieves pain in periodontal pockets, oral ulcers, and dental sores. It is also used to **emulsify** (enable mixing with water) and disperse earwax.

Benzocaine (Hurricaine, Orabase-B) is a local anesthetic, but it also forms a protective barrier over the mucosa. The patient should not eat for an hour after applying to oral mucosa. Benzocaine should not be applied to broken skin.

Eye Conditions and Ophthalmic Medications

Ophthalmic medications are used to treat the eyes. The internal structures of the eye, shown in Figure 15.11, are subject to various disorders including cytomegalovirus (CMV) retinitis, age-related macular degeneration, chronic dry eye, and conjunctivitis. Table 15.10 lists the ophthalmic agents used to treat these conditions. Agents used to treat glaucoma, another serious eye disorder, will be listed and discussed later in this chapter. Because patients and medical personnel can easily confuse the words "ophthalmic" and "otic" (the latter are medications intended to treat ear conditions), the medications should be clearly labeled. Antibiotics, some of which are used to treat eye and ear infections, were discussed in Chapter 4.

Many ophthalmic agents are supplied as liquids to be placed in the eye (eyedrops). It is important for the patient and the pharmacy technician to understand the general procedure for applying eyedrops. The first step, as with any procedure in which a substance is introduced into the body, is to wash the hands thoroughly. If the liquid needs to be mixed, shake the container. Then remove the bottle cap and draw up liquid in the eyedropper. To apply the eyedrops, tilt the head back and pull the lower eyelid down. Hold the tip of the eyedropper directly over the eye but do not allow it to

FIGURE 15.11
The Structures of the Eye

(a) The external eye
(b) Sagittal view of the internal eye

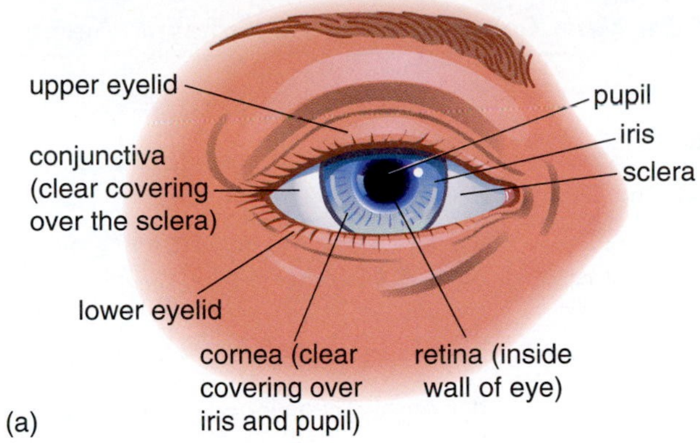

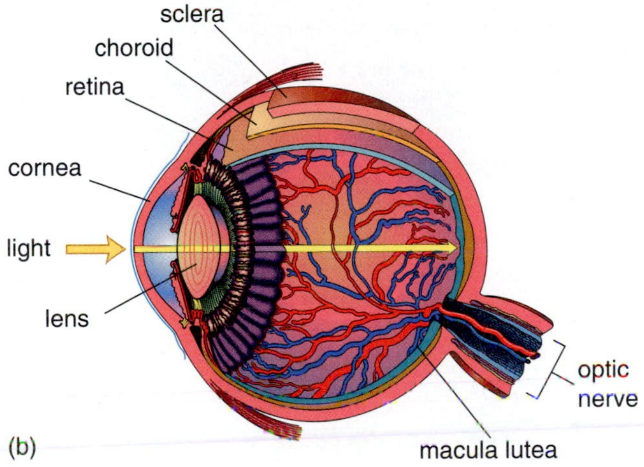

upper eyelid

pupil
iris
sclera

conjunctiva (clear covering over the sclera)

lower eyelid

cornea (clear covering over iris and pupil)

retina (inside wall of eye)

(a)

sclera
choroid
retina
cornea
light
lens

optic nerve

(b)

macula lutea

come in contact with the eye or adjacent tissues. Contact between the dropper and the body can transmit infection. With the patient looking up, place a drop in the pocket behind the lower lid. Release the eyelid. Replace the cap on the container and wash the hands again. Wait 5 or 10 minutes before applying any other medication to the eye. Ophthalmic ointments are to be placed in the pocket behind the lower eyelid in a similar manner.

For the EYE

CMV Retinitis

Cytomegalovirus (CMV) retinitis is an inflammation of the retina caused by a viral infection. Fomivirsen (Vitravene) is an intravitreal injection used to treat this condition. The drug blocks the replication of the CMV by binding to the messenger ribonucleic acid (mRNA) of the affected cells, preventing the synthesis of viral proteins. Because its mechanism of action differs from that of other antiviral agents, fomivirsen may be effective against viral isolates that have developed resistance to ganciclovir, foscarnet, or cidofovir. Because of its side effects, fomivirsen should be used only after other treatments have failed. Uveitis (inflammation of the iris, ciliary body, and choroid) is a frequent occurrence with this drug. It will also increase intraocular pressure. It is administered by intravitreal injection following the application of standard topical and/or local anesthetics and antibiotics.

TABLE 15.10 Most Commonly Used Ophthalmic Agents

Generic Name	Pronunciation	Dosage Form	Brand Name	Dispensing Status
Corticosteroids and Combinations				
bacitracin–neomycin–polymyxin B–hydrocortisone	bas-i-TRAY-sin nee-oh-MYE-sin pol-i-MIX-in B hye-droe-KOR-ti-sone	ointment	Cortisporin Ointment	Rx
dexamethasone	dex-a-METH-a-sone	solution	AK-Dex	Rx
fluorometholone	flor-oh-METH-oe-lone	suspension	FML Forte	Rx
loteprednol	loe-te-PRED-nol	suspension	Alrex, Lotemax	Rx
neomycin–polymyxin B–dexamethasone	nee-oh-MYE-sin pol-i-MIX-in B dex-a-METH-a-sone	ointment, suspension	Maxitrol	Rx
sulfacetamide-prednisolone	sul-fa-SEE-ta-mide pred-NIS-oe-lone	suspension	Blephamide	Rx
tobramycin-dexamethasone	toe-bra-MYE-sin dex-a-METH-a-sone	ointment, suspension	TobraDex	Rx
Antifungal				
natamycin	na-ta-MYE-sin	suspension	Natacyn	Rx
Decongestant				
naphazoline	naf-AZ-oh-leen	solution	AK-Con, Vasocon	Rx
			Naphcon A	OTC
Antivirals				
fomivirsen	foe-mi-VEER-sen	injection	Vitravene	Rx
ganciclovir	gan-SYE-kloe-veer	implant	Vitrasert	Rx
trifluridine	trye-FLOO-ri-deen	solution	Viroptic	Rx
Mast Cell Stabilizers				
cromolyn sodium	KROE-moe-lin SOE-dee-um	solution	Crolom	Rx
pemirolast	pe-MEER-oh-last	solution	Alamast	Rx
Antihistamines				
epinastine	ep-i-NAS-teen	solution	Elestat	Rx
ketotifen	kee-toe-TYE-fen	solution	Zaditor	Rx
olopatadine	oh-loe-PAT-a-deen	solution	Patanol	Rx
NSAIDs				
diclofenac	di-KLOE-fen-ak	solution, tablet	Voltaren	Rx
flurbiprofen	flure-BYE-proe-fen	solution	Ocufen	Rx
ketorolac	kee-toe-ROE-lak	solution	Acular	Rx
Others				
cyclosporine	SYE-kloe-spor-een	solution	Restasis	Rx
verteporfin	ver-te-POR-fin	injection	Visudyne	Rx
vitamin C–vitamin E–zinc–beta carotene	VYE-ta-min C VYE-ta-min E ZINK BAY-ta KAIR-oe-teen	tablet	Ocuvite PreserVision	OTC

Ganciclovir (Vitrasert) is approved for CMV. It must surgically be inserted and it releases ganciclovir for approximately 6 months. Patients will commonly also receive systemic therapy with this drug.

Age-Related Macular Degeneration

When light enters the eye, it is focused onto the center of the retina in an area called the macula. The macula has the highest concentration of photoreceptors in the eye and provides the high-resolution central vision that is used for reading, driving, recognizing faces, and many other tasks. For some people, as they age, the maculas deteriorate. Two types of age-related macular degeneration (AMD) are recognized. In dry AMD, the light-sensitive cells in the macula slowly break down, and vision is slowly lost. In wet AMD, new blood vessels behind the retina grow toward the macula. These new vessels are fragile and blood and other fluids leak from them under the macula. As scar tissue forms at the site of vessel rupture, damage occurs, and central vision is lost rapidly.

Pain is not a symptom of either type of AMD. Patients with dry AMD may notice visual changes such as slightly blurred vision or the need for more light for reading and other tasks. As the condition worsens, a blurred spot appears in the center of vision and enlarges with time. For wet AMD, an early symptom is a wavy appearance of truly straight lines. This effect occurs as fluids and blood leak under the macula, causing it to rise and thereby distorting vision.

The cause of AMD is unknown, but age is the greatest risk factor. Cigarette smoking may also put one at risk. Research has shown that an elevated C-reactive protein level may also be associated with increased risk of AMD. Yellow spots within the macula may indicate a risk for AMD, although the spots themselves may not affect vision. Patients usually develop problems in both eyes, but the eyes may not be equally affected.

Wet AMD can be treated with laser surgery to seal leaking vessels; this helps to stop further vision loss. Dry AMD cannot currently be treated. There is some indication, though, that high levels of antioxidants and zinc can reduce the risk of advanced AMD.

Verteporfin (Visudyne) is a light-activated drug that is injected intravenously. It is used to treat certain forms of AMD. The lesion is irradiated with a diode laser. The laser causes verteporfin to generate free radicals that damage the newly forming blood vessels without affecting the retina. This treatment can be repeated every three months as needed. The major side effects are headache, oozing, and rash at the injection site and vision changes.

Vitamins C and E, zinc, and beta carotene (Ocuvite PreserVision) may slow the progress of AMD in people who already have it. It comes in an oral tablet. Two tablets should be taken in the morning and two in the evening, both with meals. The drug provides 500 mg of vitamin C, 400 International Units of vitamin E, 15 mg of vitamin A as beta carotene, 80 mg of zinc oxide, and 2 mg of copper as daily amounts. It does not cure the disease or prevent people with early signs from contracting it. Smokers should not take beta carotene. The combination seems to increase the risk of prostate and lung cancer.

Chronic Dry Eye

Keratococonjunctivitis (dry eye) is a medical condition that can result when the eye is unable to produce sufficient tears to lubricate and nourish the eye.

Cyclosporine (Restasis) for ophthalmic use is approved for patients with chronic dry eye. It increases tears by means of anti-inflammatory and immune modulating effects. The drug is not absorbed systemically but decreases immune function in the eye. It is provided by the manufacturer as single-use vials. Patients can continue to use artificial tears but need to wait 15 minutes between applications.

Conjunctivitis

Conjunctivitis (pink eye) is another common eye disorder. It is an inflammation of the membrane that covers the inside of the eyelid and the outside of the eyeball and is evidenced by many signs and symptoms including increased tearing, itching, chemosis (conjunctival swelling), and hyperemia (redness). Conjunctivitis may be caused by infections or allergies. Treatments include topical vasoconstrictors, mast cell stabilizers, antihistamines, corticosteroids, antibiotics, and antivirals.

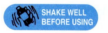

Loteprednol (Alrex, Lotemax) is an ophthalmic corticosteroid prescribed to relieve signs and symptoms of seasonal allergic conjunctivitis. It is also prescribed for the treatment of postoperative inflammation following ocular surgery. Loteprednol is less likely to increase intraocular pressure because it converts to an inactive metabolite in the eye. Patients should be reevaluated if symptoms fail to improve after 2 days of treatment. A sticker should be placed on the bottle instructing patients to shake the medication before using it. Alrex is a 0.2% solution, and Lotemax is a 0.5% solution.

Pemirolast (Alamast) is a mast cell stabilizer that inhibits the chemotaxis of eosinophils into the ocular tissue and blocks their release of mediators. Alamast is also believed to prevent the influx of calcium into mast cells that occurs following antigen stimulation. It is approved for itching due to allergic conjunctivitis. Itching may decrease within a few days, but 4 weeks of treatment are generally required for complete remission. Patients who wear soft contact lenses should be instructed to wait at least 10 minutes after administering Alamast before inserting their lenses.

Ketotifen (Zaditor) is an H_1 blocker indicated for the treatment of conjunctivitis. This drug must not be used to treat contact lens–related irritation. Contact lens wearers should allow 10 minutes between the administration of the eyedrops and the insertion of their lenses. Care should be taken not to contaminate the dropper or bottle.

Epinastine (Elestat) is an antihistamine approved for ocular itching in patients with conjunctivitis. It is selective for the H_1 receptors and does not penetrate the blood-brain barrier; therefore, epinastine is not expected to induce CNS side effects. It has a rapid onset of action, and the patient should feel relief in 3 to 5 minutes. The primary side effect of epinastine is brief burning.

Olopatadine (Patanol) is also an antihistamine approved for allergic conjunctivitis.

Gatifloxacin (Zymar) and **moxifloxacin (Vigamox)** are quinolone antibiotics indicated for the treatment of conjunctivitis.

Glaucoma

Glaucoma is the most common eye disease. Drug treatment can control glaucoma but cannot cure it. Glaucoma is a chronic disorder characterized by abnormally high internal eye pressure that destroys the optic nerve and causes partial to complete loss of vision. The increased intraocular pressure is due to an imbalance between production and drainage of the liquid (**aqueous humor**) in the front portion of the eye; obstruction of normal drainage is the main mechanism.

Three types of glaucoma are recognized: open-angle glaucoma, narrow-angle glaucoma, and secondary glaucoma. In open-angle glaucoma, the angle of the anterior chamber remains open, but filtration is gradually diminished because of the tissues of the angle. This type is usually treated with drops, but many of these medications have systemic effects. Narrow-angle glaucoma is characterized by a shallow anterior chamber and a narrow angle in which filtration is compromised as a result of the iris blocking the angle. This is an acute form and is treated as soon as possible by laser iridotomy. Open-angle and narrow-angle glaucoma occur in individuals with a hereditary predisposition. In secondary glaucoma, the increased intraocular pressure is due to disease or injury to the eye.

The goals of treatment are prompt reduction of intraocular pressure in narrow-angle closure glaucoma and stabilization of eye status in preparation for corrective surgery; gradual reduction and long-term normalization of intraocular pressure in chronic, simple, and open-angle glaucoma; and prevention of optic nerve damage and preservation of vision in all cases. Patients should be instructed to avoid OTC drugs for cold remedies, appetite suppressants, drugs for motion sickness, and sleep aids.

Table 15.11 presents the most commonly used agents for glaucoma.

Brimonidine (Alphagan P) is a selective alpha-2 agonist that lowers intraocular pressure by reducing fluid production in the eye and increasing the outflow. For some cases, the effectiveness will diminish with time.

Apraclonidine (Iopidine) is an alpha-adrenergic agonist that reduces intraocular pressure, possibly by decreasing aqueous humor production. Systemic effects are uncommon.

Warning

Betoptic and Betagan are easily confused. Also, Betoptic and Betoptic S could be confused.

TABLE 15.11   Most Commonly Used Agents for Glaucoma

Generic Name	Pronunciation	Dosage Form	Brand Name	Dispensing Status
Eyedrops				
apraclonidine	a-pra-KLON-i-deen	solution	Iopidine	Rx
betaxolol	be-TAX-oe-lawl	solution, suspension	Betoptic	Rx
bimatoprost	bye-MAT-oe-prost	solution	Lumigan	Rx
brimonidine	bri-MOE-ni-deen	solution	Alphagan P	Rx
brinzolamide	brin-ZOE-la-mide	suspension	Azopt	Rx
carbachol	KAR-ba-kawl	solution	Carbastat, Miostat	Rx
dipivefrin	dye-pi-VEF-rin	solution	Propine	Rx
dorzolamide	dor-ZOLE-a-mide	solution	Trusopt	Rx
echothiophate iodide	ek-oh-THYE-oh-fate EYE-oh-dide	powder for reconstitution	Phospholine Iodide	Rx
latanoprost	la-TAN-oe-prost	solution	Xalatan	Rx
pilocarpine	pye-loe-KAR-peen	solution	Isopto Carpine	Rx
timolol	TYE-moe-lawl	solution	Timoptic	Rx
travoprost	TRAV-oe-prost	solution	Travatan	Rx
unoprostone	yoo-noe-PROS-tone	solution	Rescula	Rx
Oral Agent				
acetazolamide	a-set-a-ZOE-la-mide	capsule, injection, tablet	Diamox	Rx

Latanoprost (Xalatan) is a prostaglandin (PG) that reduces intraocular pressure by slowing the production of aqueous humor and increasing the drainage of fluid from the eye. It is approved only for patients who cannot tolerate other treatments. Latanoprost has an unusual side effect: it causes light-colored eyes to turn brown by increasing the pigment in the iris. Although latanoprost is stable at room temperature for 6 weeks, it should be stored in the refrigerator. With administration of latanoprost there may be a little burning, and eyelashes may lengthen and darken.

Brinzolamide (Azopt) inhibits carbonic anhydrase, which decreases aqueous humor secretion and resulting in a decrease in intraocular pressure. If more than one eyedrop is prescribed, they should be administered at least 10 minutes apart. Concurrent use of acetazolamide could result in additive effects and toxicity.

Dorzolamide (Trusopt) is a reversible inhibitor of carbonic anhydrase. The drug produces an increase of renal excretion of fluids, thereby decreasing aqueous humor. Dorzolamide also inhibits carbonic anhydrase in the CNS. Most patients complain of a bitter taste after administration. The patient should be instructed to discontinue the use of the drug if any eyelid or ocular reactions, such as conjunctivitis, occur. Ocular solutions can easily become contaminated by bacteria and can then cause serious damage to the eye. Thus, the patient should be told to avoid allowing the tip of the dropper to touch any part of the eye.

Travoprost (Travatan) is a prostaglandin (PG) analog. It lowers intraocular pressure by increasing the outflow of aqueous humor. The iris may become browner in color, and there may be an intolerance to light. This drug should not be administered in the evening and not while the patient is wearing contact lenses. Travoprost may cause migraine headaches.

Bimatoprost (Lumigan) is a synthetic structural analog of prostaglandin. Like the other PG analogs, it can change the color of the eye. As when instilling any eyedrops, do not let the dropper touch the eye. Also gently apply pressure to the inside corner of the eye for approximately 2 to 3 minutes. If the patient is using other drops in the same eye, the patient should wait 5 minutes between applications.

Unoprostone (Rescula) is a prostaglandin-related compound. It is a lipid substance derived from the fatty acid docosahexaenoic acid, which is a naturally occurring substance essential in the development and functioning of the retina. Unoprostone increases the outflow of aqueous humor. It should not be used if there is intraocular inflammation. Changes in the iris color may occur over a period of months to several years. The long-term effects and the consequences of potential injury to the eye are currently unknown.

Acetazolamide (Diamox), a carbonic anhydrase inhibitor, is the oral agent used to treat glaucoma. It is also used for altitude sickness. It inhibits the conversion of carbon dioxide to bicarbonate, increasing oxygenation.

Ear Conditions and Otic Medications

Figure 15.12 shows the structural components of the ear. Disorders of the ear range from **otalgia** (ear pain), earache, to buildups of earwax (cerumen). Otalgia is usually treated with a prescription drug. The only OTC medications for the ear are earwax solvents and a product to dry water in the ear canal after swimming. Wax dissolvers are used to emulsify and disperse excessive buildup of earwax. The pain relievers and antibiotics are all prescription medications. In fact, the OTC drugs can be very painful if someone tries to self-medicate an ear infection.

FIGURE 15.12
The Structural Components of the Ear

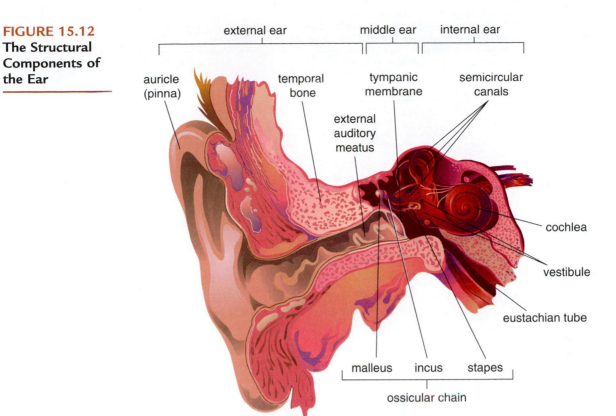

external ear   middle ear   internal ear

auricle (pinna)

temporal bone

tympanic membrane

semicircular canals

external auditory meatus

cochlea

vestibule

eustachian tube

malleus   incus   stapes

ossicular chain

Warning

It is easy to confuse an eyedrop and an eardrop. Watch the dispensing of these carefully.

Warning

Eyedrops in the ear are fine, but eardrops in the eye are not.

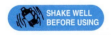

Table 15.12 lists the most commonly used otic agents. Eardrops come in solutions and suspensions. If the patient has a tube in the ear or a ruptured eardrum, a solution should not be used; only a suspension should be used. The physician may prescribe an ophthalmic agent to be used in the ear. This practice is quite common and is very effective. If an otic agent is accidentally put in the eyes, however, it is very painful. Eyedrops in the ear are fine, but eardrops in the eye are not. To avoid confusion, the pharmacy technician should clearly label all medications intended for application in the ear.

Antipyrine-benzocaine (Auralgan) is a topical anesthetic for otitis media that should be used three to four times a day. Immediate pain relief is important to the patient; physicians commonly forget this aspect of treatment. If a preparation for an otic antibiotic is not accompanied by one for pain relief, the technician should inform the pharmacist, who may choose to contact the physician. The patient and caregivers will probably be very grateful.

Ciprofloxacin-dexamethasone (Ciprodex) combines a quinolone antibiotic and a steroid to fight bacteria and reduce inflammation caused by infection. It is always a good practice to warm eardrops by holding them in the hands 1 or 2 minutes. Patients or caregivers should shake the drops just before administering. Ciprodex is used twice a day, 12 hours apart. Patients should avoid getting water in the infected ear.

TABLE 15.12   Most Commonly Used Otic Agents

Generic Name	Pronunciation	Dosage Form	Brand Name	Dispensing Status
Analgesic				
antipyrine-benzocaine	an-tee-PYE-reen BEN-zoe-kane	solution	Auralgan	Rx
Antibiotics				
ciprofloxacin-dexamethasone	sip-roe-FLOX-a-sin dex-a-METH-a-sone	suspension	Ciprodex	Rx
neomycin–polymyxin B–hydrocortisone	nee-oh-MYE-sin pol-i-MIX-in B hye-droe-KOR-ti-sone	solution, suspension	Cortisporin Otic	Rx
Wax Dissolvers				
carbamide peroxide	KAR-ba-mide per-OX-ide	solution	Debrox	OTC
triethanolamine polypeptide–oleate condensate	trye-eth-a-NOE-la-meen pol-i-PEP-tide OH-lee-ate KON-den-sate	solution	Cerumenex	Rx

Chapter Terms

acne vulgaris an inflammation of the skin, usually on the face and neck, that is caused by increased activity of the sebaceous glands at puberty

actinic keratosis a scaly skin lesion that is caused by too much sun and can lead to skin cancer

aqueous humor the liquid in the front portion of the eye

atopic eczema a chronic pruritic eruption of unknown etiology, although allergic, hereditary, and psychogenic factors may be involved; also called atopic dermatitis

basal cell carcinoma a slow-growing skin cancer that usually forms polyps and rarely metastasizes

beyond-use date the date after which a drug should not be used once it has been removed from the intact container

candidiasis a fungal infection (*Candida albicans*) most commonly involving the oral and vaginal mucosa

carbuncle a coalescent mass of infected hair follicles that are deeper than furuncles

conjunctivitis pink eye; inflammation of the membrane covering the inside of the eyelid and the outside of the eyeball

contact dermatitis an inflammatory reaction produced by contact with an irritating agent

dermatome area of the skin associated with one pair of nerves emerging horizontally from the spinal cord

dermis layer of skin below the epidermis

eczema a hot, itchy, red, oozing skin inflammation; also called dermatitis

emulsify To break a liquid that does not dissolve in water into small globules that can be suspended in water

epidermis the top layer of the skin

erysipelas a skin infection characterized by redness and warmth, local pain, edematous plaque with sharply established borders, chills, malaise, and fever; a form of cellulitis

folliculitis an inflammation of a hair follicle by a minute, red, pustulated nodule without involvement of the surrounding tissue

furuncle a boil; caused by a staphylococcal infection of a sebaceous gland and the associated hair follicle

glaucoma a chronic eye disorder characterized by abnormally high internal eye pressure that destroys the optic nerve and causes partial or complete loss of vision

impetigo a superficial, highly contagious skin infection; characterized by small red spots that evolve into vesicles, break, become encrusted, and are surrounded by a zone of erythema

keratoacanthoma an epithelial skin tumor that first grows rapidly and then regresses and heals

melanoma a highly malignant skin cancer formed from pigmented skin cells

otalgia earache

pediculosis an infestation of lice

petechiae minute red spots on the skin due to the escape of a small amount of blood

phototoxicity a property of a chemical that becomes toxic on exposure to light

photosensitivity an abnormal response of the skin or eye to sunlight

psoriasis a skin disorder characterized by patches of red, scaly skin that are slightly raised with defined margins; usually occurs on the elbows and knees but can affect any part of the body

retinoid a compound related to vitamin A that helps to regulate skin cell growth

ringworm a fungus that infects the horny (scaly) layer of skin or the nails; also called tinea

rosacea chronic dermatologic disorder involving inflammation of the skin of the face; also called acne rosacea

seborrhea a skin condition caused by excessive secretion by the sebaceous glands; gives the skin an oily appearance

squamous cell carcinoma a skin cancer that grows more rapidly than basal cell carcinoma but in which metastasis is uncommon

suppuration formation or discharge of pus

teratogenic causing birth defects

wart a virally caused epidermal tumor

Chapter Summary

Skin Ailments and Their Treatment

- The skin is a major organ in the human body and accounts for 10% of body weight. It is the main organ involved in temperature regulation.
- The dermis is composed of connective tissue with upward projections into the epidermis.
- Two types of glands receive widespread distribution in the skin: sebaceous glands and sweat glands.
- Earwax is made of secretions, squamous cells, and dust. It has antibacterial and antifungal activity.
- When filling a prescription, creams, gels, and ointments are not interchangeable.

Ultraviolet Radiation, Phototoxicity, and Photosensitivity

- A suntan may look good but can permanently damage the skin.
- A sunscreen should contain a combination of oxybenzone and para-aminobenzoic acid or other UV-absorbing agents that protect against both UV-A and UV-B rays.
- Some classes of drugs that cause photosensitivity are antidepressants, antihistamines, antibiotics, antipsychotics, chemotherapeutic agents, diuretics, hypoglycemics, NSAIDs, and cardiovascular drugs, including ACE inhibitors.

- Solagé combines the synergistic action of two drugs (mequinol and tretinoin) to treat damaged skin.

Skin Disorders and Their Pharmaceutical Treatment

- Acne is treated with tretinoin, azelaic acid, and adapalene. It is also treated systemically and topically with tetracycline, erythromycin, azithromycin, or clindamycin.
- Oral contraceptives can have a beneficial effect on acne.
- A lower dose of tretinoin, Renova, is used for wrinkles.
- Several systemic diseases, such as liver disease, uremia, Hodgkin disease, diabetes, and thyroid disease, can cause itching. Pregnancy, senility, and various psychological disorders can also cause excessive itching.
- Camphor in liniments and ointments has a cooling and antipruritic effect. Antihistamines may also be used to relieve itching.
- Warts are caused by a virus.
- Psoriasis is a chronic noncontagious condition with no cure. It is treated with corticosteroids, methotrexate, alefacept (Amevive), and calcipotriene (Dovonex).
- Dandruff is treated with selenium sulfide.
- Eflornithine (Vaniqa) is approved to treat unwanted facial hair in females.

- Actinic keratosis is a precancerous condition resulting from excessive exposure to the sun. It can be treated with fluorouracil (Efudex) and aminolevulinic acid (Levulan).
- Atopic dermatitis is a chronic pruritic eruption of unknown etiology; allergic, hereditary, and psychogenic factors may be involved. It is treated with doxepin (Zonalon), a topical tricyclic antidepressant with strong antihistaminic effects.
- Ringworm is caused by a fungus.
- Butenafine (Lotrimin) and terbinafine (Lamisil) are frequently used to treat ringworm.
- Antifungals are often administered through pulse dosing to treat conditions under the nails. Always read the generic name of these over the counter drugs, because they may not be what you think they are. Lotrimin may be butenafine, clotrimazone, or miconazole.

Skin Infections

- Skin infections are common, and most can be managed with nonprescription topical antimicrobial products.
- Impetigo is a highly contagious skin infection common in early childhood.

Topical Corticosteroids

- Topical corticosteroids should be applied sparingly as a very thin film. Significant quantities may reach the systemic circulation because they can penetrate the skin. Depending on the type of steroid, the quantity used, and the amount absorbed, suppression of the hypothalamus-pituitary axis may occur.
- Only the 0.5% hydrocortisone OTC creams should be used on children. Their skin can be easily penetrated, and the 1% creams could be too strong if used repeatedly.
- Hydrocortisone is the drug of choice for most cases of poison ivy. Severe poison ivy may require short-term treatment with oral corticosteroids.

- Creams and ointments are generally not interchangeable.
- Usually, ointments are stronger than creams, and gels are somewhere in between.
- Most superpotent topical corticosteroids have restrictions limiting their use to 2 consecutive weeks of treatment and/or a maximum of 45 g to 50 g in any one week. (Psorcon) is an exception.

External Parasites

- Head lice infestations are among the most common contagious diseases in the United States.
- The OTC drugs available are as effective as the prescription drugs when treating lice. Some products used for lice infestation are effective for treating mites.

Antiseptics and Disinfectants

- When an antiseptic is used to disinfect instruments or to maintain sterility in a clean room, it is always best to use two separate cleansers with different mechanisms of action.
- Phenytoin (Dilantin) capsules can be compounded into a mixture that will accelerate wound healing.

Eye Conditions and Ophthalmic Medications

- Conjunctivitis is a common eye disorder, and treatments include topical vasoconstrictors, mast cell stabilizers, antihistamines, corticosteroids, antibiotics, and antivirals.
- Eyedrops, as well as an oral medication, can be used to treat glaucoma.

Ear Conditions and Otic Medications

- The pharmacist should dispense only the suspension dosage form of an otic if the patient has tubes in the ears or a ruptured eardrum.

- Ophthalmics (eyedrops) are often prescribed for use in the ear, but otics (eardrops) should never be used in the eye. Antibiotic eyedrops are frequently dispensed for ear infections.

- Antipyrine-benzocaine (Auralgan) is a topical anesthetic dispensed as an eardrop; it can be very effective for ear pain.

Drug List

The following drugs were discussed in this chapter.

Sun-Damaged Skin
aloe gel
aspirin
benzocaine (Dermoplast)
hydrocortisone (Anusol-HC, Cortaid, Solu-Cortef)
lidocaine (Solarcaine)
mequinol-tretinoin (Solagé)
vitamin A
vitamin C
vitamin E

Skin Diseases and Disorders

Acne Vulgaris
adapalene (Differin)
azelaic acid (Azelex)
azithromycin (Zithromax)
benzoyl peroxide (Brevoxyl, Zoderm)
clindamycin–benzoyl peroxide (BenzaClin)
isotretinoin (Accutane, Claravis)
tazarotene (Avage, Tazorac)
tetracycline
tretinoin (Retin-A, Vesanoid)

Wrinkles
botulinum toxin type A (Botox)
tretinoin (Renova)

Psoriasis and Eczema
acitretin (Soriatane)
alefacept (Amevive)
calcipotriene (Dovonex)
coal tar (Cutar, Tarsum)
cyclosporine (Neoral)
doxepin (Zonalon)
efalizumab (Raptiva)
methotrexate (Rheumatrex, Trexall)

pimecrolimus (Elidel)*
tacrolimus (Protopic)
tazarotene (Tazorac)
urea (Carmol, Keralac)

Viral Infections
acyclovir (Zovirax)
diethyl ether (Wartner)
docosanol (Abreva)
imiquimod (Aldara)
penciclovir (Denavir)

Dandruff
selenium sulfide (Head & Shoulders Intensive Treatment, Selsun Blue)

Unwanted Facial Hair
eflornithine (Vaniqa)

Actinic Keratosis
aminolevulinic acid (Levulan)
diclofenac (Solaraze)
fluorouracil (Efudex)
imiquimod (Aldara)

Fungal Infections
amphotericin B (Fungizone)
butenafine (Lotrimin Ultra, Mentax)
ciclopirox (Loprox)
clotrimazole (Gyne-Lotrimin, Lotrimin, Mycelex)
clotrimazole-betamethasone (Lotrisone)*
econazole (Spectazole)
griseofulvin (Fulvicin-U/F, Grifulvin V)
itraconazole (Sporanox)
ketoconazole (Xolegel, Nizoral)
miconazole (Monistat)
miconazole–zinc oxide (Vusion)

nystatin (Mycostatin, Nilstat)
oxiconazole (Oxistat)
sertaconazole (Ertaczo)
sulconazole (Exelderm)
terbinafine (Lamisil, Lamisil AT)
tolnaftate (Tinactin Antifungal)

Antibiotics for Skin Infections
azelaic acid (Finacea)
bacitracin–neomycin–polymyxin B (Triple
    Antibiotic, Neosporin, Mycitracin)
clindamycin (Cleocin T)
erythromycin (Eryderm, T-Stat)
mafenide (Sulfamylon)
metronidazole (MetroGel)
mupirocin (Bactroban)*
neomycin–polymyxin B (Neosporin G.U.
    Irrigant)
retapamulin (Altabax)
silver sulfadiazine (Silvadene)
sulfur-sulfacetamide (Rosac, Rosula)

Topical Steroids
alclometasone (Aclovate)
amcinonide (Cyclocort)
betamethasone (Beta-Val, Diprolene,
    Diprosone, Luxiq)
clobetasol (Clobex, Olux, Temovate)
clocortolone (Cloderm)
desoximetasone (Topicort)
diflorasone (Florone, Psorcon)
fluocinolone (Capex, Synalar)
fluocinonide (Lidex)
fluticasone (Cutivate)*
halcinonide (Halog)
halobetasol (Ultravate)
hydrocortisone (Scalpicin)
hydrocortisone butyrate (Locoid)
hydrocortisone valerate (Westcort)
hydrocortisone-lidocaine (Lida-Mantle HC)
mometasone furoate (Elocon)
triamcinolone (Kenalog)*

Treatments for Lice
lindane
crotamiton (Eurax)
permethrin (Elimite, Nix)
pyrethrins (Rid Mousse)

Antiseptics and Disinfectants
hexachlorophene (pHisoHex)
isopropyl alcohol
povidone-iodine (Betadine)
sodium hypochlorite (Clorox)

Heavy Metal Compounds
zinc oxide (Desitin Creamy)

Orals
benzocaine (Hurricaine, Orabase-B)
carbamide peroxide (Gly-Oxide Oral)
chlorhexidine gluconate (Hibiclens)
clove oil (Eugenol)

Others
benzalkonium chloride (Zephiran)
hydrogen peroxide
phenytoin (Dilantin)

Ophthalmics

Corticosteroids and Combinations
bacitracin–neomycin–polymyxin
    B–hydrocortisone (Cortisporin Ointment)
dexamethasone (AK-Dex)
fluorometholone (FML Forte)
loteprednol (Alrex, Lotemax)
neomycin–polymyxin B–dexamethasone
    (Maxitrol)
sulfacetamide-prednisolone (Blephamide)
tobramycin-dexamethasone (TobraDex)

Antifungal
natamycin (Natacyn)

Decongestant
naphazoline (AK-Con, Naphcon A, Vasocon)

Antivirals
fomivirsen (Vitravene)
ganciclovir (Vitrasert)
trifluridine (Viroptic)

Mast Cell Stabilizers
cromolyn sodium (Crolom)
pemirolast (Alamast)

Antihistamines
epinastine (Elestat)
ketotifen (Zaditor)
olopatadine (Patanol)*

NSAIDs
diclofenac (Voltaren)
flurbiprofen (Ocufen)
ketorolac (Acular)

Others
cyclosporine (Restasis)
verteporfin (Visudyne)
vitamin C–vitamin E–zinc–beta carotene
(Ocuvite PreserVision)

Glaucoma Treatments

Eyedrops or Inserts
apraclonidine (Iopidine)
betaxolol (Betoptic)
bimatoprost (Lumigan)
brimonidine* (Alphagan P)
brinzolamide (Azopt)
carbachol (Carbastat, Miostat)
dipivefrin (Propine)
dorzolamide (Trusopt)
echothiophate iodide (Phospholine Iodide)

latanoprost (Xalatan)*
pilocarpine (Isopto Carpine)
timolol (Timoptic)
travoprost (Travatan)
unoprostone (Rescula)

Oral Agent
acetazolamide (Diamox)

Otics

Analgesic
antipyrine-benzocaine (Auralgan)

Antibiotics
ciprofloxacin-dexamethasone (Ciprodex)
neomycin–polymyxin B–hydrocortisone
(Cortisporin Otic)

Wax Dissolvers
carbamide peroxide (Debrox)
triethanolamine polypeptide–oleate conden-
sate (Cerumenex)

Chapter Review

Pharmaceuticals and Body Functions

Select the best answer from the choices given.

1. As a rule, which is most potent?
   a. ointments
   b. gels
   c. creams
   d. a and c

2. As a rule, which is least potent?
   a. ointments
   b. gels
   c. creams
   d. a and c

3. Which of the following is a topical analog
   of vitamin D used for psoriasis?
   a. methotrexate
   b. Azelex
   c. Cleocin T
   d. Dovonex

4. Which drug is used to treat dandruff?
   a. Dovonex
   b. Azelex
   c. selenium sulfide
   d. Retin-A

5. Which topical can be used to treat
   depression when taken systemically?
   a. azelaic acid
   b. povidone-iodine
   c. doxepin
   d. flurouracil

6. Which drug is a topical analgesic used in
   otitis media for pain?
   a. Debrox
   b. Ciprodex
   c. Cortisporin Otic
   d. antipyrine-benzocaine

7. Which class of drugs probably does not cause photosensitivity?
   a. beta blockers
   b. antineoplastics
   c. antifungals
   d. ACE inhibitors

8. After application of eyedrops, the time period before another eyedrop can be instilled is
   a. 1 to 2 minutes.
   b. 3 to 4 minutes.
   c. 4 to 5 minutes.
   d. 5 to 10 minutes.

9. Which eyedrop is an antifungal?
   a. AK-Con
   b. Viroptic
   c. Ocuflox
   d. Natacyn

10. Which eardrop revieves pain?
    a. antipyrine-denzocaine
    b. Ciprodex
    c. Cortisporin
    d. Debrox

The following statements are true or false. If the answer is false, rewrite the statement so it is true.

_____ 1. Folliculitis is a superficial skin infection caused by *Staphylococcus* or *Streptococcus*. It is especially contagious and is common in early childhood.

_____ 2. Impetigo involves a progressively rapid spread of infection through the superficial layers of the skin. Facial involvement may assume a butterfly distribution.

_____ 3. Erysipelas is an inflammation of a hair follicle by a minute, red, pustulated nodule without involvement of surrounding tissues.

_____ 4. Folliculitis is another name for boils.

_____ 5. Most superpotent topical corticosteroids have restrictions limiting their use to two consecutive weeks of treatment and/or a warning not to exceed 45 g to 50 g in any one week. An exception to this rule is Temovate.

_____ 6. The three types of glaucoma are open-angle, narrow-angle, and secondary.

_____ 7. Eardrops are often prescribed for use in the eye.

_____ 8. AK-Dex is an antiviral.

_____ 9. Ciprodex is an eyedrop.

_____ 10. If a patient has a tube in the ear, only solutions should be used for therapy.

Diseases and Drug Therapies

1. Define the terms fungicide, disinfectant, germicide, and antiseptic.

2. Identify the esthetic factors that may influence the choice of an antiseptic.

3. Discuss the meaning of the term acne vulgaris and its treatment.

4. List the antihistamines that cause photosensitivity.

5. Discuss the side effects of topical corticosteroids.

Dispensing Medications

1. School has just begun, and the administration has sent home a note indicating that there is a problem with head lice in the community. Which drugs should the pharmacy order from the wholesaler?

2. The very next patient who enters the pharmacy shows a skin lesion. The pharmacist verifies that it is ringworm and asks you to get a drug for the patient from the OTC shelf. Which drug will you get?

3. Mr. Brown is purchasing an OTC eyedrop. He has trouble putting eyedrops in his eye. He is also taking some prescription eyedrops. Write the instructions for him.

Internet Research

Use the Internet to complete the following activities.

1. Locate statistics on head lice. How many people are affected per year? Define the risk population. What are the most common signs and symptoms of head lice? List your Internet sources.

2. Significant research efforts are under way to find new ways to diagnose and treat glaucoma. Use the Internet to find information related to these efforts. Describe two or three current research programs: state the goal of the project (e.g., to find genes responsible for glaucoma, to develop more accurate means of detection) and provide a brief description of the product status (e.g., "Animal studies show . . .," "Phase I clinical trials completed . . .").

What Would You Do?

1. The eye clinic is using the same eyedropper on multiple patients. When you question them about this, they say it would be prohibitive, cost-wise, to open a new bottle for each patient. This is probably accurate, since eyedrops are so very expensive. However, is it worth passing an infection from one patient to another? They guarantee you that the dropper never touches the patient's eye or eyelid.

Unit

4

Chemotherapy and Miscellaneous Pharmaceutical Products

Recombinant Drugs and Chemotherapy

16

Learning Objectives

- Understand recombinant DNA and the process for producing medications in this manner.
- Identify colony-stimulating factors and their uses.
- Understand the immune system and how it works.

- Identify drugs used to treat specific disease states and the classification of drugs used in treatments.

Preview chapter terms and definitions.

The exciting, innovative field of recombinant DNA technology provides exciting new developments for managing some of the most serious diseases. These techniques re-engineer cells to manufacture specified proteins. Cancer patients are one of several groups who benefit from this biotechnology. In addition to recombinant DNA products, a wide variety of other types of chemotherapy agents are utilized in the fight against cancer and are covered here as well. Pharmacy technicians play a vital role in dispensing the drugs discussed in this chapter. Mixing and preparation can be very complicated, so education and training of the pharmacy technician are very important. Most of these drugs, which are very expensive, must be stored under refrigerated conditions. The technician must make sure that chemotherapy agents are not allowed to remain un-refrigerated for an extended period.

Recombinant DNA

Biotechnology is the application of biologic systems and organisms for industrial and technical uses. It is generally regarded as a relatively new science, but in reality it is one of the oldest. For thousands of years, microorganisms have been used to produce gases, leaven bread, ferment alcoholic liquids, and generate other desired results that are, from the perspective of the organisms, byproducts. In recent decades, an important aspect of biotechnology is the production and use of **recombinant DNA**, a technique that uses the information-processing capabilities of living cells for human purposes.

The Natural Process for Making Proteins

Proteins are large, complex organic molecules that carry out the vast number of chemical processing tasks needed to keep a cell alive. A protein molecule is composed of one or more linear chains of amino acids that, once synthesized, fold and twist into a specific three-dimensional (3-D) shape that depends on the specific sequence of **amino acid** units in the chain. This 3-D shape places various parts of these large molecules in the proper position to come into contact with, and chemically bond to, the other molecules on which the protein does its work. In other words, the shape, and thus the amino acid sequence, is responsible for protein activity. The sequence of amino acids in the protein depends in turn on the sequence of the **nucleotide** bases in deoxyribonucleic acid (DNA). Molecular machinery in the cell attaches each amino acid, corresponding to a group of three nucleotides according to a specific code, into correct position in the linear protein molecule. Figure 16.1 illustrates an example of a **DNA sequence** and the part of the protein generated from it.

Each of the four nucleotide bases can attach itself (not by a permanent chemical bond) to one and only one of the other three bases. The bases A and T can match only to each other, and the bases C and G can match only to each other. This matching characteristic enables the information in a sequence of DNA to be copied for use in a new cell as well as for translation into protein. When DNA is not being copied, it exists in two strands that run in opposite directions facing each other, each nucleotide in one strand paired to its counterpart in the other strand, and the strands twist around each other to form a double helix, protecting the bases from damage. The two strands are said to be **complementary** to each other.

The information contained in a DNA sequence is transferred by means of three distinct steps, each of which is important for biochemical processes. In one step, the

FIGURE 16.1
The DNA Sequence

A sequence of three nucleotide bases exists for each amino acid.

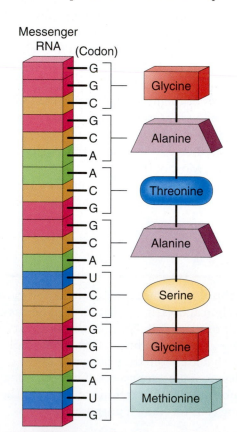

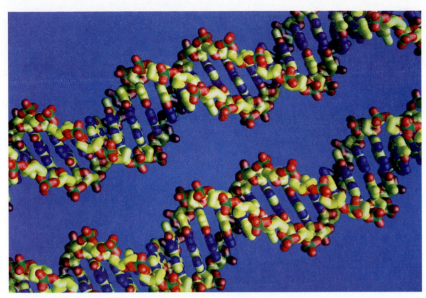

A model of two strands of the double helix of DNA. Each ball represents an atom.

DNA of a cell undergoes **replication** (direct copying onto new DNA to make a new cell). Two steps are needed to produce a protein from DNA. In the first, the DNA for the gene that codes for the protein is copied onto a molecule of ribonucleic acid (RNA), which exists in only one strand. This process is referred to as **transcription**. The newly produced RNA serves as a messenger to the molecular machinery that is to construct the protein. The final step in this process is **translation**, in which the amino acids corresponding to the groups of three nucleotide bases in the messenger RNA according to the code are strung together in the required sequence for manufacturing the desired protein.

Recombinant Process for Manufacturing Protein

In the recombinant DNA process, the DNA sequence, or gene, that codes for a valuable protein in the body is inserted into the DNA of a different kind of cell, often a bacterium, so that that cell can produce the protein and can also reproduce itself to yield a huge number of cells that produce mass quantities of a protein that may naturally exist as only a few molecules in the body.

Most frequently, the gene is transported into a host cell by means of a **plasmid**, which is a small circular ring of DNA. Plasmids have four characteristics that make them useful for recombinant DNA:

- They are present in bacteria.
- They replicate themselves.
- They move freely between bacterial cells.
- They transfer genes, including those that produce resistance to antibiotics, between bacterial cells.

After the gene of interest has been transferred into the host cells, it is necessary to determine whether the host cells are actually producing the desired protein. In this process, the same probe molecules that identify the correct amino acid sequence of the naturally occurring human protein are used as a test to identify whether the same protein is produced by the recombinant cell. The cell type selected must have a high degree of efficiency at producing the desired protein. The DNA that codes for the amino acids in the protein is not enough. A **promoter** sequence is needed to start protein production, and a **terminator** sequence is needed to stop it (see Figure 16.2). The receiving host cell must produce these controls for the inserted recombinant DNA.

FIGURE 16.2
Promoter and Terminator Controls in a Cell

These sequences of DNA must be carried on a plasmid along with the desired human gene.

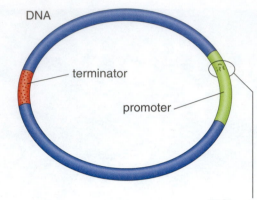

The environment of the host cell is also critical for the proper folding of the protein. Some proteins are modified by the host cell with the addition of sugar molecules and realignment of the chains themselves. Without the modifications and proper folding, the protein does not work therapeutically, and the human body rejects it by forming antibodies. Proteins generated in mammalian cells generally fold properly, those formed in yeast cells do sometimes, and proteins generated by bacterial cells rarely do, necessitating additional modification of the protein after it is collected from the bacteria. However, it is easier to insert a gene into a bacterium than into a yeast or mammalian cell.

Once a cell that expresses the proper recombinant gene (that is, produces the protein) has been identified, duplication, or **cloning,** can proceed. The organism is put into an appropriate growth medium and allowed to ferment. Cell division occurs many times over (thousands to millions to billions of times). The protein is then harvested, purified, and packaged. Figure 16.3 illustrates this process.

Through recombinant DNA technology, pure human protein can be produced in large quantities without the risk of viral contamination that is present when proteins are harvested from pooled sources of human body fluids or tissues. In addition to its uncertain purity, protein extracted from plasma or tissues is available only in small quantities from limited sources. Over the half-century since the structure of DNA and the transcription and translation processes were discovered, the techniques of molecular biology have improved to the point that virtually all known human proteins can be produced in sufficient quantities at almost 100% purity by replicating the corresponding genes. Thus, the use of biotechnology offers many advantages.

Economic Challenges

The high cost of these products may require study and analysis to determine pharmacoeconomic outcomes (i.e., cost-effectiveness, cost-benefit ratio, cost minimization, cost-utility ratio, and cost of illness). For example, in many hospitals the standard of practice supports the combination of antibiotic therapy and hospitalization for 4 to 14 days if neutropenia (a shortage of specific white blood cells known as neutrophils) develops. If the patient does not experience neutropenia, the economic impact in terms of cost savings is significant. A protein known as granulocyte-macrophage colony-stimulating factor (GM-CSF) promotes the growth of white blood cells. The hospital stay for bone marrow transplant patients might be reduced by 6 days if neutropenia can be prevented with GM-CSF. This benefit saves patients more in hospital costs than the cost of the recombinant drug itself.

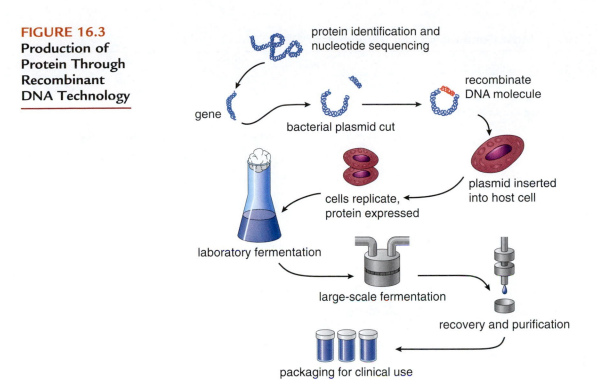

FIGURE 16.3
Production of Protein Through Recombinant DNA Technology

Figure labels:
- protein identification and nucleotide sequencing
- gene
- bacterial plasmid cut
- recombinate DNA molecule
- plasmid inserted into host cell
- cells replicate, protein expressed
- laboratory fermentation
- large-scale fermentation
- recovery and purification
- packaging for clinical use

Recombinant DNA Drugs

Table 16.1 presents the most commonly used recombinant DNA drugs.

Colony-Stimulating Factors A **colony-stimulating factor (CSF)** is an agent that stimulates the bone marrow to produce blood cells. CSFs have clinical implications, including decreasing the period of severe neutropenia after cytotoxic chemotherapy or marrow transplantation; treatment of noncancerous anemia; and treatment of other immunodeficiency states associated with cytopenia (deficiency in some particular type of blood cells). CSF agents are well tolerated. They are used in hematopoietic (red blood cells) malignancies, testicular cancer, ovarian cancer, and small-cell carcinoma of the lung. They allow higher doses of chemotherapy, which increases the likelihood of effectiveness, while reducing danger from white and red blood cell platelet levels. CSF agents are expensive, complex chemical entities with unique therapeutic indications that necessitate specific storage and preparation, utilization review standards, and outcome monitoring.

Epoetin alfa (Epogen, Procrit) is a synthetic form of erythropoietin, a glycoprotein produced by the kidneys. This drug is used in anemia associated with end-stage renal disease and other types of anemia that are unresponsive to the usual treatment modality. It stimulates the division and differentiation of bone marrow cells to produce red blood cells. Hematocrit should be monitored at least twice daily during the initiation of therapy and during any dosage adjustment; the dose should be withheld if the hematocrit exceeds 36%. Frequent blood tests are necessary to determine the correct dose. The following clinical evaluations should precede treatment and then be continued daily during treatment: CBC, differential, and platelet counts; blood chemistries (electrolytes); renal and hepatic function tests; and chest X-rays. Close monitoring of blood pressure is also recommended. Most patients also require supplemental iron therapy. There are some practice sites where it is the responsibility of the pharmacy technician to ensure the proper lab analyses have been completed before dispensing the drugs. Vigorous shaking may denature the glycoprotein, rendering it biologically inactive. This drug *cannot* be delivered through a tube system and it is stored in the refrigerator.

DO NOT SHAKE

TABLE 16.1   Most Commonly Used Recombinant DNA Drugs

Generic Name	Pronunciation	Dosage Form	Brand Name	Dispensing Status
Colony-Stimulating Factors (CSFs)				
epoetin alfa	e-POE-e-tin AL-fa	injection	Epogen, Procrit	Rx
filgrastim	fil-GRA-stim	injection, IV	Neupogen	Rx
pegfilgrastim	peg-fil-GRAS-tim	injection	Neulasta	Rx
sargramostim	sar-GRAM-oh-stim	injection, IV	Leukine	Rx
Biologic-Response Modifiers				
aldesleukin (interleukin-2)	al-des-LOO-kin	injection, IV	Proleukin	Rx
interferon alfa-2a	in-ter-FEER-on AL-fa 2A	injection	Roferon A	Rx
interferon alfa-2b	in-ter-FEER-on AL-fa 2B	injection, IV	Intron A	Rx
interferon beta-1a	in-ter-FEER-on BAY-ta 1A	injection	Avonex, Rebif	Rx
interferon beta-1b	in-ter-FEER-on BAY-ta 1B	injection	Betaseron	Rx
Secretion-Thinning Enzyme				
dornase alfa	DOR-nayse AL-fa	inhalation	Pulmozyme	Rx
Hematologic Agent				
antihemophilic factor (factor VIII)	an-tee-hee-moe-FIL-ik FAK-tor	IV	Alphanate	Rx

Filgrastim (Neupogen) increases white blood cells and granulocyte production by acting on hematopoietic cells by binding to specific cell surface receptors and stimulating proliferation, differentiation, commitment, and some end-cell functional activation. This agent is produced by inserting the human **granulocyte colony-stimulating factor G-CSF** gene into *(E. coli)* bacterial cells. A complete blood count (CBC) and platelet count should be obtained before beginning therapy with filgrastim. The agent should not be used in the period from 24 hours before to 24 hours after chemotherapy because of the potential sensitivity of rapidly dividing cells to cytotoxic chemotherapy. It is incompatible with normal saline and should be mixed in 5% dextrose. Also, when administering intravenously, the lines should not be flushed with a normal saline solution. Instead, a 5% dextrose solution should be flushed prior to administering a second drug and/or heparinizing the catheter. The pharmacy technician should make sure the dextrose flushes are dispensed with filgrastim and available for the nurses.

Warning

Neupogen and Epogen are easily confused.

Pegfilgrastim (Neulasta) is a long-acting form of filgrastim. Polyethylene glycol (PEG) is attached to filgrastim so that it has a longer duration of action and therefore the drug can be administered less frequently. Pegfilgrastim is administered to prevent infection in chemotherapy patients and to increase production of white blood cells. It is only for patients for whom chemotherapy treatments are more than 2 weeks apart. Only one dose is given after a cycle of chemotherapy. Pegfilgrastim is available in a prefilled syringe.

Sargramostim (Leukine) is granulocyte-macrophage colony-stimulating factor (GM-CSF) produced by recombinant DNA. It has been demonstrated to increase the white blood cell count in autologous bone marrow transplantation, decrease duration of antibiotic administration, reduce the incidence of infections, and shorten hospital stays. The drug stimulates proliferation and differentiation of neutrophils, eosinophils, monocytes, and macrophages. The white blood count (WBC) increases in 7 to 14 days but returns to normal within 1 week after the drug is discontinued. The drug is given daily for up to 30 days or until the absolute neutrophil count (ANC) has reached 1,000/mm³ for 3 consecutive days. A CBC with differential is recommended twice a week. Sargramostim is given subcutaneously or intravenously. When given by IV infusion, it must be infused over at least 2 hours. It should not be mixed with dextrose; rather, it should be reconstituted with sterile water. During dissolution, the water should be directed at the side of the vial and gently swirled to avoid foaming. The drug should not be shaken, and only normal saline is used for infusion.

Biologic-Response Modifiers A **biologic-response modifier** is a chemical that enhances immune system activity so that the body will attack and kill invading organisms.

Aldesleukin (Proleukin) is synthesized using *E. coli*. It promotes proliferation, differentiation, and recruitment of T and B cells, natural killer cells, and thymocytes. It can stimulate lymphokine-activated killer cells that have the ability to lyse cells resistant to natural killer cells. Orders should be written in quantities of millions of International Units. Treatment consists of two 5 day treatment cycles separated by a rest period of 9 days.

Interferon alfa-2a (Roferon A) is approved by the FDA for hairy cell leukemia and AIDS-related Kaposi's sarcoma. Chemotherapy precautions should be observed when dispensing and using this drug. This involves gowning-up appropriately and working under a ventilated chemical hood. The person who is mixing medications will wear double-gowns and double-gloves that are specifically designed for chemotherapy preparation and *must* wear eye protection.

Patients who take Interferon alfa-2a usually experience chills, fever, malaise, fatigue, tiredness, and dizziness within 4 to 6 hours. The WBC is suppressed in 7 to 10 days but recovers within 21 days. Other longer-lasting side effects are weight loss, metallic taste, nausea, vomiting, and abdominal cramps.

Interferon alfa-2b (Intron A) is used for hairy cell leukemia, AIDS-related Kaposi's sarcoma, and chronic hepatitis B and C. Baseline chest X-ray films, electrocardiogram (ECG), CBC with differential, liver function tests, electrolyte levels, platelets, and weight should be monitored. Changes in mental status are common with patients on this drug. The physician should be informed of any persistent or severe sore throat, fever, fatigue, or unusual bleeding or bruising.

Interferon beta-1b (Betaseron) and **interferon beta-1a (Avonex, Rebif)** reduce cytokines and increase the activity of T suppressor cells. They reduce the frequency of clinical exacerbations in ambulatory patients with relapsing multiple sclerosis (MS). Flu-like symptoms of myalgia, fever, chills, malaise, fatigue, and sweating are common following initiation of therapy.

Secretion-Thinning Enzyme Excessive secretion of viscous fluids causes problems in several diseases. Deoxyribonuclease is an enzyme produced by recombinant DNA technology. It reduces mucus viscosity.

Dornase alfa (Pulmozyme) is used in managing cystic fibrosis. The hallmark of this disease is the presence of purulent airway secretions composed primarily of highly polymerized DNA. The principal source of this DNA is the nuclei of degenerating neutrophils, which are present in large concentrations of lung secretions. When this DNA is cleaved, mucus viscosity is reduced and airflow in the lung is improved. Thus the risk of bacterial infection is decreased.

Hematologic Agent A **hematologic agent** is a replacement plasma protein that is necessary for blood coagulation and which is not produced in persons with hemophilia. **Antihemophilic factor (Alphanate)**, also referred to as **factor VIII**, is recombinant therapy to supply antihemophilic factor to patients not producing factor VIII. It should be refrigerated before reconstitution but should not be refrigerated after reconstitution. Antihemophilic factor should be administered within 3 hours of reconstitution.

Immune System

The human body presents three lines of defense against invasion by pathogens:

1. The **body surfaces** of intact skin and mucous membranes: infection-fighting chemicals in saliva, tears, and other body fluids; the normally harmless bacteria inhabiting body surfaces that resist pathogen invasion; and the flushing effect of tears, urination, diarrhea, vomiting, sneezing, and coughing
2. **Nonspecific internal defense**: inflammation and increase in the numbers of white blood cells, macrophages, complement proteins, blood-clotting proteins, and other infection-fighting chemicals
3. The **immune response**: the production of communicating and antigen-fighting substances by T cells and B cells

The immune system is highly complicated and protects the body from invading pathogens. The **immune response** provides resistance to disease and malignancy through the production of active phagocyte cells and antibodies, which are specialized proteins that are produced in response to the presence of an antigen. As described in earlier chapters, an antigen is any substance that the immune system cells view as "foreign" to the body.

Immune System Cells

The immune system depends on several types of white blood cells, or leukocytes, including B cells, T cells, small lymphocytes, and macrophages. The different types of cells enable the immune system to have two features: (1) specificity, or the ability to attack a particular antigen, and (2) memory, or the ability to "remember" the antigen for future invasions. The immune system has the ability to identify not only infecting agents, tumor cells, and dying and dead cells but also the products of cellular degeneration. Cells that recognize the antigen and enter the fight are effector cells, whereas those that enter a resting phase are memory cells.

A **T cell** is a lymphocyte that responds directly to antigens by forming clones. They take up residence in the lymph nodes and spleen. T cells participate in cellular immunity by stimulation of certain antigens, viruses, fungi, neoplastic cells, and foreign cells. T cells ignore major histocompatibility complex (MHC) or "self" molecules not bound to an antigen.

When activated by the combined signal, a T cell multiplies into a clone of T cells that recognize that antigen. Some of these cells are effector T cells, which releases cytokines that signal to the rest of the immune system to mobilize; some are cytotoxic T cells, which directly kill cells infected with a virus; some are regulatory T cells, which shut down the active immune response after the attack has passed; and some are memory T cells, which continue to reproduce at a sustainable level indefinitely after the attack has passed.

The cytotoxic T cells kill the pathogens or infected body cells by contact, secreting protein molecules called perforins that cause pores to form in the target cell membrane. The cytoplasm of the target cell is expelled, its organelles are disrupted, its DNA becomes fragmented, and the cell dies.

A **B cell** is also a lymphocyte. Like T cells, B cells arise from the bone marrow, but they do not enter the thymus and differentiate. Each B cell, like each T cell, recognizes a particular antigen, but unlike a T cell, a B cell produces antibody molecules specific to that antigen. The antibody has a Y shape, formed by four polypeptide chains with identical antigen-binding sites on each arm. The tail becomes embedded in the lipid layer of the cell membrane while the arms stick out. B cells are stimulated by a wider range of antigens than T cells. When a B cell contacts the antigen that its antibody recognizes, the antigen binds to the antibody. The antigen is then taken into the cell and broken into fragments, which are then complexed with surface MHC molecules. If a T cell recognizes the combination of MHC and antigen and becomes activated, the T cell may secrete interleukin, which stimulates the B cell to become a **plasma cell** and produce the antibody in massive quantities in a form that circulates freely in the bloodstream. Free circulating antibody molecules can bind to antigen, labeling or identifying it for destruction.

Clones of T and B cells also produce memory T and B cells, known as **small lymphocytes**, which are specifically committed to recognizing the particular antigen and react rapidly (more so than in the initial response) in mounting an attack.

Another type of immune system cell is the **macrophage**, which ingests the foreign substances, digests them, and display them complexed with MHC molecules on the cell surface, setting the stage for T cell and B cell interactions. Helper T cells then bind to the MHC-antigen complex. The macrophages and helper T cells secrete interleukins, which bring about rapid cell division of the T cells, producing cytotoxic T cells and memory cells. The target cytoplasm is expelled, its DNA becomes fragmented, and the cancer cell dies.

Immunoglobulins

An **immunoglobulins** (Ig), or antibody, is a glycoprotein (proteins with attached sugar molecules) that reacts to a specific antigen. Immunoglobulins are designated as IgG, IgM, IgA, IgE, and IgD.

IgG IgG is the most common of the five immunoglobulins, constituting approximately 80% of these glycoproteins in plasma. It is also found in saliva, tears, and cerebrospinal fluid. It is the smallest Ig and can cross the placental membrane. Small amounts are produced after first exposure to an antigen; large amounts are produced and released after the second and subsequent exposures to most bacteria, bacterial toxins, viruses, and fungi. IgG serves as the primary defense against pyrogenic (fever-producing) bacteria.

IgM IgM has the highest molecular weight of immunoglobulins and represents approximately 10% of the total Igs in plasma. The concentration of IgM increases as a result of chronic infection, particularly those due to viral infections. IgM is formed predominantly in the presence of gram-negative bacteria. IgM sensitive to antigens carried on the surface of red blood cells is responsible for the effects of ABO blood type mismatch. If transfusion errors are made, agglutination in the blood can cause blockage of small vessels and result in organ damage.

IgA IgA is synthesized by plasma cells associated with mucous membranes, especially of the respiratory and alimentary tracts. It aids in transport across mucosal epithelium. IgA is the main immunoglobulin in salivary and bronchial secretions, bile, and tears. It is also found in breast milk and colostrum, where it transfers immunity to a child.

IgE IgE occurs in lower concentrations than other immunoglobulins. It is bound to the membranes of basophils and mast cells in tissues. A reaction with antigens leads to disruption of these cells, which causes release of some cellular contents, particularly histamine. IgE causes certain hypersensitivity reactions. It is present in increased amounts in patients with allergic rhinitis and allergic asthma.

IgD IgD functions as a B-cell receptor and may affect B-cell maturation.

Immune Response

The immune response has two main aspects: humoral immunity and cellular (cell-mediated) immunity. **Humoral immunity** is an immune response in which secreted antibodies are transported by fluids (hence the term humoral, from the ancient concept of bodily "humors" or fluids). In contrast, **cellular (cell-mediated) immunity** is a specific response to antigens that is mediated primarily by lymphocytes and macrophages.

Humoral Immunity Humoral immunity is an antibody-mediated response in which B cells are mobilized to defend against foreign antigens. The magnitude of the antibody response depends on the nature of the antigen, the frequency of exposure, and the duration of each exposure. Antigens introduced into tissue through a wound or by injection are carried to a regional lymph node. Orally ingested antigens go to gut-associated lymphoid tissue. Antigens in the bloodstream arrive at the spleen. In these tissues the antigen stimulates the proliferation of specifically committed B lymphocytes. If the antigen has not previously been encountered, lymphocytes in a mass of proliferating cells synthesize a specific IgM against the antigen and release it into the plasma. With a single dose of antigen, there is no stimulus for continued production of lymphocytes; proliferation ceases, and the plasma level of IgM decreases.

Some lymphocytes become the memory cells that remain in peripheral lymphoid tissues. A second dose of the same antigen evokes a rapid and greater response from the now large population of memory cells capable of responding. Proliferation yields a high proportion of plasma cells and antibodies, with IgG rising rapidly in the plasma.

After the antigen-antibody reaction, the antibody may be fixed by a **complement**. A complement is a complex of lipoprotein and globulins in plasma that plays a secondary role after an antigen has bound to an antibody (IgG and IgM). Part of the complement binds to the antibody molecule after the antigen-antibody reaction, resulting in cell lysis with **opsonization** of the cellular debris, making it more susceptible to phagocytosis. Opsonization labels the antigen so that it is more readily recognized and destroyed by macrophages.

Cellular Immunity Cellular immunity is responsible for functions such as organ transplant rejection, killing of tumor or virus-infected cells, and hypersensitivity reactions. Certain antigens (e.g., tubercle bacillus and foreign cell membranes) associated with particulate matter are carried to lymphoid tissue after phagocytosis by specific immune system cells. There the antigens induce proliferation of committed T memory cells. Little or no freely circulating antibody is released because T cells rather than B cells are involved. With continued exposure to the antigen, or with a second exposure, these memory cells proliferate, are released into circulation, and accumulate in the vicinity of the source of the antigen in the tissues. Combining the T cells with antigen results in the release of a number of factors (chemical substances), including a substance (secreted by cytotoxic, or killer, T cells) that is lethal to the antigenic cells, a substance that induces lymphocyte division, and substances that mediate and cause the inflammatory reaction.

Cellular immunity provides the main-line defense against invasion by pathogenic viruses, acid-fast bacilli, fungi, and parasites. As mentioned earlier, it is also responsible for rejection of incompatible tissue grafts and the elimination of neoplastic cells.

Lymphatic System

The **lymphatic system** is a key part of the immune system. It includes (1) a network of capillaries and vessels for collecting and transporting lymph; (2) the lymph nodes; and (3) the lymphoid organs, which include the tonsils, spleen, and thymus. Figure 16.4 shows the components and flow of the lymphatic system.

Toward the end of intrauterine development, lymphocyte stem cells leave the thymus and take up stations with red cells of the bone marrow. Lymphocytes formed in the bone marrow first pass to the thymus, divide, mature, and acquire the ability to recognize and respond to specific antigens; they become T cells, which leave the thymus and establish in peripheral tissues. Lymphocytes that are formed from stem cells in bone marrow and do not migrate to the thymus are B cells.

FIGURE 16.4
Components and Flow of the Lymphatic System

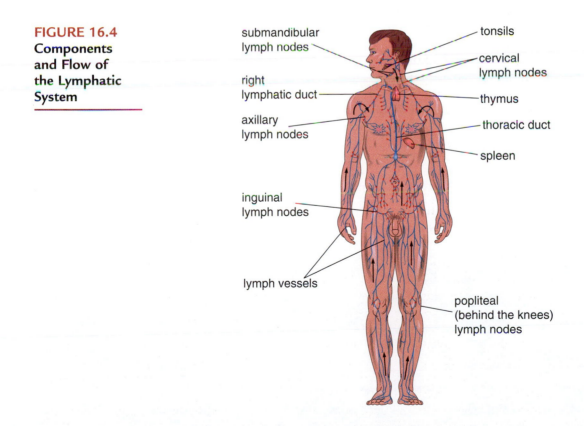

submandibular lymph nodes

tonsils

cervical lymph nodes

right lymphatic duct

thymus

axillary lymph nodes

thoracic duct

spleen

inguinal lymph nodes

lymph vessels

popliteal (behind the knees) lymph nodes

Antirejection Drugs

The immune system is very good at kicking out whatever it recognizes as not being a part of the healthy body. Consequently, medications intended to prevent rejection must be given to patients who have received a transplanted organ. This type of medication, called an **antirejection drug,** depresses the immune system. Unfortunately, antirejection drugs inhibit the critical processes by which the body fights infections, which are also foreign to the body. Table 16.2 presents the most commonly used antirejection drugs.

Azathioprine (Imuran) is used with other agents to prevent rejection of solid organ transplants. It is also used in rheumatoid arthritis. The patient should check with the physician if persistent sore throat, unusual bleeding, bruising, or fatigue occur.

Cyclosporine (Sandimmune) is an immunosuppressant drug that may be used with azathioprine and/or corticosteroids to prolong organ and patient survival in kidney, liver, heart, or bone marrow transplant. It inhibits production and release of interleukin-2. In preparing the dose, the patient should use only glass droppers and glass containers and rinse the dropper to get the full dose. It may be mixed with milk, chocolate milk, or orange juice, preferably at room temperature. The patient should stir it well and drink the entire quantity at one time. The dose should be taken at the same time each day.

Mycophenolate (CellCept) inhibits guanosine nucleotide synthesis, on which both T cells and B cells are highly dependent. As a result, it suppresses antibody formation by B cells. Mycophenolate is used to prevent kidney rejection in organ transplantation. The side effects are diarrhea, leukopenia, sepsis, and vomiting.

Tacrolimus (Prograf) is a potent immunosuppressive agent used for recipients of liver, kidney, heart, lung, or small-bowel transplants. It suppresses humoral immunity by inhibiting T lymphocyte activation. It should not be taken within 2 hours of an antacid.

> **Do not take with ANTACIDS**

Sirolimus (Rapamune) is indicated to prevent renal organ rejection. It inhibits T lymphocyte activation and proliferation in response to antigenic stimulation. Its mechanism of action differs from that of other immunosuppressants. It should not be administered with grapefruit juice and should be taken consistently either with or without food. In other words, to minimize variability, the patient should always take the drug with food or always take it on an empty stomach.

Monoclonal Antibodies

A **monoclonal antibody** (abbreviated MAb or mAb) is an antibody produced in quantity in the laboratory by a culture of B cells descended from a single memory B cell.

TABLE 16.2   Most Commonly Used Antirejection Drugs

Generic Name	Pronunciation	Dosage Form	Brand Name	Dispensing Status
azathioprine	ay-za-THYE-oh-preen	IV, tablet	Imuran	Rx
cyclosporine	SYE-kloe-spor-een	capsule, IV, oral liquid	Sandimmune	Rx
mycophenolate	mye-koe-FEN-oe-late	capsule, IV, oral liquid, tablet	CellCept	Rx
sirolimus	sir-OE-li-mus	oral liquid, tablet	Rapamune	Rx
tacrolimus	ta-KROE-li-mus	capsule, IV	Prograf	Rx

Therefore all the antibody molecules are targeted to attach to one specific substance in the body in one specific way. Monoclonal antibodies are structurally similar to natural antibodies, which are also known as immunoglobulins. Of the five immunoglobulins (IgA, IgD, IgE, IgG, and IgM), IgM is the one most commonly manipulated in the production of MAbs. Their function is to stimulate the immune system and target different types of cells. This targeting effect is put to use in a number of ways, including.

- The MAb attaches to certain parts of the cell, making it easier for the immune system to find and destroy that cell. This effect can be used against cancer cells; it can also be used against graft rejection by targeting the immune system cells that react to the graft.
- The MAb binds to a receptor to block it. For example, cancer cells make extra growth factor, one reason why they grow faster than normal cells. MAbs can block growth factor receptors and prevent the growth signal from getting through.
- A MAb can be combined with a radioactive element to deliver radiation directly to the target cell. This protects the normal cells from harm.
- A MAb can be combined with a powerful drug that will remain inactive until the MAb places it in the target cell. Again, this protects the healthy cells.

Antibodies to a specific tumor or tissue are developed by stimulating lymphocytes with antigens from the target cells and testing for a response.

The primary side effects of monoclonal antibody therapy, are dangerously low levels of red blood cells, white blood cells, and platelets. The resources of the immune system are directed toward the target cancer cells, leaving the body open for other infections. MAb medications are all administered intravenously or by injection, so site reaction can also be a problem. The Institute for Safe Medication Practices has labeled all MAbs as high-alert drugs because of the significant harm that can occur to a patient if used in error.

In addition to their use in drug therapy, MAbs are also used in diagnostic assays, localization of proteins in histochemical investigations, and cell labeling.

Monoclonal Antibody Nomenclature A nomenclature (naming) system for mono-clonal antibodies is now used by the World Health Organization and the American Medical Association. In this scheme, drug names for monoclonal antibodies include several letters that distinguish the drug (first several letters), one or several letters that indicate the target of the antibody (Table 16.3), one or several letters that indicate the source of the antibody (Table 16.4), and, finally, the name of the drug ends in "mab" (for monoclonal antibody).

As an example, the syllables in the name of abciximab signify the following:

- ab: distinctive name of the antibody
- ci: target, cardiovascular
- xi: source, combination
- mab: monoclonal antibody

For daclizumab, the syllables signify:

- dac: distinctive name
- li: immune
- zu: human
- mab: monoclonal antibody

TABLE 16.3	Monoclonal Antibody Nomenclature: Target Stems	
Target	**Identifier**
viral	vir
bacterial	bac
immune	li
infections	les
cardiovascular	ci
colon	col
melanoma	mel
mammary	mar
testis	got
ovary	gov
prostate	pr(o)
miscellaneous	tu

TABLE 16.4	Monoclonal Antibody Nomenclature: Source Stems	
Target	**Identifier**
zu	human
o	mouse
a	rat
e	hamster
i	primate
xi	combination

Prescribed Monoclonal Antibodies The most commonly prescribed monoclonal antibodies are listed in Table 16.5.

Very few MAbs are first-line treatment; often they are a last resort, and the patient usually has to have failed other drugs before MAbs are administered. Most patients must have pre-meds dispensed with them to minimize the side effects. An invaluable service the pharmacy technician can render to a patient is to make sure that pre-meds are ordered and available in a timely manner for these patients.

MAbs must be handled with extreme care. When they are mixed, they must be gently swirled, not shaken, or they will be **denatured** and lose their effectiveness. MAbs should not be sent to the floor through pneumatic tubes but carefully hand-delivered to ensure the integrity of the drug.

Alemtuzumab (Campath) is indicated for the treatment of B cell chronic lympho-cytic leukemia in patients who have not responded to alkylating agents (chemotherapy drugs described in the next section). Alemtuzumab binds to leukemic cells to cause lysis. If alemtuzumab is ordered, the pharmacy technician should check with the pharmacist to make sure the doctor has also ordered diphenhydramine and acetaminophen, which are necessary to minimize patient reaction to the monoclonal antibody. Alemtuzumab affects normal cells, so patients develop neutropenia (decrease in neutrophils) and thrombocytopenia (decrease in platelets). Patients who receive alemtuzumab should also receive anti-infective prophylaxis, a broad-spectrum antibiotic, and Bactrim. Aalemtuzamab must be filtered prior to dilution. It is mixed in either normal saline or D_5W. Once mixed, the bag must be gently inverted so as to ensure that the drug is evenly distributed. Alemtuzumab must be used within 8 hours of dilution.

Basiliximab (Simulect) is indicated for prophylaxis of acute organ rejection in renal transplantation. It is a chimeric (mirror twin) MAb that blocks the alpha chain of the interleukin-2 receptor complex. This receptor is expressed in activated T lymphocytes and is a critical pathway for activating cell-mediated allograft rejection. Intact vials should be stored under refrigeration. Basiliximab should be reconstituted

TABLE 16.5 Most Commonly Prescribed Monoclonal Antibodies

Generic Name	Pronunciation	Dosage Form	Brand Name	Approved to treat
abciximab	ab-SIK-si-mab	IV	ReoPro	cardiovascular disease
adalimumab	a-da-LIM-yoo-mab	IV	Humira	autoimmune inflammatory disorders
alemtuzumab	ay-lem-TOO-zoo-mab	IV	Campath	chronic lymphocytic leukemia
basiliximab	bas-il-IX-i-mab	IV	Simulect	transplant rejection
bevacizumab	bev-uh-SIZ-yoo-mab	IV	Avastin	colorectal cancer
cetuximab	see-TUK-see-mab	IV	Erbitux	colorectal cancer
daclizumab	da-KLIZ-yoo-mab	IV	Zenapax	transplant rejection
efalizumab	e-fa-LIZ-yoo-mab	IV	Raptiva	inflammatory diseases (psoriasis)
gemtuzumab	gem-TOO-zoo-mab	IV	Mylotarg	leukemia (AML)
ibritumomab tiuxetan	ib-ree-TYOO-mo-mab ti-UK-se-tan	IV	Zevalin	non-Hodgkin lymphoma
infliximab	in-FLIKS-e-mab	IV	Remicade	autoimmune inflammaatory diseases
muromonab-CD3	myoo-roe-MOE-nab CD3	IV	Orthoclone OKT3	transplant rejection
natalizumab	nat-uh-LIZ-yoo-mab	IV	Tysabri	autoimmune inflammatory diseases (MS)
omalizumab	o-mah-LIZ-yoo-mab	injection	Xolair	allergy related inflammatory diseases
palivizumab	pal-ee-VIZ-yoo-mab	IV	Synagis	viral infection (RSV)
panitumumab	pan-i-TOOM-yoo-mab	IV	Vectibix	colorectal cancer
ranibizumab	ra-ni-BIZ-yoo-mab	IV	Lucenetis	macular degeneration
rituximab	ri-TUK-si-mab	IV	Rituxan, Mabthera	non-Hodgkin lymphoma
tositumomab	toe-si-TOO-moe-mab	IV	Bexxar	non-Hodgkin lymphoma
trastuzumab	tras-TOO-zoo-mab	IV	Herceptin	breast cancer

REFRIGERATE with sterile water for injection and shaken gently to dissolve. It is then further diluted with normal saline or D_5W. The bag should be inverted gently to avoid foaming.

Bevacizumab (Avastin) is approved to treat colorectal cancer and small-cell lung cancer. It must be protected from light and, in contrast to the preceding two MAb drugs, *not mixed* with dextrose. Bevacizumab must not be shaken. It is a therapeutic antibody designed to inhibit vascular endothelial growth factor, a protein that plays a role in the formation and maintenance of tumor blood vessels (angiogenesis). Bevacizumab is a promising agent for the treatment of metastatic colorectal cancer. It is used in combination with chemotherapy. An uncommon but serious side effect of this drug is perforation of the colon, which generally requires surgery and sometimes leads to intra-abdominial infections, impaired wound healing, and internal bleeding.

Cetuximab (Erbitux) is approved for advanced colorectal cancer. It has not been shown to extend life, but it does shrink tumors. Cetuximab targets a natural protein receptor on the surface of cancer cells, interfering with their growth. It is intended for patients who no longer respond to irinotecan or other chemotherapy. Cetuximab can cause serious side effects, including difficulty breathing and low blood pressure. Doctors use a test kit to analyze a colon tissue sample. The kit detects a protein in the body that stimulates cancerous tissue cell growth. Presence of this protein indicates eligibility for this drug.

Daclizumab (Zenapax) is a monoclonal antibody that is part of a regimen for prophylaxis of acute organ rejection in patients who receive renal transplants. The regimen also includes cyclosporine and corticosteroids. Daclizumab inhibits the binding of interleukin-2 to the high-affinity receptor, thereby suppressing T-cell activity against allografts (transplanted tissue from a human donor). Its active ingredient is a humanized MAb.

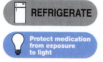

Daclizumab should be kept refrigerated and protected from light. It should be diluted only in normal saline (not D_5W) and used within 24 hours of admixture if refrigerated and within 4 hours if not refrigerated.

Gemtuzumab (Mylotarg) is approved to treat myeloid leukemia in patients under 60 years of age who are in first relapse and are not candidates for cytotoxic chemotherapy. It is a last-resort therapy. Gemtuzumab is very sensitive to light. It must be prepared in a darkened room and placed in a UV bag immediately after reconstitution. It is infused over 2 hours and is good for 20 hours after reconstitution. Gemtuzumab interferes with the growth of cancer cells and slows their spread throughout the body. When dispensing gemtuzumab, the pharmacy technician should affirm that the prescriber also ordered diphenhydramine and acetaminophen.

Ibritumomab-tiuxetan (Zevalin) acts as a delivery system to direct radioactive substances to the cell. Emission of radioactive particles damages both healthy and cancer cells. Patients need to be premedicated with diphenhydramine, acetaminophen, and an antiemetic. Ibritumomab is given in two doses, the second 7–9 days after the first dose.

Muromonab-CD3 (Orthoclone OKT3) is used to treat acute allograft rejection in renal transplant patients; it is effective in reversing acute hepatic, cardiac, and bone marrow transplant rejection episodes resistant to conventional treatment. Muromonab-CD3 binds to T cells and interferes with their function. The first dose can cause severe pulmonary edema. The patient should be monitored carefully for forty-eight hours after the first dose. It is strongly recommended that a corticosteroid precede the first dose. It is also recommended that acetaminophen and antihistamines be given concurrently. The edema is markedly reduced with subsequent administration of this drug.

Rituximab (Rituxan) targets cells that are non-Hodgkin lymphomas. It is used both for initial and re-treatment. Patients should receive acetaminophen and diphenhydramine before the infusions. Infusion must be very slow, especially the first one. Patients must be well hydrated, so fluids are to be administered with the MAb. Patients must not take blood pressure medication on the day they receive rituxan.

Trastuzumab (Herceptin) is used as monotherapy for patients with breast cancer. Typical reactions are fever and chills with the first dose. Premedications are unnecessary, but should be available as needed.

Tositumomab (Bexxar) is an IgG2a monoclonal antibody. It enters the body and kills specific cells that are positive for a form of non-Hodgin lymphoma. This drug is prepared in a nuclear pharmacy. In order to protect the thyroid gland from damage, one of the agents, SSKI, Lugol's Solution or potassium iodide, should be given to the patient at least 24 hours prior to administration of tositumomab and continued for two weeks after administration

Cancer

The division of cells, mitosis, is one of the most vital characteristics of living organisms, providing growth and repair, in addition to cell division and replication of DNA. When normal cellular growth control mechanisms become altered and cell proliferation is uncoordinated and exceeds that of normal tissue, the result is the growth of tumors and/or the onset of cancer. This situation is known as neoplasm. **Neoplastic disease** is thus a disease of uncontrolled cellular growth in which abnormal cells develop and reproduce.

Cancer, a neoplastic disease, is a leading cause of death in the United States. Regardless of the type of cancer, malignant (resulting in growths that are tumors) cells display commonalities, including:

- Structural alteration with loss of function occurs regardless of the cell type (e.g., epithelium, muscle, bone).
- Uncontrolled cellular reproduction results in the production of groups of cells that have no useful function and may increase in number at a rate faster than that of normal body cells.

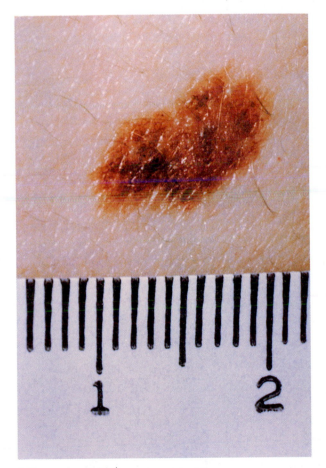

A Precancerous Mole

Malignancy is characterized by the following.

- Abnormal, uncontrolled growth threatens normal body functions and can lead to death.
- DNA and RNA synthesis is increased.
- Metabolism is altered so that as the tumor grows, it robs the body of the nutrients necessary for body cells, leading to loss of weight and vitality.
- Cells lose their contact inhibition. Normal cells have a property that prevents division if the cells become crowded together in a tissue or organ; cancer cells continue to divide even when the pressure of surrounding cell masses is considerable.

The types of cancer can be classified as follows.

- **Solid tumor:** A growth that can be palpated when it becomes significantly large or accessible.
- **Diffuse tumor:** A growth that is not restricted to one location but is scattered throughout the body, as in leukemia and Hodgkin disease.

The sites of cancer are classified as follows.

- **Primary site:** Cancer occurs at the location where disease first began to form.
- **Secondary site:** A location where detached and relocated cells have migrated from some other location and formed a new tumor (metastasis).

Agents for Chemotherapy

Several modalities are available and are commonly used in combination when treating cancer. Surgery is used to remove solid tumors that are surgically accessible; it may be followed by radiation therapy in several treatments. Radiation therapy is most commonly used after surgery or chemotherapy. Chemotherapy is used to kill cancer cells that remain after surgery or radiation or that are not readily detectable, especially in diffuse tumors.

As larger numbers of chemotherapy agents become available as oral medications, it will be more common for them to be dispensed at the retail level. Insurance companies are spearheading the administration of thse drugs outside of the institutional setting. However, because of several factors, patients can become confused. These factors include:

Warning

Cisplatin and carboplatin can be misread.

- the complicated nature of some of the regimens
- the free periods to allow the body to recover from the chemotherapy drugs
- the drugs then used to salvage the body from the effects of the chemotherapy drugs

Table 16.6 lists the most commonly used agents for chemotherapy.

Many antitumor drugs are most efficient during the period when cancer cells are synthesizing DNA and dividing rapidly. In a young tumor, most of the cells are making DNA and dividing. As the tumor ages, the growth fraction decreases; growth slows, and drug sensitivity is reduced. Treatable tumors are discovered when 30 to 100% of cells are in the growth fraction.

Many antineoplastic drugs are extremely toxic because they also destroy normal cells, especially those with a normal growth rate close to that of tumor cells, such as those in the bone marrow, the gastrointestinal (GI) tract, and the skin. Therapy often causes toxicity in these tissues, resulting in bone marrow depression (anemia, leukopenia, and thrombocytopenia), stomatitis (inflammation of the oral mucosa), skin and GI tract ulceration, and hair loss (alopecia). Therapy is generally structured to allow for a 2 to 6 week drug-free period between treatments.

The goal of most chemotherapy regimes is to put the cancer into remission. In **remission**, the tumor is in an inactive period with no active cell division and growth. Remission does not cure the disease, but it does extend the patient's life.

Resistance is a lack of responsiveness of the cancer cells to chemotherapy. Malignant cells continue to reproduce even in the presence of the drug. Combinations of agents with different mechanisms of action are used to attack different areas of the cancer cell, providing more efficient therapy.

The increasing availability of chemotherapy agents at pharmacies is placing significant responsibility on pharmacy personnel to be knowledgeable in order to handle and dispense these drugs properly.

Alkylating Agents Alkylating agents create irreversible cross-links in DNA so that the DNA and cells cannot reproduce.

Dacarbazine (DTIC-Dome) is used to treat various cancers. It interferes with cell growth and impedes the formation of new tissue. It affects normal cells as well as cancer cells. Dacarbazine is administered under the supervision of a nurse. It can be used as a single agent (monotherapy). As with other powerful drugs, the side effects are nausea, fatigue, and headache.

Oxaliplatin (Eloxatin) is approved for advanced colorectal cancer and also for ovarian cancer. It is combined with fluorouracil and leucovorin. Oxaliplatin has

TABLE 16.6 Most Commonly Used Agents for Chemotherapy

Generic Name	Pronunciation	Dosage Form	Brand Name	Dispensing Status
Alkylating Agents				
busulfan	byoo-SUL-fan	tablet	Myleran	Rx
carboplatin	KAR-boe-plat-in	IV	Paraplatin	Rx
carmustine	kar-MUS-teen	IV	BiCNU	Rx
cisplatin	sis-PLAT-in	IV	Platinol	Rx
cyclophosphamide	sye-kloe-FOS-fa-mide	IV, tablet	Cytoxan	Rx
dacarbazine	da-KAR-ba-zeen	IV	DTIC-Dome	Rx
ifosfamide	eye-FOS-fa-mide	IV	Ifex	Rx
lomustine	loe-MUS-teen	capsule	CeeNU	Rx
oxaliplatin	ox-ah-li-PLAT-in	IV	Eloxatin	Rx
streptozocin	strep-toe-ZOE-sin	IV	Zanosar	Rx
temozolomide	tem-oh-ZOHL-oh-mide	capsule	Temodar	Rx
Antibiotics				
bleomycin	blee-oh-MYE-sin	injection, IV	Blenoxane	Rx
dactinomycin	dak-ti-noe-MYE-sin	injection, IV	Cosmegen	Rx
daunorubicin	daw-noe-ROO-bi-sin	IV	Cerubidine	Rx
doxorubicin	dox-oh-ROO-bi-sin	IV	Adriamycin PFS	Rx
epirubicin	ep-i-ROO-bi-sin	IV	Ellence	Rx
idarubicin	eye-da-RUE-bi-sin	IV	Idamycin	Rx
mitomycin	mye-toe-MYE-sin	IV	Mutamycin	Rx
plicamycin	plye-ka-MYE-sin	IV	Mithracin	Rx
valrubicin	val-ROO-bi-sin	injection (into bladder)	Valstar Preservative Free	Rx
Antimetabolites				
capecitabine	ka-pe-SYE-ta-been	tablet	Xeloda	Rx
cytarabine	sye-TAIR-a-been	injection, IV	Cytosar-U	Rx
floxuridine	flox-YOOR-i-deen	IV	FUDR	Rx
fludarabine	floo-DAIR-a-been	IV	Fludara	Rx
fluorouracil	floo-roe-YOOR-a-sil	cream, injection, IV, solution	Efudex	Rx
hydroxyurea	hye-drox-ee-yoo-REE-ah	capsule	Hydrea	Rx
mercaptopurine	mer-kap-toe-PYOOR-een	tablet	Purinethol	Rx
methotrexate	meth-o-TREX-ate	tablet	Rheumatrex	Rx
thioguanine	thye-oh-GWON-een	tablet	Tabloid	Rx
Hormones				
abarelix	a-ba-REL-ix	injection	Plenaxis	Rx
aminoglutethimide	a-mee-noe-gloo-TETH-i-mide	tablet	Cytadren	Rx
bicalutamide	bye-ka-LOO-ta-mide	tablet	Casodex	Rx

TABLE 16.6 Most Commonly Used Agents for Chemotherapy (continued)

Generic Name	Pronunciation	Dosage Form	Brand Name	Dispensing Status
flutamide	FLOO-ta-mide	capsule	Eulexin	Rx
goserelin	GOE-se-rel-in	implant	Zoladex	Rx
leuprolide	loo-PROE-lide	implant, injection	Eligard, Lupron Depot, Viadur	Rx
megestrol	me-JES-trole	suspension, tablet	Megace	Rx
mitotane	MYE-toe-tane	tablet	Lysodren	Rx
triptorelin	trip-toe-REL-in	injection	Trelstar	Rx
Nitrogen Mustards				
chlorambucil	klor-AM-byoo-sil	tablet	Leukeran	Rx
estramustine	es-tra-MUS-teen	capsule	Emcyt	Rx
mechlorethamine	me-klor-ETH-a-meen	IV	Mustargen	Rx
melphalan	MEL-fa-lan	IV, tablet	Alkeran	Rx
thiotepa	thye-oh-TEP-a	IV	(none)	Rx
Plant Alkaloids				
docetaxel	doe-se-TAX-el	IV	Taxotere	Rx
etoposide	e-toe-POE-side	capsule, IV	VePesid	Rx
paclitaxel	pak-li-TAX-el	IV	Taxol	Rx
vinblastine	vin-BLAS-teen	IV	Velban	Rx
vincristine	vin-KRIS-teen	IV	Oncovin, Vincasar PFS	Rx
Topoisomerase I Inhibitors				
irinotecan	eye-ri-noe-TEE-kan	IV	Camptosar	Rx
topotecan	toe-poe-TEE-kan	IV	Hycamtin	Rx
Tyrokinase Inhibitors				
dasatinib	da-SAT-i-nib	tablet	Sprycel	Rx
erlotinib	er-LOE-ti-nib	tablet	Tarceva	Rx
imatinib	eye-MAT-i-nib	tablet	Gleevec	Rx
nilotinib	nye-LOE-ti-nib	capsule, tablet	Tasigna	Rx
Miscellaneous Agents				
alitretinoin	al-i-TRET-i-noe-in	gel	Panretin	Rx
altretamine	al-TRET-a-meen	capsule	Hexalen	Rx
arsenic trioxide	AR-sen-ik trye-OX-ide	IV	Trisenox	Rx
asparaginase	a-SPAIR-a-ji-nase	injection, IV	Elspar	Rx
bortezomib	bor-TEZ-oe-mib	injection	Velcade	Rx
denileukin diftitox	DEN-i-loo-kin DIF-ti-tox	IV	ONTAK	Rx
gefitinib	ge-FI-ti-nib	tablet	Iressa	Rx
mitoxantrone	mye-toe-ZAN-trone	IV	Novantrone	Rx

TABLE 16.6   **Most Commonly Used Agents for Chemotherapy (continued)**

Generic Name	Pronunciation	Dosage Form	Brand Name	Dispensing Status
pemetrexed	pem-ah-TREX-ed	IV	Alimta	Rx
procarbazine	pro-KAR-ba-zeen	capsule	Matulane	Rx
Cytoprotective (Rescue) Agents				
amifostine	am-i-FOS-teen	IV	Ethyol	Rx
dexrazoxane	dex-ray-ZOX-ayn	IV	Zinecard	Rx
leucovorin	loo-koe-VOR-in	injection, IV, tablet	(none)	Rx

shown promising results after surgery for stage II and III colorectal cancer. It interrupts cell growth and slows the spread of cancer cells in the body. Oxaliplatin may be effective in shrinking tumors resistant to cisplatin and carboplatin.

Temozolomide (Temodar) is a prodrug that undergoes rapid nonenzymatic conversion at physiological pH to alkylate DNA. The mechanism of the drug is similar to that of dacarbazine, but temozolomide is administered orally, whereas dacarbazine is given intravenously. Temozolomide was approved by the FDA in 1999—the first new drug for the treatment of brain cancer to be approved in more than 20 years. The dose-limited adverse event associated with temozolomide is myelosuppression.

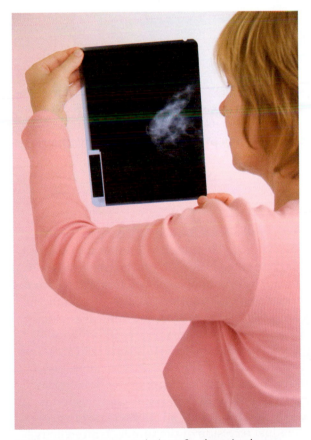

Mammograms are one technique for detecting breast cancer. Treatment commonly involves chemotherapy.

Antibiotics Antibiotics inhibit DNA-dependent RNA synthesis or delay or inhibit mitosis.

Doxorubicin (Adriamycin) depresses the number of blood cells in bone marrow. It slows or stops the growth of cancer cells in the body. Doxorubicin should be administered through a central line and not into a peripheral vein. If doxorubicin leaks into surrounding tissue (**extravasation**), most of that tissue will have to be surgically removed.

Epirubicin (Ellence) is an anthracycline cytotoxic agent related to doxorubicin. It is able to penetrate into cells more readily because it is more lipophilic. Epirubicin is indicated as adjuvant therapy in patients with axillary node tumor following resection of primary breast cancer. It kills cancer cells in any part of the cell cycle. Epirubicin treatments are repeated in 3 and 4 week cycles. This drug can be given in higher doses than related drugs such as doxorubicin because it causes less nausea, neutropenia, and cardiotoxicity, though cardiotoxicity is still a major risk. Epirubicin must be protected from light.

Valrubicin (Valstar Preservative Free), a semi-synthetic analog of doxorubicin, is indicated for intravesical therapy of the urinary bladder. The powder has a red color, and red-tinged urine is typical for the first 24 hours after administration of the drug.

Valrubicin should be stored in the refrigerator. If a waxy form precipitates from the solution, the vial should be warmed until it is clear. The drug should be prepared and stored in glass and it is diluted with normal saline. A urethral catheter is inserted into the patient's bladder after it is drained, and the diluted valrubicin solution is instilled slowly. The patient will then need to retain the drug for 2 hours.

Antimetabolites Antimetabolite cancer drugs inhibit the normal function of a key enzyme and render them nonfunctional. Most of the antimetabolites used in cancer chemotherapy are modified forms of nucleotides or nucleotide bases that prevent DNA replication or transcription.

Capecitabine (Xeloda) is enzymatically converted to 5-fluorouracil. This is a three-step process in which the last step is to catalyze the drug by an enzyme that is present in higher concentrations in carcinogenic cells than normal tissue. Because the drug is absorbed and metabolized in a higher concentration for tumor tissue than normal tissue, there is less risk of systemic toxicity than with standard fluorouracil. Capecitabine is indicated in cases of breast cancer that have shown resistance to regimens of other agents.. The most prominent side effects of this drug are nausea and vomiting. When diarrhea occurs, it can usually be controlled with loperamide. Capecitabine is given daily with food over a period of 2 weeks. This period is followed by a 1 week rest period. Therapy is therefore given in 3 week cycles. The daily dosage is administered in two divided doses, 12 hours apart.

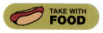

Hormones Hormones are modified forms of steroid hormones. They are useful against neoplasms of reproductive tissues. These drugs and their target neoplasms are:

- **Abarelix (Plenaxis)**: prostate
- **Aminoglutethimide (Cytadren)**: breast, prostate
- **Bicalutamide (Casodex)**: prostate
- **Flutamide (Eulexin)**: prostate
- **Goserelin (Zoladex)**: prostate, metastatic breast cancer in premenopausal women. It acts by suppressing estrogen production to postmenopausal levels to reduce the growth of estrogen-responsive tumors. It is also used to treat endometriosis.
- **Leuprolide (Eligard, Lupron Depot, Viadur)**: prostate carcinoma, endometriosis, central precocious puberty
- **Megestrol**: breast, endometrial
- **Mitotane (Lysodren)**: adrenal cortex
- **Triptorelin (Trelstar)**: prostate

Abarelix (Plenaxis) is approved for the palliative treatment of advanced prostate cancer for patients who have no alternative therapy. It reduces the amount of testosterone produced in the body. Abarelix is distributed only to approved physicians and hospital pharmacies and is not available through retail pharmacies. It is injected into the muscles of the buttocks every 2 weeks. Patients should wait at least 30 minutes in the doctor's office after receiving this drug, because there are some immediate side effects, such as fainting. Patients are asked to read and sign a patient information leaflet before receiving the drug. Abarelix is provided by the manufacturer in a vial for injection and may be stored at room temperature.

Triptorelin (Trelstar) is approved for treatment of prostate cancer. It increases testosterone levels, so the cancer may worsen at first. After chronic and continuous administration, usually for 2–4 weeks after initiation, a sustained decrease of estrogen and testosterone begins to occur with gradual recession of the tumor. Triptorelin is injected intramuscularly once a month.

Nitrogen Mustards Nitrogen mustards bind irreversible cross-links in cellular DNA and RNA, disrupting normal nucleic acid function so that it cannot reproduce. They have their name because they are chemically related to mustard gas, a chemical weapon used during World War I. The damage to the DNA of cells is similar to radiation damage. Nitrogen mustards are used on specific tumors and produce the best results when the cell is in a resting phase (not dividing and growing).

Plant Alkaloids Plant alkaloids inhibit the formation of spindle fibers, arresting the metaphase of cell division.

Paclitaxel (Taxol, Abraxane) is indicated for metastatic ovarian cancer after failure of first-line chemotherapy with a platinum alkylating agent and for breast carcinoma after failure of combination chemotherapy with doxorubicin and cyclophosphamide. Patients should be warned to avoid pregnancy because of harm to the fetus and should be told that alopecia occurs in almost all patients. A patient should alert the physician if tingling, burning, or numbness occurs in the extremities, as the dosage may need to be reduced if these symptoms occur. It must be dispensed in glass, and PVC tubing must be avoided.

The new formulation, Abraxane, is better tolerated by patients. Abraxane is bound to albumin and therefore patients can take higher doses without the need of pre-medication. Other advantages are that no special tubing is needed for IV administration, and infusions require much less time. However, one drug cannot be substituted for the other, because the dosing is very different. Abraxane must be protected from light. It is reconstituted with 20 mL of normal saline. To ensure proper wetting it must set for at least 5 minutes, then the vial should be gently swirled or inverted for a minimum of 2 minutes. If there is any foaming of clumping, let it set for 15 minutes. Unlike Taxol, which must be dispensed in glass, Abraxane is then injected into an IV bag of normal saline.

Topoisomerase I Inhibitors Topoisomerase I inhibitors cause DNA damage when cells attempt to replicate. These drugs and their target neoplasms are as follows:

- **Irinotecan (Camptosar):** colorectal cancer. A second-line drug, it can cause severe diarrhea. It is often combined with centuximab (Erbitax). The combination of irinotecan and cetuximab has been shown to be more effective than irinotecan alone.
- **Topotecan (Hycamtin):** ovarian (second-line after paclitaxel)

Tyrokinase Inhibiting Agents A tyrokinase (tyrosine kinase) is an enzyme that promotes growth and multiplication of a cell in response to growth factors. Many enzymes in the body have a tyrokinase activity. By blocking an ATP-binding site, tyrokinase-inhibiting agents inhibit cellular growth and decrease proliferation of cells. Tyrokinase inhibitors appear to be as effective as other chemotherapy agents, but with fewer and less severe side effects.

Dasatinib (Sprycel) is an oral drug for certain forms of leukemia. It is intended only for patients who have shown resistance to other forms of therapy. Dasatinib reduces the activity of one or more proteins responsible for the uncontrolled growth of the leukemia cell. It is taken without regard to food and the primary side effects are anemia, thrombocytopenia, and neutropenia

Erlotinib (Tarceva) is approved as a single-agent treatment for locally advanced or metastatic non-small-cell lung cancer, the most common lung cancer, in patients in whom another chemotherapy regime has failed. It is to be taken on an empty stomach. It received "fast track" status by the FDA. It has come to be preferred to gefitinib for non-small-cell lung cancer and has been approved in combination with gemcitabine for pancreatic cancer.

Gefitinib (Iressa) was approved to treat advanced non-small-cell lung cancer in patients whose cancer has continued to progress despite treatment with platinum-based and docetaxel chemotherapy. Common side effects are nausea, vomiting, diarrhea, rash, acne, and dry skin. Gefitinib was approved through the FDA's accelerated process, and it has since been found to be less effective than erlotinib. Since 2007, in the United States, gefitinib has been prescribed only for patients who already had a positive response to it.

Imatinib (Gleevec) is approved for three stages of chronic myeloid leukemia. Myeloid leukemia occurs when two different chromosomes break off and reattach on the opposite chromosome, forming the "Philadelphia" chromosome. The chromosome translocation leads to a combined protein that acts as a blood cell enzyme—a tyrokinase—that is turned on all the time. Life-threatening levels of white blood cells are produced in the bone marrow and blood. Imatinib blocks this combined protein that stimulates proliferation of abnormal white blood cells only, so it does not injure healthy cells.

Nilotinib (Tasigna) can be taken 1 hour before or 2 hours after meals. It was designed to overcome imatinib resistance in Philadelphia chromosome syndrome. It binds to and inhibits abnormal tyrokinase as well as the tyrokinase receptor. It affects both the cancer and human cells, but slows tumor growth.

Miscellaneous Agents A number of anticancer drugs do not fit into the previously discussed categories. These miscellaneous agents have different mechanisms of action and destroy malignant cells in a variety of ways.

Alitretinoin (Panretin) is related to vitamin A. It is indicated for the treatment of skin lesions in patients with AIDS-related Kaposi sarcoma. It inhibits the growth of Kaposi sarcoma cells in vitro. Lesions should be covered with a generous coating of the gel. It should be allowed to dry for 3 to 5 minutes before covering the treated areas. Application of the drug to normal skin should be avoided. The adverse events associated with this drug occur almost exclusively at the site of application. Most reactions are mild to moderate in severity. Patients should be advised to minimize exposure of treated areas to sunlight and sunlamps. Following topical application, little alitretinoin is absorbed systemically.

Denileukin diftitox (ONTAK) is a recombinant protein that combines the activity of interleukin-2 and diphtheria toxin. If a cell has an interleukin-2 receptor, the drug can bind to the receptor and kill the cell with the toxin. Denileukin diftitox was developed for treatment of lymphomas and leukemias and has also shown effectiveness against late-stage melanoma. It is supplied as a solution that must remain frozen during storage. Before the dose is prepared, the solution must be brought to room temperature. Preparations should be administered within 6 hours of thawing. The solution must never be heated and must not be shaken vigorously, though it can be mixed by swirling gently. The concentration of denileukin difititox must be at least 15 mcg/mL during all steps in the preparation of the infusion. This can best be accomplished by withdrawing the calculated dose from the vials and injecting it into an empty IV infusion bag. For each 1 mL of the solution from the vial, no more than 9 mL of sterile saline without preservative should be added to the IV bag. The diluted solution should be prepared in soft IV bags, because the drug may be adsorbed onto glass when it is in its diluted state. This drug should not be physically mixed with other drugs or come into contact with other drugs within the IV line.

Pemetrexed (Alimta) is an antifolate that, when given with cisplatin, is approved for malignant pleural mesothelioma cases for which surgery is not an option. It has shown a benefit in survival and tumor repression with less neutropenia and hair loss than some of the other drugs used to treat this malignancy. It disrupts the folate-dependent metabolic processes essential for cell replication. The patient should also receive folic acid and vitamin B_{12} when taking this drug. The side effects are decreased renal function and bone marrow suppression.

Procarbazine (Matulane) is used to treat Hodgkin disease. It has side effects of bone marrow depression, leukopenia, thrombocytopenia, ulceration of the skin and GI tract, hair loss, nausea, vomiting, nephrotoxicity, and teratogenicity.

Biologic-Response Modifiers

Biologic-response modifiers were introduced earlier in this chapter, in the discussion of recombinant DNA agents. These substances can alter the host immune response in ways that promote destruction of human malignancies. Three types of agents are discussed here, including interferon, interleukin-2, and tumor necrosis factor.

Interferon Interferon is the name for a group of small proteins produced by immune system cells in response to foreign agents, such as viruses and parasites, and tumor cells. Interferon inhibits viral replication and binds to specific cell receptors, which cause intracellular changes that induce antitumor enzymes. They also stimulate macrophages and render tumor cells more susceptible to immune responses. Interferons used medically are produced by recombinant DNA in *Escherichia coli*. Roferon A (alfa-2a) differs from Intron A (alfa-2b) in only one amino acid. Interferon is approved for use in hairy cell leukemia. Additional studies are being done with melanoma, non-Hodgkin lymphoma, other leukemias, and tumors, but the results are not as encouraging. Side effects include flu-like symptoms, such as fever, chills, fatigue, myalgias, confusion, and hypotension. Symptoms are dose related and diminish with continued use.

Interleukin-2 Interleukin-2 is secreted by T cells. Increased doses activate lymphocytes and enhance their ability to lyse a broad variety of tumor cells. Extremely high doses are administered for several days, followed by removal of activated lymphocytes, which are incubated for 3 to 4 days, then reinfused along with additional high doses. Treatment is highly toxic. Response occurs in 25% of patients with renal cell carcinoma or melanoma, with lesser percentages for other common malignancies. The side effects can be hypotension, fluid retention, arthralgia, dyspnea, malignant hyperthermia, myocardial infarction, delirium, and coma.

Tumor-Necrosis Factor Tumor-necrosis factor is secreted by some macrophages in response to endotoxin, which is released when cells are disrupted by certain bacteria. Tumor-necrosis factor directly causes lysis of susceptible tumor cells.

Cytoprotective (Rescue) Agents

A **cytoprotective agent** is a compound administered to reduce the side effects and toxicity of chemotherapy agents. Timing is critical in the administration of these agents. The chemotherapy agent must be active in the body long enough to kill the malignant cells, and the antidote or "rescue agent" must be administered in time to prevent destruction of the healthy cells.

Amifostine (Ethyol) is a prodrug that is converted primarily in tumor tissue to an active form. It may also tie up free radicals in healthy cells. When used with cisplatin, it reduces kidney toxicity. It is adjunctive therapy for use with chemotherapeutic agents. Side effects are reduced blood pressure, nausea, vomiting, flushing, feeling of warmth, chills, dizziness, somnolence, hiccups, and sneezing.

Dexrazoxane (Zinecard) interferes with the iron radical thought to be responsible for cardiomyopathy. It is used to reduce the incidence and severity of cardiomyopathy associated with doxorubicin administration in women with metastatic breast cancer. The side effects include alopecia, nausea, vomiting, fatigue, stomatitis, fever, diarrhea, pain of injection, and kidney toxicity.

Leucovorin, also called folinic acid, reduces the toxicity of agents that antagonize folic acid. It is used as a rescue agent in methotrexate administration.

Complications of Cancer and Chemotherapy

Cancer patients who are undergoing chemotherapy experience various complications, including pain, nausea and vomiting, and oral complications. Treatments have been developed to reduce these negative effects.

Pain   Cancer patients commonly suffer needlessly because their pain is not adequately controlled. Pain also weakens the patient's appetite, interferes with sleep, and increases fear and anxiety. There is little need to worry about a cancer patient becoming addicted to pain medication. Studies indicate that where there is real pain, there is little, if any, risk of addiction. Treatment should deal with the immediate problem of controlling the pain. If the patient survives and the need for pain medication is eliminated, the issue of physical dependence can be dealt with at that time.

Nausea and Vomiting   The primary side effects of chemotherapy are nausea and vomiting. Despite many advances in treatment, incomplete control of emesis remains a major problem for patients undergoing chemotherapy. Drugs used to control emesis were discussed in Chapter 10.

Oral Complications   Cells of the mucous membranes such as those of the mouth are among the normal cells that divide most rapidly and therefore suffer the most from chemotherapy and radiation. **Oral complications** are common manifestations of toxicity and tissue injury associated with the administration of certain anticancer drugs and radiation. The most common of these oral complications are mucositis and concomitant ulceration and infection. Similar problems are encountered with irradiation to the head and neck.

Oral mucositis and ulceration, with the accompanying pain and discomfort, can interfere with the patient's ability to eat, can necessitate use of potent analgesics, and can create favorable conditions for a local infection that can lead to septicemia and compromise the entire treatment protocol and prognosis. Although oral mucositis and ulceration cannot be prevented, proper management can minimize the duration, discomfort, and potential for infection. Table 16.7 lists the most commonly used agents for mucositis.

Cevimeline (Evoxac) is a cholinergic agonist that binds to muscarinic receptors, a specific type of cell membrane receptor. This leads to an increase in exocrine gland secretions, including saliva and sweat. Cevimeline is available in a hard gel capsule and is indicated for the treatment of dry mouth. Dry mouth may be treated for various reasons; one is to prevent infections of the oral cavity following radiation to the salivary

TABLE 16.7 Most Commonly Used Agents for Mucositis

Generic Name	Pronunciation	Dosage Form	Brand Name	Dispensing Status
cevimeline	se-VIM-e-leen	capsule	Evoxac	Rx
chlorhexidine gluconate	klor-HEX-i-deen GLOO-koe-nate	dental solution	Peridex	Rx
hydrogen peroxide	HYE-dro-jen per-OX-ide	solution	Peroxyl	OTC
lidocaine-diphenhy-dramine-Maalox	LYE-doe-kayn dye-fen-HYE-dra-meen MAY-lox	solution	"Magic Swizzle"	Rx
phenol–sodium borate–sodium bicarbonate–glycerin	FEE-nole SOE-dee-um BOR-ate SOE-dee-um bye-KAR-boe-nate GLIS-er-in	solution	Ulcerease	OTC
pilocarpine	pye-loe-KAR-peen	tablet	Salagen	Rx

glands during treatment of head and neck cancers. In addition, Sjögren syndrome is an autoimmune disorder that results in the inflammation of the salivary and lacrimal (tear) glands, which then progresses to dry mouth and dry eyes. The most common side effect of this drug is increased sweating. It should be taken three times a day.

Hydrogen peroxide has some antibacterial effects, but its primary benefit is the nonmechanical cleansing action produced by the nascent oxygen. It should never be used full-strength for oral cleansing of irritated tissues, but should be diluted with water or saline, preferably in a ratio of one part hydrogen peroxide to one or more parts diluent. **Peroxyl** is a ready-to-use form and should be used at the recommended strength of 1.5%. This pleasant, mint-flavored, aqueous solution is well accepted. Twice-daily brushing and a 30 second rinsing are recommended.

Lidocaine-diphenhydramine-Maalox ("Magic Swizzle") provides some relief for patients. The solution is held in the mouth, swished around, and then spat out. This formula has many names ("Pink Magic" for one). It does not need to be refrigerated and may be made with an antacid other than Maalox. There are many formulas for this and many names for this mixture. Some contain nystatin, tetracycline, hydrocortisone, and/or sulcralfate, so the prescriber must specify the ingredients. Magic Swizzle, or Pink Magic, or whichever name the prescriber uses, is commonly made by the pharmacy technician by combining the three agents in equal parts. For example, if it is written for 120 mL with three ingredients, it will be 40 mL of each, but if it has four ingredients, then it will be 30 mLs of each.

Phenol–sodium borate–sodium bicarbonate–glycerin (Ulcerease) provides topical desensitization and some antimicrobial effect. It contains 0.6% phenol. It may be used as the primary rinse of an oral care regimen to reduce the discomfort of the other cleansing measures.

Pilocarpine (Salagen), artificial saliva, stimulates the salivary glands (muscarinic agonist), alleviating chronic dry mouth, which is painful and makes it difficult to eat or speak. It can lead to tearing, sweating, and runny nose. The patient should be told to drink plenty of fluids when taking this medication.

TAKE WITH
FLUIDS

Prevention of Breast Cancer Recurrence

As shown in Table 16.8, hormonal therapies used to prevent recurrence of breast cancer include two classes of drugs: estrogen receptor antagonists and aromatase inhibitors. Many breast cancers have estrogen receptors, and tumor growth is stimulated by estrogen. Drugs that intercept the production of estrogen therefore prevent cancer growth. All of these drugs cause hot flashes, nausea, and weight gain.

Anastrozole (Arimidex) is used in women with early stage disease after surgical removal of the cancer. It prevents the conversion of adrenally generated androstenedione to estrone in peripheral tissues. It is first-line treatment for postmenopausal women with hormone-receptor-positive breast cancer. Although this drug results in less weight gain, thrombosis, and endometrial cancer than some of the others, there is more risk of bone fracture.

Exemestane (Aromasin) inhibits the endogenous conversion of androgens to estrogens and therefore prevents estrogen from reaching the tumor cells. It is indicated only for women with hysterectomies. It is approved for cancer that progressed while the patient was taking tamoxifen (discussed below). It may have a role in postmenopausal early-stage breast cancer. It is suggested that women be switched to this drug after 2 to 3 years of tamoxifen treatment.

Warning

Faslodex and Zoladex are two injectables that could be easily confused.

Fulvestrant (Faslodex) is a true estrogen receptor antagonist. There are no agonist effects. It is taken for metastatic breast cancer if tumors progress. The most common side effects are gastrointestinal. It is indicated only for second-line use.

Letrozole (Femara) suppresses estrogen synthesis. It is approved to prevent recurrent breast cancer. In addition to reducing the risk of breast cancer recurrence, it decreases the risk of endometrial cancer and blood clots. However, the risk of bone loss increases. The physician should make sure that women on this drug consume vitamin D, calcium, and a bisphosphonate.

Tamoxifen (Nolvadex) blocks estrogen receptors in only some tissue; unlike other common breast cancer drugs, it prevents bone fractures. This latter attribute is due to the estrogenic effects of tamoxifen in bone cells that decrease bone loss. A 5 year course of this agent after lumpectomy or mastectomy significantly reduces the risk of recurrence and improves survival. Over time, however, the tumors can become resistant to tamoxifen therapy. Consequently, the National Cancer Institute is now alerting oncologists to limit tamoxifen use to 5 years. New evidence indicates that longer use does not improve survival and might even be detrimental by increasing the risk of uterine cancer. Tamoxifen also increases the possibility of endometrial cancer, vaginal bleeding, and blood clots. Patients usually begin by using tamoxifen, but after the benefits of tamoxifen decrease, the patient is often switched to letrozole.

TABLE 16.8 Most Commonly Used Drugs for Prevention of Breast Cancer Recurrence

Generic Name	Pronunciation	Dosage Form	Brand Name	Dispensing Status
Estrogen Receptor Antagonists				
fulvestrant	fool-VES-trant	injection	Faslodex	Rx
tamoxifen	ta-MOX-i-fen	tablet	Nolvadex	Rx
Aromatase Inhibitors				
anastrozole	an-AS-troe-zole	tablet	Arimidex	Rx
exemestane	ex-uh-MES-tane	tablet	Aromasin	Rx
letrozole	LET-roe-zole	tablet	Femara	Rx

Chapter Terms

amino acid the basic unit of a protein molecule; there are 20 different amino acids used in proteins, each having a specific set of shape, electrical charge, and water or fat affinity characteristics

antirejection drug a medication that prevents the body from rejecting foreign solid organ transplants

B cell antibody-producing lymphocyte involved in humoral immunity

biologic-response modifiers agents that alter the expression and response to surface antigens and enhance immune cell activities in ways that promote destruction of human malignancies

biotechnology the application of biologic systems and organisms for agricultural, industrial, and medical purposes

cellular (cell-mediated) immunity a specific response to antigens that is mediated primarily by T lymphocytes and macrophages

cloning reproducing identical copies of a gene by DNA technology

colony-stimulating factor (CSF) a chemical that stimulates the bone marrow to produce blood cells

complement lipoproteins and globulins in blood plasma that react with the antigen-antibody complex

complementary of a nucleic acid strand, having each nucleotide base paired up with its counterpart in the other strand

cytoprotective agent an agent administered to reduce the side effects and toxicity of chemotherapy agents

denatured disruption of the structure

diffuse tumor a cancerous growth that is widely distributed and is not localized

DNA sequence order of nucleotide bases in the DNA molecule; a group of three nucleotides translates into one amino acid

extravasation the escape of IV fluids into the surrounding tissue

granulocyte colony-stimulating factor (G-CSF) an agent that stimulates the bone marrow to produce specific white cells, such as the granulocytes

hematologic agent a replacement plasma protein that is necessary for blood coagulation and is not produced in a person with hemophilia

humoral immunity an immune response in which secreted antibodies are transported by bodily fluids

immune response the immune system's way of providing resistance to disease and malignancy through the production of antibodies and phagocytes

immunoglobulin (Ig) a protein that responds to a specfic antigen; also known as an antibody

lymphatic system a network of vessels that carry lymph, the lymph nodes, and the lymphoid organs including the tonsils, spleen, and thymus; a system for filtering body fluids by nodes, vessels, and lymphocytes before the fluid returns to general circulation

MAb (monoclonal antibody) an antibody produced in the laboratory by a culture derived from a single B cell

macrophage a large white blood cell that engulfs antigens, toxins, and cellular debris, and digests it, and displays peptides complexed with MHC for recognition by T cells

neoplastic disease a disorder that occurs when normal cellular control mechanisms become altered; characterized by uncontrolled cellular growth and the development of abnormal cells; also referred to as cancer

nucleotide the basic unit of a DNA molecule, containing one of four possible bases

opsonization labeling antigenic material so that it is more readily identified and destroyed by macrophages

oral complications tissue injury to the oral cavity associated with chemotherapy and radiation

plasma cell a B cell that produces freely circulating antibody in very large quantities

plasmid a small circular ring of DNA that can insert itself into bacterial genes and can carry genes from one bacterial cell to another

primary site the original site where a cancer tumor develops

promoter the part of plasmid DNA where protein production starts

recombinant DNA artificial DNA produced in a laboratory by inserting strands of DNA from one organism into that of another organism

remission the condition in which a tumor is inactive with no cell division or growth; typically, a goal of chemotherapy

replication the process of copying the DNA of a cell into a new set of DNA molecules to produce a new cell

resistance lack of responsiveness of cancer cells to chemotherapy

secondary site a new cancer tumor site to which malignant cells have spread from the original site

small lymphocyte T and B memory cells, which carry and preserve information for the recognition of specific antigens

solid tumor a tumor that forms a solid mass and can be palpated

T cell lymphocyte that responds to antigens presented on the surface of other cells; involved in cellular immunity

terminator the portion of plasmid DNA where protein production stops

transcription the copying of information from a DNA strand onto an RNA strand, which then serves as a messenger to the molecular systems that use it to assemble a protein

Chapter Summary

Recombinant DNA

- Biotechnology is the method of applying biologic systems and organisms to industrial and technical use.
- In the recombinant DNA process, the DNA that codes for a valuable protein in the body is inserted into the DNA of a different organism so that that cell can multiply and produce the protein in large quantities.
- The desired gene may be introduced into a bacterial, fungal, or mammalian cell.
- Plasmids are small circular rings of DNA found in bacteria. They replicate themselves and move freely between bacterial cells. Plasmids can carry genes such as those that make a bacterium resistant to antibiotics.
- Cloning produces identical copies of the gene of interest.

- The environment of the host cell is critical for the proper folding of the protein.
- Producing protein through recombinant DNA technology offers many advantages: protein can be produced in large quantities without the risk of contamination that is present when protein is harvested from human sources.
- Some studies are showing that the expense saved by curtailing hospital stays, shortening the duration of illnesses, and decreasing the incidence of disease more than pays for recombinant DNA drugs.
- The positive clinical implications of colony-stimulating factors (CSFs) include decreasing the period of severe neutropenia after cytotoxic chemotherapy or marrow transplantation, treatment of aplastic anemia,

and treatment of other immunodeficiency states associated with cytopenia.

- Epoetin alfa (erythropoietin) increases RBCs; filgrastim and pegfilgrastin increase WBCs.
- Biologic-response modifiers reduce cytokines and increase T-suppressor cell activity. They reduce the frequency of clinical exacerbations in ambulatory patients with relapsing multiple sclerosis.
- Alteplase (Activase) is a tissue plasminogen activator that catalyzes the conversion of tissue plasminogen to plasmin in the presence of fibrin.
- Dornase alfa (Pulmozyme) reduces sputum thickness in cystic fibrosis.
- Antihemophilic factor, also called factor VIII, is used to treat hemophilia.

Immune System

- The body presents three lines of defense: (1) surfaces of intact skin and mucous membranes, (2) a nonspecific defense, and (3) the immune response.
- The immune response has two features: specificity, or the ability to attack a specific antigen, and memory, or the ability to remember the antigen for future invasion.
- Opsonization is the enhancing of phagocytosis of bacteria.
- There are several types of immunoglobulins. IgG is the smallest and most common. IgM has the highest molecular weight. IgA is the main Ig in salivary and bronchial secretions, bile, and tears; it is also found in breast milk and colostrum. IgE is responsible for hypersensitivity reactions and is present in increased amounts in patients with allergic rhinitis and allergic asthma; IgD functions as a B cell receptor and may affect B cell maturation.
- The magnitude of an antibody response depends on the nature of the antigen, the frequency of exposure, and the duration of each exposure.
- A lack of humoral immunity, as in inherited disorders in which B cells are deficient or absent, increases susceptibility to bacterial infections, but not to viral infections or neoplastic disease. Conversely, attenuation of cellular immunity without a corresponding reduction in the reactive capacity of B cells increases susceptibility to viral infection and neoplasm, but not to bacterial infection.
- CellCept, Imuran, Prograf, Sandimmune, and Orthoclone OKT3 are antirejection drugs.
- Monoclonal antibodies (MAbs) are laboratory-produced antibodies (immunoglobulins), produced by a culture derived from a single B cell, that can be targeted to attack specific substances in the body.
- MAbs can be put to work in several ways: to bind to defective cells to help the immune system find those cells; to bind to receptors so as to block growth signals; to deliver radioactive elements to specific cells; and to slip drugs into specific cells.
- MAbs are named in a unique way.
- MAbs must be handled gently and not shaken.

Cancer

- Neoplastic disease occurs when cells become resistant to normal growth controls and growth patterns are altered.
- Generally the side effects of chemotherapy are bone marrow depression, leukopenia, thrombocytopenia, stomatitis, ulceration of the skin and GI tract, hair loss, nausea, vomiting, nephrotoxicity, and teratogenicity.
- Remission puts the tumor into an inactive period when there is no active cell division and growth. It does not cure the disease, but it does extend the patient's life.
- Alkylating agents prevent cell division by binding cross-links in DNA strands, which leads to death within the cell.
- Antibiotics inhibit DNA-dependent RNA synthesis or delay or inhibit mitosis.
- Antimetabolites incorporate into normal cell constituents, making them nonfunctional, or inhibit the normal function of a key enzyme.

- Hormones inhibit the synthesis of adrenal steroids and the actions of hormones on specific tissues.

- Nitrogen mustards bind irreversible cross-links in cellular DNA; thus, DNA and RNA cannot reproduce.

- Plant alkaloids inhibit the formation of spindle fibers, arresting the metaphase of cell division.

- Topoisomerase I inhibitors lead to DNA damage when cells replicate. Other agents work by producing toxic metabolites and inhibiting RNA and protein synthesis.

- Interferon inhibits viral replication.

- Tumor necrosis factor is secreted by macrophages in response to endotoxin.

- Colony-stimulating factors increase the host's ability to produce blood cells, which enhances production of granulocytes, monocytes, or RBCs.

- Monoclonal antibodies are used to direct attacks against specific objectives.

- Tyrokinase inhibiting agents block tyrosine kinase activity, which promotes cell growth. They seem to be as effective as other chemo agents with fewer and less severe side effects.

- Rescue agents reduce the side effects and toxicity of chemotherapy. Timing is critical to prevent destruction of healthy cells.

- Many cancer patients do not get adequate pain relief.

- Oral complications are common manifestations associated with chemotherapy.

- The pharmacy technician can provide an invaluable service to patients by making sure they get their pre-meds and checking for fluids for hydration.

Drug List

The following drugs were discussed in this chapter. Each generic drug name is followed in parentheses by one or more brand names.

Recombinant DNA Agents

Colony-Stimulating Factors
epoetin alfa (Epogen, Procrit)
filgrastim (Neupogen)
pegfilgrastim (Neulasta)
sargramostim (Leukine)

Biologic-Response Modifiers
aldesleukin (Proleukin)
interferon alfa-2a (Roferon A)
interferon alfa-2b (Intron A)
interferon beta-1a (Avonex, Rebif)
interferon beta-1b (Betaseron)

Secretion-Thinning Enzyme
dornase alfa (Pulmozyme)

Hematologic Agent
antihemophilic factor (Alphanate)

Antirejection Drugs
azathioprine (Imuran)
cyclosporine (Sandimmune)
mycophenolate (CellCept)
sirolimus (Rapamune)
tacrolimus (Prograf)

Monoclonal Antibodies

abciximab (ReoPro)
adalimumab (Humira)
alemtuzumab (Campath)
basiliximab (Simulect)
bevacizumab (Avastin)
cetuximab (Erbitux)
daclizumab (Zenapax)
efalizumab (Raptiva)
gemtuzumab (Mylotarg)
ibritumomab tiuxetan (Zevalin)
infliximab (Remicade)
muromonab-CD3 (Orthoclone OKT3)
natalizumab (Tysabri)
omalizumab (Xolair)
palivizumab (Synagis)
panitumumab (Vectibix)
ranibizumab (Lucenetis)
rituximab (Rituxan, Mabthera)
tositumomab (Bexxar)
trastuzumab (Herceptin)

Agents for Chemotherapy

Alkylating Agents

busulfan (Myleran)
carboplatin (Paraplatin)
carmustine (BiCNU)
cisplatin (Platinol)
cyclophosphamide (Cytoxan)
dacarbazine (DTIC-Dome)
ifosfamide (Ifex)
lomustine (CeeNU)
oxaliplatin (Eloxatin)
streptozocin (Zanosar)
temozolomide (Temodar)

Antibiotics

bleomycin (Blenoxane)
dactinomycin (Cosmegen)
daunorubicin (Cerubidine)
doxorubicin (Adriamycin PFS)
epirubicin (Ellence)
idarubicin (Idamycin)
mitomycin (Mutamycin)
plicamycin (Mithracin)
valrubicin (Valstar Preservative Free)

Antimetabolites

capecitabine (Xeloda)
cytarabine (Cytosar-U)

floxuridine (FUDR)
fludarabine (Fludara)
fluorouracil (Efudex)
hydroxyurea (Hydrea)
mercaptopurine (Purinethol)
methotrexate (Rheumatrex)
thioguanine (Tabloid)

Hormones

abarelix (Plenaxis)
aminoglutethimide (Cytadren)
bicalutamide (Casodex)
flutamide (Eulexin)
goserelin (Zoladex)
leuprolide (Eligard, Lupron Depot, Viadur)
megestrol (Megace)
mitotane (Lysodren)
triptorelin (Trelstar)

Nitrogen Mustards

chlorambucil (Leukeran)
estramustine (Emcyt)
mechlorethamine (Mustargen)
melphalan (Alkeran)
thiotepa

Plant Alkaloids

docetaxel (Taxotere)
etoposide (VePesid)
paclitaxel (Taxol, Abraxane)
vinblastine (Velban)
vincristine (Oncovin, Vincasar PFS)

Topoisomerase I Inhibitors

irinotecan (Camptosar)
topotecan (Hycamtin)

Tyrokinase Inhibitors

dasatinib (Sprycel)
erlotinib (Tarceva)
imatinib (Gleevec)
nilotinib (Tasigna)

Miscellaneous Agents

alitretinoin (Panretin)
altretamine (Hexalen)
arsenic trioxide (Trisenox)
asparaginase (Elspar)
bortezomib (Velcade)
denileukin diftitox (ONTAK)
gefitinib (Iressa)
mitoxantrone (Novantrone)

pemetrexed (Alimta)
procarbazine (Matulane)

Cytoprotective (Rescue) Agents
amifostine (Ethyol)
dexrazoxane (Zinecard)
leucovorin

Agents for Mucositis
cevimeline (Evoxac)
chlorhexidine gluconate (Peridex)
hydrogen peroxide (Peroxyl)
lidocaine-diphenhydramine-Maalox ("Magic Swizzle")
phenol–sodium borate–sodium bicarbonate–glycerin (Ulcerease)
pilocarpine (Salagen)

Drugs to Prevent Recurrence of Breast Cancer
Estrogen Receptor Antagonists
fulvestrant (Faslodex)
tamoxifen (Nolvadex)

Aromatase Inhibitors
anastrozole (Arimidex)
exemestane (Aromasin)
letrozole (Femara)

Chapter Review

Pharmaceuticals and Body Functions

Select the best answer from the choices given.

1. Betaseron is used to treat
   a. infections.
   b. multiple sclerosis.
   c. Kaposi sarcoma.
   d. chronic hepatitis.

2. A secretion thinning enzyme used in cystic fibrosis is
   a. Imuran
   b. Prograf
   c. Pulmozyme
   d. Sandimmune

3. The most common protein with antibody activity is
   a. IgG.
   b. IgM.
   c. IgE.
   d. IgD.

4. MAbs work by
   a. helping the immune system find defective cells
   b. blocking growth signals
   c. slipping drugs into specific cells
   d. all of the above

5. Which class of drugs seems to be as effective as the other chemotheraeutic agents with fewer side effects?
   a. nitrogen mustards
   b. plant alkaloids
   c. topoisomerase I inhibitors
   d. tyrokinase inhibitors

6. As a product source identifier for a MAb, the syllable "zu" represents
   a. human
   b. mouse
   c. combination
   d. none of the above

7. What steps are required to produce protein?
   a. replication
   b. transcription
   c. translation
   d. both b and c

8. More and more chemo and salvage agents are being dispensed outside the hospital setting. The pharmacy technician needs to be aware of the following
   a. regimens
   b. free periods
   c. salvage therapy
   d. all of the above

9. "Vir" is the symbol to identify which target?
   a. infections
   b. ovary
   c. circulation
   d. virus

10. Remission
    a. puts a tumor into an inactive period.
    b. cures the disease.
    c. gives the patient less time.
    d. results in active cell division.

The following statements are true or false. If the answer is false, rewrite the statement so it is true.

_____ 1. The side effects of most chemotherapy are bone marrow depression, leukopenia, nausea, and vomiting.

_____ 2. The technician can provide an invaluable service to the patient when dispensing the drugs discussed in this chapter by making sure the patients gets the pre-meds.

_____ 3. Epogen must be shaken well.

_____ 4. Colony-stimulating factors decrease the period of severe neutropenia.

_____ 5. Neoplastic disease occurs when cells become resistant to normal growth controls and growth patterns are altered.

_____ 6. Interferon increases the host's ability to produce blood cells.

_____ 7. Interleukin is secreted by some macrophages in response to endotoxin.

_____ 8. Tumor-necrosis factor inhibits viral replication.

_____ 9. Alkylating agents inhibit DNA-dependent RNA synthesis or delay or inhibit mitosis.

_____ 10. Antimetabolites are incorporated into normal cell constituents, making them nonfunctional, or inhibit the normal function of a key enzyme.

Diseases and Drug Therapies

1. List the disadvantages of extracting protein from plasma or tissue.

2. List the three lines of defense the human body has against invasion by pathogens.

3. Define remission.

4. Define resistance.

Complete the following chart

MAb	Target	Source
abciximab		
alemtuzumab		
daclizumab		
gemtuzumab		
ibritumomab		

Dispensing Medications

1. Mrs. Brown brings in the following prescription. She has been taking the drug for at least 5 years. What should be done?

2. A patient brings the following prescription into the pharmacy. What should the pharmacy technician do?

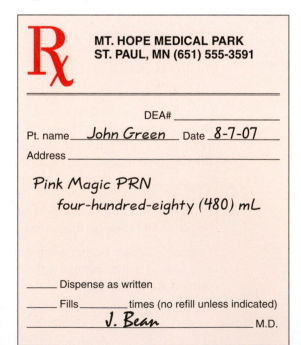

℞ MT. HOPE MEDICAL PARK
ST. PAUL, MN (651) 555-3591

DEA# _____

Pt. name _Sue Brown_ Date _8-7-07_

Address _____

Tamoxifen ten (10) mg bid
sixty (60)

____ Dispense as written
✓ Fills _twelve_ times (no refill unless indicated)
_J. Bean_____ M.D.

℞ MT. HOPE MEDICAL PARK
ST. PAUL, MN (651) 555-3591

DEA# _____

Pt. name _John Green_ Date _8-7-07_

Address _____

Pink Magic PRN
four-hundred-eighty (480) mL

____ Dispense as written
____ Fills _____ times (no refill unless indicated)
_J. Bean_____ M.D.

Internet Research

Use the Internet to complete the following activities.

1. The antirejection drugs covered in this chapter are an important component of successful organ transplantation. Find data on common organ transplantation procedures. Create a table giving an overview of three procedures. Include the number of transplants done per year, the disease states/conditions that lead to the need for transplantation, the cost of the procedure, and the Internet sites from which you obtained your information.

2. New chemotherapeutics are being developed continuously. Research new chemotherapeutics, focusing on one particular type of cancer (e.g., colorectal, breast, liver, lung). Create a table listing three new agents. If you include drugs that are currently in clinical trials, indicate what phase of testing has been completed. Be sure to include the type of cancer researched in your table. List your Internet sources.

What Would You Do?

1. Orders came down for rituximab (Rituxan). There are no orders for premeds or hydration for this patient. What should the pharmacy technician do?

Vitamins, OTC Supplements, Antidotes, and Miscellaneous Topics

17

Learning Objectives

- Understand how the body uses vitamins and electrolytes.
- Understand enteral and parenteral nutrition, including its purposes, ingredients, stability, and complications.
- Recognize herbs, their values, uses, and dangers.
- Become familiar with the supportive therapy and antidotes used to treat occurrences of poisoning.

- Understand the importance of the Blue Alert cart, its supplies, and its maintenance.
- Be aware of the role of the pharmacy technician in the event of a bioterrorist attack.

Preview chapter terms and definitions.

Consumption of food and other nondrug substances has far-reaching effects on the healthy body and in recuperation after an illness. Foods contain vitamins, minerals, and other nutrients that maintain body function and aid in disease prevention and treatment. Electrolytes regulate electrical activity of the body and need to be kept in balance with body fluids. Plant substances such as herbs can affect the body, and many of them have medicinal applications. Ingestion of some substances can result in poisoning, causing critical states and necessitating use of lavage measures, antidotes, and supportive therapy. Recent improvements have been made in dealing with life-threatening diseases and emergencies. The pharmacy technician plays an important role by understanding a hospital Code Blue emergency system and the use and maintenance of the Blue Alert carts. Furthermore, pharmacy technicians are trained to be primary responders in the event of a bioterrorist attack.

Vitamins, Fluid Levels, and Electrolytes

Vitamins are organic substances that are necessary for normal metabolic functioning but that are not synthesized in the body in sufficient amounts. Usually a vitamin is a **coenzyme** (a chemical other than a protein needed by an enzyme to assist in performing a metabolic function) or is converted to a coenzyme in the body. If dietary intake of any of these substances is inadequate, a deficiency results; such deficiencies can lead to serious illness. Vitamins occur in many foods and can be supplemented artificially.

In humans, vitamin deficiencies occur as five major diseases. Most signs and symptoms can be reversed by administering the appropriate vitamin.

- Keratomalacia is a vitamin A deficiency that causes softening of the cornea.
- Rickets is a vitamin D deficiency that causes bending of the bones.
- Beriberi is a vitamin B_1 deficiency that causes polyneuritis, edema, and cardiac problems.
- Pellagra is a vitamin B_3 (niacin) deficiency that causes dermatitis and diarrhea.
- Scurvy is a vitamin C deficiency that causes anemia, spongy gums, hemorrhages, and brawny hardening of calf and leg muscles.

Vitamins

Vitamins are classified as either fat-soluble or water-soluble. Vitamins are listed in Table 17.1.

Fat-Soluble Vitamins **Fat-soluble vitamins** are absorbed with dietary fats and are maintained in stores by the body, mainly in the liver. Deficiency develops only after several months of restricted intake. As excessive amounts collect, signs of toxicity develop.

Vitamin A, retinol, is present in milk, butter, cheese, liver, fish oils, and other foods. It can be formed in the body from plant pigments and carotene from fruits and vegetables; the conversion occurs in the wall of the small intestine. Impaired ability to absorb lipids affects absorption of vitamin A. The body uses vitamin A for normal growth, bone formation, shedding and repair of epithelial tissue, retinal function, male and female reproductive functions, and stability of cell membranes.

TABLE 17.1 **Vitamins**

Vitamin	Function in human body	Vitamin type
A	bones, skin, eyes, reproduction	fat-soluble
B1 (thiamine)	metabolism, mental, cardiac	water-soluble
B2 (riboflavin)	hair, skin, nails	water-soluble
B3 (niacin)	cholesterol levels, brain cells, skin, bowel	water-soluble
B5 (pantothenic acid)	growth, normal physiological functions and energy production	water-soluble
B6 (pyridoxine)	nerves	water-soluble
B7 (biotin)	hair, energy production, growth	water-soluble
B9 (folic acid)	red blood cells, depression	water-soluble
B12 (cyanocobalamin)	red blood cells	water-soluble
C	immunity	water-soluble
D	bones	fat-soluble
E	eyes, immunity, dementia	fat-soluble
K	blood clotting	fat-soluble

Vitamin D (D_2, ergocalciferol; D_3, cholecalciferol) is found in butter, milk, cheese, egg yolk, and fish oils. In the body, vitamin D is transported in lipoprotein particles into the lymphatic system; bile is necessary for its absorption. It is normally formed by ultraviolet irradiation of the skin, which converts precursors into active forms. Calciferol is formed from D_2 and D_3 and is then rapidly absorbed into the bloodstream. The major effects of vitamin D are seen in calcium and phosphate balance. Deficiency in children causes rickets; long bones of the legs and bones of the pelvis and spine become distorted because of poor mineralization of newly formed bone. Deficiency in adults causes **osteomalacia**, which is the demineralization and weakening of the skeleton.

Vitamin E comprises the **tocopherol** group of compounds. Sources include soybean oil, wheat germ, rice germ, cottonseed, nuts, corn, butter, eggs, liver, and leafy green vegetables. Vitamin E acts as an antioxidant for unsaturated fatty acids, preventing or delaying their deterioration by the oxygen in the air. Vitamin E requirements increase with increased intake of fatty acids. Only the amount on the bottle should be taken, because taking too much vitamin E can be bad for the heart. The body uses this vitamin to prevent cataracts, enhance the immune response (especially against prostate cancer), prevent cardiovascular disease, and slow the onset of dementia.

Vitamin K, **phytonadione**, functions in the formation of prothrombin in the liver and thus plays a role in blood clotting. Its sources are leafy green vegetables, wheat bran, and soybean products.

Water-Soluble Vitamins **Water-soluble vitamins**—the B complexes and vitamin C —are present in extracellular fluids, which are readily excreted by the kidneys. Because these vitamins are not stored in the body and the kidneys rapidly remove any excess, a deficiency quickly becomes apparent if dietary sources are inadequate, but an overdose is unlikely to be as serious as with fat-soluble vitamins.

Vitamin C, ascorbic acid, is found in green plants, tomatoes, citrus fruits, and potatoes, with smaller amounts in animal tissues. It is the most powerful natural reducing agent (antioxidant) in living tissue. Vitamin C increases the phagocytic functioning of leukocytes, has anti-inflammatory activity, promotes healing, and plays an important role in the function of the immune system.

Vitamin B is not a single vitamin, but a group of vitamins. Sources are yeast, meats, whole meal flour, peas, and beans.

B_1, thiamine, acts as a coenzyme in carbohydrate metabolism. Sources include pork, liver, kidney, whole cereal, grains, peas, beans, and yeast. Deficiency results in beriberi. Alcoholics commonly have a vitamin B_1 deficiency; thus, they frequently receive B_1 supplements. Thiamine is necessary for energy production, normal functioning of the heart, nervous system, and muscles. The biggest impact of deficiency is on mental and cardiac function.

B_2, riboflavin, is needed for metabolic energy pathways and for phosphorylation in intestinal mucosa, which functions to maintain the integrity of mucous membranes. Sources are milk, meat, cereals, green vegetables, and intestinal synthesis. It is important for growth, nerve function, and red blood cell production, but the primary impact is on the hair, skin, and nails.

B_3, nicotinic acid or **niacin**, is involved in fat synthesis, electron transport, and protein metabolism. It occurs in yeast, liver, lean meats, peanuts, peas, beans, whole wheat, rice grains, and, in lesser amounts, potatoes and vegetables. The three Ds of a vitamin B_3 deficiency are diarrhea, dementia (depression, memory loss, confusion), and dermatitis (a dark red coloration on all areas of the skin exposed to air and light). Niacin lowers cholesterol.

B$_5$, pantothenic acid, is found in most vegetables, cereals, yeast, and liver. Deficiency symptoms include fatigue, headache, sleepiness, nausea, GI pain, muscle spasms, and impaired coordination. It is a coenzyme in numerous chemical reactions in all cells. It is essential for growth, normal physiological functions, and energy production.

B$_6$, pyridoxine, is a coenzyme in amino acid and fatty acid metabolism. It is found in practically all foods of plant and animal origin. Vitamin B$_6$ is given to alcoholics who have nerve damage. Tuberculosis patients who take isoniazid (INH) and hypertension patients who take hydralazine have depleted B$_6$, which may lead to peripheral neuropathies.

B$_7$, biotin (also known as vitamin H) is a water-soluble vitamin found in yeast, egg yolk, vegetables, nuts, and cereals. It is a coenzyme required for the synthesis of fatty acids and amino acids and to metabolize carbohydrates, fats, and proteins for energy. It promotes healthy nerve tissue, bone marrow, and sweat glands. It can improve fingernail and toenail health. Deficiencies are uncommon because biotin is found in many foods, is recycled by the body, and is also formed by intestinal flora.

B$_9$, folic acid, occurs in liver and fresh green vegetables. Together, vitamins B$_{12}$ and B$_9$ provide for production of healthy red blood cells. It is especially important that sexually active women of child-bearing age get the minimum daily requirement of folic acid. This is because during the first few weeks of pregnancy, which is before women generally know they are pregnant, folic acid is critical to healthy fetal development. Insufficient folic acid is associated with birth defects. Folic acid is also commonly given to alcoholics. If the cause of an anemia is unknown, the treatment of choice is usually B$_{12}$ with folic acid. The lack of folic acid may be associated with depression more than any other nutrient deficiency.

B$_{12}$, cyanocobalamin, occurs in animal tissues and most multivitamin preparations. It is a cofactor and combines with the intrinsic factor (a protein produced in the stomach) in the production of red blood cells. The deficiency is exhibited as pernicious anemia. When treating deficiency, it is recommended that B$_{12}$ be given intramuscularly or intravenously because it is poorly absorbed orally. B$_{12}$ is absorbed from the GI tract only in the presence of intrinsic factor, which is produced by the gastric mucosa. If intrinsic factor is deficient, B$_{12}$ must be given by injection because it will not be absorbed orally. If taken orally, it must be consumed in very large amounts to have any effect whatsoever.

Medical Foods

According to the Food and Drug Administration, a **medical food** is a "food formulated to be consumed or administered enterally under the supervision of a physician and which is intended for the specific dietary management of a disease or condition for which distinctive nutritional requirements, based on recognized scientific principles, are established by

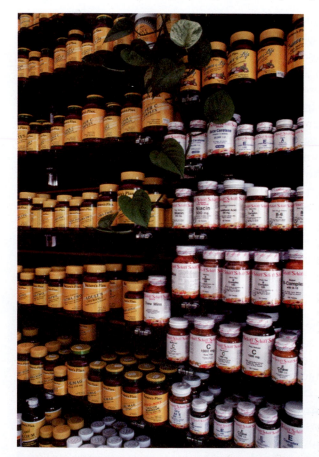

Self-medicating with large doses of vitamins can cause problems. A well-balanced diet is the best way to ensure good health.

medical evaluation." Products on the market for which manufacturers are allowed to make medical claims to help a particular disease are designated as medical foods. They do not require a prescription, but the manufacturer may decide they are to be dispensed only with a prescription. They do not undergo FDA review. Medical food products are used for burn victims, kidney dialysis patients, and individuals with cardiovascular disease or osteoporosis. The most common medical foods are listed in Table 17.2.

Flavocoxid (Limbrel), is marketed for the clinical management of osteoarthritis. Flavocoxid contains plant pigments that naturally occur in some fruits, vegetables, teas, wines, nuts, and seeds. It may have antioxidant and anti-inflammatory activity, which the manufacturer contrasts with the single activitiy of COX-2 inhibitors.

L-methylfolate (Deplin) is intended for the dietary management of low plasma and/or low red blood cell folate. The manufacturers emphasize the utility of L-methylfolate for those who have a major depressive disorder and have not responded to antidepressant medication. L-methylfolate is the primary active isomer of folate and the form of folate in circulation in the body.

L-methylfolate/methylcobalamin/N-acetylcysteine (Cerefolin NAC) is a vitamin combination high in folic acid. It provides folate and vitamin B_{12}, reduces oxidative stress, and lowers homocysteine levels.

Probiotics

Just as an antibiotic reduces harmful bacteria in the body, a **probiotic** stimulates the growth of "good" bacteria in the body—the normal bacterial flora of the body, especially of the the intestinal tract, which can be depleted by antibiotic treatment.

Yogurt is a probiotic; however, not all yogurt contains the right combination. It would take about 8 ounces of yogurt twice a day to prevent antibiotic-associated diarrhea. The eating of the yogurt and taking of the antibiotic should be separated by at least 2 hours. It is very important to watch the expiration dates on these products. Table 17.3 lists some probiotic products and their uses.

Body Fluids

Water is the major constituent of living cells. Body fluids are divided into two compartments: intracellular (inside cells) and extracellular (outside cells; that is, in the spaces between cells and in the lymph and plasma). Furthermore, body fluids are in equilibrium across the capillary walls. In fact, the chemical and physical processes that proceed in an effort to maintain equilibrium are some of the most important processes in the human body.

TABLE 17.2   The Most Common Medical Foods

Generic Name	Pronunciation	Dosage Form	Brand Name	Use
flavocoxid	flav-oe-KOX-id	capsule	Limbrel	osteoarthritis
L-methylfolate	ell-meth-ill-FOE-late	tablet	Deplin	low red blood cells
L-methylfolate/ methylcobalamin/ N-acetylcysteine	ell-meth-ill-FOE-late/ meth-ill-koe-BAL-a-min/ en-a-see-til-SIS-teen	tablet	Cerefolin	lowers homocysteine

TABLE 17.3   The Most Common Probiotic Products

Probiotic	Species	Form	Use
acidophilus (generic)	*Lactobacillus acidophilus*	capsule, liquid, powder, suppository	diarrhea, vaginitis
Activia	*Bifidobacterium animalis*	yogurt	constipation
Align	*Bifidobacterium infantis*	capsule	irritable bowel syndrome
Culturelle	*Lactobacillus GG*	capsule	diarrhea
Flora-Q	*Lactobacillus acidophilus, Bifidobacterium, L. paracasei, Streptococcus thermophilus*	capsule	irritable bowel syndrome
Lactinex	*Lactobacillus acidophilus, L. helveticus*	tablet, granules	diarrhea, cold sores

FIGURE 17.1
Average Water Percentage of Body Weight for Adult Men and Women

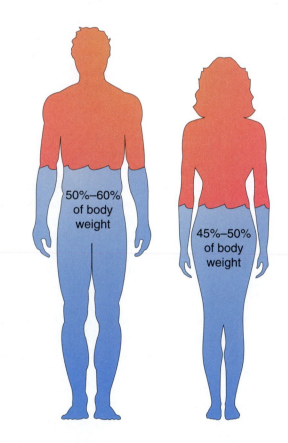

50%–60% of body weight

45%–50% of body weight

The human body consists of 40 to 70% water by weight. Total body water varies between men and women. Figure 17.1 shows the average percentage of body weight that is made up of water in adult men and women. The difference is due to skeletal weight and the inverse relation of water to adipose tissue.

The percentage of body water (that is, fluid levels) varies according to conditions, weight, sex, and age. Fatty tissue holds little water. Therefore, the proportion of water in obese persons may be as little as 55%, whereas in lean, well-muscled persons it may be as much as 70%. Women have more fat than men; therefore, they have proportionally less body water. The body loses water with aging. Newborns may have as much as 75% or more; the elderly have 60% or less.

Water deficits are caused by loss of body fluids as a result of such disorders as vomiting, diarrhea, edema, and excessive sweating from fever; large urine output; and acute weight loss (more than 5% of body weight). A water deficit can cause dry skin and mucous membranes, longitudinal wrinkling of the tongue, hypotension, tachycardia, and lowered body temperature. A loss of 25% of body water can lead to death.

Electrolytes

An **electrolyte** is a compound that separates into ions when dissolved in water. Ions are electrically-charged particles; positive ions are called cations and negative ions are called anions. Thus, when electrolytes are in solution, they transport an electrical charge. Electrolyte concentrations relevant to healthcare are measured in milliequivalents (mEq) of an ion per liter of solution. One equivalent of an ion in grams is equal to the atomic or molecular weight divided by the charge of the ion. For example, sodium ion (Na^{1+}) has an atomic weight of 23 and a charge of +1, so 1 mEq of sodium is 23 mg. Calcium (Ca^{2+}) has an atomic weight of 40 and a charge of +2, so 1 mEq of calcium is 20 mg. Appendix E shows normal lab values.

Sodium (Na^{1+}) Sodium is the primary cation of extracellular fluid. Sodium has a variety of crucial functions, including retaining fluid in the body, generating and transmitting nerve impulses, maintaining acid-base balance, regulating enzyme activities, and regulating osmolarity and electroneutrality of cells. The kidneys are responsible for maintaining normal sodium concentrations in plasma and other body fluids. Significant losses of sodium can occur through vomiting or diarrhea, either of which reduces extracellular fluid volume. Fluids then move out of the cells in an effort to maintain blood volume. If water and sodium are not replaced, blood volume and blood pressure are reduced, and circulatory collapse may occur. The average diet provides sufficient sodium to meet the body's requirements.

Potassium (K^{1+}) Potassium is the primary cation of intracellular fluid. Potassium is important in the regulation of the acid-base and water balance of the body, in protein synthesis and carbohydrate metabolism, in muscle building, and in the function of the nervous system. Potassium depletion produces loss of muscle tone, weakness, and paralysis; potassium excess, on the other hand, can produce cardiac arrhythmias and heart block. Intravenous potassium solutions should be diluted to a concentration no greater than 100 mEq/L. More concentrated solutions may cause phlebitis (irritation of the vein), and rapid infusions can result in lethal cardiac arrhythmias. Klor-Con is a brand name for oral potassium. It is probably the most commonly prescribed potassium supplement. Klor-Con is commonly used by patients who take diuretics.

Calcium (Ca^{2+}) Calcium is important in bone formation and dynamics, muscle contraction, and blood coagulation. Deficiency results in hyperexcitability of nerves and muscle fibers (tetany). An excess may cause muscle weakness leading to cardiac and respiratory failure. When a patient's blood test shows low calcium, the albumin levels should be checked. Low albumin will result in low calcium levels, as calcium is highly bound to this protein.

Warning

The various calcium salts are used for different purposes.

Various calcium salts are used for different purposes. Four calcium salts currently in use are calcium chloride, calcium carbonate, calcium acetate, and calcium gluconate.

Calcium chloride is the fastest of the calcium salts to diffuse into the bloodstream, so it is the salt primarily used in cardiac emergencies. It moderates nerve and muscle performance through regulation of the action potential excitation threshold. If infused directly into an IV line or mixed in too high a concentration with phosphate, calcium will precipitate. IV is the only available dosage form of calcium chloride.

Calcium carbonate is usually used as an antacid and is sold under many brand names, such as Tums. It is also used as a dietary supplement to prevent a negative calcium balance. Calcium carbonate is taken only by mouth. Calcium cannot penetrate bone without the aid of vitamin D, so most of these supplements have vitamin D added to them.

Calcium acetate is used to control hyperphosphatemia in end-stage renal failure. It binds to the phosphorus in the GI tract more efficiently than other calcium salts. This efficient binding is due to its lower solubility and subsequent reduced absorption and increased formation of calcium phosphate. Calcium acetate is also used in parenteral nutrition. It can be administered as a capsule, tablet, or injection.

Calcium gluconate is used to prevent negative calcium balances. It moderates muscle and nerve performance and allows normal cardiac function. It is used in total parenteral nutrition and can be taken by mouth or parenterally.

Hydrogen (H^{1+}) The concentration of hydrogen ions determines the acid-base nature of fluids. Hydrogen ion concentrations determine the acidity or alkalinity of body fluids. The common method of reporting H^{1+} concentration is by pH. A low pH is acidic and a high pH is basic (alkaline). A pH of 7.0 is a neutral solution (neither acidic nor basic). Blood pH is usually 7.4, mildly basic. **Acidosis** (blood pH below 7.35) is a metabolic condition due to excessive loss of bicarbonate or sodium as a result of diarrhea, starvation, or diabetic coma. In the respiratory system, the carbon dioxide concentrations increase. **Alkalosis** (blood pH above 7.45) is a metabolic condition due to excessive loss of potassium or chloride and is most often caused by vomiting or diarrhea. Respiratory system manifestations are hyperventilation and lowered carbon dioxide levels.

Magnesium (Mg^{2+}) Magnesium is the second most abundant cation in intracellular fluids. Most body magnesium occurs in bones and within cells. Many body enzymes and enzyme systems need magnesium for activation. It helps maintain normal nerve and muscular function, the transmission of impulses across neuromuscular junctions, and steady heart rhythms. Magnesium can be lost as a result of alcohol abuse, stress, and the taking of medications that cause electrolytes to be eliminated from the body. Medications that increase magnesium excretion include digoxin, estrogen, and diuretics. Poor GI absorption can also result in deficiency. Magnesium sulfate is the drug of choice for preeclampsia and eclampsia. It is administered intravenously for acute prevention of uterine contractions in preterm labor. Magnesium sulfate can delay labor for 1 to 2 days.

Chloride (Cl^{1-}) In the body, chloride functions to transport carbon dioxide, form hydrochloric acid in the stomach, retain potassium, and maintain osmolarity of the cells. The main effect of a chloride ion excess or deficiency is on acid-base balance. The concentration of chloride ions in parenteral nutrition solutions should usually be adjusted to equal that of sodium ions by adding nonchloride salts of sodium and potassium.

IV Therapy

The goal of IV fluids is to provide the patient with sufficient water and electrolytes to maintain intracellular and extracellular fluids and excrete the end products of metabolism. In IV solutions, the solvent (the liquid that dissolves the substance) is water. The substance dissolved in a solvent is called the solute. The solutes in IV solutions include minerals, which exist as acids, bases, and salts and are dissolved in body fluids.

A common measurement of solution concentration is percent composition of grams of solute per 100 cc (cc =mL) of solution. Thus, a 5% dextrose solution contains 5 g of dextrose in 100 cc of water.

IV fluids can be classified according to their tonicity. **Tonicity** is the relationship of a solution to the body's own fluids and is measured by determining the number of dissolved particles in solution. A **hypotonic solution** has a lower concentration of particles than body fluids contain, so water from the solution enters the body cells by osmotic pressure and causes them to swell. A **hypertonic solution** has a higher concentration of particles than body fluids contain, so the solution draws water from the cells and causes them to shrink. An **isotonic solution** has the same tonicity—the same level of each type of particle—as the body fluids; for example, 0.9% sodium chloride. Therefore, body cells can be bathed in an isotonic solution without net flow of water across the semi-permeable cell membrane.

Enteral Nutrition

When oral feeding is not possible but the patient's GI tract can still function, the patient may be fed through a tube that leads to the GI system; this is called **enteral nutrition**. The word **"enteral"** means "by way of, or pertaining to, the intestine." In an enteral feeding, liquid food is introduced into the GI tract (the stomach or intestines) through a tube. It may be administered as a bolus or drip or with an enteral pump. The tube may be introduced through the nose and run to the stomach (nasogastric tube) or small intestine (nasoenteric tube), or the tube may be introduced surgically through incisions in the abdominal wall and the stomach (gastrostomy tube) or small intestine (jejunostomy tube). Enteral nutrition is indicated for patients with disorders such as partial obstruction in the bowel, short-bowel syndrome, and Crohn disease and is preferred to feeding through the veins because the GI system will remain functional if a patient is on enteral feedings. Specialized formulas are available for patients with specific disease states.

Enterals are prepared by the pharmacy technician in some settings. In other settings they may be prepared by the nutrition services department. Sometimes a blue dye is added to the enteral to enable the physician to differentiate it from other body fluids. Some type of fiber is generally added to the feeding, because these patients become constipated very easily. It is very important to place a sticker on all enteral preparations warning that they are not for intravenous use. Table 17.4 lists some of the formulations used for enteral nutrition.

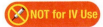

TABLE 17.4   Most Commonly Used Enteral Nutrition Formulations

Enteral Feeding	Population Receiving
Fibersource HN, Jevity Plus, Probalance	patients with high nitrogen needs, noninjured patients, nursing home patients
Fibersource, Jevity, Ultracal	patients with intact GI tracts who are unable to eat for various reasons
Isosource VHN, Promote, Replete	patients with very high nitrogen needs, trauma victims, burn victims
Magnacal Renal, Nepro, Novasource Renal	renal patients on dialysis
Impact, Impact Glutamine, Perative	immune-compromised patients, abdomen trauma victims, seriously ill patients
Choice DM, Glucerna, Resource Diabetic	diabetic patients

Parenteral Nutrition

In **parenteral nutrition (PN),** the patient is fed through a vein. **Total parenteral nutrition (TPN)** provides the patient with all the nutritional requirements through the parenteral route, in contrast to providing nutrition through the usual route of the alimentary canal. The availability of PN is important to the survival and well-being of some patients. The system itself has evolved over more than 300 years.

The provision of parenteral nutritional support has become increasingly more complex. Although PN can be lifesaving, careless administration, caused by inadequate understanding or poor supervision, can have devastating consequences. Proportions of water, electrolytes, carbohydrates, and protein must be maintained within a narrow range through a combination of dietary intake, metabolism, and excretion. Imbalances can be caused by disease or injury and can be determined by blood analysis. It is much easier to maintain body cell mass or restore small deficiencies through PN than to restore a seriously ill patient.

Patients receiving PN should have blood drawn for lab analysis on a regular basis (at least weekly, daily for some patients), in order to monitor the patient's nutritional state. The timing of these tests will depend on the patient's nutritional state and disease state. It is important that lab results are reviewed before the next PN bag is mixed, because the formulation may need to be changed as the status of the patient changes. It is commonly the pharmacy technician's responsibility to retrieve these lab results (by phone, fax, etc.) and make sure the pharmacist has reviewed them.

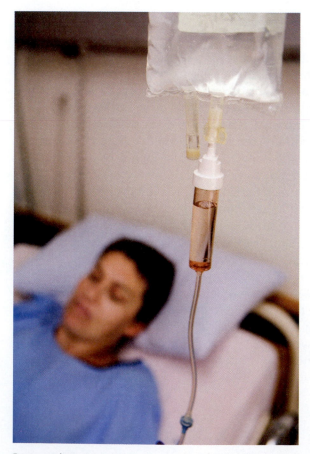
Parenteral nutrition is administered intravenously.

Malnutrition

Parenteral nutrition can be of particular benefit in helping patients avoid malnutrition. **Malnutrition** is any disorder of nutrition, and moderate-to-severe malnutrition has been demonstrated in as much as 20% of all hospitalized patients. Malnutrition can affect many parts of the body. A malnourished patient heals slowly and is much more prone to serious infection, because malnutrition is associated with poor wound healing and an increase in the number of infections. The malnourished body destroys its red blood cells in order to use their protein as a source of energy. In severe malnutrition, organ failure can occur in the cardiovascular, renal, and GI systems. Because the lungs require a lot of energy to function correctly, the malnourished patient may experience respiratory failure. The body needs a sufficient percentage of body fat to offset high stresses and to help the body deal with a crisis; malnutrition decreases these fat stores. In addition, malnutrition decreases glycogen stores—carbohydrate reserves that, in healthy patients, provide quick energy between meals.

The effects of protein malnutrition can be especially devastating. The body contains two types of protein stores: somatic and visceral. Somatic protein stores are skeletal muscle protein. Visceral protein stores are plasma proteins, which make up 5% of body mass. In malnutrition, these protein stores decrease, as do energy stores and lean body mass. A 20% reduction in body mass is considered moderate malnutrition; a 40% reduction is considered severe malnutrition.

Indications for Parenteral Nutrition

The indications for PN are poor wound healing, infections, anemia, specific GI disease, and hypermetabolic states (states of increased metabolism). It may also be used when the patient does not tolerate enteral nutrition.

The following patients may require parenteral nutrition.

- Patients who cannot eat at all because of GI problems, a complete obstruction, or a tumor.
- Patients who cannot eat enough because they have abnormal nutrition requirements.
- Patients who have severe burns or short-bowel syndrome and therefore need almost three times the normal nutritional allotment.
- Patients who can eat, but refuse to do so because of eating disorders such as anorexia nervosa.
- Patients who can eat, but should not. This includes those with pancreatitis, severe gallbladder disease, inflammatory bowel disease, or severe diarrhea.

Complications of Parenteral Nutrition

Patients may experience various complications as a result of PN including the following:

- acid-base imbalance
- dehydration
- elevated serum triglycerides
- failure to induce anabolism
- high serum lipid concentrations
- hyperammonemia
- hyperglycemia or hypoglycemia
- hypoalbuminemia
- imbalance of electrolytes
- liver toxicity

Even nondiabetic patients may show increased blood sugar when on PN; therefore, insulin may be added to the solution even for the nondiabetic.

Infections are frequently a problem for patients receiving parenteral nutrition. PN solutions are rich in nutrients and therefore capable of hosting many types of bacteria and fungi. Aseptic technique should be used, and the solution should be tested for growth around the line. The area around the central line often becomes infected, and the line has to be pulled and another put in to clear the infection. PN may be held during this time and sometimes reformulated when restarted.

Preparing Parenteral Nutrition Solutions

Parenteral nutrition solutions are formulated to ensure adequate absorption of nutrients from circulation, providing fluids, carbohydrates, and protein while maintaining osmolarity. Cell membranes are the primary barriers to the movement of solute in the body. All membranes are permeable to water (through which water passes freely). Small solutes may diffuse through all membranes at a rate slower than that of water. The large size of lipoprotein molecules restricts lipoprotein crossing. Lipid-soluble gases—oxygen and carbon dioxide—and lipid-soluble urea pass readily. Small hydrophilic ions and glucose use aqueous channels, moving slower than lipid-soluble substances; the movement is a passive process from areas of higher concentration to those of lower concentration.

Two types of PN solutions are available: (1) a type of solution that contains lipids in addition to amino acids and dextrose, known as a **total nutrient admixture (TNA)** or a **three-in-one,** and (2) a type of solution that does not contain lipids but only amino acids and dextrose (a **two-in-one**). Both three-in-ones and two-in-ones have electrolytes added. The three-in-one formula offers these advantages:

- lower cost of preparation and delivery
- less nursing time needed for administration
- potentially reduced risk of sepsis with fewer violations (breaks, points of entry) of the administration line

The three-in-one formulations also have two disadvantages. First, if precipitation of the electrolytes occurs, it cannot be seen. Second, the formulations are not stable for as long a period of time as PNs prepared without lipids.

PNs without lipids last about three times as long as those with lipids. If stored properly, a two-in-one may have an expiration date as long as 21 days after being mixed, compared to only 7 days for a three-in-one (with lipids). The lipid emulsions in a three-in-one formula will separate with prolonged or incorrect storage. Producing a compatible three-in-one formulation has been challenging, requiring the amino acid products to be buffered at a higher pH.

With either type of PN solution, the electrolytes are added to the mixture during initial preparation, but the vitamins are always added just before administration. This mixture is stable for 24 hours after addition of the vitamins. Both types of PN solution may remain at room temperature for 24 hours (usually a parenteral bag is hung this long). Otherwise the solution is always stored in the refrigerator.

When mixing a three-in-one PN, electrolytes should be added carefully. **Pooling** saves considerable time, but this method is controversial because precipitation is more common when it is used. In pooling, all the electrolytes except phosphate are put into a small-volume parenteral bag and then transferred into each batch. Cysteine is sometimes added to prevent precipitation of the electrolytes. If pooling is used, be sure to separate the phosphates from the calcium and magnesium. The phosphates should be injected into the bag first; next the amino acids, dextrose, lipids, and water should be added; and then the pooled electrolytes. When the PN is mixed in this way, precipitates are very unlikely to occur.

Solutions that contain lipids should be carefully inspected in the pharmacy and before infusion for **cracking,** or separation. Cracking can be demonstrated by adding hydrochloric acid to the PN solution. The result is a distinct separation of the oil that is easily visible.

To provide all nutrients intravenously, parenteral nutrition solutions must contain a large number of different components in a relatively small volume of fluid. The possibility of component interactions and microprecipitation is quite high and must be considered when mixing each batch. Solutions that do not contain lipids should be inspected during preparation against both black and white backgrounds with proper lighting. All bags with precipitates should be refiltered or discarded. It is advantageous to look for particulate matter before adding insulin or albumin, because particles can be removed by passing the mixture through a filter into another bag, but albumin and insulin cannot pass through microfilters.

Albumin (Albuminar) is a major plasma protein used clinically to reduce edema by osmotic effect; it shifts fluid volume from the tissues into the circulation and increases serum protein levels in hypoproteinemia (plasma protein lost in the urine). It is also used to increase plasma volume by osmotic effect to diminish red blood cell aggregation and reduce blood viscosity. Antigenic reactions can cause problems. Renal involvement, due to high specific gravity, may make albumin toxic to the kidneys. This may lead to prolongation of clotting time, which could lead to disseminated intravascular coagulation.

Calcium and phosphorus are the electrolytes that cause the most problems with precipitation. The phosphate ion should always be added to the bag first and mixed thoroughly with other ingredients; after the PN is mixed, the calcium ion is added with constant swirling. Calcium chloride should not be used; calcium acetate is preferred. The sulfate salt is the preferred form for magnesium. The actual concentration of magnesium depends on the amount of calcium, because both are divalent cations (having a charge of +2) and destabilize the lipid emulsion.

Regular insulin is often added to the parenteral nutrition. As little as 10 units per liter has been found to be clinically effective in lowering mild elevations of blood glucose.

Table 17.5 lists the recommended multivitamin additions for PN. These come in one bottle and are added to the PN as close to the time of administration as possible because vitamins degrade more rapidly than other components. Tables 17.6 and 17.7 list other additions that may vary according to the product.

All of the items in the above charts will be based on the labs and will differ per those values.

After the PN solution is mixed and given a final inspection, each batch should be clearly labeled with the patient's name, address or hospital unit, solution name, concentration and volume, and additives. Instructions for the additives, such as vitamins, should be given on the label, and an expiration date must be included on any IV product. In both the hospital setting and the home infusion pharmacy, it is the pharmacy technician who mixes PN. It is then checked by the pharmacist and sent out to the patient.

Warning

All IV products must be labeled with expiration dates.

TABLE 17.5   Recommended Multivitamin Additions for PN

Vitamin	Pronunciation	Daily Adult Dose
ascorbic acid (vitamin C)	a-SKOR-bik AS-id	60 mg
biotin (vitamin B_7)	BYE-oh-tin	150 mcg
cyanocobalamin (vitamin B_{12})	sye-an-oh-koe-BAL-a-min	2 mcg
ergocalciferol (vitamin D_2)	er-goe-kal-SIF-e-rawl	200 mg
folic acid (vitamin B_9)	FOE-lik AS-id	180 mcg
niacin (vitamin B_3)	NYE-a-sin	15 mg
pyridoxine HCl (vitamin B_6)	peer-i-DOX-een	1.6 mg
retinol (vitamin A)	RE-tin-awl	800 mg
riboflavin (vitamin B_2)	RYE-boe-flay-vin	1.3 mg
thiamine (vitamin B_1)	THYE-a-min	1.1 mg
tocopherol (vitamin E)	to-KOF-er-awl	12 mg

TABLE 17.6   Recommended Trace Element Additions for TPN

Vitamin	Daily Adult Dose
chromium	10 to 15 mcg
copper	0.5 to 1.5 mg
manganese	0.15 to 0.80 mg

TABLE 17.7   Standard per Liter Additions for TPN

Additive	Amount per Liter
acetate	limited by cation
calcium	9 mEq
chloride	limited by cation
insulin, regular	30 units (dependent on blood glucose level)
magnesium	12 mEq
phosphate	21 mEq
potassium	80 mEq
sodium	patient tolerance
zinc	2.5 to 4.0 mg

Alternative Supplements

Various terms are used in the literature to describe **herbs.** The term generally refers to plants or plant parts extracted or dried and valued for their savory, aromatic, or medicinal qualities. The use of herbs to treat various complaints is one type of what is referred to as alternative medicine. Herbs have been used for centuries for medicinal purposes. They were the original sources of many important drugs and have served as models for many synthetic agents. Most references can be traced back to one original source, *Gerard's Herbal*, written in the sixteenth century. Pharmacopeias in most developing countries include herbal materials.

Alternative Supplement Safety Issues

For some people, there is a false sense of security when it comes to plants and herbs. In reality, the safety issues surrounding alternative medicine are complex.

As for the safety of herbs, the poison laws of the Food and Drug Administration (FDA) prevent many relatively poisonous plants from being sold. Furthermore, many herbs are used in small amounts, in dilute form, or for short periods, so the risk of toxicity is minimal. Herbs are generally less toxic on a weight basis than manufactured pharmaceutical drugs because more of the inert portion of a plant, by weight, is included compared to a drug.

Nevertheless, herbs raise some safety concerns. Healthcare professionals identify three issues in particular: (1) the possibility that one herb may be mistaken for another, resulting in serious side effects or an allergic response; (2) the potential for interactions with other herbs and drugs; and (3) the possibility that a patient will initially treat a disease with herbs and forgo effective pharmaceutical treatment until the disease is too far advanced to realize the full benefits of drug therapy. It should be noted, though, that there is relatively little cooperation or agreement between herbalists and healthcare professionals in the United States. Whereas some herbalists believe that herbs are natural to the body, lack side effects, and are beneficial, most medical practitioners believe that the more desirable drugs are single entities that have been approved by FDA standards. With such drugs, if there is an adverse event, it is more likely that the causative agent can be identified.

A major problem with herbs is the lack of regulation and standardization. Although consumers may believe that the FDA regulates herbal products in the same way that it regulates pharmaceutical drugs, this is not true. Federal regulations permit the sale of herbs as foods, so they are labeled as to content, but not as to medical uses, doses, and dangers. No FDA quality control currently exists, and false claims for herbs are common and numerous. The content of herbal products also varies widely. The composition of an herb will vary depending on how the plant is grown, harvested, extracted, and stored. Standardizing products would require that the manufacturer ensure that each bottle contains the same quantity of active ingredients, but sometimes it is not even clear which ingredients within a particular herb cause the desired effect. This lack of information, combined with the variations inherent in herbal farming methods, makes standardization across manufacturers almost impossible.

A second problem is that accurate information may be hard to find. Consumers obtain most of their information about herbal products from the companies that sell the products or from books and pamphlets written and sold by these companies. In addition, the available information can be confusing. Several different plants may have the same common name. Consumers have difficulty evaluating the safety of herbal products because they do not know the scientific name of the material in question or because the product contains a mixture of materials.

Even when the product is known, determining its toxicity can be difficult. Despite the common belief that plants are "natural" and "nontoxic," some of the most toxic chemicals are obtained from plants. Thus, herbs may be as toxic as synthetic drugs. The belief that herbs are not toxic, coupled with increased dosages, has led to incidents of toxicity from herbs that were considered safe in smaller amounts. Furthermore, the "natural" ingredients in herbs can interact with prescribed or OTC drugs the patient is taking.

Again, the lack of information is a problem. Healthcare professionals are expected to warn patients about the side effects and potential interactions of prescription drugs, but as explained earlier, herbs are sold as food and are not required to list their side effects on the label or in the promotional literature. Hence, interactions between herbs and other medications can pose potential dangers. There is a considerable difference not only in one brand to another, but in batches made by the same company.

Certainly, many people report beneficial effects from herbs. Nevertheless, health-care professionals point out that the herbs may not have been responsible for the "cures." Most people survive many illnesses, such as colds and coughs, that run their course without medical treatment. Infections usually are terminated when the body's defense mechanisms are mobilized; cuts, bruises, and broken bones heal by themselves. Most patients with chronic and debilitating illnesses such as cancer or arthritis have "good days" and "bad days" because spontaneous periods of regression occur in the normal course of the disease. Positive reinforcement and a desire to be cured may account for some positive response, even with a placebo.

Most Commonly Used Alternative Supplements

Table 17.8 presents common herbs that are in widespread use for medicinal purposes. The most commonly used herbs are St. John's wort for depression, ginseng for energy, ginkgo for memory improvement, feverfew for migraines, saw palmetto for prostate disease, valerian as a tranquilizer, and echinacea, also called Siberian ginseng, for the common cold. Non-herbal alternative supplements include melatonin for sleep, chromium picolinate for weight loss, and glucosamine for arthritis.

Chamomile, used for GI complaints, may inhibit some cytochrome enzymes, thus causing toxicity with calcium channel blockers and some lipid-lowering agents. It may also have an additive effect when taken with sedative drugs and/or alcohol. It has some antiflatulent activity. A patient may steep 3 g in 250 mL hot water for 15 minutes. The patient drinks this tea three to four times daily.

Chondroitin interferes with the enzymes that break down cartilage. This agent is often combined with glucosamine and is widely used as a supplement to promote joint health. Chondroitin is not as effective as glucosamine.

Chromium picolinate improves glucose tolerance and has been shown to benefit diabetics by improving the efficiency of their insulin metabolism. It is also used widely for weight loss,.

Coenzyme Q10 is used for cardiovascular disorders and congestive heart failure (CHF). It can reduce the anticoagulant effect of warfarin.

Dong quai is used for menopausal symptoms.

Echinacea, used for the common cold, inhibits cytochrome enzymes that metabolize calcium channel blockers, benzodiazepines, and protease inhibitor (HIV) drugs. Echinacea is used orally to stimulate the immune system of the body. It is used topically in the treatment of wounds and burns.

Feverfew is used for the same disorders that aspirin would be used to treat. It may be used for disease caused by chronic inflammation such as arthritis. It inhibits the release of two inflammatory substances, serotonin and prostaglandins, that are believed to contribute to the onset of migraines. Feverfew interacts with anticoagulants and NSAIDs.

Garlic is used for hyperlipidemia, hypertension, and other cardiovascular conditions and should be avoided by patients taking protease inhibitors (HIV drugs). It is used orally as an antioxidant. Garlic can be used topically to treat corns, warts, and calluses, as well as arthritis.

Ginger is used for motion sickness, flatulence, stomach disorders, anorexia, and postsurgical nausea and vomiting, among other things. It is possibly effective for motion

TABLE 17.8   Most Commonly Used Alternative Supplements and Their Uses

Common Name	Purported Use	Safety/Efficacy
chamomile	anti-inflammatory, antispasmodic, anti-infective	may be effective as an antiflatulant
chondroitin	arthritis	possibly effective
chromium picolinate	weight loss, improve insulin metabolism	benefits diabetes by improving insulin metabolism
coenzyme Q10	congestive heart failure	insufficient evidence
dong quai	menstrual cramps	does not work
echinacea	common cold	probably as effective as anything on the market
enada, NADH	mental clarity and alertness, chronic fatigue syndrome	insufficient evidence
feverfew	migraine prophylaxis	safe and possibly effective
garlic	high blood pressure and hyperlipidemia	insufficient evidence
ginger	antiemetic	safe; may work for motion sickness
ginkgo	circulatory stimulant	safe and effective
ginseng	energy	safe, but not very efficacious
glucosamine	arthritis	may help osteoarthritis
hawthorn	cardiovascular problems	possibly effective, but insufficient evidence
kava	anxiety, psychosis, induces relaxation	possibly effective
melatonin	sleep	may work for some people
saw palmetto	prostate	may relieve some symptoms
St. John's wort	depression	may work for mild depression with few side effects
valerian	sleep	possibly effective as bath additive
yohimbe	impotence	possibly effective

sickness but is not effective for postsurgical nausea and vomiting. It interacts with anti-coagulant and antiplatelet drugs. A common dosage is 1 g to 2 g three times daily.

Ginkgo is indicated for peripheral vascular disease and cerebral insufficiency. A number of well-regarded studies support the use of ginkgo. It is said to relieve twelve symptoms in elderly persons that supposedly are typical of cerebral insufficiency: difficulty concentrating, absentmindedness, confusion, lack of energy, tiredness, decreased physical performance, depressive mood, anxiety, dizziness, tinnitus, head-ache, and memory difficulties. Ginkgo is used for Alzheimer disease. It inhibits plate-let aggregation, thus having an additive effect with anticoagulants.

Ginseng is used to enhance well-being, improve the immune system, and boost energy. It is also sometimes used to reduce the symptoms of a hangover. It may cause hypoglycemia in adults using insulin. It can potentiate the stimulant effects of caffeine.

Glucosamine, a combination of glucose and the amino acid glutamine, is produced naturally in the body. Glucosamine stimulates the biosynthesis of a cartilage-building compound and can thereby help restore damaged tissue through the synthesis of cartilage, tendons, and synovial fluid. This supplement may also provide some anti-inflammatory effects. Some research suggests that glucosamine might slow the progression of osteoarthritis; It has no effect on rheumatoid arthritis. Patients with osteoarthritis who take glucosamine experience less pain and have reduced knee joint deterioration. It seems to work as well as nonsteroidal anti-inflammatory drugs (NSAIDs) for pain and is better tolerated by many patients. The patient may not feel the effects of glucosamine for 4 to 6 weeks after the initiation of therapy. This agent can cause GI discomfort, but this effect is minimal compared to that of the NSAIDs.

Hawthorn can potentiate digoxin and is used for cardiovascular problems. It increases the force of contractions of the myocardium.

Kava is used for anxiety, psychosis, and depression. It induces relaxation.

Melatonin is a hormone produced naturally in the body during the hours of darkness. It helps the body adjust to night and day. This is a function of the circadian rhythm. Young people have much more melatonin in their bodies than older persons. Some researchers think this may help to explain why young people fall asleep so much easier than older people. Travelers use melatonin as an antidote to jet lag, stress, and insomnia. With traditional sleeping pills, one can be groggy the next day, but this is not the case with melatonin. Some stomach discomfort has been the only reported side effect.

St. John's wort, sometimes called "nature's Prozac," is used for mild-to-moderate depression, anxiety, and insomnia. A dose of 300 mg three times a day may work as well as prescription antidepressants for some people. Contrary to popular belief, it does not interact with some foods, as is the case for monoamine oxidase inhibitors (MAOIs). However, one should be very careful not to combine St. John's wort with an antidepressant. It causes photosensitivity and interacts with some prescription drugs. It may also cause irregular bleeding in women taking oral contraceptives and can reduce the effectiveness of the contraceptives.

NADH or **Enada** is supported by a reputable study as a treatment for chronic fatigue syndrome. NADH is an essential coenzyme in the cellular process that generates energy. This agent reportedly increases energy and mental concentration. NADH is claimed to improve mental clarity and alertness. NADH has no known interactions with other drugs.

Saw palmetto is used for benign prostate hyperplasia. It does not affect the overall prostate size but shrinks the inner epithelium. It is a mild diuretic and increases urine flow. It can be used as hormone therapy in postmenopausal women. Conflicting findings on efficacy of saw palmetto have been reported. However, the fact that it acts as a diuretic would account for the relief of prostate hyperplasia and symptoms of menopause. Saw palmetto interacts with hormones.

Valerian is used for sleep. Currently, it is used most frequently as a bath additive. Taken orally, it also may ease menstrual cramps and help with mood disorders. It can interact with alcohol, barbiturates, benzodiazepines, and any drugs that have a sedative effect.

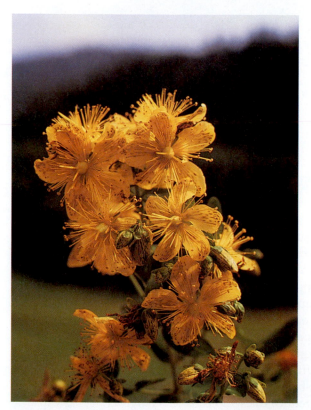

St. John's wort is a popular dietary herbal supplement, but researchers have discovered that it can reduce the effectiveness of some oral contraceptives. Patients should consult with their physician before taking herbal supplements such as St. John's wort.

Yohimbe causes vasodilation, increasing genital blood flow, and can act as an aphrodisiac. It is used for sexual impotence, but its use has declined since sildenafil (Viagra) became available. The active ingredient is found in the bark of the tree. Yohimbe causes excitation, insomnia, tremor, and anxiety. It can increase blood pressure and decrease the effects of hypertensive drugs, and it interacts with caffeine and MAOIs.

Poisons and Antidotes

Prevention of accidental poisoning should be a major concern of healthcare professionals. More than two-thirds of accidental poisonings occur in children under 6 years of age, and in many of these cases the child ingests compounds in household use. Drugs in particular present a danger to children. Several drugs cause the most childhood poisonings.

- Iron tablets are the leading cause of fatal poisonings in children. Just a few iron or prenatal supplement tablets can kill a small child.
- Tricyclic antidepressants are extremely toxic in children. Small amounts can cause heart arrhythmias, seizures, and shock.
- Calcium channel blockers are becoming a major problem; they lead to low blood pressure and heart failure.
- Opiates (even Lomotil) can cause respiratory failure.
- Aspirin poisoning is down dramatically because of childproof caps and the increased use of nonaspirin OTC pain relievers. Symptoms of aspirin poinsoning include tinnitus, nausea, and vomiting. Nausea and vomiting occur with doses greater than 150 mg/kg.
- Alcohol is often overlooked, but small amounts can cause low blood sugar, coma, and seizures. Some mouthwashes contain enough alcohol to harm a child.

Warning

The national poison hotline is 800-222-1222.

Poisoning also frequently occurs among older persons who mistake household chemicals for medication. It also happens as a result of occupational exposure to noxious chemicals.

Skin contamination is the most important external route of exposure to industrial poisons. When skin has been exposed to a toxic chemical, the area should be properly irrigated. Chemicals may not only damage skin but may also produce systemic toxicity if absorbed through the skin. Inhalation poisoning can cause damage to the respiratory tract by systemic absorption as well as local irritation. The patient should be immediately carried into fresh air, and breathing support should be provided if necessary. Eye contamination is treated by immediate irrigation of the eye with water or an eye flush solution to diminish the strength of the poison.

Ingestion is the most common route of poisoning. Once a toxic substance is ingested, there are two concerns: (1) eliminating it from the patient's GI tract to prevent absorption, and (2) diminishing the effects of the dose absorbed. In addition, **supportive therapy** consists of establishing the airway and providing cardiopulmonary resuscitation (CPR); maintaining body temperature, nutritional status, and fluid and electrolyte balance; and preventing circulatory collapse, hypoglycemia, uremia, and liver failure.

Poison Elimination

The first step in handling ingestion is to remove as much of the ingested poison as possible from the patient's GI tract before it can be absorbed. Emptying the stomach, administering an adsorbent (such as activated charcoal), and catharsis (vomiting) are potential treatments that should be considered when a sufficient amount of a potentially toxic substance has been ingested within a specific time.

The patient's stomach may be emptied by inducing vomiting or by a **gastric lavage**, commonly known as a stomach pump, a procedure to wash out or irrigate a patient's stomach. This procedure involves passing a tube into the stomach, pumping warm water or saline in, and pumping stomach contents out until the fluid withdrawn is clear. Gastric lavage should not be used, and vomiting should not be induced, if the poison is corrosive or volatile. Gastric lavage should not be performed if 60 minutes or more have elapsed since ingestion. For patients in coma, convulsing, or with no gag reflex, a tube should first be passed into the patient's trachea to ensure an open airway.

Activated charcoal has become the primary emergency room treatment for preventing absorption of poison from the GI tract.It is administered as a powder dispersed in water. Like gastric lavage, activated charcoal should not be used for patients at risk for aspiration.

Cathartics are used in conjunction with activated charcoal to decrease the absorption of the ingested agent further. Speeding the travel and elimination of gastric contents decreases the likelihood of absorption. Saline cathartics, such as magnesium sulfate and magnesium citrate, or hyperosmotic cathartics, such as sorbitol, are the agents of choice.

Pharmacologic Antagonists (Antidotes)

Usually, it is not possible to eliminate the poison completely, so three steps are taken next to diminish the effective dose of the ingested absorbed poison.

Step 1. Pharmacologic antagonists (specific antidotes) are given to counteract the effects of the poison.

Step 2. Large quantities of fluid are given orally, rectally, or intravenously to cause forced diuresis. This is even more effective if the pH can be adjusted appropriately: acidifiers are given for an alkaline poisoning, and alkalizers are given for an acid poisoning.

Step 3. Dialysis and exchange transfusion are needed if the patient has ingested a very large dose of a water-soluble poison. They are contraindicated if the patient has ingested a fat-soluble, protein-bound, or tissue-bound substance.

A variety of drugs serve as antidotes. An **antidote** is a drug that reduces the harmful effects of a poison. Some antidotes are chelating agents. A **chelating agent** is an organic molecule that chemically bonds to a metal ion, which prevents the ion from interacting with biological molecules as it circulates through the body and is eventually removed through the kidney or the liver. Table 17.9 lists the most commonly used antidotes.

Acetylcysteine (Acetadote, Mucomyst) is used for acetaminophen overdose.

Atropine is used in poisoning from cholinergic agents to treat drug-induced bradycardia.

A **cyanide antidote kit** contains amyl nitrite inhalers, sodium nitrite ampules for injection, and sodium thiosulfate ampules for injection.

Dapsone may be useful in tissue disorders caused by spiders or insects, for example, bites from the brown recluse spider. It is also used in the treatment of leprosy.

TABLE 17.9   Most Commonly Used Antidotes

Generic Name	Pronunciation	Dosage Form	Brand Name	Dispensing Status	Chemical It Binds or Reverses
acetylcysteine	a-se-teel-SIS-teen	inhalation, IV, oral liquid	Acetadote, Mucomyst	Rx	acetaminophen
activated carbon, charcoal	AK-ti-vay-ted KAR-bon	oral liquid	(many)	OTC	contaminants in the GI tract
amyl nitrite	AY-mil NYE-trite	inhalation	(none)	Rx	cyanide
antivenin	an-tye-VEN-in	IV	(none)	Rx	snake bites
atropine	AT-roe-peen	injection, IV, tablet	(none)	Rx	cholinergic agents
dapsone	DAP-sone	tablet	(none)	Rx	spider bites
deferoxamine	dee-fer-OX-a-meen	injection, IV	Desferal	Rx	iron
digoxin immune Fab	di-JOX-in im-MYOON FAB	IV	Digibind	Rx	digoxin, digitoxin
dimercaprol, British Anti-Lewisite	dye-mer-KAP-role	injection	BAL in Oil	Rx	lead, arsenic, mercury, gold, bismuth, chromium, nickel, copper
edetate calcium disodium	ED-e-tate KAL-see-um dye-SOE-dee-um	IV	Calcium Disodium Versenate	Rx	lead
flumazenil	floo-MAZ-e-nil	IV	Romazicon	Rx	benzodiazepines
fomepizole	foe-MEP-i-zole	IV	Antizol	Rx	ethylene glycol, methanol
glucagon	GLOO-ka-gon	injection, IV	GlucaGen	Rx	insulin, beta blockers, possibly calcium channel blockers
methylene blue	METH-i-leen BLOO	IV, tablet	Urolene Blue	Rx	cyanide
naloxone	nal-OX-one	IV	Narcan	Rx	narcotics
octreotide	ok-TREE-oh-tide	injection, IV	Sandostatin	Rx	oral sulfonylureas
penicillamine	pen-i-SIL-a-meen	capsule, tablet	Cuprimine	Rx	copper, zinc, mercury, lead
phentolamine	fen-TOLE-a-meen	IV	Regitine	Rx	extravasations
physostigmine	fye-zoe-STIG-meen	IV	(none)	Rx	atropine and other belladonna alkaloids
phytonadione, vitamin K	fye-toe-na-DYE-one	injection, IV, tablet	Aqua-MEPHYTON	Rx	warfarin
polyethylene glycol	pol-ee-ETH-il-een GLYE-kawl	oral liquid	GoLYTELY, HalfLytely, MiraLax	Rx	contaminants in the GI tract
pralidoxime	pral-i-DOX-eem	injection, IV	Protopam	Rx	organophosphates
protamine sulfate	PROE-ta-meen SUL-fate	IV	(none)	Rx	heparin
pyridoxine, vitamin B_6	peer-i-DOX-een	injection, IV, tablet	(many)	OTC, Rx	isoniazid (INH), hydralazine

TABLE 17.9   Most Commonly Used Antidotes (continued)

Generic Name	Pronunciation	Dosage Form	Brand Name	Dispensing Status	Chemical It Binds or Reverses
sodium nitrite	SOE-dee-um NYE-trite	injection	none		cyanide
sodium thiosulfate	SOE-dee-um thye-oh-SUL-fate	injection, IV	Versiclear	Rx	arsenic, cyanide

Digoxin immune Fab (Digibind) treats life-threatening digoxin overdose, referred to as dig toxicity (see Chapter 12). It is often used to treat chronic ingestions leading to toxic steady-state concentrations, or for acute ingestions of digoxin in children.

Glucagon (GlucaGen) is an antidote for hypoglycemia.

Methylene Blue (Urolene Blue) is used to treat cyanide poisoning.

Naloxone (Narcan) reverses narcotic respiratory depression.

Octreotide (Sandostatin) is an analog of somatostatin. It is used to counteract oral sulfonylureas.

Pralidoxime (Protopam) is an acetylcholinesterase reactivator used for acetylcholinesterase-inhibiting agents (organophosphates) such as certain pesticides (parathion or malathion) and nerve gas war agents. It is given after atropine in life-threatening situations.

Protamine sulfate is the antidote for heparin overdose. It forms a stable complex with heparin, neutralizing the anticoagulant effects.

Pyridoxine, **vitamin B$_6$**, releases glycogen stored in the liver and muscles. Pyridoxine acts as an antidote to isoniazid, hydralazine, and cycloserine toxicity.

Physostigmine is a cholinesterase inhibitor used to reverse toxic effects of drugs that block acetylcholine receptors (i.e., atropine and other belladonna alkaloids).

Phytonadione (AquaMEPHYTON) is **vitamin K** (previously discussed in this chapter), which promotes formation of clotting factors; it is an antagonist for warfarin.

Fomepizole (Antizol) is a competitive inhibitor for the metabolism of methyl alcohol and ethylene glycol. It is used to reverse ethylene glycol and methanol toxicity. It complexes with and inactivates alcohol dehydrogenase, thus preventing the formation of formaldehyde and the other toxic metabolites of the alcohols. Fomepizole is diluted in normal saline and dextrose and is stable for at least 48 hours when refrigerated. The solution may become solid in the bottle, and in this case, it should be warmed by rotating it in the hand or running it under warm water.

Edetate calcium disodium (Calcium Disodium Versenate) is a chelating agent for injection that enhances the mobilization and excretion of lead from the body.

Dimercaprol, also called **British Anti-Lewisite (BAL in Oil)**, forms a stable chelate with lead, arsenic compounds (such as lewisite, a chemical weapon used in World War II), mercury compounds, gold salts, bismuth, chromium, nickel, and copper. It also reactivates enzymes shut down by these metals.

Deferoxamine (Desferal) is a chelator for ferric iron and is used in acute iron poisoning.

Penicillamine (Cuprimine) is a chelator of copper, zinc, mercury, and lead. It promotes the excretion of these metals in the urine.

Antivenoms

An **antivenin** is a material used to treat poisoning by animal venom and is produced by hyperimmunization of a host. Hyperimmunization produces very high levels of circulating antibodies. The dose required may be large. A high percentage of patients experience serum sickness (an immune reaction to a foreign protein) from the antivenin.

Antivenin was originally developed to treat bites from two species of North American rattlesnakes (a type of pit viper). The antivenin has been shown to be clinically effective against venoms of all pit vipers, whose bites are deadly. The drug must be on hand at the time of the emergency, together with epinephrine 1:1000, IV antihistamine, and hydrocortisone. First a very small dose of the antivenin is pretested, and if a reaction occurs, the value of giving the antivenin must be weighed against the risk of reaction.

Warning

Diprolene, dantrolene, and dapsone can be easily confused.

In North America, the two most common bites from poisonous spiders are those from black widow and brown recluse spiders. Most healthy adults will survive the bite of a black widow spider with only supportive care. However, antivenin is indicated for patients under 12 years of age or for those older than 65 years with medical problems such as hypertension and cardiovascular disease. For a brown recluse spider bite, some physicians prescribe **dapsone** in an attempt to preserve the skin around the bite. Dapsone is a sulfone antimicrobial. It causes photosensitivity, and the physician should be notified if persistent sore throat, fever, malaise, or fatigue occurs.

Emergency Procedures

The emergency procedures to deal with the conditions that may lead to sudden death are to stabilize the patient at the scene and then transport to a site of continuing care. Basic life support involves measures to prevent circulatory or respiratory arrest or provide external support for circulation and respiration if they have failed. Advanced cardiac life support ensures ready access to adjunctive equipment to support ventilation, give IV infusions, administer drugs, and provide cardiac monitoring, defibrillation, arrhythmic control, and post-resuscitation care. The objectives are to

Warning

Blue Alert carts must be checked regularly by the pharmacist. The technician should always make sure the pharmacist has checked the cart before it is returned to the hospital floor. When a cart has been returned to the pharmacy, the drugs must be restocked and the expiration dates checked. The technician must remove and replace any expired drugs and any that will expire in the next 1 to 2 months.

- correct hypoxia
- reestablish spontaneous circulation
- optimize cardiac function
- suppress sustained ventricular arrhythmias
- correct acidosis
- relieve pain
- treat congestive heart failure

A patient in cardiac arrest has a flat ECG tracing. Various terms are used to categorize the causes of death. Sudden cardiac death is death that occurs within 24 hours of the onset of illness or injury. Most patients have no symptoms immediately before collapse. The aim of treatment is to prevent ventricular fibrillation or to treat the arrest itself.

Sudden arrhythmic death is the loss of consciousness and pulse without prior circulatory collapse. It is *not* preceded by circulatory impairment, but is preceded by chronic heart failure. Death results from ventricular fibrillation associated with myocardial infarction (MI), transient myocardial ischemia, and underlying myocardial abnormalities (usually from previous MI).

Myocardial failure is a gradual circulatory failure and collapse before loss of pulse. It is due to hemorrhage, trauma, infarction, stroke, or respiratory failure.

The American Heart Association has recommended guidelines for use of oxygen. The aim is to increase the oxygen level of the blood, thereby raising levels in organs and tissues. Indications include acute chest pain due to suspected or confirmed heart attack, suspected hypoxia of any cause, and cardiopulmonary arrest.

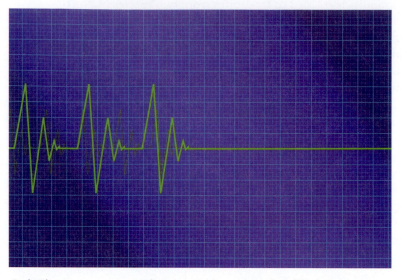

Code Blue emergency procedures are set in motion when life-threatening situations arise

Hospitals use a system of codes to alert staff of various emergency situations. A **Code Blue** is set in motion when a patient is in a life-threatening situation, such as when a patient's heart has stopped or breathing has ceased. In response to a blue alert emergency, hospital personnel respond with appropriate emergency procedures.

Table 17.10 presents the most commonly used agents for cardiac emergencies.

Amiodarone (Cordarone) is used for first-line management of life-threatening recurrent ventricular fibrillation. It is an antiarrhythmic agent that inhibits adrenergic stimulation, prolongs the action potential and refractory period in myocardial tissue, and decreases atrioventricular conduction and sinus node function. During a Code Blue emergency, amiodarone may be mixed and infused in a plastic container. If the patient is put on a drip, however, it must be mixed in a glass container unless the hospital uses polyolefin bags. It is incompatible with most drugs and must be protected from light.

Atropine blocks vagus nerve stimulation, which slows the heart, allowing the sympathetic system to speed the rate. It is most useful in bradycardia for rates less than 60 beats per minute and in asystole (a state of no cardiac electrical activity). However, atropine increases oxygen demand on the heart during arrhythmias and hypotension.

Calcium chloride is used for cardiac resuscitation when epinephrine fails to improve myocardial contractions.

Dextrose 50% is included for diabetic coma.

Digoxin (Lanoxin) acts by direct suppression of the atrioventricular node conduction to increase effective refractor period and decrease conduction velocity.

Diltiazem (Cardizem) is used for atrial fibrillation or flutter and paroxysmal supraventricular tachycardia.

Dobutamine is a beta-1 selective sympathomimetic adrenergic agonist. It increases heart rate with little action on beta-2 or alpha receptors. Dobutamine is used to increase cardiac output in the short-term treatment of patients who have a very weak heartbeat because of organic heart disease, cardiac surgical procedures, or acute myocardial infarction. It is compatible with dopamine, epinephrine, isoproterenol, and lidocaine. The drug is stable for 48 hours after mixing if refrigerated and for 6 hours if not refrigerated. It may turn a slight pink color, but this color change does not indicate a significant loss of potency.

TABLE 17.10 Drugs Recommended by Advanced Cardiac Life Support Guidelines for Cardiac Emergencies and Blue Alert Carts

Generic Name	Pronunciation	Dosage Form	Brand Name	Dispensing Status
amiodarone	am-ee-OH-da-rone	IV	Cordarone	Rx
atropine	A-troe-peen	injection, IV	(none)	Rx
calcium chloride	KAL-see-um KLOR-ide	IV	(none)	Rx
dextrose 50%	DEX-trohs	IV	(none)	Rx
digoxin	di-JOX-in	IV	Lanoxin	Rx
diltiazem	dil-TYE-a-zem	IV	Cardizem	Rx
dobutamine	doe-BYOO-ta-meen	IV	Dobutrex	Rx
dopamine	DOE-pa-meen	IV	Intropin	Rx
epinephrine	ep-i-NEF-rin	IV	Adrenalin	Rx
etomidate	e-TOM-i-date	IV	Amidate	Rx
flumazenil	FLOO-may-ze-nil	IV	Romazicon	Rx
ibutilide	i-BYOO-ti-lide	IV	Corvert	Rx
lidocaine	LYE-doe-kane	IV	(none)	Rx
magnesium sulfate	mag-NEE-zee-um SUL-fate	IV	(none)	Rx
naloxone	nal-OX-one	IV	Narcan	Rx
nimodipine	nye-MOE-di-peen	capsule	Nimotop	Rx
norepinephrine	nor-ep-i-NEF-rin	IV	Levophed	Rx
procainamide	proe-KANE-a-mide	IV	Pronestyl	Rx
vasopressin	vay-soe-PRES-in	IV	(none)	Rx
verapamil	ver-AP-a-mil	IV	Isoptin	Rx

Warning

In an emergency situation it would be very easy to confuse dobutamine and dopamine. Be sure they are not stored side by side on the emergency cart or box.

Dopamine (Intropin) increases blood pressure by causing constriction of peripheral vessels while maintaining blood flow to internal organs and kidneys. It is used to support blood pressure. Dopamine is also used as adjunctive treatment of left ventricular failure secondary to acute myocardial infarction, and in hypertensive crisis from sympathomimetic amines.

Epinephrine (Adrenalin) is the most commonly used agent in cardiopulmonary arrest. A strong heart stimulant, it increases contractility and excitability. It is used in any form of cardiopulmonary standstill and helps to convert fine ventricular fibrillations to a coarser form that is easier to defibrillate. Epinephrine must be used cautiously in the presence of liver disease, low cardiac output, or allergy.

Etomidate (Amidate) is used to calm the patient and prevent resistance to intubation. Another anesthetic inducer may be used, but if the patient must be intubated to begin breathing again, the process is easier if some form of anesthesia is available. Etomidate acts very quickly and is safe enough to be used in children.

Flumazenil (Romazicon) is used for benzodiazepine overdoses.

Ibutilide (Corvert) is used for acute termination of atrial fibrillation or flutter. It prolongs the action potential in cardiac tissue. It is stable for 24 hours at room temperature and for 48 hours if refrigerated.

Lidocaine stabilizes ventricular arrhythmias and should be administered directly into the heart after defibrillation and epinephrine.

Magnesium sulfate is used to treat cardiac arrhythmias and prevent seizures. It slows the rate of sinoatrial node impulse formation and prolongs conduction time.

Naloxone (Narcan) is used to reverse narcotic overdose.

Nimodipine (Nimotop) is a calcium channel blocker with a greater effect on blood vessels of the brain than on heart cells. It is used to treat blood vessel spasm after subarachnoid hemorrhage in patients in good neurologic condition. Between days 4 and 14 after hemorrhage, cerebral arterial spasm is common, with frequent severe ischemic neurologic deficits or death. Use of this drug may result in headache, nausea, bradycardia, flushing, and fluid retention.

Norepinephrine (Levophed) causes increased contractility and heart rate as well as vasoconstriction, thereby increasing systemic blood pressure and coronary blood flow.

Procainamide (Pronestyl) decreases the fibrillation threshold and prevents recurrence; it is used to suppress arrhythmias not responsive to lidocaine or in lidocaine allergy. It is not used in ventricular fibrillation because of the slow onset of activity. This drug can cause hypotension, ECG changes, and kidney disease.

Vasopressin is an antidiuretic hormone injected into the superior mesenteric artery (which branches off of the abdominal aorta). It is used as an adjunct with an esophageal inflation device to control bleeding.

Verapamil (Isoptin) is a calcium channel blocker (slows the movement of calcium ions through slow channels). It slows sinoatrial node action, slows atrioventricular node conduction, and dilates coronary artery smooth muscle. It is used in atrial fibrillations and/or flutters that result in fast ventricular rates. Use of this drug may result in hypotension and heart block.

Bioterrorism

Bioterrorism is an attack or threatened attack by terrorists whereby the weapons are biologic agents and emerging infectious diseases. Potential biologic agents include both microorganisms and toxins. Disease-causing microorganisms may **propagate** (grow and spread) either in the environment or in a living host. Toxins are the product of living organisms, including those derived from plants, bacteria, or fungi. The major difference between toxins and microorganisms is that toxins do not reproduce.

The threat posed by biologic agents, particularly bacteria and viruses, is increased by the fact that once they are released, containment will be very difficult and potentially impossible.

For obvious security reasons, limited information is available as to how a bioterrorist attack would be dealt with by government and emergency preparedness officials.. Although a bioterrorism attack could potentially be unlike any disaster that the response community has faced before, a terrorist attack would present many of the same challenges as a natural disaster.

Bacterial Diseases with Potential for Bioterrorism

Among the diseases that might be used in a bioterrorist attack are anthrax, plague, tularemia, and smallpox. As a member of the response team, the pharmacy technician will have several important responsibilities in dealing with an outbreak.

Before dispensing medications to treat or prevent an outbreak, it will be important to identify patient allergies. This will be a role for the pharmacy technician. Technicians will document drug allergies and dispense drugs. Keeping records of who receives which drugs will be a massive task, and one that pharmacy technicians are well-equipped to perform.

Anthrax There are three forms of anthrax:

- cutaneous
- inhalation
- oropharyngeal and gastrointestinal

Anthrax is treated with antibiotics. A vaccine is available for anthrax; once a person is exposed, the vaccine may be administered.

Plague Typically, plague (the Black Death of the Middle Ages) is transmitted when an infected flea bites its host, but infection can also be introduced directly into the lungs through inhalation. There are three forms of plague: bubonic, septicemic, and pneumonic. Plague is very contagious in any form.

Antibiotics will be dispensed to the population as both prophylaxis and treatment.

Tularemia Tularemia is not contagious, but it is useful as a biologic weapon because of its debilitating effects and because only a few organisms are required to cause an infection. There are six forms of tularemia: ulceroglandular, oculoglandular, oropharyngeal, typhoidal, pneumonic, and septic. In the event of an attack in which tularemia is dispersed, antibiotics would be dispensed. An investigational vaccine is available, but its use is restricted to high-risk groups.

Smallpox Even though smallpox was eradicated in 1979, stocks of this virus exist in highly secured vaults in the United States and Russia. In the event of exposure, vaccination should be given within 1 to 4 days. Care would be simply supportive.

Viral Hemorrhagic Fevers (VHFs) These fevers are caused by a diverse group of viruses. The mode of transmission, clinical course, and mortality of these illnesses vary with the specific virus, although most outbreaks have involved the *Ebola* and *Marburg* viruses. Treatment is mainly supportive. Ribavirin (Rebetol, Virazole) is under investigation for some of them. Hemorrhage should be treated with the usual blood products. Disseminated intravascular coagulation with complications of

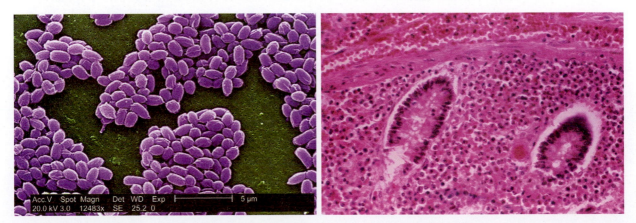

Anthrax bacteria at medium (left) and high (right) magnification

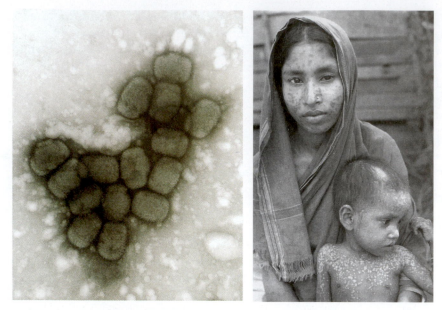

Smallpox was responsible for millions of deaths throughout history. These photos show smallpox bacteria under high magnification (left) and victims with the conspicuous blisters (right).

ischemia may be treated with heparin. Infections should be aggressively managed.

Toxins **Botulin toxin** is a neurotoxin that blocks the release of acetylcholine at the neuromuscular junction and at receptors in the autonomic nervous system, resulting in muscular paralysis. As a biological weapon, it may be spread by ingestion, inhalation, or injection. It is treated with an antitoxin. (See Chapter 15 for its medical use.)

Ricin is a toxin that is derived from the castor bean. It acts by disabling the molecular machinery for protein synthesis. There is no known treatment and no antidote, but a vaccine has been developed. Ricin is easy to produce in large amounts. If a person is exposed to as little as 3 mcg by inhalation or injection, it can be lethal. If ricin is ingested, charcoal lavage should be used; contaminated patients should have their clothes removed and be decontaminated prior to treatment.

The Role of the Pharmacy Technician

The U.S. government is currently stockpiling antibiotics and vaccines to prepare for a bioterrorist emergency. As mentioned, the pharmacy technician will play a very important supportive role in responding to a bioterrorist attack.

In that event, healthcare providers will need to be aware of unusual symptoms in a group of people. Agents will most likely be spread by inhalation. However they are spread, the pharmacy technician, as a dispenser of medication, will be a vital part of the team that disseminates the medications necessary to take care of the populace. Technicians are already involved in many of the top secret programs across the country, and this will continue. As healthcare professionals, pharmacy technicians will be a major contributor in this process. Dispensing drugs, maintaining patient profiles, and documenting patient allergies will be critical components of the response to a bioterrorist attack. Pharmacy technicians will be on the front line of defense if there is ever a biological terrorist attack against this country.

Chapter Terms

acidosis a blood pH below 7.35; a metabolic condition due to excessive loss of bicarbonate or sodium

alkalosis a blood pH above 7.45; a metabolic condition due to excessive loss of potassium or chloride

antidote a drug that counters the harmful effects of a poison

antivenin a material used in treatment of poisoning by animal venom

botulin toxin a neurotoxin that blocks the release of acetylcholine at the neuromuscular junction, resulting in muscular paralysis

chelating agent a drug that bonds to a metal ion to prevent it from reacting with biological compounds

Code Blue a system to communicate that a patient is in a life-threatening situation

coenzyme a chemical other than a protein that is needed to assist an enzyme in performing a metabolic function

cracking separation of lipid from a parenteral nutrition solution

electrolyte a substance that dissociates into ions in solution and is thus capable of conducting electricity

enteral by way of, or pertaining to, the intestine

enteral nutrition feeding a patient liquid food through a tube that leads to the gastrointestinal system

fat-soluble vitamins vitamins that are absorbed along with dietary fat and are maintained in large stores by the body; vitamins A, D, E, and K

gastric lavage a procedure to wash out or irrigate the patient's stomach, commonly known as a stomach pump

herbs plants or plant parts extracted and valued for their savory, aromatic, or medicinal qualities

hypertonic solution a solution with a higher concentration of particles than body fluids contain

hypotonic solution a solution with a lower concentration of particles than body fluids contain

isotonic solution a solution with the same level of particles, and thus the same tonicity, as body fluids

malnutrition any disorder of nutrition

medical food a preparation taken orally consisting of nutrients specifically required to treat some disease or condition

osteomalacia demineralization and weakening of the skeleton, caused by a deficiency of vitamin D in adults

parenteral nutrition feeding a patient by supplying a nutrient solution through a vein

phytonadione vitamin K_1

pooling a time-saving process used when preparing a three-in-one TPN, in which all electrolytes except phosphate are put into a small-volume parenteral bag and then transferred into each batch

probiotic a product to restore or promote the growth of normal bacterial flora in the body

propagate reproduce

ricin a toxin derived from the castor bean that acts by disabling the molecular machinery for protein synthesis

supportive therapy therapy for poisoning that consists of establishing the airway and providing cardiopulmonary resuscitation (CPR); maintaining body temperature, nutritional status, and fluid and electrolyte balance; and preventing circulatory collapse, hypoglycemia, uremia, and liver failure

three-in-one see total nutrient admixture

tocopherol one of the alcohols that constitute vitamin E

tonicity the relationship of a solution to the body's own fluids; measured by determining the number of dissolved particles in solution

total nutrient admixture (TNA) an amino acid–dextrose–lipid formulation used for parenteral nutrition; often called three-in-one

total parenteral nutrition (TPN) feeding a patient through the veins only

two-in-one a formulation for parenteral nutrition that contains only amino acids and dextrose

vitamin an organic substance that is necessary for the normal metabolic functioning of the body but that the body does not synthesize, so it must be obtained from food

water-soluble vitamins vitamins that are excreted in the urine and are not stored in the body; vitamin C and the B vitamins

Chapter Summary

Vitamins, Fluid Levels, and Electrolytes

- Vitamins are classified as water-soluble or fat-soluble. The B vitamins and vitamin C are water-soluble; A, D, E, and K are fat-soluble.
- Water is the major constituent of living cells. Body fluids are divided into two compartments, intracellular and extracellular.
- Water deficits are caused by loss of body fluids as a result of such disorders as vomiting, diarrhea, edema, and excessive sweating from fever; large urine output; and acute weight loss of more than 5% of body weight. Water loss can cause dryness of skin and mucous membranes, longitudinal wrinkling of the tongue, hypotension, tachycardia, and lowered body temperature. A loss of 25% of body water can result in death.
- Sodium is the primary cation of extracellular fluid.
- With a loss of water and sodium in the body, blood volume is reduced, blood pressure is reduced, and circulatory collapse may occur.
- Potassium is the primary cation of intracellular fluid.
- Calcium is associated with bone formation and dynamics, muscle contraction, and blood coagulation.
- Each calcium salt has a specific use.

- Hydrogen ions regulate the acidity or alkalinity of body fluids.
- An isotonic solution has the same level of each type of particles as the body fluids; e.g., 0.9% sodium chloride.
- Medical foods are not approved by the FDA, but the manufacturer may determine that they must have a prescription in order to be dispensed. Some diseases for which they are used are osteoarthritis, low red blood cells, and to lower homocysteine.
- Probiotics stimulate the growth of beneficial bacteria in the body. They are "good" bacteria. They are used to prevent vaginitis and diarrhea caused by antibiotics, speed gut transit time, IBS, diarrhea, lactose intolerance and ulcerative colitis.

Enteral Nutrition

- Enterals, which are fed through a tube directly into the stomach or small intestine, are preferred to feeding by vein (parenteral nutrition) because the lower abdomen continues to function. A blue dye is sometimes added to the enteral feeding fluid to differentiate it from other body fluids. The pharmacy technician should always label enteral preparations so that they are not confused with intravenous preparations.

Parenteral Nutrition

- It is much easier to maintain body cell mass or restore small deficiencies through PN than to restore a seriously ill patient.
- Malnutrition can lead to poor wound healing, infections, anemia, organ system failure, and decreased body stores of protein and calories.
- The advantages of three-in-one formulations are lower costs of preparation and delivery, less nursing time needed for administration, and potentially reduced risk of sepsis with fewer violations of the administration line.
- The disadvantages of three-in-ones are their short stability and the inability to see precipitants if they occur.

Alternative Supplements

- Herbs were the original source of many important drugs and have served as models for many synthetic drugs.
- Herbs have many drug interactions.
- Three potential major problems with herbs are (1) mistaken identity, (2) forgoing professional treatment, and (3) interactions with other drugs.

Poisons and Antidotes

- The drugs that cause the most childhood poisonings are iron tablets, tricyclic antidepressants, calcium channel blockers, opiates, aspirin, and alcohol.
- Once a poison is ingested, there are two concerns: (1) removing it from the GI tract before it can be absorbed, and (2) diminishing the effects of poison that has been absorbed.

- Activated charcoal has become the primary emergency room treatment to prevent absorption of poison from the GI tract.

Emergency Procedures

- The pharmacy technician is responsible for keeping the Blue Alert carts/boxes stocked. All medications must be kept up to date. An out-of-date medication could cost someone his or her life.
- Advanced cardiac life support guidelines should be followed when determining which drugs will be on a Blue Alert cart.

Bioterrorism

- Bioterrorism may include biologic agents and emerging infectious diseases.
- A bioterrorist attack would be a disaster unlike any the response community has faced before.
- The pharmacy technician will be a primary responder.

Drug List

Vitamins

Vitamin A
retinol

Vitamin B
B_1, thiamine
B_2, riboflavin
B_3, nicotinic acid, niacin
B_5, pantothenic acid
B_6, pyridoxine
B_9, folic acid
B_{12}, cyanocobalamin

Vitamin C
ascorbic acid

Vitamin D
D_2, ergocalciferol
D_3, cholecalciferol

Vitamin E
tocopherol

Vitamin K
phytonadione

Medical Foods
flavocoxid (Limbrel)
L-methylfolate (Deplin)
L-methylfolate,
    L-methylcobalamin/N-acetylcysteine
    (Cerefolin)

Probiotics
acidophilus
Activia
Align
Culturelle
Flora Q
Lactinex

Electrolytes
calcium, Ca^{2+} (calcium acetate, calcium
    carbonate, calcium chloride, calcium
    gluconate)
chloride, Cl^{1-}
hydrogen ions, H^{1+}
magnesium, Mg^{2+}

potassium, K^{1+} (Klor-Con)*
sodium, Na^{1+}

Enteral Nutrition Formulations
Choice DM
Fibersource
Fibersource HN
Glucerna
Impact
Impact Glutamine
Isosource VHN
Jevity
Jevity Plus
Magnacal Renal
Nepro
Novasource Renal
Perative
Probalance
Promote
Replete
Resource Diabetic
Ultracal

Alternative Supplements
chamomile
chondroitin
chromium picolinate
coenzyme Q10
dong quai
echinacea
enada, NADH
feverfew
garlic
ginger
ginkgo
ginseng
glucosamine
hawthorn
kava
melatonin
saw palmetto
St. John's wort
valerian
yohimbe

Antidotes

acetylcysteine (Acetadote, Mucomyst)
activated carbon, charcoal
amyl nitrite
antivenin
atropine
dapsone
deferoxamine (Desferal)
digoxin immune Fab (Digibind)
dimercaprol, British Anti-Lewisite (BAL in Oil)
edetate calcium disodium (Calcium Disodium Versenate)
flumazenil (Romazicon)
fomepizole (Antizol)
glucagon (GlucaGen)
methylene blue (Urolene Blue)
naloxone (Narcan)
octreotide (Sandostatin)
penicillamine (Cuprimine)
phentolamine (Regitine)
physostigmine
phytonadione, vitamin K (AquaMEPHYTON)
polyethylene glycol (GoLYTELY, HalfLytely, MiraLax)
pralidoxime (Protopam)
protamine sulfate
pyridoxine, vitamin B_6
sodium nitrite
sodium thiosulfate (Versiclear)

Code Blue Emergencies

amiodarone (Cordarone)
atropine
calcium chloride
dextrose 50%
digoxin (Lanoxin)
diltiazem (Cardizem)
dobutamine
dopamine (Intropin)
epinephrine (Adrenalin)
etomidate (Amidate)
flumazenil (Romazicon)
ibutilide (Corvert)
lidocaine
magnesium sulfate
naloxone (Narcan)
nimodipine (Nimotop)
norepinephrine (Levophed)
procainamide (Pronestyl)
vasopressin
verapamil (Isoptin)

Chapter Review

Pharmaceuticals and Body Functions

Select the best answer from the choices given.

1. All of the following are advantages of three-in-one parenteral nutrition formulas except
   a. decreased costs of preparation and delivery.
   b. reduced nursing time for administration.
   c. longer stability.
   d. potentially reduced risk of sepsis with fewer violations of the administration line.

2. A three-in-one formula contains
   a. protein, dextrose, lipids, electrolytes, and vitamins.
   b. protein, dextrose, lipids, and vitamins.
   c. protein, dextrose, electrolytes, and vitamins.
   d. protein, dextrose, and electrolytes.

3. Water-soluble vitamins are
   a. B and C.
   b. A and D.
   c. A and B.
   d. C and D.

4. Vitamin A is found in
   a. milk.
   b. fish oils.
   c. cheese.
   d. all of the above

5. The body uses vitamin A for
   a. normal growth.
   b. shedding and repair of epithelial tissue.
   c. reproductive function in males and females.
   d. all of the above

6. Which vitamin is normally formed by ultraviolet radiation in the skin?
   a. A
   b. B
   c. C
   d. D

7. Which vitamin is the most powerful reducing agent to occur naturally in living tissue?
   a. A
   b. B
   c. C
   d. D

8. Which vitamin is used in treating and preventing colds?
   a. A
   b. B
   c. C
   d. D

9. Which vitamin helps calcium move into the bone?
   a. A
   b. B
   c. C
   d. D

10. Which vitamin is usually purchased as a complex of vitamins?
    a. A
    b. B
    c. C
    d. D

The following statements are true or false. If the answer is false, rewrite the statement so it is true.

_____ 1. The leading cause of childhood poisoning is iron tablets.

_____ 2. Some indications for PN are poor wound healing, infections, and anemia.

_____ 3. Causes of water loss are large weight loss and large urine output.

_____ 4. An isotonic solution has fewer particles than body fluids.

_____ 5. Ginkgo is recommended as an anti-emetic.

_____ 6. Melatonin is a hormone produced naturally in our bodies.

_____ 7. Feverfew is an anti-inflammatory, antispasmodic, and anti-infective.

_____ 8. Ginseng is recommended for increasing circulation.

_____ 9. There are no major problems with herbs.

_____ 10. Opiates can cause respiratory failure.

Diseases and Drug Therapies

1. List three specific gastrointestinal diseases and/or hypermetabolic states that could be an indication for PN.

2. List ten complications of PN.

3. What is the phone number of the national poison prevention center?

4. Which alternative medicines are touted to treat which conditions, fill in the blanks.

   Impotence: _____

   Common cold: _____

   Antiemetic: _____

   Sleep: _____

   Prostate: _____

5. Match the following

Medical Food/Probiotic

1. Limbrel   (a) lowers homocysteine

2. Deplin   (b) low red blood cells

3. Activia   (c) osteoarthritis

4. Culturelle   (d) speeds gut transit time

5. Cerefolin   (e) diarrhea

Dispensing Medications

1. The pharmacy technician is told to add morphine and midazolam to the automated dispensing machine because an order for conscious sedation has been given. What other drugs should also be added?

2. What drugs must be in the emergency room before administering snake antivenin? The technician must get these together.

Internet Research

Use the Internet to complete the following activities.

1. Create a table listing tips for adults on preventing accidental poisonings in the home and instructions for dealing with a case of suspected poisoning. In a third column include a list of useful resources for parents concerned about the potential for accidental poisoning (e.g., phone numbers, Web sites). List your Internet sources.

2. Herbal medicines have become increasingly popular. Use the Internet to research two of the herbal remedies covered in this chapter. List two or three medicinal benefits as well as precautions of use for each. List your Internet sources.

What Would You Do?

Write an oath for technicians to take at graduation. The pharmacist's oath, reproduced below, may be used as a guide.

Oath of a Pharmacist

At this time, I vow to devote my professional life to the service of all humankind through the profession of pharmacy.

I will consider the welfare of humanity and relief of human suffering my primary concerns.

I will apply my knowledge, experience, and skills to the best of my ability to assure optimal drug therapy outcomes for the patients I serve.

I will keep abreast of developments and maintain professional competency in my profession of pharmacy. I will maintain the hightest principles of moral, ethical and legal conduct.

I will embrace and advocate change in the profession of pharmacy that improves patient care.

I take these vows voluntarily with the full realization of the responsibility with which I am entrusted by the public.

(Oath of Pharmacist at school graduation and Code of Ethics are practicing pharmacists' guidelines)

Appendix A
Most Commonly Prescribed Drugs

Table A presents the most commonly prescribed drugs in the United States. The drugs are listed by their generic name. This table, as well as a table organized by brand names, appears on the Internet Resource Center for this textbook at www.emcp.net/pharmacology4e.

TABLE A: Most Commonly Prescribed Drugs

Generic Name	Pronunciation	Category	Brand Name	Table Reference
acetaminophen	a-seat-a-MIN-oh-fen	analgesic	Tylenol	13.2
acetaminophen-codeine	a-seat-a-MIN-oh-fen KOE-deen	analgesic	Phenaphen With Codeine, Tylenol With Codeine	6.12
acyclovir	ay-SYE-kloe-veer	systemic antifungal	Zovirax	14.9
albuterol	al-BYOO-ter-ole	bronchodilator	Proventil, Proventil HFA, Ventolin HFA, ProAir HFA	9.1
alendronate	a-LEN-droe-nate	bone resorption inhibitor	Fosamax, Fosamax Plus D	14.10
alfuzosin	al-FYOO-zoe-sin	alpha blocker	Uroxatral	12.9
allopurinol	al-oh-PURE-i-nawl	antigout agent	Zyloprim	13.6
alprazolam	al-PRAZ-oh-lam	antianxiety agent, sleep agent	Xanax	7.11, 7.13
amitriptyline	a-mee-TRIP-ti-leen	antidepressant	Elavil	7.3
amlodipine	am-LOE-di-peen	antihypertensive	Norvasc	12.1
amlodipine-benazepril	am-LOE-di-peen ben-AYE-ze-pril	antihypertensive	Lotrel	12.9
amlodipine-atoravastatin	am-LOE-di-peen a-tor-va-STAT-in	antihypertensive-statin	Caduet	12.15
amoxicillin	a-mox-i-SIL-in	systemic antibacterial	Amoxil, Trimox	4.3, 10.3, 11.4
amoxicillin-clavulanate	a-mox-i-SIL-in klav-yoo-LAN-ate	systemic antibacterial	Augmentin	4.4, 11.14
aripiprazole	air-i-PIP-ra-zole	antipsychotic	Abilify	7.10
aspirin-dipyridamole	AS-pir-in dye-peer-ID-a-mole	stroke prevention agent	Aggrenox	12.4
atenolol	a-TEN-oh-lawl	antihypertensive	Tenormin	12.1

TABLE A: Most Commonly Prescribed Drugs (continued)

Generic Name	Pronunciation	Category	Brand Name	Table Reference
atenolol-hydrochlorothiazide	a-TEN-oh-lawl hye-droe-klor-oh-THYE-a-zide	beta-blocker-diuretic	Tenorectic	12.9
atomoxetine	at-oh-MOX-e-teen	ADHD therapy agent	Strattera	8.5
atorvastatin	a-tor-va-STAT-in	antihyperlipidemic	Lipitor	12.15
azithromycin	az-ith-roe-MYE-sin	systemic antibacterial	Zithromax	4.9, 14.9, 15.3
benazepril	ben-AZ-eh-pril	antihypertensive	Lotensin	12.5
benazapril-hydrochlorothiazide	ben-AZ-eh-pril hye-droe-klor-oh-THYE-a-zide	antihypertensive-diuretic	Lotensin HCTZ	12.9
bisoprolol-hydrochlorothiazide	bis-OE-proe-lawl hye-droe-klor-oh-THYE-a-zide	beta-blocker-diuretic	Ziac	12.9
brimonidine	bri-MOE-ni-deen	antiglaucoma agent	Alphagan P	15.11
budesonide	byoo-DES-oh-nide	antiasthmatic	Entocort EC, Pulmicort Respules, Pulmicort Turbuhaler, Rhinocort	9.1
bupropion	byoo-PROE-pee-on	antidepressant, smoking cessation adjunct	Wellbutrin, Zyban	7.6, 9.13
buspirone	byoo-SPYE-rone	antianxiety	BuSpar	7.11
calcitonin-salmon	kal-si-TOE-nin SAM-en	bone resorption inhibitor	Miacalcin	14.10
candesartan	kan-de-SAR-tan	antihypertensive	Atacand	12.9
carisoprodol	kar-eye-soe-PROE-dawl	skeletal muscle relaxant	Soma	13.1
carvedilol	KAR-ve-dil-ole	antihypertensive	Coreg	12.5
cefdinir	sef-DI-neer	systemic antibacterial	Omnicef	4.5
cefprozil	sef-PROE-zil	systemic antibacterial	Cefzil	4.5
celecoxib	sel-a-KOX-ib	analgesic, antirheumatic NSAID	Celebrex	13.4
cephalexin	sef-a-LEX-in	systemic antibacterial	Keflex	4.5
cetirizine	se-TEER-a-zeen	antihistaminic, H_1 receptor	Zyrtec	9.9
cetirizine-pseudoephedrine	se-TEER-a-zeen soo-doe-e-FED-rin	antihistaminic, H_1 receptor–decongestant	Zyrtec-D	9.7
ciprofloxacin	sip-roe-FLOX-a-sin	ophthalmic antibacterial	Occuflox, Ciprodex, Ciloxan	4.17
		systemic antibacterial	Cipro	4.11, 9.4, 11.4
citalopram	sye-TAL-oh-pram	antidepressant	Celexa	7.1
clarithromycin	kla-rith-roe-MYE-sin	systemic antibacterial, antimycobacterial	Biaxin	4.9, 10.3

TABLE A: Most Commonly Prescribed Drugs (continued)

Generic Name	Pronunciation	Category	Brand Name	Table Reference
clindamycin	klin-da-MYE-sin	antibiotic	Cleocin	4.15
clonazepam	kloe-NAZ-e-pam	anticonvulsant	Klonopin	8.1
clonidine	KLON-i-deen	antihypertensive	Catapres, Catapres-TTS	12.9
			Duraclon	12.9
clopidogrel	kloh-PID-oh-grel	antithrombotic, platelet aggregation inhibitor	Plavix	12.11
clotrimazole-betamethasone	kloe-TRIM-a-zole bay-ta-METH-a-sone	antifungal, corticosteroid	Lotrisone	15.3
conjugated estrogen	CON-ju-gate-ed ES-troe-jen	antineoplastic, systemic estrogen, osteoporosis prophylactic, ovarian hormone therapy agent	Cenestin, Enjuvia, Premarin	14.5
conjugated estrogen–medroxyprogesterone	CON-ju-gate-ed ES-troe-jen me-DROX-ee-proe-JES-te-rone	estrogen-progestin, osteoporosis prophylactic, ovarian hormone therapy agent	Premphase, Prempro	14.5
cyclobenzaprine	sye-kloe-BEN-za-preen	skeletal muscle relaxant	Flexeril	13.1
desloratadine	des-lor-AT-a-deen	antihistaminic, H_1 receptor	Clarinex	9.9
dextroamphetamine-amphetamine	dex-troe-am-FET-a-meen am-FET-a-meen	CNS stimulant, ADHD therapy	Adderall	8.5
diazepam	dye-AZ-e-pam	amnestic, antianxiety agent, anticonvulsant, antipanic agent, anti-tremor agent, sedative-hypnotic, skeletal muscle relaxant adjunct	Valium	6.2, 7.13 8.1, 13.1
diclofenac-misoprostol	dye-KLOE-fen-ak mye-soe-PROST-awl	NSAID	Arthrotec	13.4
digoxin	di-JOX-in	antiarrhythmic, cardiotonic	Lanoxicaps	12.3
			Lanoxin	12.3, 17.10
diltiazem	dil-TYE-a-zem	antianginal, antiarrhythmic, antihypertensive	Cardizem	12.1, 17.10
			Dilacor XR	12.1
divalproex	dye-VAL-pro-ex	anticonvulsant, antimanic, migraine headache prophylactic	Depakote	7.7, 8.1
donepezil	don-EP-a-zil	dementia symptoms treatment adjunct	Aricept	8.8
doxycycline	dox-i-SYE-kleen	systemic antibacterial, antiprotozoal	Vibramycin, Oracea, Adoxa, Doryx	4.7, 10.12, 14.9

TABLE A: Most Commonly Prescribed Drugs (continued)

Generic Name	Pronunciation	Category	Brand Name	Table Reference
enalapril	e-NAL-a-pril	antihypertensive, vasodilator	Vasotec	12.5
escitalopram	es-sye-TAL-oh-pram	antianxiety agent, antidepressant	Lexapro	7.1
esomeprazole	es-oh-MEP-ray-zole	gastric acid pump inhibitor, antiulcer agent	Nexium	10.1
estradiol	es-tra-DYE-awl	estrogen only hormone replacement	Alora, Climara, Elestrin, Eselim, Estrace, Estraderm, Estrasorb, Estring, Evamist, Femring, Menostar, Vivelle, Vivelle Dot	14.5
eszopiclone	es-zo-PIK-lone	hypnotic	Lunesta	7.13
ethinyl estradiol–desogestrel	ETH-in-il es-tra-DYE-awl des-oh-JES-trel	antiendometriotic, systemic contraceptive, gonadotropin inhibitor	Cyclessa, Desogen, Kariva, Mircette, Ortho-Cept	14.6
ethinyl estradiol–drospirenone	ETH-in-il es-tra-DYE-awl droh-SPYE-re-none	systemic contraceptive	Yasmin, Yaz	14.6
ethinyl estradiol–levonorgestrel	ETH-in-il es-tra-DYE-awl LEE-voe-nor-jes-trel	antiendometriotic, systemic postcoital contraceptive, systemic contraceptive, estrogen progestin, gonadotropin inhibitor	Aviane, Levlen, Lybrel, Nordette, Seasonale, Tri-Levlen, Triphasil, Trivora-28	14.6
ethinyl estradiol–norelgestromin	ETH-in-il es-tra-DYE-awl nor-el-JES-troe-min	systemic contraceptive	Ortho Evra	14.6
ethinyl estradiol–norethindrone	ETH-in-il es-tra-DYE-awl nor-eth-IN-drone	antiacne agent, antiendometriotic, systemic contraceptive, estrogen progestin, gonadotropin inhibitor	Estrostep Fe, femhrt, Loestrin Fe, Loestrin 24 Fe Ovcon	14.5, 14.6
ethinyl estradiol–norgestimate	ETH-in-il es-tra-DYE-awl nor-JES-ti-mate	antiacne agent, antiendometriotic, systemic contraceptive, estrogen progestin, gonadotropin inhibitor	Ortho Tri-Cyclen, Ortho Tri-Cyclen Lo	14.6
ethinyl estradiol-norgestrel	ETH-in-il es-tra-DYE-awl nor-JES-trel	antiacne agent, antiendometriotic, systemic contraceptive, estrogen progestin, gonadotropin inhibitor	Lo/Ovral, Low-Ogestral, Ovral	14.6
ezetimibe	ee-ZET-e-mib	antihyperlipidemic	Zetia	12.15

TABLE A: Most Commonly Prescribed Drugs (continued)

Generic Name	Pronunciation	Category	Brand Name	Table Reference
ezetimbe-simvastatin	ee-ZET-e-mib sim-va STAT-in	antihyperlipidemic-statin	Vytorin	12.15
famotidine	fa-MOE-ti-deen	H-2 Histamine receptor antagonist	Pepcid	10.1
fenofibrate	fen-oh-FYE-brate	antihyperlipidemic	TriCor	12.15
fentanyl	FEN-ta-nil	analgesic	Duragesic	6.9
		analgesic, anesthesia adjunct	Actiq, Sublimaze	6.2, 6.9
fexofenadine	fex-o-FEN-a-deen	antihistaminic, H_1 receptor	Allegra	9.9
fexofenadine-pseudoephedrine	fex-o-FEN-a-deen soo-doe-e-FED-rin	antihistaminic, H_1 receptor–decongestant	Allegra-D	9.7
finasteride	fin-AS-tur-ide	benign prostatic hyperplasia therapy agent, hair growth stimulant	Propecia, Proscar	11.6
fluconazole	floo-KOE-na-zole	systemic antifungal	Diflucan	5.2, 14.9
fluoxetine	floo-OX-e-teen	antidepressant, antiobsessional agent, antibulemic agent	Prozac, Sarafem	7.1
fluticasone	floo-TIK-a-sone	steroidal nasal anti-inflammatory, nasal corticosteroid	Flonase, Flovent	9.1
fluticasone-salmeterol	floo-TIK-a-sone sal-ME-te-role	antiasthmatic, inhalation anti-inflammatory, bronchodilator	Advair Diskus	9.1
furosemide	fur-OH-se-mide	antihypercalcemic, antihypertensive, renal disease diagnostic aid adjunct, diuretic	Lasix	11.7
gabapentin	gab-a-PEN-tin	anticonvulsant, antineuralgic	Neurontin	8.1
gemfibrozil	jem-FI-broe-zil	antihyperlipidimic	Lopid	12.15
glimepiride	GLYE-me-pye-ride	antidiabetic	Amaryl	14.17
glipizide	GLIP-i-zide	antidiabetic	Glucotrol, Glucotrol XL	14.17
glyburide	GLYE-byoo-ride	antidiabetic	DiaBeta, Glynase, Micronase	14.17
glyburide-metformin	GLYE-byoo-ride met-FOR-min	antidiabetic	Glucovance	14.17
guaifenesin	gwye-FEN-e-sin	expectorant	Mucinex	9.6
guaifenesin-codeine	gwye-FEN-e-sin KOE-deen	expectorant	Robitussin A-C	9.6
guaifenesin-pseudoephedrine	gwye-FEN-e-sin soo-doe-e-FED-rin	expectorant-decongestant	Mucinex D	9.6

Generic Name	Pronunciation	Category	Brand Name	Table Reference
hydrochlorothiazide	hye-droe-klor-oh-THYE-a-zide	antihypertensive, diuretic, antiurolithic	Esidrix	11.7
hydrocodone-acetaminophen	hye-droe-KOE-done a-seat-a-MIN-oh-fen	analgesic	Lortab, Vicodin	6.12
hydrocodone-chlorpheniramine	hye-droe-KOE-done klor-fen-EER-a-meen	antihistaminic, H_1 receptor–antitussive	Tussionex	9.5
ibandronate	eye-BAN-droh-nate	bone resorption inhibitor	Boniva	14.10
ibuprofen	eye-byoo-PROE-fen	analgesic	Advil, Motrin	13.4
insulin glargine	IN-soo-lin GLARE-jeen	antidiabetic	Lantus	14.16
insulin lispro	IN-soo-lin LYE-sproe	antidiabetic	Humalog	14.16
insulin regular	IN-soo-lin re-gyoo-lar	antidiabetic	Humilin R, Novolin R	14.15
ipratropium	i-pra-TROE-pee-um	antiasthmatic	Atrovent	9.1
ipratropium-albuterol	i-pra-TROE-pee-um al-BYOO-ter-ole	antiasthmatic-bronchodilator	Combivent	9.2
irbesartan	ir-be-SAR-tan	antihypertensive	Avapro	12.9
irbesartan-hydrochlorothiazide	ir-be-SAR-tan hye-droe-klor-oh-THYE-a-zide	antihypertensive, diuretic	Avalide	12.9
isosorbide-hydralazine	eye-soe-SOR-bide hye-DRAL-a-zeen	vasodilator	BiDil	12.5
lamotrigine	la-MOE-tri-jeen	anticonvulsant	Lamictal	8.1
lansoprazole	lan-SOE-pra-zole	gastric acid pump inhibitor, antiulcer agent	Prevacid	10.1
latanoprost	la-TAN-oe-prost	antiglaucoma agent, ocular antihypertensive	Xalatan	15.11
levofloxacin	lee-voe-FLOX-a-sin	systemic antibacterial	Levaquin	4.11
levothyroxine, T_4	lee-voe-thye-ROX-een	antineoplastic, thyroid function diagnostic aid, thyroid hormone	Levothroid, Synthroid	14.1
lisinopril	lyse-IN-oh-pril	antihypertensive, vasodilator	Prinivil, Zestril	12.5
lisinopril-hydrochlorothiazide	lyse-IN-oh-pril hye-droe-klor-oh-THYE-a-zide	antihypertensive, diuretic	Zestoretic	12.9
lorazepam	lor-AZ-e-pam	amnestic, antianxiety agent, anticonvulsant, antiemetic, antipanic agent, antitremor agent, sedative-hypnotic, skeletal muscle relaxant	Ativan	6.2, 7.11, 7.13, 8.1
losartan	loe-SAR-tan	angiotensin II–receptor antagonist, antihypertensive	Cozaar	12.9

TABLE A: Most Commonly Prescribed Drugs (continued)

Generic Name	Pronunciation	Category	Brand Name	Table Reference
losartan-hydrochlorothiazide	loe-SAR-tan hye-droe-klor-oh-THYE-a-zide	antihypertensive-diuretic	Hyzaar	12.9
lovestatin	loe-ve-STAT-in	lipid-lowering agent	Mevacor	12.15
meclizine	MEK-li-zeen	antiemetic, antivertigo agent	Antivert	7.9, 9.9, 10.8
meloxicam	mel-OX-i-kam	antirheumatic (NSAID)	Mobic	13.4
memantine	MEM-an-teen	treatment of dementia	Namenda	8.8
metaxalone	me-TAX-a-lone	skeletal muscle relaxant	Skelaxin	13.1
metformin	met-FOR-min	antihyperglycemic	Glucophage, Riornet	14.17
methylphenidate	meth-il-FEN-i-date	CNS stimulant, ADHD therapy	Concerta, Daytrana, Metadate, Metadate ER, Methylin, Ritalin-SR, Ritalin	8.5
methylprednisolone	meth-il-pred-NIS-oh-lone	steroidal anti-inflammatory, corticoid steroid, immunosuppressant	Medrol, Solu-Medrol	9.1, 14.12
metoclopromide	met-oh-KLOE-pra-mide	anti-emetic	Reglan	10.4
metolazone	me-TOLE-a-zone	thiazide diuretic	Zaroxolyn	11.7
metronidazole	me-tro-NYE-da-zole	systemic antibiotic	Flagyl	4.15
metoprolol	met-TOE-proe-lawl	antiadrenergic, antianginal, antianxiety therapy adjunct, antiarrhythmic, antihypertensive, anti-tremor agent, hypertrophic cardiomyopathy therapy adjunct, myocardial infarction therapy, neuroleptic-induced akathisia therapy, pheochromocytoma therapy adjunct, thyrotoxicosis therapy adjunct, vascular headache prophylactic	Lopressor, Toprol-XL	12.1
minocycline	mi-noe-SYE-kleen	systemic antibacterial	Minocin Soladyne	4.7
mirtazapine	meer-TAZ-a-peen	antidepressant	Remeron	7.3
mometasone	moe-MET-a-sone	nasal steroidal anti-inflammatory, nasal corticosteroid	Nasonex	9.10
montelukast	mon-te-LOO-kast	antiasthmatic, leukotriene receptor antagonist	Singulair	9.1

Generic Name	Pronunciation	Category	Brand Name	Table Reference
moxifloxacin	mox-i-FLOX-a-sin	ophthalmic antibacterial	Vigamox	4.17
		systemic antibacterial	Avelox	4.11
mupirocin	myoo-PEER-oe-sin	topical antibacterial	Bactroban	15.4
naproxen	na-PROX-en	analgesic, nonsteroidal anti-inflammatory, anti-dysmenorrheal, antigout agent, antipyretic, non-steroidal anti-inflammatory antirheumatic, vascular headache prophylactic, vascular headache suppressant	Aleve, Anaprox, Naprosyn	13.4
nifedipine	nye-FED-i-peen	antianginal, antihypertensive	Procardia	12.1
nisolidipine	nye-SOLE-di-peen	calcium channel blocker	Sular	12.1
nitrofurantoin	nye-troe-fyoor-AN-toyn	systemic antibacterial	Macrobid, Macrodantin	4.2, 11.4
nitroglycerin	nye-troe-GLISS-er-in	antianginal, congestive heart failure vasodilator	Minitran, Nitrolingual, Nitrostat, NitroDur	12.1
olanzapine	oh-LAN-za-peen	antipsychotic	Zyprexa	7.10
olmesartan	ohl-me-SAR-tan	Angiotensin II receptor antagonist	Benicar	12.9
olopatadine	oh-loe-PAT-a-deen	ophthalmic antihistaminic, H_1 receptor; ophthalmic mast cell stabilizer; ophthalmic antiallergic	Patanol	15.10
omeprazole	oh-MEP-ra-zole	gastric acid pump inhibitor, antiulcer agent	Prilosec, Prilosec OTC	10.1
oxybutynin	ox-i-BYOO-ti-nin	urinary tract antispasmodic	Ditropan, Oxytrol	11.3
oxycodone	ox-i-KOE-done	analgesic	OxyContin	6.9
oxycodone-acetaminophen	ox-i-KOE-done a-seat-a-MIN-oh-fen	analgesic	Endocet, Percocet, Tylox	6.12
pantoprazole	pan-TOE-pra-zole	gastric acid pump inhibitor, antiulcer agent	Protonix	10.1
paroxetine	pa-ROX-e-teen	antianxiety agent, antidepressant, antiobsessional agent, antipanic agent, posttraumatic stress disorder agent, social anxiety disorder agent	Paxil	7.1, 7.11
penicillin V	pen-i-SIL-in V	systemic antibacterial	Veetids	4.3

Generic Name	Pronunciation	Category	Brand Name	Table Reference
phenytoin	FEN-i-toyn	antiarrhythmic, anticonvulsant, trigeminal neuralgic antineuralgic, skeletal muscle relaxant	Dilantin	8.1, 12.3
pimecrolimus	pim-e-KROW-li-mus	immunomodulator	Elidel	15.3
pioglitazone	pye-oh-GLIT-a-zone	antidiabetic	Actos	14.17
polyethylene glycol	pol-ee-ETH-il-een GLYE-kawl	hyperosmotic laxative	MiraLax	10.6, 17.9
potassium chloride	poe-tass-EE-um KLOR-ide	antihypokalemic, electrolyte replenisher	Klor-Con	17.7
pravastatin	PRA-va-sta-tin	antihyperlipidemic, HMG-CoA reductase inhibitor	Pravachol	12.15
prednisone	PRED-ni-sone	steroidal inflammatory, cancer chemotherapy antiemetic, corticosteroid, immunosuppressant	Deltasone	9.1, 14.12
pregabalin	pree-GAB-a-lin	antiseizure	Lyrica	8.1
promethazine	proe-METH-a-zeen	antiemetic; antihistaminic, H_1 receptor; antivertigo agent; sedative-hypnotic	Phenergan	9.9, 10.8
promethazine-codeine	proe-METH-a-zeen KOE-deen	antihistaminic, H_1 receptor-antitussive	Phenergan with codeine	9.5
propoxyphene-acetaminophen	proe-POX-i-feen a-seat-a-MIN-oh-fen	analgesic	Darvocet-N 100	6.12
propranolol	proe-PRAN-oh-lawl	antiadrenergic, antianginal, antianxiety therapy adjunct, antiarrhythmic, antihypertensive, antitremor agent, hypertrophic cardiomyopathy therapy adjunct, myocardial infarction prophylactic, myocardial infarction therapy, neuroleptic-induced akathisia therapy, pheochromocytoma therapy adjunct, thyrotoxicosis therapy adjunct, vascular headache prophylactic	Inderal	6.13, 7.11, 12.1
quetiapine	kwe-TYE-a-peen	antipsychotic	Seroquel	7.10
quinapril	KWIN-a-pril	antihypertensive, vasodilator	Accupril	12.5
rabeprazole	ra-BEP-ra-zole	gastric acid pump inhibitor, antiulcer agent	Aciphex	10.1

TABLE A: Most Commonly Prescribed Drugs (continued)

Generic Name	Pronunciation	Category	Brand Name	Table Reference
raloxifene	ral-OX-i-feen	selective estrogen receptor modulator, osteoporosis prophylactic	Evista	14.10
ramipril	RA-mi-pril	antihypertensive, vasodilator	Altace	12.5
ranitidine	ra-NIT-i-deen	histamine H_2-receptor antagonist, antiulcer agent, gastric acid secretion inhibitor	Zantac, Zantac 75	10.1
risedronate	ris-ED-roe-nate	bone resorption inhibitor	Actonel	14.10
risperidone	ris-PAIR-i-done	antipsychotic	Risperdal	7.10
ropinirole	ro-PIN-a-role	anti-parkinson agent	ReQuip	8.3
rosiglitazone	ros-e-GLIT-a-zone	antidiabetic	Avandia	14.17
rosurvastatin	roe-soo-va-STAT-in	HmgCoA reductase inhibitor	Crestor	12.15
sertraline	SER-tra-leen	antianxiety agent, antidepressant, antiobsessional agent, antipanic agent, posttraumatic stress disorder therapy agent, premenstrual dysphoric disorder therapy agent	Zoloft	7.1
sildenafil	sil-DEN-a-fil	systemic impotence therapy agent	Viagra	14.4
simvastatin	SIM-va-STAT-in	antihyperlipidemic, HMG-CoA reductase inhibitor	Zocor	12.15
spironolactone	speer-on-oh-LAK-tone	aldosterone antagonist, antihypertensive, antihypokalemic, primary hyperaldosteronism diagnostic aid, diuretic	Aldactone	11.7
sulfamethoxazole-trimethoprim	sul-fa-meth-OX-a-zole trye-METH-oh-prim	systemic antibacterial, antiprotozoal	Bactrim, Bactrim DS, Cotrim, Cotrim DS, Septra, Septra DS	4.2, 10.11, 11.4
sumatriptan	soo-ma-TRIP-tan	antimigraine agent	Imitrex	6.13
tadalafil	tah-DAL-a-fil	male impotence	Cialis	14.4
tamsulosin	tam-SOO-loh-sin	benign prostatic hyperplasia therapy agent	Flomax	11.6
telmisartan	tel-me-SAR-tan	Antihypertensive - ARB	Micardis	12.9
temazepam	tem-AZ-e-pam	sedative-hypnotic	Restoril	7.13
terazosin	ter-AYE-zoe-sin	antihypertensive, benign prostatic hyperplasia therapy agent	Hytrin	11.6, 12.9

TABLE A: Most Commonly Prescribed Drugs (continued)

Generic Name	Pronunciation	Category	Brand Name	Table Reference
timolol	TYE-moe-lawl	ophthalmic antiglaucoma agent	Timoptic	15.11
tiotropium	tye-oh-TRO-pee-um	bronchodilator	Spiriva	9.1
tobramycin-dexamethasone	toe-bra-MYE-sin dex-a-METH-a-sone	ophthalmic corticosteroid, ophthalmic steroidal anti-inflammatory, ophthalmic antibacterial	TobraDex	15.10
tolterodine	tole-TAIR-oh-deen	urinary bladder antispasmodic	Detrol	11.3
topiramate	toe-PYRE-a-mate	anticonvulsant, antimigraine headache	Topamax	7.16, 8.1
tramadol	TRA-ma-dawl	analgesic	Ultram	6.13, 13.4
tramadol-acetaminophen	TRA-ma-dawl a-seat-a-MIN-oh-fen	analgesic	Ultracet	13.4
trandolapril-verapamil	tran-DOE-la-pril ver-AP-a-mil	calcium channel blocker	Tarka	12.9
trazodone	TRAZ-oh-done	antidepressant, antineuralgic	Desyrel	7.6
triamcinolone	trye-am-SIN-oh-lone	inhalation anti-inflammatory, antiasthmatic	Azmacort	9.1
		nasal steroidal anti-inflammatory, nasal corticosteroid	Aristocort, Nasacort AQ	9.1, 9.10, 14.12
triamterene-hydrochlorothiazide	trye-AM-ter-een hye-droe-klor-oh-THYE-a-zide	antihypertensive, antihypokalemic, diuretic	Dyazide, Maxzide	11.7
valacyclovir	val-ay-SYE-kloe-veer	systemic antiviral	Valtrex	5.3, 14.9
valproic acid	val-PRO-ik AS-id	anticonvulsant	Depakene	7.7
valsartan	val-SAR-tan	antihypertensive	Diovan	12.9
valsartan-hydrochlorothiazide	val-SAR-tan hye-droe-klor-oh-THYE-a-zide	antihypertensive	Diovan HCT	12.9
venlafaxine	ven-la-FAX-een	antidepressant, antianxiety agent	Effexor	7.2, 7.11
verapamil	ver-AP-a-mil	antianginal, antiarrhythmic, antihypertensive, hypertrophic cardiomyopathy therapy adjunct, vascular headache prophylactic	Calan, Covera HS, Verelan	12.1
			Isoptin	12.1, 17.10
warfarin	WOR-far-in	anticoagulant	Coumadin	12.10
zolpidem	ZOLE-pi-dem	sedative hypnotic	Ambien	7.13

SOURCE: Adapted from RxList, The Top 200 Prescriptions for 2007 by Number of U.S. Prescriptions Dispensed (www.rxlist.com, accessed 11/17/08). Category information from the U.S. National Library of Medicine and National Institutes of Health MedlinePlus Web site Lexicom 2008-2009 (www.nlm.nih.gov/medlineplus, accessed 11/17/08).

Appendix B
Common Look-Alike and Sound-Alike Medications

While manufacturers have an obligation to review new trademarks for error potential before use, there are some actions that prescribers, pharmacists, and pharmacy technicians can do to help prevent errors with products that have look- or sound-alike names. The Institute for Safe Medication Practices (ISMP) provides several types of tools that are designed to prevent dispensing errors. These include the following recommended actions as well as the list of look-alike and sound-alike drugs presented in Table B.

- **Use electronic prescribing** to prevent confusion with handwritten drug names.
- **Encourage physicians to write prescriptions that clearly specify the dosage form, drug strength, and complete directions.** They should include the product's indication on all outpatient prescriptions and on inpatient *prn* orders. With name pairs known to be problematic, reduce the potential for confusion by writing prescriptions using both the brand and generic name. Listing both names on medication administration records and automated dispensing cabinet computer screens also may be helpful.
- **Whenever possible, determine the purpose of the medication** before dispensing or administering it. Many products with look-alike or sound-alike names are used for different purposes.
- **Accept verbal or telephone orders only when truly necessary.** Require staff to read back all orders, spell the product name, and state its indication. Like medication names, numbers can sound alike, so staff should read the dosage back in numerals (eg. "one five" for 15 milligrams) to ensure clear interpretation of dose.
- **When feasible, use magnifying lenses and copyholders** under good lighting to keep prescriptions and orders at eye level during transcription to improve the likelihood of proper interpretation of look-alike product names.
- **Change the appearance of look-alike product names** on computer screens, pharmacy and nursing unit shelf labels, and bins (including automated dispensing cabinets), pharmacy product labels, and medication administration records by highlighting, through bold face, color, and/or capital letters, the parts of the names that are different (e.g., hydr**OXY**zine, hydr**ALA**zine).
- **Install a computerized reminder** (also placed on automated dispensing cabinet screens) for the most serious confusing name pairs so that an alert is generated when entering prescriptions for either drug. If possible, make the reminder auditory as well as visual.
- **Affix "name alert" stickers** in areas where look-alike or sound-alike products are stored (available from pharmacy label manufacturers).
- **Store products with look-alike or sound-alike names in different locations.** Avoid storing both products in the fast-mover area. Use a shelf sticker to help locate the product that is moved.

- **Continue to employ an independent check in the dispensing process** (one person interprets and enters the prescription into the computer and another reviews the printed label against the original prescription and the product).
- **Open the prescription bottle or the unit dose package in front of the patient** to confirm the expected product appearance and review the indication. Caution patients about error potential when taking products that have a look-alike or sound-alike counterpart. Take the time to fully investigate the situation if a patient states he or she is taking an unknown medication.
- **Monitor reported errors caused by look-alike and sound-alike medication names** and alert staff to mistakes.
- **Look for the possibility of name confusion when a new product is added to the formulary.** Have a few clinicians handwrite the product name and directions, as they would appear in a typical order. Ask frontline nurses, pharmacists, technicians, unit secretaries, and physicians to view the samples of the written product name as well as pronounce it to determine if it looks or sounds like any other drug product or medical term. It may be helpful to have clinicians first look at the scripted product name to determine how they would interpret it before the actual product name is provided to them for pronunciation. Once the product name is known, clinicians may be less likely to see more familiar product names in the written samples. If the potential for confusion with other products is identified, take steps to avoid errors as listed below.
- **Encourage reporting of errors** and potentially hazardous conditions with look-alike and sound-alike product names and use the information to establish priorities for error reduction. Also maintain awareness of problematic product names and error prevention recommendations provided by ISMP (www.ismp.org and also listed on the quarterly *Action Agenda*), FDA (www.fda.gov), and United States Pharmacopoeia (USP; www.usp.org).
- **Review Table B for look-alike and sound-alike drug name pairs in use at your practice location.** Decide what actions might be warranted to prevent medication errors. Stay current with alerts from ISMP, FDA, and USP in case new problematic name pairs emerge.

TABLE B: Common Look-Alike and Sound-Alike Medications

Medication Name	Look- or Sound-Alike Name
Abelcet	amphotericin B
Accupril	Aciphex
acetazolamide	acetohexamide
acetohexamide	acetazolamide
Aciphex	Aricept
Aciphex	Accupril
Activase	TNKase
Actonel	Actos
Actos	Actonel
Adderall	Inderal
Advicor	Altocor
Aggrastat	argatroban

TABLE B: Common Look-Alike and Sound-Alike Medications (continued)

Medication Name	Look- or Sound-Alike Name	
Aldara	Alora	
Alkeran	Leukeran	Myleran
Allegra	Viagra	
Alora	Aldara	
Altocor	Advicor	
Amaryl	Reminyl	
AmBisome	amphotericin B	
amphotericin B	Abelcet	
amphotericin B	Ambisome	
antacid	Atacand	
Antivert	Axert	
Anzemet	Avandamet	
argatroban	Aggrastat	
Aricept	Aciphex	
aripiprazole	rabeprazole	
Asacol	Os-Cal	
Atacand	antacid	
Atrovent	Natru-Vent	
Avandamet	Anzemet	
Avandia	Prandin	
Avandia	Coumadin	
Avinza	Invanz	
Avinza	Evista	
Axert	Antivert	
BayHep B	BayRab	BayRho-D
BayRab	BayRho-D	BayHep B
BayRho-D	BayHep B	BayRab
Bicillin C-R	Bicillin L-A	
Bicillin L-A	Bicillin C-R	
Brethine	Methergine	
camphorated tincture of opium (paregoric)	opium tincture	
carboplatin	cisplatin	
Cedax	Cidex	
Celexa	Zyprexa	
chlorpromazine	chlorpropamide	
chlorpropamide	chlorpromazine	
Cidex	Cedax	
cisplatin	carboplatin	
Claritin-D	Claritin-D 24	
Claritin-D 24	Claritin-D	

TABLE B: Common Look-Alike and Sound-Alike Medications (continued)

Medication Name	Look- or Sound-Alike Name
Clozaril	Colazal
Colace	Cozaar
Colazal	Clozaril
colchicine	Cortrosyn
Comvax	Recombivax HB
Cortrosyn	colchicine
Coumadin	Avandia
Cozaar	Colace
Cozaar	Zocor
dactinomycin	daptomycin
daptomycin	dactinomycin
Darvon	Diovan
daunorubicin	idarubicin
Denavir	Indinavir
Depakote	Depakote ER
Depakote ER	Depakote
Depo-Medrol	Solu-Medrol
Diabenese	Diamox
DiaBeta	Zebeta
Diamox	Diabenese
Diatex (diazepam in Mexico)	Diatx
Diatx	Diatex (diazepam in Mexico)
Dilacor XR	Pilocar
Dilaudid	Dilaudid-5
Dilaudid-5	Dilaudid
Dioval	Diovan
Diovan	Dioval
Diovan	Zyban
Diovan	Darvon
Diprivan	Ditropan
Ditropan	Diprivan
dobutamine	dopamine
dopamine	dobutamine
doxorubicin hydrochloride	liposomal doxorubicin (DOXIL)
Duricef	Ultracet
Endocet	Indocin
Engerix-B adult	Engerix-B pediatric/adolescent
Engerix-B pediatric/adolescent	Engerix-B adult
ephedrine	epinephrine
epinephrine	ephedrine

TABLE B: Common Look-Alike and Sound-Alike Medications (continued)

Medication Name	Look- or Sound-Alike Name
Estratest	Estratest H.S.
Estratest H.S.	Estratest
ethambutol	Ethmozine
Ethmozine	ethambutol
Evista	Avinza
Femara	Femhrt
Femhrt	Femara
fentanyl	sufentanil
folic acid	folinic acid (leucovorin calcium)
folinic acid (leucovorin calcium)	folic acid
Foradil	Toradol
gentamicin	gentian violet
gentian violet	gentamicin
Granulex	Regranex
Healon	Hyalgan
heparin	Hespan
Hespan	heparin
Humalog	Humulin
Humalog Mix 75/25	Humulin 70/30
Humulin	Humalog
Humulin 70/30	Humalog Mix 75/25
Hyalgan	Healon
hydromorphone	morphine
idarubicin	daunorubicin
Inderal	Adderall
indinavir	Denavir
Indocin	Endocet
infliximab	rituximab
Invanz	Avinza
iodine	Lodine
Isordil	Plendil
isotretinoin	tretinoin
K-Phos Neutral	Neutra-Phos K
Kaletra	Keppra
Keppra	Kaletra
Ketalar	ketorolac
ketorolac	Ketalar
Lamictal	Lamisil

TABLE B: Common Look-Alike and Sound-Alike Medications (continued)

Medication Name	Look- or Sound-Alike Name
Lamisil	Lamictal
lamivudine	lamotrigine
lamotrigine	lamivudine
Lanoxin	levothyroxine
Lantus	Lente
Lasix	Luvox
Lente	Lantus
leucovorin calcium	Leukeran
Leukeran	Myleran Alkeran
Levbid	Levsin
levothyroxine	Lanoxin
Levsin	Levbid
Lexapro	Loxitane
Lipitor	Zyrtec
liposomal doxorubicin (Doxil)	doxorubicin hydrochloride
Lodine	iodine
Lotronex	Protonix
Loxitane	Lexapro
Lupron Depot-3 Month	Lupron Depot-Ped
Lupron Depot-Ped	Lupron Depot-3 Month
Luvox	Lasix
Maxzide	Microzide
Metadate	methadone
Metadate CD	Metadate ER
Metadate ER	Metadate CD
Metadate ER	methadone
methadone	Metadate ER
methadone	Metadate
Methergine	Brethine
Micronase	Microzide
Microzide	Maxzide
Microzide	Micronase
mifepristone	misoprostol
Miralax	Mirapex
Mirapex	Miralax
misoprostol	mifepristone
morphine	hydromorphone
morphine, oral liquid concentrate	morphine, non-concentrated oral liquid
MS Contin	OxyContin
Mucinex	Mucomyst

TABLE B: Common Look-Alike and Sound-Alike Medications (continued)

Medication Name	Look- or Sound-Alike Name
Mucomyst	Mucinex
Myleran	Alkeran Leukeran
Narcan	Norcuron
Natru-Vent	Atrovent
Navane	Norvasc
Neulasta	Neumega
Neumega	Neupogen
Neumega	Neulasta
Neupogen	Neumega
Neurontin	Noroxin
Neutra-Phos K	K-Phos Neutral
Norcuron	Narcan
Noroxin	Neurontin
Norvasc	Navane
Novolin 70/30	NovoLog Mix 70/30
NovoLog Mix 70/30	Novolin 70/30
Occlusal-HP	Ocuflox
Ocuflox	Occlusal-HP
opium tincture camphorated	tincture of opium (paregoric)
Os-Cal	Asacol
oxycodone	OxyContin
OxyContin	MS Contin
OxyContin	oxycodone
Pamelor	Panlor DC
Panlor DC	Pamelor
Patanol	Platinol
Paxil	Taxol
Paxil	Plavix
Percocet	Procet
Pilocar	Dilacor XR
Platinol	Patanol
Plavix	Paxil
Plendil	Isordil
pneumococcal 7-valent vaccine	pneumococcal polyvalent vaccine
pneumococcal polyvalent vaccine	pneumococcal 7-valent vaccine
Prandin	Avandia
Precare	Precose
Precose	Precare
Prilosec	Prozac
probenecid	Procanbid

TABLE B: Common Look-Alike and Sound-Alike Medications (continued)

Medication Name	Look- or Sound-Alike Name
Procanbid	Probenecid
Procardia XL	Protain XL
Procet	Percocet
propylthiouracil	Purinethol
Protain XL	Procardia XL
protamine	Protonix
Protonix	Lotronex
Protonix	protamine
Prozac	Prilosec
Purinethol	propylthiouracil
quinine	quinidine
quinidine	quinine
rabeprazole	aripiprazole
Recombivax HB	Comvax
Regranex	Granulex
Reminyl	Robinul
Reminyl	Amaryl
Retrovir	ritonavir
Rifater	Rifidin
Rifidin	Rifater
Ritalin	ritodrine
Ritalin LA	Ritalin-SR
Ritalin-SR	Ritalin LA
ritodrine	Ritalin
ritonavir	Retrovir
rituximab	infliximab
Robinul	Reminyl
Roxanol	Roxicodone Intensol
Roxanol	Roxicet
Roxicet	Roxanol
Roxicodone Intensol	Roxanol
saquinavir (free base)	saquinavir mesylate
saquinavir mesylate	saquinavir (free base)
Saquinivir	Sinequan
Sarafem	Serophene
Serophene	Sarafem
Seroquel	Serzone
sertraline	Soriatane
Serzone	Seroquel
Sinequan	Saquinivir

TABLE B: Common Look-Alike and Sound-Alike Medications (continued)

Medication Name	Look- or Sound-Alike Name
Solu-Medrol	Depo-Medrol
Soriatane	sertraline
sufentanil	fentanyl
sumatriptan	zolmitriptan
Taxol	Taxotere
Taxol	Paxil
Taxotere	Taxol
Tegretol	Tequin
Tegretol	Tegretol XR
Tegretol XR	Tegretol
Tequin	Tegretol
Tequin	Ticlid
Testoderm	Testoderm w/ Adhesive
Testoderm w/ Adhesive	Testoderm
tetanus diptheria toxoid (Td)	tuberculin purified protein derivative (PPD)
tiagabine	tizanidine
Tiazac	Ziac
Ticlid	Tequin
tizanidine	tiagabine
TNKase	Activase
TNKase	t-PA
Tobradex	Tobrex
Tobrex	TobraDex
Topamax	Toprol-XL
Toprol-XL	Topamax
Toradol	Foradil
t-PA	TNKase
Tracleer	TriCor
tramadol hydrochloride	trazodone hydrochloride
trazodone hydrochloride	tramadol hydrochloride
tretinoin	isotretinoin
TriCor	Tracleer
tuberculin purified protein derivative (PPD)	tetanus diptheria toxoid (Td)
Tylenol	Tylenol PM
Tylenol PM	Tylenol
Ultracet	Duricef
valacyclovir	valganciclovir
Valcyte	Valtrex
valganciclovir	valacyclovir
Valtrex	Valcyte

TABLE B: Common Look-Alike and Sound-Alike Medications (continued)

Medication Name	Look- or Sound-Alike Name
Varivax	VZIG
Vexol	VoSol
Viagra	Allegra
vinblastine	vincristine
vincristine	vinblastine
Viokase	Viokase 8
Viokase 8	Viokase
Viracept	Viramune
Viramune	Viracept
VoSol	Vexol
VZIG	Varivax
Wellbutrin SR	Wellbutrin XL
Wellbutrin XL	Wellbutrin SR
Xeloda	Xenical
Xenical	Xeloda
Zantac	Zyrtec
Zebeta	DiaBeta
Zebeta	Zetia
Zestril	Zetia
Zetia	Zebeta
Zetia	Zestril
Ziac	Tiazac
Zocor	Cozaar
zolmitriptan	sumatriptan
Zostrix	Zovirax
Zovirax	Zyvox
Zovirax	Zostrix
Zyban	Diovan
Zyprexa	Zyrtec
Zyprexa	Celexa
Zyrtec	Zyprexa
Zyrtec	Zantac
Zyrtec	Lipitor
Zyvox	Zovirax

This list of confused drug names is based on information reported in the ISMP Medication Safety Alert! AccuteCare Edition, published by the Institute for Safe Medication Practices (www.ismp.org). This master is used with permission of ISMP.

Numerous abbreviations were introduced in this textbook. For quick reference, these are listed in Table C along with the word or phrase represented by the abbreviation.

TABLE C: Abbreviations

ACE	antiotensin-converting enzyme inhibitors	CDC	Centers for Disease Control
ACh	acetylcholine	CF	cystic fibrosis
ACTH	adrenocorticotrophic hormone	CFCs	chlorofluorocarbons
ADA	American Dental Association	CHF	congestive heart failure
ADD	attention-deficit disorder	CMV	cytomegalovirus
ADH	antidiuretic hormone	CNS	central nervous system
ADHD	attention-deficit hyperactivity disorder	COMT	catechol-o-methyl transferase
ADME	absorption, distribution, metabolism, and elimination	COPD	chronic obstructive pulmonary disease
		COX-1	cyclooxygenase-1
ADP	adenosine diphosphate	COX-2	cyclooxygenase-2
ADR	adverse drug reaction	CPAP	continuous positive airway pressure machine
AIDS	acquired immune deficiency syndrome		
ALS	amyotrophic lateral sclerosis	CPhT	certified pharmacy technician
AMD	age-related macular degeneration	CPR	cardiopulmonary resuscitation
ANC	absolute neutrophil count	CRF	corticotrophin-releasing factor
ANDA	Abbreviated New Drug Application	CSF	cerebrospinal fluid
ANS	autonomic nervous system	CSF	colony-stimulating factors
APhA	American Pharmaceutical Association	CTZ	chemotrigger zone
ARBs	angiotensin receptor blockers	CV	cardiovascular
ASHP	American Society of Health-System Pharmacists	CVA	cardiovascular accident
		D_5W	5% dextrose solution
ATP	adenosine triphosphate	DAW	dispense as written
AUC	area under the curve	DEA	Drug Enforcement Administration
AV	atrioventricular	DMARD	disease-modifying antirheumatic drug
BMI	body mass index	DNA	deoxyribonucleic acid
BP	blood pressure	DOC	drug of choice
BPH	benign prostatic hyperplasia or hypertrophy	DRIs	direct renin inhibitors
BUN	blood urea nitrogen	DTs	delirium tremens
CBC	complete blood count; complete blood [cell] count	DVT	deep vein thrombosis
		ECG	electrocardiographic

TABLE C: Abbreviations (continued)

EPS	extrapyramidal symptoms	LH	luteinizing hormone
ER	extended release	LSD	lysergic acid diethylamide
ESR	erythrocyte sedimentation rate	MAb	monoclonal antibody
ESRD	end-stage renal disease	MAOI	monoamine oxidase inhibitor
FDA	Food and Drug Administration	MCA	monoclonal antibody
FSH	follicle-stimulating hormone	MDI	metered dose inhaler
GABA	gamma-aminobutyric acid	MHC	major histocompatability complex
G-CSF	granulocyte colony-stimulating factor	MI	myocardial infarction
GERD	gastroesophageal reflux disease	MLWH	low-molecular-weight heparin
GH	growth hormone	MMA	Medicare Modernization Act
GHRF	growth hormone releasing factor	MMR	measles, mumps, rubella
GI	gastrointestinal	MPA	Michigan Pharmacists Association
GM-CSF	granulocyte-macrophage colony-stimulating factor	MRSA	methicillin-resistant *S. aureus*
		MS	multiple sclerosis
GMP	good manufacturing practice	NABP	National Association Boards of Pharmacy
GnRH	gonadotropin-releasing hormone	NDA	New Drug Application
hBNP	human B-type natriuretic peptide	NGU	nongonococcal urethritis
HCG	human chorionic gonadotropin	NKA	no known allergies
HDL	high-density lipoprotein	NNRTI	non-nucleoside reverse transcriptase inhibitor
HFA	hydrofluoroalkane		
HIPAA	Health Insurance Portability and Accountability Act	NREM	nonrapid eye movement
		NRTI	nucleoside reverse transcriptase inhibitor
HIV	human immunodeficiency virus	NS	normal saline
HPV	human papillomavirus	NSAID	nonsteroidal anti-inflammatory drug
IBS	irritable bowel syndrome	NtRTI	nucleotide reverse transcriptase inhibitor
IBW	ideal body weight		
ICHP	Illinois Council of Health-System	OC	oral contraceptive
ICU	intensive care unit	OCD	obsessive-compulsive disorder
Ig	immunoglobulin	OR	operating room
IgE	immunoglobulin E	OROS	osmotic-controlled release oral delivery system
IgG	immunoglobulin G		
IL-2	interleukin-2	OTC	over-the-counter
IM	intramuscular	PABA	para-aminobenzoic acid
IND	Investigational New Drug Application	PCA	patient-controlled analgesia
INH	isoniazid	PE	pulmonary embolism
INR	International Normalized Ratio	PEFR	peak expiratory flow rate
ISMP	Institute for Safe Medication Practices	PEP	post-exposure prophylaxis
IV	intravenous	PG	prostaglandin
JCAHO	Joint Commission on the Accreditation of Healthcare Organizations	pH	acid-base balance
		PI	protease inhibitor
		PID	pelvic inflammatory disease
LDL	low-density lipoprotein	PMDD	premenstrual dysphoric disorder
		PMS	premenstrual syndrome

TABLE C: Abbreviations (continued)

PN	parenteral nutrition	SPF	sunburn protection factor
PNS	peripheral nervous system	SQ	subcutaneous
PO	peroral, by mouth	SSRI	selective serotonin reuptake inhibitor
POE	physician order entry	STD	sexually transmitted disease
PPD	purified protein derivative	TB	tuberculosis
PPI's	proton pump inhibitors	TCA	tricyclic antidepressant
PT	prothrombin time	TIA	transient ischemia attack
PTCB	Pharmacy Technician Certification Board	TIM	topical immunomodulators
PTSD	post-traumatic stress disorder	TNA	total nutrient admixture
PTT	partial thromboplastin time	TNF	tumor necrosis factor
PTU	propylthiouracil	TPN	total parenteral nutrition
PVC	premature ventricular contraction	TSH	thyroid stimulating hormone
RA	rheumatoid arthritis	USAN	United States Adopted Name
RDA	recommended daily allowance	USP	United States Pharmacopoeia
RDS	respiratory distress syndrome	USP-NF	United States Pharmacopoeia and the National Formulary
REM	rapid eye movement		
RF	rheumatoid factor	UTIs	urinary tract infections
RIND	reversible ischemic neurologic deficit	UV	ultraviolet
RNA	ribonucleic acid	UV-A	ultraviolet-A
RSV	respiratory syncytial virus	VHF	viral hemorrhagic fever
SA	sinoatrial	VLDL	very-low-density lipoprotein
SAD	seasonal affective disorder	VRE	vancomycin-resistant *E. faecium*
SEDDS	self emulsifying drug delivery system	WBC	white blood cell; white blood [cell] count
SNRI	serotonin norepinephrine reuptake inhibitor		

Appendix D

Greek Alphabet

Greek letters are commonly employed in science, medicine, and pharmacology. For convenience, the Greek alphabet is listed in Table D.

TABLE D: Greek Alphabet

Capital	Low-case	Greek Name	English
A	α	alpha	a
B	β	beta	b
Γ	γ	gamma	g
Δ	δ	delta	d
E	ε	epsilon	e
Z	ζ	zeta	z
H	η	eta	h
Θ	θ	theta	th
I	ι	iota	i
K	κ	kappa	k
Λ	λ	lambda	l
M	μ	mu	m
N	ν	nu	n
Ξ	ξ	xi	x
O	o	omicron	o
Π	π	pi	p
P	ρ	rho	r
Σ	σ	sigma	s
T	τ	tau	t
Y	υ	upsilon	u
Φ	φ	phi	ph
X	χ	chi	ch
Ψ	ψ	psi	ps
Ω	ω	omega	o

Appendix E

Lab Values

In the course of their work, pharmacy technicians need to look up reference lab values for various chemical components of the human body. Table E presents normal ranges for adults for some of the most commonly discussed lab values. These values are for reference only; laboratories that obtain and report values for specific tests will provide normal ranges for the provided results.

TABLE E: Lab Values

Serum Plasma
- Albumin 3.2–5 g/dL
- Bicarbonate 19–25 mEq/L
- Calcium 8.6–10.3 mg/dL
- Chloride 98–108 mEq/L
- Creatinine 0.5–1.4 mg/dL
- Glucose 80–120 mg/dL
- Hemoglobin, glycosylated 4–8%
- Magnesium 1.6–2.5 mg/dL
- Potassium 3.5–5.2 mEq/L
- Sodium 134–149 mEq/L
- Urea nitrogen (BUN) 7–20 mg/dL

Cholesterol
- Total <200 mg/dL
- LDL 65–170 mg/dL
- HDL 40–60 mg/dL
- Triglycerides 45–150 mg/dL

Liver Enzymes
- GGT
  - Male 11–63 International Unit/L
  - Female 8–35 International Unit/L
- SGOT (AST) <35 International Unit/L
- SGPT (ALT) <35 International Unit/L

CBC
- Hgb (hemoglobin)
  - Male 13.5–16.5 g/dL
  - Female 12.0–15.0 g/dL
- Hct (hematocrit or "crit")
  - Male 41–50 mL/dL
  - Female 36–44 mL/dL
- WBC with differential 4.5–11.0 ∞ 10^3 per microliter

Glossary

A

AB rated of a generic drug, rated as bioequivalent to the branded drug by the FDA as shown by an experimental study

absence seizure a type of generalized seizure characterized by a sudden, momentary break in consciousness; formerly often called petit mal seizure

absorption the process whereby a drug enters the circulatory system

acetylcholine (ACh) a neurotransmitter that binds to ACh receptors on the membranes of muscle cells, beginning a process that ultimately results in muscle contraction

acidosis a blood pH below 7.35; a metabolic condition due to excessive loss of bicarbonate or sodium

acne vulgaris an inflammation of the skin, usually on the face and neck, that is caused by increased activity of the sebaceous glands at puberty

actinic keratosis a scaly skin lesion that is caused by too much sun and can lead to skin cancer

action potential the electrical signal that causes a muscle to contract

active immunity protection against disease that occurs as a result of coming into contact with an infectious agent or an inactivated part of such an agent administered by a vaccine

acute renal failure rapid reduction in kidney function resulting in accumulation of nitrogen and other wastes

acute viral infection an infection that quickly resolves with no latent infection

addiction a compulsive disorder that leads to continued use of a drug despite harm to the user; a dependence characterized by a perceived need to take a drug to attain the psychological and physical effects of mood altering substances

Addison disease a life-threatening deficiency of glucocorticoids and mineralocorticoids that is treated with the daily administration of corticosteroid

adjunct a drug used with another drug

adverse drug reaction reaction to a drug that is harmful to the well-being of the patient

aerobic needing oxygen to survive

afferent system the nerves and sense organs that bring information to the CNS; part of the peripheral nervous system

affinity the strength by which a particular chemical messenger binds to its receptor site on a cell

afterload arterial impedance, or the force against which cardiac muscle shortens; along with preload and contractility, determines cardiac output

agonist drugs that bind to a particular receptor site and trigger the cell's response in a manner similar to the action of the body's own chemical messenger

alkalosis a blood pH above 7.45; a metabolic condition due to excessive loss of potassium or chloride

allergen substance that produces an allergic response

allergic disease a disease caused by an allergic reaction

allergic response an instance in which the immune system overreacts to an otherwise harmless substance

allergy a state of heightened sensitivity as a result of exposure to a particular substance

alopecia hair loss

alpha receptors (alpha-adrenergic receptors) nerve receptors that control vasoconstriction, pupil dilation, and relaxation of the GI smooth muscle in response to epinephrine

alternative medicine use of herbs, dietary supplements, and homeopathic remedies rather than pharmaceuticals

Alzheimer disease a degenerative disorder of the brain that leads to progressive dementia and changes in personality and behavior

amide a compound containing a –CONH– group; a longer-acting local anesthetic that is metabolized by liver enzymes

amino acid the basic unit of a protein molecule; there are 20 different amino acids used in proteins, each having a specific set of shape, electrical charge, and water or fat affinity characteristics

aminoglycoside a class of antibiotics that inhibit bacterial protein synthesis by binding to ribosomal subunits; commonly used to treat serious infections

amyotrophic lateral sclerosis (ALS) a degenerative disease of the motor nerves; also called Lou Gehrig disease

anabolic treatment muscle building

anaerobic capable of surviving in the absence of oxygen

analgesic a drug that alleviates pain; pain relieving

analgesic ladder a guideline for selecting pain-relieving medications according to the severity of the pain and whether agents lower on the ladder have been able to control the pain

anaphylactic reaction a severe allergic response resulting in immediate life-threatening respiratory distress, usually followed by vascular collapse and shock and accompanied by hives

androgen hormone that promotes development and maintenance of male characteristics

anesthesiologist a physician who oversees administration of anesthesia during surgery

angina pectoris spasmodic or suffocating chest pain caused by an imbalance between oxygen supply and oxygen demand

angioedema abnormal accumulation of fluid in tissue

anorexia loss of appetite for food

antagonists drugs that bind to a receptor site and block the action of the endogenous messenger or other drugs; drugs used to reverse the effects of other drugs, such as in treatment of benzodiazepine or narcotic overdoses

antibiotic a chemical substance with the ability to kill or inhibit the growth of bacteria by interfering with bacteria life processes

anticholinesterase a drug that potentiates the action of acetylcholine by inhibiting the enzyme acetylcholinesterase, which breaks down acetylcholine

anticoagulant a drug that prevents clot formation by affecting clotting factors

anticonvulsant a drug to control seizures

antidote a drug that counters the harmful effects of a poison

antiemetic a drug that inhibits impulses that cause vomiting from going to the stomach

antigen a specific molecule that stimulates an immune response; the molecule that an antibody recognizes

antihistamines common term for drugs that block the H1 receptors

antiplatelet a drug that reduces the risk of clot formation by inhibiting platelet aggregation

antipsychotics drugs that are used to treat schizophrenia; reduce symptoms of hallucinations, delusions, and thought disorders; also called neuroleptics

antipyretic fever reducing

antirejection drug a medication that prevents the body from rejecting foreign solid organ transplants

antiretroviral a drug that limits the progression of HIV or other retrovirus infections

antiseptic a substance that kills or inhibits the growth of microorganisms on the outside of the body

antitussives drugs that block or suppress the act of coughing

antivenin a material used in treatment of poisoning by animal venom

antiviral an agent that prevents virus replication in a host cell without interfering with the host's normal function

anxiety a state of uneasiness characterized by apprehension and worry about possible events

apothecary forerunner of the modern pharmacists; the name also refers to the shop

aqueous humor the liquid in the front portion of the eye

area under the curve (AUC) a measure of drug concentration in the blood

arrhythmia any variation from the normal heartbeat; irregular heartbeat

arthritis joint inflammation; persistent pain due to functional problems of the joints

ascites the accumulation of fluids in the abdominal organs and the lower extremities

aspiration inhalation of fluids from the mouth and throat

asthma a reversible lung disease with intermittent attacks in which inspiration is obstructed; provoked by airborne allergens

ataxia irregular muscle movements

atherosclerosis accumulation of lipoproteins and fats on the inner surfaces of arteries, eventually clogging the arteries and leading to MI, stroke, or gangrene

atonic seizure a type of generalized seizure characterized by sudden loss of both muscle tone and consciousness

atopic eczema a chronic pruritic eruption of unknown etiology, although allergic, hereditary, and psychogenic factors may be involved; also called atopic dermatitis

atrioventricular (AV) node part of the conduction system of the heart that carries the action potential from the atria to the ventricles with a delay

attention-deficit hyperactivity disorder (ADHD) a neurologic disorder characterized by hyperactivity, impulsivity, and distractibility

aura a subjective sensation or motor phenomenon that precedes and marks the onset of a migraine headache

autism a disorder that first appears in childhood, characterized by repetitive behavior and impairment in social interaction and communication; it can be expressed through mood swings, irritability, tantrums, aggression, and self-injury

autoimmune disease illness in which the immune system attacks and destroys healthy tissue within the body

autonomic nervous system (ANS) the part of the efferent system of the PNS that regulates activities of body structures not under voluntary control

B

B cell antibody-producing lymphocyte involved in humoral immunity

bacteria small, single-celled microorganisms that exist in three main forms: spherical (i.e., cocci), rod shaped (i.e., bacilli), and spiral (i.e., spirilla)

bactericidal agent a drug that kills bacteria

bacteriostatic agent a drug that inhibits the growth or multiplication of bacteria

basal cell carcinoma a slow-growing skin cancer that usually forms polyps and rarely metastasizes

basal nuclei symmetric, subcortical masses of gray matter embedded in the lower portions of the cerebral hemisphere; part of the extrapyramidal system; also called basal ganglia

Beers List a list of drugs for which monitoring is especially important in elderly patients

benign prostatic hyperplasia (BPH) abnormal enlargement of the prostate gland, usually associated with aging

beta blocker a Class II antiarrhythmic drug that competitively blocks response to beta adrenergic stimulation and therefore lowers heart rate, myocardial contractility, blood pressure, and myocardial oxygen demand; used to treat arrhythmias, MIs, and angina

beta-1 receptors nerve receptors on the heart that control the rate and strength of the heartbeat in response to epinephrine

beta-2 receptors nerve receptors that control vasodilation and relaxation of the smooth muscle of the airways in response to epinephrine

beyond-use date the date after which a drug should not be used once it has been removed from the intact container

bioavailability the degree to which a drug or other substance becomes available to the target tissue after administration

biologic-response modifiers agents that alter the expression and response to surface antigens and enhance immune cell activities in ways that promote destruction of human malignancies

biopharmaceutical a drug produced by recombinant DNA technology

biotechnology the application of biologic systems and organisms for agricultural, industrial, and medical purposes

bipolar disorder a condition in which a patient presents with mood swings that alternate between periods of major depression and periods of mild to severe chronic agitation

Black Box warning information printed on a drug package to alert prescribers to potential problems with the drug

blastocyst the stage in development at which a fertilized egg has divided into 70–100 cells and is ready to implant, consisting of the inner embryoblast and an outer layer that will become the placenta

blood pressure (BP) the result of the heart forcing the blood through the capillaries; measured in millimeters of mercury, both when the heart is contracting and forcing the blood (systolic) and when the heart is relaxed and filling with blood (diastolic)

blood-brain barrier a barrier that prevents many substances from entering the cerebrospinal fluid from the blood; formed by glial cells that envelope the capillaries in the central nervous system, presenting a barrier to many water-soluble compounds though they are permeable to lipid-soluble substances

body mass index (BMI) a guide to use in determining whether to initiate pharmacologic treatment for obesity; calculated by dividing the patient's weight (in kilograms) by the patient's height (in meters) squared (kg/m2)

boost one drug given to increase the serum concentration of another drug

botulin toxin a neurotoxin that blocks the release of acetylcholine at the neuromuscular junction, resulting in muscular paralysis

bowel evacuant an agent used to empty the colon prior to GI examination or after toxic ingestion

bradycardia abnormally slow heart rate (below 60 beats per minute)

brand name the name under which the manufacturer markets a drug; also known as the trade name

broad-spectrum antibiotic an antibiotic that is effective against multiple organisms

bronchitis a condition in which the inner lining of the bronchial airways becomes inflamed, causing the expiration of air from the lungs to be obstructed

bronchodilator an agent that relaxes smooth-muscle cells of the bronchioles, thereby increasing airway diameter and improving the movement of gases into and out of the lungs

bronchospasm spasmodic contraction of the smooth muscles of the bronchiole

buccal to be placed between the cheek and the gums

bursitis inflammation of a bursa

C

calcium channel blocker a Class IV antiarrhythmic drug that prevents the movement of calcium ions through slow channels; used for most supraventricular tachyarrhythmias and in angina

candidiasis a fungal infection (*Candida albicans*) most commonly involving the oral and vaginal mucosa

capsid a protein shell that surrounds and protects the nucleic acid within a virus particle

carbonic anhydrase inhibitor a diuretic that acts in the proximal tubule to increase urine volume and change the pH to alkaline

carbuncle a coalescent mass of infected hair follicles that are deeper than furuncles

cardiomegaly enlargement of the heart due to overwork from overstimulation

cardiovascular (CV) pertaining to the heart and blood vessels

cataplexy short periods of muscle weakness and loss of muscle tone associated with sudden emotions such as joy, fear, or anger; a symptom of narcolepsy

catechol-O-methyl transferase (COMT) an enzyme that metabolizes levodopa in the body; inhibited by certain anti-Parkinson agents

ceiling effect a point at which no clinical response occurs with increased dosage

cellular (cell-mediated) immunity a specific response to antigens that is mediated primarily by T lymphocytes and macrophages

central nervous system (CNS) the brain and spinal cord

cephalosporin a class of antibiotics with a mechanism of action similar to that of penicillins, but with a different antibacterial spectrum, resistance to beta-lactamase, and pharmacokinetics; divided into first-, second-, third-, and fourth-generation agents

cerebral hemorrhage bleeding in the cerebellum

chancre small, usually painless, highly infectious ulcer; the primary lesion of syphilis

chelating agent a drug that bonds to a metal ion to prevent it from reacting with biological compounds

chelation combination of an organic molecule such as a drug with a metal in complexes in which the metal ion is part of a ring

chemical name a name that describes a drug's chemical composition in detail

chemokine coreceptor a drug that prevents a strain of HIV from attaching to an immune system cell

chemoreceptor trigger zone (CTZ) an area below the floor of the fourth ventricle of the brain that can trigger nausea and vomiting when certain signals are received

cholesterol an odorless, white, waxlike, powdery substance that is present in all foods of animal origin but not in foods of plant origin; circulates continuously in the blood for use by all body cells; a eukaryotic sterol that in higher animals is the precursor of bile acids and steroid hormones and is a key constituent of cell membranes

chronic viral infection an infection that has a protracted course with long periods of remission interspersed with recurrence

C-I schedule I controlled substance, a drug with the highest potential for abuse, which may be used only for research under a special license

C-II schedule II controlled substance, a drug with a high potential for abuse, for which dispensing is severely restricted and prescriptions may not be refilled

C-III schedule III controlled substance, a drug with a moderate potential for abuse, which can be refilled no more than 5 times in 6 months and only if authorized by the physician for this time period

C-IV schedule IV controlled substance, a drug dispensed under the same restrictions as schedule III but having less potential for abuse

circadian regularly recurring on cycles of 24 hours

clearance the rate at which a drug is eliminated from a specific volume of blood per unit of time

climacteric the syndrome of endocrine, somatic, and psychic changes occurring at the end of the reproductive period in females

clinical trial drug testing on humans, used to determine drug safety and efficacy

cloning reproducing identical copies of a gene by DNA technology

clotting cascade a series of events that initiate blood clotting, or coagulation

Code Blue a system to communicate that a patient is in a life-threatening situation

coenzyme a chemical other than a protein that is needed to assist an enzyme in performing a metabolic function

colony-stimulating factor (CSF) a chemical that stimulates the bone marrow to produce blood cells

community-acquired contracted outside of the hospital

complement lipoproteins and globulins in blood plasma that react with the antigenantibody complex

complementary of a nucleic acid strand, having each nucleotide base paired up with its counterpart in the other strand

compliance a patient's adherence to the dose schedule and other particular requirements of the specified regimen

congestive heart failure (CHF) a condition in which the heart can no longer pump adequate blood to the body's tissues; results in engorgement of the pulmonary vessels

conjunctivitis pink eye; inflammation of the membrane covering the inside of the eyelid and the outside of the eyeball

contact dermatitis an inflammatory reaction produced by contact with an irritating agent

contractility the cardiac muscle's capacity for becoming shorter in response to a stimulus; along with preload and afterload, determines cardiac output

contraindication a disease, condition, or symptom for which a drug will not be beneficial and may do harm

controlled substance a drug with potential for abuse; organized into five categories or schedules that specify whether and how the drug may be dispensed

convulsion involuntary contraction or series of contractions of the voluntary muscles

corticosteroid a drug that chemically resembles substances produced by the adrenal gland and acts as an anti-inflammatory agent to suppress the immune response by stimulating adenylate cyclase; steroid hormone produced by the adrenal cortex

cotinine a major metabolite of nicotine

cough reflex a coordinated series of events, initiated by stimulation of receptors in the lungs and airways, that results in a cough

cracking separation of lipid from a parenteral nutrition solution

Crohn disease an inflammatory bowel disease affecting the entire GI tract from mouth to anus

Cushing disease a disease caused by overproduction of steroids or by excessive administration of corticosteroids over an extended period

C-V schedule V controlled substance, a drug with a slight potential for abuse; some of which may be sold without a prescription depending on state law, but the purchaser must sign for the drug and show identification

cyclic lipopeptide a new class of antibiotics that bind to bacterial membranes and cause the cell membrane to depolarize, thus leading to an inhibition of DNA and RNA synthesis

cyclooxygenase-1 (COX-1) an enzyme that is present in most body tissues and produces protective prostaglandins to regulate physiological processes such as GI mucosal integrity

cyclooxygenase-2 (COX-2) an enzyme that is present in the synovial fluid of arthritis patients and is associated with the pain and inflammation of arthritis

cystic fibrosis (CF) a hereditary disorder of infants, children, and young adults that involves widespread dysfunction of the gastrointestinal and pulmonary systems

cytoprotective agent an agent administered to reduce the side effects and toxicity of chemotherapy agent

D

D₅W dextrose 5% in water

decongestant an agent that causes the mucous membranes to shrink, thereby allowing the sinus cavities to drain

delirium tremens (DTs) a condition caused by cessation of alcohol consumption in which coarse, irregular tremors are accompanied by vivid hallucinations

denatured disruption of the structure

dependence a state in which a person's body has adapted physiologically and psychologically to a drug and cannot function without it; a physical and emotional reliance on a drug

depolarization reversal of the negative voltage across a heart or nerve cell membrane, caused by an inflow of positive ions

depression a condition characterized by the feeling that life has no meaning, pessimism, intense sadness, loss of concentration, and problems with eating and sleeping

dermatome area of the skin associated with one pair of nerves emerging horizontally from the spinal cord

dermis layer of skin below the epidermis

diastolic blood pressure the blood pressure measurement that measures the pressure during the dilation of the heart

diffuse tumor a cancerous growth that is widely distributed and are not localized

diplopia the perception of two images of a single object

disease-modifying antirheumatic drugs (DMARDs) agents that can modify the progression of rheumatoid arthritis

disinfectant an agent that frees inanimate objects from infection

Dispense As Written (DAW) instruction in a prescription to prevent substitution of generic drugs for the branded drug

distribution the process by which a drug moves from the blood into other body fluids and tissues and ultimately to its sites of action

diuretic a substance that rids the body of excess fluid and electrolytes by increasing the urine output

diverticular disease formation and inflammation of an outpocketing from the colon wall

DNA sequence order of nucleotide bases in the DNA molecule; a group of three nucleotides translates into one amino acid

dose the quantity of a drug administered at one time

double blind study a clinical trial in which neither the trial participants nor the study staff know whether a particular participant is in the control group or the experimental group

drug a medicinal substance or remedy used to change the way a living organism functions; also called a medication

Drug Enforcement Administration (DEA) the branch of the U.S. Justice Department that is responsible for regulating the sale and use of specified drugs, especially controlled substances

drug sponsor the entity, usually a pharmaceutical company, responsible for testing the efficacy and safety of a drug and proposing the drug for approval

duodenal ulcer a peptic lesion situated in the duodenum

duration of action the length of time a drug gives the desired response or is at the therapeutic level

dysarthria imperfect articulation of speech

dyskinesia impairment of the power of voluntary movement

dyspareunia a condition of the female in which normal intercourse is painful

dysphagia difficulty in swallowing

E

ectopic pacemaker a pacemaker other than the SA node

eczema a hot, itchy, red, oozing skin inflammation; also called dermatitis

efferent system the nerves that dispatch information out from the CNS; part of the peripheral nervous system

electrolyte a substance that dissociates into ions in solution and is thus capable of conducting electricity

elimination removal of a drug or its metabolites from the body by excretion

emesis vomiting

emphysema an irreversible lung disease characterized by destruction of the alveoli in the lungs, which allows air to accumulate in tissues and organs

empirical treatment treatment begun before a definite diagnosis can be obtained

empty stomach 2 hours before or after eating

emulsify to break a liquid that does not dissolve in water into small globules that can be suspended in water

endocrine system glands and other structures that elaborate internal secretions, called hormones, that are released directly into the circulatory system

endogenous anxiety anxiety caused by factors within the organism

endometrium the lining of the uterus, which grows in the early part of the menstrual cycle to be ready to receive a fertilized egg and breaks down at the end of the cycle, leading to menstruation

endotracheal intubation insertion of a tube into the trachea to keep it open

enteral by way of, or pertaining to, the intestine

enteral nutrition feeding a patient liquid food through a tube that leads to the gastrointestinal system

envelope membrane surrounding the capsid in some viruses and carrying surface proteins that attach to cell surface receptors

epidermis the top layer of the skin

epilepsy a neurologic disorder involving sudden and recurring seizures

E-prescribing the process which allows a prescriber's computer system to talk to the pharmacy's computer system and the medication order/prescription is transmitted to the pharmacy

ergosterol a form of lipid found in the cell membrane of fungi where higher animals have cholesterol

erysipelas a skin infection characterized by redness and warmth, local pain, edematous plaque with sharply established borders, chills, malaise, and fever; a form of cellulitis

ester a compound containing a –COO– group; a short-acting local anesthetic, metabolized by pseudocholinesterase of the plasma and tissue fluids

estrogen one of the group of hormones that stimulate the growth of reproductive tissue in females

eukaryotic having a defined nucleus, such as an animal or fungal cell

exogenous anxiety anxiety caused by factors outside the organism

expectorant an agent that decreases the thickness and stickiness of mucus, enabling the patient to rid the lungs and airway of mucus when coughing

extrapyramidal symptoms disorders of muscle movement control caused by blocking dopamine receptors in the basal ganglia

extravasation the escape of IV fluids into the surrounding tissue

F

fat-soluble vitamins vitamins that are absorbed along with dietary fat and are maintained in large stores by the body; vitamins A, D, E, and K

feedback mechanism the return of some of the output of a system as input so as to exert some control on the process

fiber the undigested residue of fruits, vegetables, and other foods of plant origin that remains after digestion by the human GI enzymes; characterized by fermentability and may be either water soluble or insoluble

fibrinolytic an agent that dissolves clots

filtration the removal of substances from the blood as part of the formation of urine by the renal tubules

first-order depending directly on the concentration of the drug; elimination of most drugs is a first-order process in which a constant fraction of the drug is eliminated per unit of time

first-pass effect the extent to which a drug is metabolized by the liver before reaching systemic circulation

flu influenza, a common viral infection

folliculitis an inflammation of a hair follicle by a minute, red, pustulated nodule without involvement of the surrounding tissue

Food and Drug Administration (FDA) the agency of the federal government that is responsible for ensuring the safety of drugs and food prepared for the market

fungus a single-cell eukaryotic organism (similar to a human cell rather than to bacteria); marked by a rigid cell wall, the absence of chlorophyll, and reproduction by spores

furuncle a boil; caused by a staphylococcal infection of a sebaceous gland and the associated hair follicle

fusion inhibitor a drug that prevents HIV from entering the immune cells

G

gastric lavage a procedure to wash out or irrigate the patient's stomach, commonly known as a stomach pump

gastric stasis lack of stomach motility

gastric ulcer a local excavation in the gastric mucosa

gastritis irritation and superficial erosion of the stomach lining

gastroesophageal reflux disease (GERD) a GI disease characterized by radiating burning or pain in the chest and an acid taste, caused by backflow of acidic stomach contents across an incompetent lower esophageal sphincter; also referred to as heartburn

gastrointestinal (GI) tract a continuous tube that begins in the mouth and extends through the pharynx, esophagus, stomach, small intestine, and large intestine to end at the anus

general anesthesia a condition characterized by reversible unconsciousness, analgesia, skeletal muscle relaxation, and amnesia on recovery

generalized seizure a seizure that involves both hemispheres of the brain simultaneously and has no local origin; can be a tonicclonic (grand mal), absence (petit mal), myoclonic, or atonic seizure

generalized viral infection an infection that has spread to other tissues by way of the bloodstream or the central nervous system

generic name a name that identifies a drug independently of its manufacturer; sometimes denotes a drug that is not protected by a trademark; also referred to as a USAN (United States Adopted Name)

gestational diabetes diabetes that occurs during pregnancy when insufficient insulin is produced

ghost empty shell of an OROS tablet, excreted in the stool after the drug has dissolved

GI transit time the time it takes for material to pass from one end of the GI tract to the other; the slower the GI transit time, the greater the amounts of nutrients and water absorbed

glaucoma a chronic eye disorder characterized by abnormally high internal eye pressure that destroys the optic nerve and causes partial or complete loss of vision

glucocorticoid corticosteroid involved in metabolism and immune system regulation

glycoprotein antagonist an antiplatelet agent that binds to receptors on platelets, preventing platelet aggregation as well as the binding of fibrinogen and other adhesive molecules

gouty arthritis a disease resulting from the improper excretion of uric acid; also called gout

Gram staining a staining technique that divides bacteria into gram-positive (purple) or gram-negative (red) based on the properties of their cell walls

grand mal seizure see tonic-clonic seizure

granulocyte colony-stimulating factor(G-CSF) an agent that stimulates the bone marrow to produce specific white cells, such as the granulocytes

growth hormone (GH) a fundamental hormone that affects metabolism, skeletal growth, and somatic growth; deficiency causes growth retardation

growth hormone releasing factor (GHRF) a neuropeptide secreted by the hypothalamus that stimulates the secretion of growth hormone by the pituitary

gynecomastia excessive development of the male mammary glands, with or without tenderness

H

H2 histamine receptor antagonist an agent that blocks acid and pepsin secretion in response to histamine, gastrin, foods, distention, caffeine, or cholinergic stimulation; used to treat GERD and *H. pylori*

half-life the time necessary for the body to eliminate half of the drug in the body at any time; written as T1/2

HbA1C glycosylated hemoglobin (Hb stands for hemoglobin), an "average" of the sugar measured in blood glucose over a period of time

Helicobacter pylori (H. pylori) a bacterium that contributes to the development of many gastric ulcers

hematocrit the proportion of volume of red blood cells to the total volume of blood

hematologic agent a replacement plasma protein that is necessary for blood coagulation and is not produced in a person with hemophilia

hemorrhoids engorgements of the vascular cushions situated within the sphincter muscles; result from pressure exerted on anal veins while straining to pass a stool

hepatitis a disease of the liver that causes inflammation, can be acute or chronic, and has several forms A through G

hepatitis A a viral form of hepatitis that is usually mild and transient and can be spread from one person to another

hepatitis B the most dangerous form of hepatitis, accompanied by jaundice and easily spread from one person to another

hepatitis C an infection of the liver that cannot be spread from one person to another by contact; most commonly transmitted by blood transfusions or illicit drug use

herbs plants or plant parts extracted and valued for their savory, aromatic, or medicinal qualities

hiatal hernia a protrusion through the esophageal hiatus of the diaphragm

high-density lipoproteins (HDLs) lipoproteins containing 5% triglyceride, 25% cholesterol, and 50% protein; "good cholesterol"

hirsutism abnormal hairiness, especially in women

histamine a chemical produced by the body that evokes the symptoms of an allergic reaction and is blocked by antihistamines

histoplasmosis a respiratory tract infection caused by a fungus, most often found in accumulated droppings from birds and bats; often called the summer flu

homeopathy a system of therapeutics in which diseases are treated by administering minute doses of drugs that, in healthy patients, are capable of producing symptoms like those of the disease being treated

homeostasis stability of the organism

hormone therapy (HT) replacement of deficient hormones such as estrogen

host the animal on which a parasite feeds

human immunodeficiency virus (HIV) a retrovirus transmitted in body fluids that causes acquired immune deficiency syndrome (AIDS) by attacking T lymphocytes

humoral immunity an immune response in which secreted antibodies are transported by bodily fluids

hypercholesterolemia excessive cholesterol in the blood

hyperglycemia elevated blood sugar level

hyperlipidemia elevation of the levels of one or more of the lipoproteins in the blood

hypertension elevated blood pressure, where systolic blood pressure is greater than 140 mm Hg and diastolic pressure is greater than 90 mm Hg

hyperthyroidism a condition caused by excessive thyroid hormone and marked by increased metabolic rate; also called thyrotoxicosis

hypertonic solution a solution with a higher concentration of particles than body fluids contain

hypnotic a drug that induces sleep

hypoglycemia low blood glucose level (less than 70 mg/dL)

hypogonadism a deficiency of hormone production and secretion

hypotension low blood pressure

hypothyroidism a deficiency of thyroid activity that results in a decreased metabolic rate, tiredness, and lethargy in adults and causes cretinism in children

hypotonic solution a solution with a lower concentration of particles than body fluids contain

I

idiosyncratic reaction an unusual or unexpected response to a drug that is unrelated to the dose given

immune response the immune system's way of providing resistance to disease and malignancy through the production of antibodies and phagocytes

immunization the process by which the immune system is stimulated to acquire protection against a specific disease; usually achieved by use of a vaccine

immunocompromised having a deficiency in the immune response system

immunoglobulin (Ig) a protein that responds to a specific antigen; also known as an antibody

immunoglobulin an antibody that reacts to a specific foreign substance or organism and may prevent its antigen from attaching to a cell receptor or may destroy the organism

impetigo a superficial, highly contagious skin infection; characterized by small red spots that evolve into vesicles, break, become encrusted, and are surrounded by a zone of erythema

impotence failure of the male to initiate or to maintain an erection until ejaculation in the body

indication a disease, symptom, or condition for which a drug is known to be of benefit

induction the process whereby a drug increases the concentration of certain enzymes that affect the pharmacologic response to another drug

infection a condition in which bacteria grow in body tissues and cause tissue damage to the host either by their presence or by toxins they produce

inhalation administration of a medication through the respiratory system

inhibition the process whereby a drug blocks enzyme activity and impairs the metabolism of another drug

inscription part of a prescription that identifies the name of the drug, the dose, and the quantities of the ingredients

insomnia difficulty falling asleep or staying asleep or not feeling refreshed on awakening

instillation administration of a medication drop by drop

integrase inhibitor a drug that prevents DNA produced by the reverse transcriptase of HIV from becoming incorporated into the patient's DNA

interaction a change in the action of a drug caused by another drug, a food, or another substance such as alcohol or nicotine

interferon a substance that exerts virus-nonspecific but host-specific antiviral activity by inducing genes coding for antiviral proteins that inhibit the synthesis of viral RNA

International Normalized Ratio (INR) a method of standardizing the prothrombin time (PT) by comparing it to a standard index

intradermal to be injected into the skin

intramuscular to be injected into a muscle; abbreviated IM

intraspinal to be injected into the spinal column

intrathecal see intraspinal

intravenous administration of a medication through a vein, thereby avoiding the first-pass effect; abbreviated IV

irritable bowel syndrome (IBS) a functional disorder in which the lower GI tract does not have appropriate tone or spasticity to regulate bowel activity

irritant receptor a nerve cell in the lungs and airways that responds to coarse particles and chemicals to trigger a cough

ischemic stroke a cerebral infarction, in which a region of the brain is damaged by being deprived of oxygen

isomer one of two or more compounds that contain the same number and type of atoms but have different molecular structures

isotonic solution a solution with the same level of particles, and thus the same tonicity, as body fluids

IVIG the notation for immune globulin that is given intravenously

K

keratoacanthoma an epithelial skin tumor that first grows rapidly and then regresses and heals

ketolide a class of antibiotics that block protein synthesis by binding to ribosomal subunits and may also inhibit the formation of new ribosomes; used primarily to treat bacterial infections in the lungs and sinuses

L

latency the ability of a virus to lie dormant and then, under certain conditions, reproduce and again behave like an infective agent, causing cell damage

legend drug a drug that may be sold only by prescription and must be labeled "Caution: Federal law prohibits dispensing without prescription" or "Rx only"

leukotriene inhibitor an agent that blocks the body's inflammatory responses to the leukotrienes or blocks their synthesis

lipid a fatty molecule, an important constituent of cell membranes

lipoprotein a spherical particle containing a core of triglycerides and cholesterol, in varying proportions, surrounded by a surface coat of phospholipids that enables it to remain in solution

loading dose amount of a drug that will bring the blood concentration rapidly to a therapeutic level

local anesthesia the production of transient and reversible loss of sensation in a defined area of the body

local effect an action of a drug that is confined to a specific part of the body

local infection an infection restricted to or pertaining to one area of the body

local viral infection a viral infection affecting tissues of a single system such as the respiratory tract, eye, or skin

loop diuretic a drug that inhibits reabsorption of sodium and chloride in the loop of Henle, thereby causing increased urinary output

Lou Gehrig disease see amyotrophic lateral sclerosis (ALS)

low-density lipoproteins (LDLs) lipoproteins containing 6% triglycerides and 65% cholesterol; "bad cholesterol"

lymphatic system a network of vessels that carry lymph, the lymph nodes, and the lymphoid organs including the tonsils, spleen, and thymus; a system for filtering body fluids by nodes, vessels, and lymphocytes before the fluid returns to general circulation

M

MAb (monoclonal antibody) an antibody produced in the laboratory by a culture derived from a single B cell

macrolide a class of bacteriostatic antibiotics that inhibit protein synthesis by combining with ribosomes; used primarily to treat pulmonary infections caused by *Legionella* and gram-positive organisms

macrophage a large white blood cell that engulf antigens, toxins, and cellular debris, and digest it, and display peptides complexed with MHC for recognition by T cells

maintenance dose amount of a drug administered at regular intervals to keep the blood concentration at a therapeutic level

malabsorption syndrome impaired intestinal absorption of nutrients

malaria an infectious febrile disease caused by the protozoan *Plasmodium* and transmitted by the *Anopheles* mosquito

malignant hyperthermia a rare, but serious, side effect of anesthesia associated with an increase in intracellular calcium and a rapid rise in body temperature

malnutrition any disorder of nutrition

mania a mood of extreme excitement, excessive elation, hyperactivity, agitation, and increased psychomotor activity

mast cell stabilizer an agent that stabilizes mast cell membranes against rupture caused by antigenic substances and thereby reduces the amount of histamine and other inflammatory substances released in airway tissues

medical food a preparation taken orally consisting of nutrients specifically required to treat some disease or condition

medication guide specific information about certain types of drugs that is required by the FDA to be made available to the patient

medication reconciliation the providing of a complete and accurate drug profile to each health care provider who cares for a patient

melanoma a highly malignant skin cancer formed from pigmented skin cells

membrane stabilizing agent a Class I antiarrhythmic drug that slows the movement of ions into cardiac cells, thus reducing the action potential and dampening abnormal rhythms and heartbeats

metabolic pathway the sequence of chemical steps that convert a drug into a metabolite

metabolism the process by which drugs are chemically converted to other compounds

metabolite a substance into which a drug is chemically converted in the body

metered dose inhaler (MDI) a device that delivers a specific amount of medication (as for asthma) in a fine enough spray to reach the innermost parts of the lungs using a puff of compressed gas

migraine headache a severe, throbbing, unilateral headache, usually accompanied by nausea, photophobia, phonophobia, and hyperesthesia

mineralocorticoid corticosteroid involved in electrolyte and water balance

monoamine oxidase inhibitor (MAOIs) an antidepressant drug that inhibits the activity of the enzymes that break down catecholamines (such as norepinephrine) and serotonin

monoclonal antibody an antibody produced in a laboratory from an isolated specific lymphocyte that produces a pure antibody against a known, specific antigen

morbid obesity a state in which an individual's weight is two or more times the ideal body weight (IBW)

morbidity rate of occurrence of a diseased state or condition

mortality death rate from a particular disease

motor end plate the neuromuscular junction, where the nervous system and muscular system meet to produce or stop movement

mucolytic an agent that destroys or dissolves mucus

multiple sclerosis (MS) an autoimmune disease in which the myelin sheaths around nerves degenerate

muscle fasciculation a small, local, involuntary muscular contraction visible under the skin

muscle relaxant a drug that reduces or prevents skeletal muscle contraction

muscle spasticity a condition whereby muscle fibers are in a state of involuntary, continuous contraction that causes pain

myasthenia gravis an autoimmune disorder of the neuromuscular junction in which the ACh receptors are destroyed at the motor end plate, preventing muscles from responding to nerve signals to move them

myocardial hypertrophy thickening of the heart muscle in response to overstimulation

myocardial infarction (MI) a heart attack; occurs when a region of the heart muscle is deprived of oxygen

myoclonic seizure a type of generalized seizure characterized by sudden muscle contractions with no loss of consciousness

N

naked virus a virus without an envelope covering the capsid

narcolepsy a sleep disorder in which inappropriate attacks of sleep occur during the daytime hours

narcotic analgesic pain medication containing an opioid

nebulizer a device used in the administration of inhaled medications, using air flowing past a liquid to create a mist

neoplastic disease a disorder that occurs when normal cellular control mechanisms become altered; characterized by uncontrolled cellular growth and the development of abnormal cells; also referred to as cancer

nephron glomerulotubular units that are the working units of the kidney

nephrotoxicity ability to damage the kidneys

neuroleptics see antipsychotics

neuromuscular blocking skeletal muscle paralysis

neuron a nerve cell that transmits information

neurotransmitter a chemical substance that is selectively released from a neuron and stimulates or inhibits activity in the neuron's target cell; a chemical produced by a nerve cell and involved in transmitting information

New Drug Application (NDA) the vehicle through which drug sponsors formally propose that the FDA approve a new pharmaceutical for sale and marketing in the United States

nicotine the addictive component of tobacco

nocturia urinary frequency at night

noncompliance failure to adhere to an appropriate drug regimen

nonnarcotic analgesic a drug used for pain, inflammation, and fever that is not a controlled substance

non-nucleoside reverse transcriptase inhibitor (NNRTI) a drug that inhibits HIV reverse transcriptase by preventing the enzyme from working mechanically

nonpathologic not related to disease

nonsteroidal anti-inflammatory drugs (NSAIDs) anti-inflammatory, analgesic, and antipyretic drugs that are not controlled substances or steroids; used to treat arthritis and for other indications such as pain and inflammation; a drug such as aspirin or ibuprofen that reduces pain and inflammation

nosocomial acquired by patients in the hospital

NS normal saline

nucleoside reverse transcriptase inhibitor (NRTI) a drug that inhibits HIV reverse transcriptase by competing with natural nucleic acid building block substrates, causing termination of the DNA chain

nucleotide reverse transcriptase inhibitor (NtRTI) a drug that inhibits HIV reverse transcriptase by competing with natural nucleic acid building block substrates, causing termination of chain formation, and is more nearly in the form used by the body than an NRTI

nucleotide the basic unit of a DNA molecule, containing one of four possible bases

O

obesity a state in which an individual's total body weight includes greater quantities of fat than is considered normal (25% of total body weight for men and 35% for women)

obsessive-compulsive disorder (OCD) a mental disorder characterized by recurrent, persistent urges to perform repetitive acts such as hand washing

on-off phenomenon a wide fluctuation between abnormally increased and abnormally diminished motor function, present in many Parkinson patients after about 5 years of levodopa therapy

ophthalmic to be administered through the eye; to be used in the eye

opiate a narcotic that is either derived from opium or synthetically produced to resemble opium derivatives chemically

opioid a substance, whether a drug or a chemical naturally produced by the body, that acts on opioid receptors to reduce the sensation of pain

opsonization labeling antigenic material so that it is more readily identified and destroyed by macrophages

oral complications tissue injury to the oral cavity associated with chemotherapy and radiation

oral contraceptive (OCs) a combination of one or more hormonal compounds taken orally to prevent the occurrence of pregnancy

oral see peroral (PO)

order a prescription issued in an institutional setting

osmotic diuretic a drug that increases the osmotic pressure of glomerular filtrate, thereby inhibiting tubular reabsorption of water and electrolytes and increasing urinary output

osmotic laxative an organic substance that draws water into the colon and thereby stimulates evacuation

osmotic-controlled release oral delivery system (OROS) a drug delivery system that allows the drug to dissolve through pores in the tablet shell; the empty shell, called a ghost, is passed in the stool

osteoarthritis a degenerative joint disease resulting in loss of cartilage, elasticity, and thickness

osteoblast a cell that forms bone

osteoclast a cell that resorbs bone

osteomalacia demineralization and weakening of the skeleton, caused by a deficiency of vitamin D in adults

osteoporosis the condition of reduced bone mineral density, disrupted microarchitecture of bone structure, and increased likelihood of fracture

otalgia earache

otic administered in the ear; to be used in the ear

ototoxicity ability to damage the organs of hearing

over-the-counter (OTC) drug a drug that may be sold without a prescription

oxytocic agent a drug that promotes contraction of uterine muscle at term of pregnancy

P

pain the activation of electrical activity in afferent neurons with sensory endings in peripheral tissue with a higher firing threshold than those of temperature or touch; a protective signal to warn of damage or presence of disease; the fifth vital sign; classified as acute, chronic nonmalignant, and chronic malignant

panic intense, overwhelming, and uncontrollable anxiety

parasite an organism that lives on or in another organism (known as the host), surviving by drawing nourishment from the food or the tissues of the host; the parasite lives within the intermediate host during the larval stage and within the definitive host at maturity

parenteral administered by injection rather than by way of the alimentary canal

parenteral nutrition feeding a patient by supplying a nutrient solution through a vein

Parkinson disease a neurologic disorder characterized by akinesia, resting tremor, and muscular rigidity

partial seizure an abnormal electrical discharge centered in a specific area of the brain; usually caused by a trauma

partial thromboplastin time (PTT) a test that measures the function of the intrinsic and common pathways in blood clotting; affected by heparin

passive immunity protection against a disease as the result of receiving antibodies that were formed by another person or animal who developed them in response to being infected with the disease

patent a government grant that gives a drug company the exclusive right to manufacture a drug for a certain number of years; protects the company's investment in developing the drug

patient-controlled analgesia (PCA) pump a means of pain control whereby the patient can regulate, within certain limits, the administration of pain medication

peak expiratory flow rate (PEFR) the maximum flow rate generated during a forced expiration, measured in liters per minute

peak flow meter a device used to measure the PEFR as an indication of respiratory status; usually used twice a day by asthma patients

peak the top or upper limit of a drug's concentration in the blood

pediculosis an infestation of lice

penicillin a class of antibiotics obtained from *Penicillium chrysogenum*; kill bacteria by preventing them from forming a rigid cell wall, thereby allowing an excessive amount of water to enter through osmosis and cause lysis of the bacterium cell

peptic disease disorders of the upper GI tract caused by the action of acid and pepsin; includes mucosal injury, erythema, erosions, and frank ulceration

peptic ulcer an ulcer formed at any part of the GI tract exposed to acid and the enzyme pepsin

peptide a string of amino acid molecules bound together, usually a fragment of a larger protein molecule

percussion a therapy used for cystic fibrosis (CF) patients involving a tapping movement to induce cough and expectoration of sputum from the lungs; usually preceded by nebulizer therapy during which nebulized sterile water or normal saline is breathed to liquefy pulmonary secretions

peripheral nervous system (PNS) the nerves and sense organs outside the CNS

permeability the ability of a material to allow molecules or ions to pass through it

peroral (PO) administration of a medication by mouth in either solid form, as a tablet or capsule, or in liquid form, as a solution or syrup; often referred to as oral

petechiae minute red spots on the skin due to the escape of a small amount of blood

petit mal seizure see absence seizure

pH a measurement of acidity or alkalinity. pH 7 is neutral; a solution with a pH above 7 is alkaline; a solution with a pH below 7 is acidic

pharmacist one who is licensed to prepare and sell or dispense drugs and compounds and to fill prescriptions

pharmacognosy the study and identification of natural sources of drugs

pharmacokinetic modeling a method of describing the process of absorption, distribution, metabolism, and elimination of a drug within the body mathematically

pharmacokinetics the activity of a drug within the body over a period of time; includes absorption, distribution, metabolism, and elimination

pharmacologic effect the action of a drug on a living system

pharmacology the science of drugs and their interactions with the systems of living animals

pharmacopoeia an official listing of medicinal preparations

pharmacy technician an individual working in a pharmacy who, under the supervision of a licensed pharmacist, assists in activities not requiring the professional judgment of a pharmacist

Pharmacy Technician Certification Board (PTCB) a national organization that develops pharmacy technician standards and serves as a credentialing agency for pharmacy technicians

pharmakon a Greek word meaning a magic spell, remedy, or poison that was used in early records to represent the concept of a drug

phenothiazine a drug, related to the typical antipsychotics, that controls vomiting by inhibiting the CTZ

photosensitivity an abnormal response of the skin or eye to sunlight

phototoxicity a property of a chemical that becomes toxic on exposure to light

phytonadione vitamin K1

placebo an inactive substance with no treatment value

plasma cell a B cell that produces freely circulating antibody in very large quantities

plasmid a small circular ring of DNA that can insert itself into bacterial genes and can carry genes from one bacterial cell to another

pneumonia a common lung infection, caused by microorganisms that gain access to the lower respiratory tract

polypharmacy the concurrent use of multiple medications

pooling a time-saving process used when preparing a three-in-one TPN, in which all electrolytes except phosphate are put into a small-volume parenteral bag and then transferred into each batch

post-exposure prophylaxis (PEP) the administration of antiretrovirals after exposure to HIV

posttraumatic stress disorder (PTSD) a disorder characterized by persistent agitation or persistent, recurrent fear after the end of a traumatic event and lasting for over a month or impairing work or relationships

potassium-sparing diuretic a drug that promotes excretion of water and sodium but inhibits the exchange of sodium for potassium

preload the mechanical state of the heart at the end of diastole; along with afterload and contractility, determines cardiac output

prescription a direction for medication to be dispensed to a patient, written by a physician or a qualified licensed practitioner and filled by a pharmacist; referred to as an order when the medication is requested in a hospital setting

priapism abnormal penile erection including frequent or prolonged, or painful

primary site the original site where a cancer tumor develops

probiotic a product to restore or promote the growth of normal bacterial flora in the body

prodrug a compound that, on administration and chemical conversion by metabolic processes, becomes an active pharmacological agent

progesterone the hormone that prepares the uterus for the reception and development of the fertilized ovum

progestin a synthetic hormone that emulates the effects of progesterone

prokaryotic not having a defined nucleus, like bacteria

promoter the part of plasmid DNA where protein production starts

propagate reproduce

prophylactic drug a drug that prevents or decreases the severity of a disease

prophylaxis effect of a drug in preventing infection or disease

protease inhibitor (PI) a drug that prevents the cleavage of certain HIV protein precursors needed for the replication of new infectious virions

prothrombin time (PT) a test that assesses the function of the extrinsic pathways of the coagulation system; affected by warfarin

proton pump inhibitor a drug that blocks gastric acid secretion by inhibiting the enzyme that pumps hydrogen ions into the stomach

protozoan single-celled animal

pruritus itching sensation

psoriasis a skin disorder characterized by patches of red, scaly skin that are slightly raised with defined margins; usually occurs on the elbows and knees but can affect any part of the body

ptosis paralytic drooping of the upper eyelid

pulmonary embolism (PE) sudden blocking of the pulmonary artery by a blood clot

pulse dosing a regimen of dosing one week per month; commonly used for treating fungal nail infections

Q

QT interval the time between depolarization and repolarization of the ventricles of the heart during a heartbeat, as shown on the electrocardiogram

quinolone a class of antibiotics with rapid bactericidal action against most gram-negative and many gram-positive bacteria; work by causing DNA breakage and cell death; cross the blood-brain barrier

R

reabsorption the process by which substances are pulled back into the blood after waste products have been removed during the formation of urine

receptor a protein molecule on the surface of or within a cell that recognizes and binds with specific molecules, thereby producing some effect within the cell

recombinant DNA artificial DNA produced in a laboratory by inserting strands of DNA from one organism into that of another organism

reflux backflow; specifically in GERD, the backflow of acidic stomach contents across an incompetent lower esophageal sphincter

remission the condition in which a tumor is inactive with no cell division or growth; typically, a goal of chemotherapy

replication the process of copying the DNA of a cell into a new set of DNA molecules to produce a new cell

repolarization restoration of the negative voltage across a heart or nerve cell membrane, caused by an outflow of positive ions

resistance lack of responsiveness of cancer cells to chemotherapy

respiratory distress syndrome (RDS) a syndrome occurring in newborns that is characterized by acute asphyxia with hypoxia and acidosis

restless leg syndrome an overpowering urge to move the legs, especially at rest

reticulocytes immature red blood cells

retinoid a compound related to vitamin A that helps to regulate skin cell growth

retrovirus a virus that can copy its RNA genetic information into the host's DNA

reverse transcriptase a retroviral enzyme that makes a DNA copy from an RNA original

reversible ischemic neurologic deficit (RIND) a neurologic change, caused by a temporary shortage of oxygen, that reverses spontaneously but less rapidly than a TIA

Reye syndrome a condition that can develop in children who have been exposed to chicken pox or other viral infections and are given aspirin; characterized by amnesia, lethargy, disorientation, and agitation that can culminate in coma and respiratory failure

rheumatoid arthritis (RA) an autoimmune disease in which the body's immune system attacks its own connective tissue; characterized by inflammation of the synovial membrane of the joints

rhinitis medicamentosa a condition of decreased response that results when nasal decongestants are used over prolonged periods

ricin a toxin derived from the castor bean that acts by disabling the molecular machinery for protein synthesis

ringworm a fungus that infects the horny (scaly) layer of skin or the nails; also called tinea

rosacea chronic dermatologic disorder involving inflammation of the skin of the face; also called acne rosacea

S

salicylates a class of nonnarcotic analgesics that have both pain-relieving and antipyretic (fever-reducing) properties

salicylism mild salicylate intoxication, characterized by ringing in the ears, dizziness, headache, and mental confusion

saline laxative an inorganic salt that attracts water into the hollow portion (lumen) of the colon, increasing intraluminal pressure to cause evacuation

schizophrenia a chronic psychotic disorder manifested by retreat from reality, delusions, hallucinations, ambivalence, withdrawal, and bizarre or regressive behavior

seasonal affective disorder (SAD) a form of depression that recurs in the fall and winter and remits in the spring and summer

seborrhea a skin condition caused by excessive secretion by the sebaceous glands; gives the skin an oily appearance

secondary diabetes diabetes caused by drugs

secondary site a new cancer tumor site to which malignant cells have spread from the original site

secretion the release of cell products, including hydrogen and potassium ions and acids and bases, into urine being formed

seizure abnormal electrical discharges in the cerebral cortex caused by sudden, excessive firing of neurons; result in a change in behavior of which the patient is not aware

selective serotonin reuptake inhibitor (SSRI) an antidepressant drug that blocksthe reuptake of serotonin, with little effect on norepinephrine and fewer side effects than other antidepressant drugs

sepsis a systemic inflammatory response to infection resulting from blood-borne infections

serotonin and norepinephrine reuptake inhibitor (SNRI) an antidepressant drug that blocks the reabsorption of both serotonin and norepinephrine, increasing the levels of both neurotransmitters

serotonin syndrome a possibly fatal condition caused by combining antidepressants that increase serotonin levels with other medications that also stimulate serotonin receptors

side effect a secondary response to a drug other than the primary therapeutic effect for which the drug was intended

signa part of a prescription that provides directions to be included on the label for the patient to follow in taking the medication

sinoatrial (SA) node the normal pacemaker area of the heart

slow viral infection an infection that maintains a progressive course over months or years with cumulative damage to body tissues, ultimately ending in the host's death

small lymphocyte T and B memory cells, which carry and preserve information for the recognition of specific antigens

solid tumor a tumor that forms a solid mass and can be palpated

solubility a drug's ability to dissolve in body fluids

somatic nervous system the part of the efferent system of the PNS that regulates the skeletal muscles

somatic pain dull, throbbing pain from skin, muscle, and bone

spacer a device used with a metered dose inhaler (MDI) to decrease the amount of spray deposited on the back of the throat and swallowed

specificity the property of a receptor site that enables it to bind only with a specific chemical messenger; to bind with a specific cell type, the messenger must have a chemical structure that is complementary to the structure of that cell's receptors

squamous cell carcinoma a skin cancer that grows more rapidly than basal cell carcinoma but in which metastasis is uncommon

stable angina a type of angina characterized by effort-induced chest pain from physical activity or emotional stress; usually predictable and reproducible

statin an HMG-CoA reductase inhibitor, a drug that inhibits the rate-limiting step in cholesterol formation

status asthmaticus a medical emergency that begins as an asthma attack but does not respond to normal management; can result in loss of consciousness and death

status epilepticus a serious disorder involving tonic-clonic convulsions that last at least 30 minutes

Stevens-Johnson syndrome a sometimes fatal form of erythema multiforme (an allergic reaction marked by red blotches on the skin)

stimulant laxative a laxative that increases gut activity by irritating the mucosa

streptogramin one of a class of antibiotics that inhibit protein synthesis within the bacterial ribosomes; useful in the treatment of vancomycin- and methicillin-resistant infections

stress incontinence urine leakage during physical movements

stress ulcer a peptic ulcer, usually gastric, that occurs in a clinical setting; caused by a breakdown of natural mucosal resistance

stretch receptor a nerve cell in the lungs and airways that responds to elongation of muscle to trigger a cough

stroke the result of an event (finite, ongoing, or protracted occurrences) that interrupts oxygen supply to an area of the brain; usually caused by cerebral infarction or cerebral hemorrhage

subcutaneous to be injected into the tissue just beneath the skin

sublingual to be placed under the tongue

substance P a potent neurotransmitter mediating sensations of pain, touch, and temperature

substantia nigra a layer of gray substance separating parts of the brain

sulfonamides sulfa drugs; a class of bacteriostatic antibiotics that work by blocking a specific step in the biosynthetic pathway of folic acid in bacteria

superinfection a new infection complicating the course of therapy of an existing infection

supportive therapy therapy for poisoning that consists of establishing the airway and providing cardiopulmonary resuscitation (CPR); maintaining body temperature, nutritional status, and fluid and electrolyte balance; and preventing circulatory collapse, hypoglycemia, uremia, and liver failure

suppuration formation or discharge of pus

surfactant a fluid that reduces surface tension between the air in the alveoli and the inner surfaces of the alveoli, allowing gas to be exchanged between the lung and the air

surfactant laxative a stool softener that has a detergent activity that facilitates mixing of fat and water, making the stool soft and mushy

systemic effect an action of a drug that has a generalized, all-inclusive effect on the body

systemic pertaining to or affecting the body as a whole

systolic blood pressure a blood pressure measurement that measures the pressure during contraction of the heart

T

T cell lymphocyte that responds to antigens presented on the surface of other cells; involved in cellular immunity

tachycardia excessively fast heart rate

tachypnea very rapid respiration causing a flushed appearance; a characteristic of emphysema

tardive dyskinesia involuntary movements of the mouth, lips, and tongue

target a cell, tissue, or organ that is affected by a particular hormone

teratogenic causing birth defects

terminator the portion of plasmid DNA where protein production stops

testosterone a hormone that is responsible for sperm production, sexual potency, and the maintenance of muscle mass and strength, among other functions

tetracyclines a class of broad-spectrum bacteriostatic antibiotics that are produced by soil organisms and inhibit protein synthesis by binding to bacterial ribosomes

therapeutic drug a drug that relieves symptoms of a disease

therapeutic effect the desired action of a drug in the treatment of a particular disease state or symptom

therapeutic level the amount of drug in a patient's blood at which beneficial effects occur

therapeutic range the optimum dosage, providing the best chance for successful therapy; dosing below this range has little effect on the healing process, while overdosing can lead to toxicity and death

thiazide diuretic a drug based on benzothiadiazine that blocks a pump that removes sodium and chloride together from the distal tubule

three-in-one see total nutrient admixture

thrombocytopenia a decrease in the bone marrow production of blood platelets

thrombus blood clot

thyroid gland a gland that produces hormones that stimulate various body tissues to increase their activity level

thyroid storm a life-threatening medical emergency with the symptoms of thyrotoxicosis, but more exaggerated

titer concentration of an antibody in the bloodstream

tocolytic agent a drug that slows labor in pregnancy, used to treat premature labor

tocopherol one of the alcohols that constitute vitamin E

tolerance a decrease in response to the effects of a drug as it continues to be administered

tonic-clonic seizure a type of generalized seizure characterized by body rigidity followed by muscle jerks; formerly called a grand mal seizure

tonicity the relationship of a solution to the body's own fluids; measured by determining the number of dissolved particles in solution

tophus a deposit of sodium urate around a joint

topical applied to the surface of the skin or mucous membranes

total nutrient admixture (TNA) an amino acid–dextrose–lipid formulation used for parenteral nutrition; often called three-in-one

total parenteral nutrition (TPN) feeding a patient through the veins only

transcription the copying of information from a DNA strand onto an RNA strand, which then serves as a messenger to the molecular systems that use it to assemble a protein

transient ischemic attack (TIA) temporary neurologic change that occurs when part of the brain lacks sufficient blood supply over a brief period of time; may be a warning sign and predictor of imminent stroke

traveler's diarrhea diarrhea caused by ingesting contaminated food or water; so called because it is often contracted by travelers in countries where the water supply is contaminated

tricyclic antidepressant (TCA) one of a class of antidepressant drugs, developed earlier than the SSRIs and SNRIs, that also prevent neuron reuptake of norepinephrine and/or serotonin

triglycerides a neutral fat stored in animal adipose tissue which releases free fatty acids into the blood

troche a small lozenge

trough the lowest level of a drug in the blood

tuberculosis (TB) a disease of the lungs and other body tissues and organs caused by *Mycobacterium tuberculosis*

two-in-one a formulation for parenteral nutrition that contains only amino acids and dextrose

type I diabetes insulin-dependent diabetes, in which the pancreas has no ability to produce insulin

type II diabetes a type of diabetes characterized by insulin insufficiency or by the resistance of the target tissues to the insulin produced

U

ulcer a local defect or excavation of the surface of an organ or tissue

ulcerative colitis irritation and inflammation of the large bowel, causing it to look scraped; characterized by bloody mucus leading to watery diarrhea containing blood, mucus, and pus

unipolar depression major depression with no mania

unstable angina a type of angina characterized by chest pain that occurs with increasing frequency, diminishes the patient's ability to work, and has a decreasing response to treatment; may signal an oncoming MI

uremia the clinical syndrome resulting from renal dysfunction in which excessive products of protein metabolism are retained in the blood

urinary tract infection (UTI) an infection caused by bacteria, usually *E. coli,* that enter via the urethra and progress up the urinary tract; characterized by the presence of bacteria in the urine with localized symptoms

urinary tract the group of organs that include the kidneys, ureters, bladder, and urethra, and that is involved in the production and transportation of urine

urticaria hives, itching sensation

V

vaccination the introduction of a vaccine, a component of an infectious agent, into the body to produce immunity to the actual agent

vaccine a suspension of disease-causing organisms or fragments of them, administered to induce active immunity to the disease

variant angina a type of angina characterized by chest pain due to coronary artery spasm; usually not stress induced

vascular theory a theory that proposes that migraine headaches are caused by vasodilation and the concomitant mechanical stimulation of sensory nerve endings

vasomotor affecting constriction and dilation of blood vessels

vector an animal that transfers a parasite to a host

vertigo the sensation of the room spinning when one gets up or changes positions; can be treated with anticholinergic agents

very-low-density lipoproteins (VLDLs) lipoproteins containing 60% triglycerides and 12% cholesterol

virilization the development of male characteristics

virion an individual viral particle capable of infecting a living cell; consists of nucleic acid surrounded by a capsid (protein shell)

virus a minute infectious agent that does not have all the components of a cell and thus can replicate only within a living host cell

visceral pain sharp, stabbing pain from the organs

vitamin an organic substance that is necessary for the normal metabolic functioning of the body but that the body does not synthesize, so it must be obtained from food

volume of distribution mathematical relationship between the blood concentration attained and the amount of drug administered

W

wart a virally caused epidermal tumor

water-soluble vitamins vitamins that are excreted in the urine and are not stored in the body; vitamin C and the B vitamins

wheals slightly elevated, red areas on the body surface

X

xanthine derivative a drug that causes relaxation of airway smooth muscle, thus causing airway dilation and better air movement

Z

zero-order not depending on the concentration of the drug in the body; elimination of alcohol is a zero-order process in which a constant quantity of the drug is removed per unit of time

Index

Note: Page numbers in italic refer to figures and those followed by a "*t*" indicate that the reference is to a table.

baclofen, 212, 391
bacteria, 67
  aerobic, 68
  of anthrax disease, *575*
  antibiotic-resistant, 70–71
  shapes, *68*, 69*t*
  types of, 68
bacterial infections
  superinfection, 70
  symptoms of, 69
  treatment with antibiotics, 69
bactericidal agents, 69
bacteriostatic agents, 69
Bacteroides fragilis, 84
balsalazide, 278
barbiturates, 133–134, 183
basal cell carcinoma, 469
basal nuclei, 204
basiliximab, 524–525
B cell, 519
BCG (Bacille Calmette-Guerin)
  vaccine, 53
becaplermin gel, 447
benign prostatic hyperplasia (BPH),
  320–323
benzalkonium chloride, 492
benzocaine, 477*t*, 492
benzodiazepines, 130–134
  for alcohol withdrawal, 23
  for anxiety, 177, 178*t*
  side effects of, 177
benzonatate, 243
benzoyl peroxide, 474
benztropine, 175, 205–206
beractant, 237
beta agonists, 235*t*
beta blocker, 337–339, 338*t*
beta-lactamase inhibitors, 74
beta-lactam drugs, 77, 77*t*
beta receptors, 128
bethanechol, 273, 316
bevacizumab, 525
bicalutamide, 532
biguanides, 453
bile acids, 283
bile acid sequestrants, 373
bile duct, *278*
bimatoprost, 498
binding of drugs
  to cellular constituents, 27
  to plasma proteins, 26
bioavailability, defined, 33
biochemistry, defined, 23
biologic-response modifiers, 517
  interferon, 535
  interleukin-2, 535
  tumor-necrosis factor, 535
biopharmaceutical drugs, 9

biotechnology, 540
bioterrorism, 574
  bacterial diseases and, 574–575
  role of pharmacy technician, 576
bipolar disorder
  symptoms and cause, 164
  treatment, 171–172, 171*t*
bisacodyl, 285
bismuth subcitrate potassium-
  metronidazole-tetracycline,
  275
bismuth subsalicylate, 279–280
bismuth subsalicylate–metronidazole–tetracycline, 275
bisoprolol-hydrochlorothiazide, 325
bisphosphonates, 439–440, 440*t*
bivalirudin, 362
Black Box Warning, 14
  of atripla, 116
  of clozapine, 176
  of lamotrigine, 201
  of phenothiazine, 290
  of tipranavir, 114
  of valganciclovir, 109
blood-brain barrier, 27
blood clots, 359
  anticoagulant agents and. *See*
    anticoagulant agents
  antiplatelet agents and. *See* anti-
    platelet agents
  fibrinolytic agents, 365, 365*t*
blood pressure (BP)
  in adults, staging of, 351*t*
  definition of, 350
  regimen for reducing, 352*t*
B-lymphocytes, 106
body fluids, 553–555
body lice, 487, 488
body mass index (BMI), 292
body weight
  aging, effect of, 48
  children, 50
  obesity and, 291
  water, percentage of, 554
bone
  disease, 438
  microscopic view of, *439*
  skeletal system, 387
botulin toxin, 576
botulinum toxin type A, 475
bowel evacuants, 286
bradycardia, 288, 337
brain, structure of, *204*
brand names, 9
breast cancer recurrence, prevention
  of, 537–538, 538*t*
brimonidine, 497
brinzolamide, 498

broad-spectrum antibiotics, 69, 70
bromocriptine, 206
bronchitis
  causes of, 233
  symptoms of, 233
  treatment, 235
bronchodilators, 234
  albuterol, 228, 229
  arformoterol, 234
  bronchioles, smooth-muscle cells
    of, 226
  epinephrine, 226
  formoterol, 229, 234
  ipratropium-albuterol, 234–235
  isoproterenol, 229
  levalbuterol, 229
  metaproterenol, 229
  pirbuterol, 229
  salmeterol, 229–230
  terbutaline, 230
  tiotropium, 235
  ways to use, 226
bronchospasm, 223
budesonide, 278–279
budesonide-formoterol, 232
bulk-forming agents, 285
buprenorphine, 143
buprenorphine-naloxone, 143
bupropion, 169–170
bursitis, 397
buspirone, 178
butenafine, 478
butorphanol, 146, 153

C

calcipotriene, 478
calcitonin-salmon, 441
calcium, 441, 457
calcium acetate, 556
calcium (Ca^{2+}) ions, 555
calcium carbonate, 556
calcium carbonate–famotidine–
  magnesium hydroxide, 273
calcium channel blockers, 338*t*, 340,
  567
calcium chloride, 556, 572
calcium gluconate, 556
calcium salts, 555
calfactant, 237–238
Canadian list of drugs, 49
cancer, 527
  biologic-response modifiers of,
    535–536
  chemotherapy, agents for. *See*
    chemotherapy
  complications in treatment,
    536–538

diazepam, 49, 191, 392
diclofenac, 399–400, 480
didanosine, 110
dietary fibers
    for colon cancer, 283
    for constipation, 282
    fermentability of, 281
    insoluble fiber, 281
    soluble fiber, 282
    therapeutic use of. *See* fiber
        supplementation
diet therapy
    empty stomach, 299
    fibers. *See* dietary fibers
    for obesity, 291–292
diethyl ether, 479
diethylpropion, 292
difenoxin-atropine, 280
diffuse tumor, 527
digoxin, 346–347, 572
digoxin immune Fab, 347, 570
diltiazem, 572
dimercaprol, 570
dinoprostone, 433
Dioscorides, 4
diphenhydramine, 175, 184, 243
diphenoxylate-atropine, 280
dipyridamole, 368
direct renin inhibitor, 357
dirithromycin, 80
disease-modifying antirheumatic
        drugs (DMARDs), 402–404,
        403t
disinfectants, 71, 491t
disintegration, 25
disopyramide, 344
Dispensatorium (Cordis), 5
Dispense As Written (DAW), 417
dissolution, 25
disulfiram, 187
diuretics, 323–325, 324t
    carbonic anhydrase inhibitor, 323
    for hypertension, 353
    loop, 323
    osmotic, 325
    potassium-sparing, 323
    purpose of using, 323
    thiazide, 323
divalproex, 172, 200
diverticular disease, 286–287. *See also*
        colon cancer
DMARDs. *See* disease-modifying
        antirheumatic drugs
        (DMARDs)
DNA sequence, 512, *512*
    cloning, 514
    promoter sequence, 513, *514*
    terminator sequence, 513, *514*

dobutamine, 572
docosanol, 478
docusate, 285
docusate-senna, 285
dofetilide, 346
dolasetron, 290
Domagk, Gerhardt, 6
donepezil, 213–214
dong quai, 564
dopamine, 573
dopamine receptors, 128, 172
doripenem, 77
dornase alfa, 237, 517
dorzolamide, 498
dosage forms, 45t
    ophthalmic, 88t
    selection of, 43–44
dosage routes
    common, 43, 44t
    parenteral, 45–46
    peroral, 44–45
    topical, 46
dose/dosages
    defined, 27
    loading dose, 29
    maintenance dose, 29
    metabolic changes, 48–49
    volume of distribution, 29
dose-response curve, *28*
double blind study, 12
doxazosin, 322, 356
doxepin, 168, 476
doxorubicin, 531
doxycycline, 297, 438
drotrecogin alfa, 87, 88t
drug absorption, 25–26
drug abuse, 31. *See also* alcoholism
drug actions
    allergic diseases, 54–55
    allergic response and, 54
    chemical messengers, 24
    in children, 50–51
    in elderly patients, 47–50
    immune responses, 47
    immunization and. *See* immuni-
        zation
    mechanism of, 24–25
    patient's disease state, impact of,
        47
    psychological and genetic factors,
        47
    receptors, 24
drug addiction, 31
    and dependence, 142
    treatment of, 143t
drug administration,
    common dosage forms, 43–46, 45t
    oral. *See* peroral (PO) routes

"rights" of, 42–43, *42*
drug allergy, 31
drug approval process
    clinical trials, phases of, 12
    intensive testing process, 11
    postmarketing surveillance, 13
drug-body interactions, 26–27
drug concentrations, 28, 29. *See also*
        therapeutic level
drug delivery system. *See* osmotic-
        controlled release oral delivery
        system (OROS)
drug dependence, 31
drug effects, 30–31
    on nervous system, 128–129
    toxic. *See* side effects
drug elimination, 27
Drug Enforcement Administration
        (DEA), 14
Drug Enforcement Agency, 40
drugs, history of
    ancient Greek and Roman, 4
    discovery of, 1, 6
    Middle Ages, 4–5
    modern age, 5
drug interactions, 31–32
drug levels, 26
drug metabolism, 49. *See also* first-
        pass effect
drug regulation, 10–17
    drug approval process, 11
    Black Box Warning, 14
    controlled substances, 14
    by FDA, 10–13
    generic drugs, 15
    medication guides, 11
    removing drugs from market, 14
drug relationships, 30t. *See also* drug
        interactions
drugs. *See also* over-the-counter drugs
        (OTCs); prescriptions
    allergic responses. *See* drug allergy
    biopharmaceutical, 9
    chemistry of, 23
    discovery of, 3
    expiration date, 78–79
    forms of, 43–45
    generic drugs, 15–16
    half life, 29–30
    insulins, 448t
    ionization of, 48
    marketing of, 9
    naming and classifications, 9–10
    origins and sources, 9
    pharmacologic effect, 8
    poisoning, 567
    removal of from the market, 14
    routes of administration, 43–50

letrozole, 538
leucovorin, 536
leukotriene inhibitors
    functions of, 230
        montelukast, 230
        zafirlukast, 230
        zileuton, 230
leuprolide, 322, 532
levalbuterol, 229
levetiracetam, 201
levocarnitine, 315
levodopa, 205, 206–207
levodopa-carbidopa, 207
levodopa-carbidopa-entacapone, 207
levonorgestrel, 430
levothyroxine, 417
lice, human. *See* human lice
Li Che Ten, 4
lidocaine, 136, 138, 344, 470, 574
lidocaine-diphenhydramine-Maalox,
    537–538
lindane, 488
linezolid, 86
lipase inhibitor, 293
lipid-lowering agents
    commonly used, 371, 371*t*
        fibric acid derivatives, 372–373
        HMG-CoA reductase inhibitors,
        372
        and other cholesterol-lowering
        agents, 373–374
lipids, 24
lipid solubility, 24
lipoproteins, 369
liquid antibiotics, 86, 87*t*
lisinopril-hydrochlorothiazide, 325
lithium, 171–172
liver disease, 26
L-methylfolate, 553
loading dose, 29
local anesthetics, 137*t*
    advantages, 136
    adverse reactions, 138
    classification, 137
local effect, 30
local viral infection, 105
long-term care facility, 47
loop diuretic, 323
loperamide, 280
Loracarbef, 77
loratadine, 250
lorazepam, 134, 177, 178*t*, 201
losartan, 356
losartan-hydrochlorothiazide, 325
loteprednol, 496
Lou Gehrig disease. *See* amyotrophic
    lateral sclerosis (ALS)

lovastatin, 372
low-density lipoproteins (LDLs), 369
lower respiratory tract, *222*
low-molecular-weight heparin
    (LMWH), 362–363
lubiprostone, 286
lung, 222
    inflammation due to smoking,
    233
    natural defense system, impor-
    tance of, 233–234
    penetration of the drug into, 225
lung diseases
    asthma. *See* Asthma
    COPD. *See* Chronic obstructive
    pulmonary disease (COPD)
    cystic fibrosis, 236–237
    histoplasmosis, 240
    measures for prevention of, 236
    pneumonia, 236
    RDS, 237–238
    tuberculosis, 238–240
luteinizing hormone (LH), 419
lymphatic system, 521, *521*

M

macrolides, 79
    commonly used, 80*t*
    side effects of, 79–80
    therapeutic uses of, 79
macrophage, 519
mafenide, 483
magnesium hydroxide, 270, 285
magnesium (Mg^{2+}) ions, 556
magnesium sulfate, 433, 556, 574
maintenance dose, 29
malabsorption syndrome, 276
malaria, 296–297
male hormones
    androgen in, role of, 419
    and impotence. *See* male impo-
    tence
    scrotal transdermal systems, 420
    testosterone in, role of, 419
male impotence, 419–422
male reproductive system, 320, *320*
malignancy, characteristics of, 528
malignant hyperthermia, 130–131
malnutrition, 559
mania, 164
mannitol, 25, 325
maprotiline, 168
maraviroc, 114
mast cells, 223
mast cell stabilizers, 232, 276
mebendazole, 295
meclizine, 175, 249, 289
medical foods, 552–553, 553*t*

Medicare Modernization Act (MMA),
    58
medication errors, 41, 58
medication guides, 11, 164
medication labels, 43, *43*, 55–56, *55*, *56*
medication management
    administration instructions,
    importance of, 5
    medication labels, 55–56, *56*
    medication program, benefit of, 56
    OTC drugs, information on, 56
    patient's history, importance of, 55
    patient's noncompliance of
    instructions, tackling, 56–57
    pharmacy technicians, role of, 55
medication reconciliation, 58
medication safety
    e-prescribing, 57–58
    medication reconciliation, 58
    pharmacy technician, role in,
    46–47, 57
    physical order entry, 58
    tamper-resistant pads, 58
medroxyprogesterone, 425–426, 430
mefenamic acid, 401
mefloquine, 297
megestrol, 322, 532
meglitinides, 453
melanoma, 469
melatonin, 566
meloxicam, 401
memantine, 214
membrane-stabilizing agents (class I),
    344–346
meperidine, 147
meprobamate, 179
mequinol-tretinoin, 470
meropenem, 77
mesalamine, 277
messengers, chemical, 24
metabolic modifier, 338*t*, 340–341
metabolic pathway, 27
metabolites, defined, 27
metaproterenol, 229
metaxalone, 392
metered dose inhalers (MDIs), 225
metformin, 453
methadone, 143
methamphetamine, 293
methenamine, 319
methicillin-resistant *Staphylococcus
    aureus* (MRSA), 84
methimazole, 418
methocarbamol, 392
methohexital, 133
methotrexate, 404, 478
methoxy polyethylene glycol–epoetin
    beta, 315

natural process, manufacturing of, 512–513

recombinant process, manufacturing of, 513–514, *515*

prothrombin time (PT), 360

proton pump inhibitors (PPIs), 272–273

protozoan infections
cause of, 295
drug therapy, *295*

pseudoephedrine, 247

pseudomembranous colitis, 85

pseudoparkinsonism, 174

psoriasis, *477*, 477–478

psychosis, 172. *See also* schizophrenia

psychotherapy, 179

psyllium, 285–286, 374

pubic lice, 487, 488

pulmonary diseases, 221

pulmonary embolism (PE), 359

pulse dosing, 101

purified protein derivative (PPD), 238

pyrantel, 295

pyrethrin, 488

pyridostigmine, 209

pyridoxine, 315. *See also* vitamin B$_6$

Q

quetiapine, 176

quinidine, 345

quinine, 297

quinolones, 81–82

R

rabeprazole, 273

radiation therapy, 528

radioactive iodine, ^{131}I, 417

raloxifene, 441

raltegravir, 114–115

ramelteon, 184

ranitidine, 272

ranolazine, 340–341

rasagiline, 207

receptors, defined, 24

recombinant DNA, 511
of a cell, 513
economic challenges of, 514–515
in manufacturing proteins, 513–514
sequence, 512, *512*

recombinant DNA drugs, 516*t*
biologic-response modifiers, 517
colony-stimulating factors, 515–517
hematologic agent, 517
secretion-thinning enzyme, 517

recombivax HB, 298

rectal route of medication, 46

red blood cells (RBCs), 296

regular insulin, 449

remission, 531

renal disease, 311–313

renal drug therapy
medications used in, 314–315, 314*t*
purpose of, 313

renal failure, causes of, 310–313

renal insufficiency, 311

renal system
drug therapy of. *See* renal drug therapy
formation of urine, 309
function of, 309–310
infectious disease. *See* renal disease
structure of, *310*

renal transplant, 315–316, 315*t*

repaglinide, 453

replication, 513

repolarization, 334

resistant penicillins, 74, 74*t*

respiratory distress syndrome (RDS), 237
beractant, 237
calfactant, 237–238
colfosceril palimate, 237
drug therapy, 237*t*
poractant alfa, 238
symptoms of, 237

respiratory synctial virus (RSV), 299

respiratory system
alveolus and capillary blood supply, *234*
oxygen and carbon dioxide, exchange of, *222*
respiratory tracts, upper and lower, 222, *222*

restless leg syndrome, 207

retapamulin, 483

retinoid, 470

retrovirus, 109. *See also* human immunodeficiency virus (HIV)

reverse transcriptase, 109

reversible ischemic neurologic deficit (RIND), 364

Reye syndrome, 406

rheumatoid arthritis, 397

rhinitis medicamentosa, 245

ribavirin, 108–109, 299

riboflavin. *See* vitamin B$_2$

ribonucleic acid (RNA), and protein formation, 513

ricin, 576

rifampin, 240

rifapentine, 240

rifaximin, 281

"rights" of drug administration, 42–43

riluzole, 211

rimantadine, 109

ringworm, 480

risedronate, 440

risperidone, 176

ritonavir, 113

rituximab, 526

rivastigmine, 214

ropinirole, 207

rosacea, 482

rosiglitazone, 453

rosuvastatin, 372

routes of administration, 43–46

Rx number (prescription), 40

S

safety
in medication. *See* medication safety
and herbal medicine, 563–564

salicylates
aspirin and, 395
dosages, 394
for pregnancy, 394
side effects of, 394–395

saline laxatives, 285

salmeterol, 229–230

salsalate, 395

saquinavir, 113

sarafem, 165

sargramostim, 516–517

saw palmetto, 566

scabies, 485, 488–489, *489*

schizophrenia, 172

seasonal affective disorder (SAD), 164

sebaceous glands, disorders of, 474

seborrhea, 474

secondary diabetes, 445

secondary glaucoma, 497

secondary site, of cancer cells, 527

second-generation sulfonylurea, 451

secretion-thinning enzyme, 517

sedatives. *See* antianxiety drugs

seizure, 196
types of, 197

selective serotonin reuptake inhibitors (SSRIs), 164, 165–166, 165*t*

selegiline, 169, 207

sepsis, 82

serotonin, 128

serotonin and norepinephrine reuptake inhibitors (SNRIs), 164, 166–167, 167*t*

serotonin receptor antagonists, 290

serotonin syndrome, 164

sertaconazole, 481

sertraline, 166

sevelamer, 315

valacyclovir, 109, 438
valerian, 566
valganciclovir, 109
valproates, 172
valproic acid, 172, 200
valrubicin, 531
valsartan, 356
vancomycin, 84
vancomycin-resistant *Enterococcus faecium* (VRE), 82
vardenafil, 422
varenicline, 254
variant angina, 336
vasodilators, 349, 356
vasomotor symptoms, 423
vasopressin, 574
vectors, 294
venereal diseases. *See* sexually transmitted diseases (STDs)
venlafaxine, 166, 178*t*
ventricular contraction, premature, *343*
veramyst, 250
verapamil, 340, 574
verteporfin, 495
vertigo, 289
very low density lipoproteins (VLDLs), 373
viral hemorrhagic fevers (VHFs), 575–576
viral infections, *104,* 105–106
virilization, 419

virion, 104
viruses, 104–105
visceral pain, 406
vitamin A, 550
vitamin B, 551
vitamin B_1, 551
vitamin B_2, 551
vitamin B_3, 551
vitamin B_5, 552
vitamin B_6, 552, 570
vitamin B_7, 552
vitamin B_9, 552
vitamin B_{12}, 552
vitamin C, 551
vitamin D, 551
vitamin E, 112, 551
vitamin H. *See* vitamin B_7
vitamin K, 551, 570
vitamins, 550–553
Vivelle Dot, 424
Vivitrol, 186–187
volume of distribution, 29, 34
vomiting, 288–289
vomiting center, 146, *286*
voriconazole, 101*t*, 103

W

warfarin, 361*t*
   antidote for, 363
warnings
   Black Box, 14
   on drug labels, 53

wart, 478–479
water deficits, 555
water, percentage in body, *554*
water-soluble vitamins, 551
weight loss, 291
women, estrogen deficiency, 423, 438
World Health Organization (WHO)
   analgesic ladder, 141, *141*
   nomenclature system for monoclonal antibodies, 523
wrinkles, 472*t*, 475

X

xanthine derivatives, 230

Y

yogurt, 553
yohimbe, 567

Z

zafirlukast, 230
zaleplon, 184, 190
zanamivir, 109
zero-order, 34
Z hypnotics, 183
zidovudine, 111
zileuton, 230
zinc oxide, 492
ziprasidone, 176–177
zolpidem, 184
zonisamide, 203